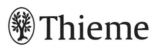

Lymphedema Management

The Comprehensive Guide for Practitioners

Fourth Edition

Joachim E. Zuther, CDT Clinical Instructor, CLT-LANA
Founder, Director
Academy of Lymphatic Studies
Founding member
North American Lymphedema Education Association (NALEA)
Sebastian, Florida, United States

Steve Norton, CDT Clinical Instructor, CLT-LANA
Founder, Executive Director
Norton School of Lymphatic Therapy
Founding member
North American Lymphedema Education Association (NALEA)
Jamesburg, New Jersey, United States

466 illustrations

Thieme
New York • Stuttgart • Delhi • Rio de Janeiro

Executive Editor: Anne M. Sydor
Managing Editor: Elizabeth Palumbo
Director, Editorial Services: Mary Jo Casey
Production Editor: Torsten Scheihagen
International Production Director: Andreas Schabert
Editorial Director: Sue Hodgson
International Marketing Director: Fiona Henderson
International Sales Director: Louisa Turrell
Director of Institutional Sales: Adam Bernacki
Senior Vice President and Chief Operating
    Officer: Sarah Vanderbilt
President: Brian D. Scanlan
Printer: Beltz Grafische Betriebe

Library of Congress Cataloging-in-Publication Data
Names: Zuther, Joachim E., author. | Norton, Steve, 1962- author.
Title: Lymphedema management : the comprehensive guide for practitioners / Joachim E. Zuther, CDT Clinical Instructor, CLT-LANA Founder, Director, Academy of Lymphatic Studies, Founding member, North American Lymphedema Education Association (NALEA), Sebastian, Florida, United States, Steve Norton, CDT Clinical Instructor, CLT-LANA Founder, Executive Director, Norton School of Lymphatic Therapy, Founding Member, North American Lymphedema Education Association (NALEA), Jamesburg, New Jersey, United States.
Description: Fourth edition. | New York : Thieme, [2018] | Includes bibliographical references.
Identifiers: LCCN 2017035764 (print) | LCCN 2017036999 (ebook) | ISBN 9781626234345 (ebook) | ISBN 9781626234338 (hardback) | ISBN 9781626234345 (ebook)
Subjects: LCSH: Lymphedema. | BISAC: MEDICAL / Allied Health Services / Physical Therapy.
Classification: LCC RC646.3 (ebook) | LCC RC646.3 .Z88 2018 (print) | DDC 616.4/2–dc23
LC record available at https://lccn.loc.gov/2017035764

Copyright © 2018 by Thieme Medical Publishers, Inc.
Thieme Publishers New York
333 Seventh Avenue, New York, NY 10001 USA
+1 800 782 3488, customerservice@thieme.com

Thieme Publishers Stuttgart
Rüdigerstrasse 14, 70469 Stuttgart, Germany
+49 [0]711 8931 421, customerservice@thieme.de

Thieme Publishers Delhi
A-12, Second Floor, Sector-2, Noida-201301
Uttar Pradesh, India
+91 120 45 566 00, customerservice@thieme.in

Thieme Publishers Rio de Janeiro, Thieme Publicações Ltda.
Edifício Rodolpho de Paoli, 25º andar
Av. Nilo Peçanha, 50 – Sala 2508
Rio de Janeiro 20020-906 Brasil
+55 21 3172-2297 / +55 21 3172-1896

Cover design: Thieme Publishing Group
Typesetting by DiTech Process Solutions

Printed in Germany by Beltz Grafische Betriebe   5 4

ISBN 978-1-62623-433-8

Also available as an e-book:
eISBN 978-1-62623-434-5

Important note: Medicine is an ever-changing science undergoing continual development. Research and clinical experience are continually expanding our knowledge, in particular our knowledge of proper treatment and drug therapy. Insofar as this book mentions any dosage or application, readers may rest assured that the authors, editors, and publishers have made every effort to ensure that such references are in accordance with **the state of knowledge at the time of production of the book.**

Nevertheless, this does not involve, imply, or express any guarantee or responsibility on the part of the publishers in respect to any dosage instructions and forms of applications stated in the book. **Every user is requested to examine carefully** the manufacturers' leaflets accompanying each drug and to check, if necessary in consultation with a physician or specialist, whether the dosage schedules mentioned therein or the contraindications stated by the manufacturers differ from the statements made in the present book. Such examination is particularly important with drugs that are either rarely used or have been newly released on the market. Every dosage schedule or every form of application used is entirely at the user's own risk and responsibility. The authors and publishers request every user to report to the publishers any discrepancies or inaccuracies noticed. If errors in this work are found after publication, errata will be posted at www.thieme.com on the product description page.

Some of the product names, patents, and registered designs referred to in this book are in fact registered trademarks or proprietary names even though specific reference to this fact is not always made in the text. Therefore, the appearance of a name without designation as proprietary is not to be construed as a representation by the publisher that it is in the public domain.

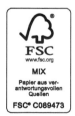

Contents

1 Anatomy

Joachim E. Zuther

2 Physiology

6   Administration

Joachim E. Zuther

Foreword to the Fourth Edition

When Steve Norton and Joachim E. Zuther asked me to write the foreword to the fourth edition of their book *Lymphedema Management: The Comprehensive Guide for Practitioners,* I was humbled by the request but immediately accepted because they are both such knowledgeable clinicians and outstanding educators we are fortunate to have in our field. It is an honor and great pleasure that I can assist them.

I first started working in the field of basic lymphatic research and then quickly transitioned to interests in multimodal lymphatic system imaging and the treatment and evaluation of patients in the lymphedema-angiodysplasia clinic (with Charles and Marlys Witte at the University of Arizona in 1989). It has been interesting to watch as the field has continued to grow (particularly in the United States) with increased recognition of patients with lymphedema and the problems they may present, by both physicians and therapists. There is still a long way to go; even in my own medical school, patients with lymphedema/lipedema and those with complicated, underappreciated, and sometimes life-threatening lymphatic system abnormalities are still not referenced in the medical curriculum. And this pervades despite our world-renowned clinician/educator and state-of-the-art imaging and research available on-site. The lymphatic system gets minimal coverage except for some anatomy. The growth in the number of therapists has been encouraging, and both Joe and Steve have contributed greatly to this with their highly rated schools and the many exceptionally trained, motivated, and successful therapists (and physicians!) they have instructed. They both greatly deserve a place of honor in the success of the growth of lymphology, the treatment community in the United States, and ultimately the patients that are served.

The book continues its clean design of color-coded sections for anatomy, physiology, and pathophysiology, which are followed by an enlarged section on comprehensive treatment and finally a practical section on administration for use in clinics. This book is written for education as well as everyday use in the clinic by practitioners. The sections flow well and are led by Steve and Joe with the addition of many experts in the field contributing their particular expertise in concise and informative fashion that interdigitates into a compendium. The book is easy to read and covers topics in a depth that may surprise in its handy to carry and use size.

In the fourth edition, the previous chapters have been updated and modified to recognize the growth in understanding that has occurred while still striving to keep the book at a manageable size. Importantly, more advanced topics such as lymphedema of the head and neck and breast and trunk are enhanced. Complications such as obesity, complete decongestive therapy (CDT) for cancer survivors, as well as relevant discoveries in exercise guidelines are included. Practical sections on imaging and genetics, as well as quality of life and other research areas, are revised, as are updates on ICD-10 codes. The new edition includes over 140 new images and over 30 new tables and includes contributions from experts such as Karen Louise Herbst, MD, who expanded the discussion on Lipedema and other related disorders (Dercum's disease, Madelung's disease), and Jay W. Granzow, MD, describing surgical options as part of an integrated treatment system for lymphedema, including vascularized lymph node transfer (VLNT), anastomosis and bypass techniques, suction-assisted protein lipectomy (SAPL), and combined and staged surgeries. Frank Aviles, PT, shares advanced wound care options as part of an integrated treatment system and Nicole L. Stout, DPT, contributes a section on early intervention and conservative therapy to highlight the growing importance of identifying lymphedema through prospective surveillance and modifying therapy appropriately. Julie M. Soderberg, PT, adds integration of conventional therapies and techniques in working closely with surgeons using specialized lymphatic procedures, and the team of Susan Struckhoff Allen, OT, Dawn Fries Brinkmann, OT, and Sandra Elizabeth Harkins, PT, present "Lymphedema Therapy in the Home," which is aimed at the growing ranks of home care–focused practitioners encountering lymphedema, and other combined edemas with tips about the required adaptations to therapy. Joy C. Cohn, PT, adds a new section called "Fitting Garments upon Delivery," which addresses the all-important transition from intensive to self-management phases and the critical aspects of proper fit, manufacture, and function of garments as well as patient autonomy, and John Beckwith, PT, expands his section on "Edema Solutions for Wound Specialists" with discussions on the "Rationale for Manual Lymphatic Drainage in

Wound Healing" and compression while using a "Negative Pressure Wound Therapy" (NPWT) vacuum. Finally, both the editors expanded this edition, with Steve contributing two new advanced sections focusing on pediatric lymphedema and adapting CDT to the pediatric patient and Joe broadening the (sometimes controversial) section on sequential intermittent pneumatic compression including its contraindications and how these devices may be integrated into the management of lymphedema.

This exciting and updated edition will be a valuable resource and guide for all levels of lymphatic knowledge. For students training to be therapists, this book is a relevant and useful source for information and training. For health professionals and researchers needing concise, clearly written, and informative sections as well as seasoned clinicians in need of a quick, well-referenced guide, this book should find an important place to keep handy on their shelf. Congratulations to Steve and Joe for their efforts!

Michael Bernas, MS

Foreword to the Third Edition

As a nurse researcher focusing on secondary lymphedema following cancer treatment, it is my privilege to write this foreword to the third edition of *Lymphedema Management: The Comprehensive Guide for Practitioners.*

It is estimated that more than 1 million men, women, and children in the United States are living with lymphedema. Although it is a long-term condition, with support and adequate treatment, there is much that can be done to decrease swelling and manage other symptoms. During the last 20 years, more and more health care professionals, including physicians from various disciplines, have made lymphedema management part of their practice.

In addition to all of the features presented in the first two editions of Joachim E. Zuther's *Lymphedema Management,* which have been updated (complete anatomy, physiology, and pathology of the lymphatic system; a comprehensive guide to the management of lymphedema and its related conditions (venous insufficiencies, lipedema, axillary web syndrome, and wounds); descriptions of the components of complete decongestive therapy (CDT); and detailed treatment sequences), the following topics have been extensively revised, with contributions from internationally recognized authors. Expanded features include: filariasis; surgical and pharmaceutical options for lymphedema; edema versus lymphedema; obesity as it relates to lymphedema; radiation-induced brachial plexopathy; nutritional aspects of lymphedema; lowlevel laser therapy; intermittent compression therapy; care for compression garments; exercises; truncal lymphedema; and diagnosis. New contributors to the third edition include co-editor Steve Norton, John Beckwith, Michael Bernas, Joy C. Cohn, Janice N. Cormier, Kate D. Cromwell, Marga F. Massey, Maureen McBeth, Linda McGrath Boyle, Judith Nudelman, Nicolle Samuels, Brad Smith, Sarah A. Stolker, and myself.

Lymphedema Management is written and edited by Joachim E. Zuther and Steve Norton, both of whom are highly respected educators of lymphedema in the United States and abroad. Each, as acting director of his respective school (Academy of Lymphatic Studies, Norton School of Lymphatic Therapy), has trained numerous practicing lymphedema therapists in the United States, championing CDT from its introduction more than 20 years ago. The additional contributors assembled include highly respected practicing clinicians, many of whom conduct specialized workshops for treating patients with less common kinds of lymphedema (e.g., truncal, head and neck, genital, neurologic impairment, stage 3 limbs), and researchers in the field.

Practicing therapists require tangible and practical tips for adapting the basics of CDT to advanced patients with complicated diagnoses. The third edition of this book is a valuable addition to the limited resources that are available. The authors offer current empirical and evidence- based techniques for clinical success. As a companion book for the CDT certification courses offered by both of these leading schools, this publication is designed to act as a teaching manual for newly minted lymphedema specialists. Thus, the third edition includes newtopics that are likely to be of great interest to practicing therapists, updates to previously published topics, and practical guidelines for the application and adaptation of CDT for patients with limb edema as well as other less common types of swelling and those in the palliative care setting. The authors incorporate "how to" technique guidelines for several topic areas. I believe practicing lymphedema specialists will gravitate to this book and find it accurate and evidence-based, yet less burdensome and less scientifically dense than the alternatives. It will act as a bridge from the classroom to the clinic and become a continuing reference for practice.

In addition to providing practical guidelines for the adaptation of CDT for basic and complex cases, the text provides a sound overview for researchers, physicians, and other health care professionals in understanding the issues and complexities of lymphedema care. The numerous full-color drawings, figures, and photos highlight several key points to enhance the understanding for therapists, clinicians, educators, and researchers alike. The depth of knowledge, diversity, and rich experience of the editors is evident throughout the book.

Whatever the therapist's background and circumstance, the main aim of lymphedema management is to better understand the condition of lymphedema and to help the patient attain his or her optimal health and functional status. I am sure the authors share this same main objective. I applaud my respected colleagues Joachim E. Zuther and Steve Norton for this fine contribution to the medical literature.

Jane M. Armer, RN, PhD, CLT, FAAN

Preface to the Fourth Edition

Our publisher's petition for a fourth edition of *Lymphedema Management: The Comprehensive Guide for Practitioners* was a clear indication that awareness and treatment for lymphedema are rapidly expanding in the United States and the English-speaking world. Recently the third edition was translated and published in Japanese, which is tremendously exciting since it furthers access to this expert knowledge base toward reaching patients and clinicians in Asia, while secondarily strengthening the Japanese Lymphedema Framework project. As is always the case, what follows complete decongestive therapy (CDT) education is the application of universally proven, practical treatment solutions that yield unparalleled results. Access to this treatment, applied systematically and with skill, always serves a desperate, misdiagnosed, and poorly understood patient population suffering from the same causes of lymphedema that occur throughout the developed world. It is always heartwarming to know that sound, accurate, evidence-based, and practical knowledge is reaching emerging global resources.

As educators, our respective lymphedema management schools have seen steadily increasing enrollment of well-trained rehabilitation professionals, as further proof of a slow but undeniable trend toward broader adoption of this standard of care. CDT "is that standard of care" and as the ever-increasing literature base grows, CDT remains the benchmark by which all other approaches are measured.

For over two decades, it has been a shared vision of Joachim E. Zuther, myself, and other respected CDT educators to continue establishing this solid foundation. But as is reflected in this book, we fully embrace the future by welcoming advancements in science, technology, patient education, surveillance, and potential prevention strategies in the hope that lymphedema detection and management intervene before the chronic, labor-intensive, and disfiguring stages. That said, although modernized and refined invasive treatment approaches have shown great promise and are welcome additions to our field as well as to this book, as editors we choose to remain cautious toward adopting these therapies into our educational models until further broad-based and long-range efficacy can be determined.

The fourth edition remains unique in its practicality as our clinician readers can immediately absorb and employ tangible advanced and modified treatment strategies for patient presentations rarely mentioned in other writings. The majority of the third editions' specific subject content has been updated and expanded by each of our subject matter experts/authors. New to this edition are highly adaptable approaches to treating patients in the home environment where so little need has been systematically addressed. Content has been added on the topic of the surgical certified lymphedema therapist (CLT) to address patients who have received autologous tissue transfers while still relying on CLTs for the support of select CDT modalities.

For clinicians encountering advanced venous disease, a vast amount of new information has been provided to bolster core knowledge of wound pathology for lymphedema specialists treating edema in the presence of wounds. Our knowledge of fat disorders and their relevance to edema formation is expanding quickly, so we are excited to highlight a major expansion of content in this area chiefly related to the lipedema patient so commonly seen in lymphedema clinics. Very little has been written about the importance of CDT for pediatric patients. In particular, staged modifications to therapy based on age, development, and most importantly parental/caregiver ability and inclination are discussed in great detail. For those who encounter pediatric limb enlargements related to lymphatic and vascular syndromes, it is helpful to consider these more complex and refined diagnoses and the contraindications and precautions they derive for safe application of select CDT modalities, as well as any revisions in our expectations for optimal outcomes.

From 2017, we look forward to a time in the near future when current scientific research yields new insights that inform our decisions about best practices, patient by patient, tailoring care and simplifying self-care with marked improvement in quality of life. We are tremendously grateful for the growing focus of so many investigators.

Steve Norton

Joachim E. Zuther

Preface to the Third Edition

This book represents an exciting step forward for the field of lymphedema therapy and, in particular, as a muchneeded aid to practicing lymphedema therapists and those affected by lymphedema. The first and second editions have enjoyed wide distribution, aiding thousands of therapists and patients worldwide. Notably, there is no such resource available for the American therapist that contains tangible and highly specific guidance for treating a variety of clinical presentations with proven and effective adaptations of complete decongestive therapy (CDT). Various exceptional and highly experienced contributors have been assembled for this edition, each with hundreds of patient cases to draw upon, as is reflected in their extensive, sound, and generous advice. New subject areas include: lymphedema taping, genetics and imaging, compression strategies for patients with wounds, paralyzed limbs, and advanced-stage involvement. Treatment of the head and neck, trunk-involved, morbidly obese and palliative patient types has been added, with additional specific treatment adaptations for a multitude of nuanced primary and secondary lymphedemas. There is a section dedicated to lymphatic microsurgery as well as an overview of surgical treatment outcomes for lymphedema. In addition considering the ever-changing landscape of cancer survivorship, a section discussing oncology rehabilitation for the certified lymphedema therapist (CLT) will prove an essential addition. Lastly, quality of life, metrics for edema detection/ documentation along with current research perspectives are included and reflect our excitement for future developments and the well-being of the multitude of current and yet undiagnosed patient beneficiaries. Topics that have been expanded upon include: bandaging with foam padding for the upper and lower extremities, clinical considerations and care instructions for compression garments and bandages, step-by-step genital manual lymphatic drainage (MLD) and bandaging techniques, as well as insights for compression garment selection and application. CDT adaptations for various universal complications associated with effective treatment of lymphedema have been expanded and patient evaluation, early detection/surveillance, risk reduction, exercise, and lymphedema diagnosis from a physician perspective have been extensively updated. Further updates on lymphatic filariasis, axillary web syndrome, Klippel-Trénaunay and Parkes Weber syndromes, and wound care are also part of this new edition. We find it difficult to express how heartwarming and rewarding it is to co-author this third edition having been respectful colleagues for the last 20 years, training many of the nation's therapists. With a shared vision, our two schools will align in using this textbook as our respective course guides. With this statement we hope to strongly reflect our unity in reverence to the gold standard of CDT and the collective evidence base it has amassed thus proving its unparalleled performance. We also hope that our alliance strengthens clinician relationships as well as the commitment, to advancement within closely related lymphedema-centered establishments, which rely heavily on the collaboration, commitment and cooperation of educators to continue certifying highly skilled lymphedema therapists. As such, we both remain keenly aware of the fragility of lymphedema therapy as a specialty within the larger realm of rehabilitation medicine. To that end, we remain focused on the chief objective, that of ensuring the future of competent and safe therapy for patients and continuing to prove CDT's effectiveness at reducing this form of human suffering.

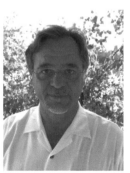 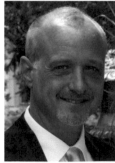

Joachim E. Zuther   *Steve Norton*

Acknowledgments

I would like to express my sincere gratitude to everybody using this book as a resource and guide for the treatment and management of lymphedema. The initial goal in writing this book was to provide clear information on the anatomy and physiology of the lymphatic system, the circumstances that lead to the development of lymphedema, and the inclusion of a comprehensive description of the currently available treatment modalities for lymphedema and related conditions.

I am proud and happy that the success of the previous three editions is proof that this book serves its purpose as a valuable tool for all health care professionals interested in learning more about the lymphatic system, and also provides individuals affected by lymphedema with extensive information on how to effectively self-manage this condition.

It has been a long and exciting road since the first edition of this textbook was published in 2005. My heartfelt thanks go to all the colleagues and friends who provided support, offered comments, and furnished exceptional contributions to the previous three editions and the new edition of *Lymphedema Management,* especially to Steve Norton, one of the outstanding lymphedema educators in this country. Steve is a longtime respected colleague and friend, who collaborated with me as a coauthor and coeditor for the third edition and this new fourth edition. His extensive experience in the field, combined with our shared vision, greatly enhances the overall content of the previous, current, and forthcoming editions.

I am very grateful to all the contributors of the first three editions, who updated and expanded on their existing topics to reflect up-to-date research and best practices in the treatment and management of lymphedema. Heartfelt thanks to the new contributors for this edition: Susan Struckhoff Allen, Frank Aviles, Dawn Fries Brinkmann, Jay Granzow, Sandra Harkins, Karen Herbst, Julie Soderberg, Rebecca Spigel, and Nicole Stout. The valuable new content these well-known and respected specialists in the field of lymphedema management provided greatly enhanced the quality of this new edition.

Many thanks to the editors at Thieme Publishers, New York, for the collaboration and guidance throughout the productions of the first three editions, and this fourth edition.

Great appreciation to Jane Armer for providing outstanding content for the past two editions and for writing the foreword to the third edition.

Finally, I would like to thank Michael Bernas for dedicating time out of his very busy schedule to provide the foreword, in addition to his other valuable contributions, to this fourth edition.

The collaboration of all involved was crucial in making this book a valuable resource for the lymphedema community!

Joachim E. Zuther

Contributors

Susan Struckhoff Allen, OTR/L, CLT-LANA
Primary Instructor
Norton School of Lymphatic Therapy
President
Lymph Logic, LLC
Cocoa, Florida, United States

Jane M. Armer, RN, PhD, CLT, FAAN
Professor
Sinclair School of Nursing
University of Missouri
Director
American Lymphedema Framework Project
Columbia, Missouri, United States

Frank Aviles, Jr., PT, CWS, FACCWS, CLT
Wound Care Service Line Director
Natchitoches Regional Medical Center
Wound Care Consultant
Louisiana Extended Care Hospital
Wound Care Consultant
Faculty, Medical Advisor, and Instructor
Academy of Lymphatic Studies
Care River Therapy Services, LLC
Natchitoches, Louisiana, United States

John Beckwith, PT, CLT-LANA
Lymphedema Specialist
Primary Instructor
Norton School of Lymphatic Therapy
Sacred Heart Medical Center
Springfield, Oregon, United States

Michael Bernas, MS
Associate Scientific Investigator
Department of Surgery
University of Arizona
Tucson, Arizona, United States

Linda McGrath Boyle, PT, DPT, OCS, CLT-LANA
Clinical Team Leader Oncology
Lehigh Valley Health Network
Primary Instructor
Norton School of Lymphatic Therapy
Allentown, Pennsylvania, United States

Dawn Fries Brinkman, OTR/L, CLT-LANA
Associate Instructor
Norton School of Lymphatic Therapy
Lymphedema Specialist
Orlando Health, Health Central Hospital Outpatient
    Rehabilitation Services
Ocoee, Florida, United States

Joy C. Cohn, PT CLT-LANA
Primary Instructor
Norton School of Lymphatic Therapy
Team Leader-Lymphedema Services
Penn Therapy and Fitness - Good Shepherd Penn Partners
Philadelphia, Pennsylvania, United States

Teresa Conner-Kerr, PT, PhD, MBA
Dean and Professor
College of Health Sciences & Professions
University of North Georgia
Dahlonega, Georgia, United States

Jay W. Granzow, MD, MPH, FACS
Assistant Chief
Division of Plastic Surgery
Harbor-UCLA Medical Center
Associate Professor of Surgery
David Geffen School of Medicine at UCLA
Hawthorne, California, United States

Sandra Elizabeth Harkins, PT, CLT/LANA
Lead Physical Therapist
Florida Hospital Home Care Services, Inc.
Orlando, Florida, United States

Karen Louise Herbst, PhD, MD
Associate Professor of Medicine
University of Arizona College of Medicine
Director
TREAT Program
Tucson, Arizona, United States

Linda Koehler, PhD, PT, CLT-LANA
Assistant Professor
Division of Physical Therapy
Department of Rehabilitation Medicine
Medical School
University of Minnesota
Minneapolis, Minnesota, United States

Maureen McBeth, MPT, CLT-LANA
Primary Instructor
Norton School of Lymphatic Therapy
M. McBeth Consulting, LLC
Hunt Valley, Maryland, United States

Steve Norton, CDT Clinical Instructor, CLT-LANA
Founder, Executive Director
Norton School of Lymphatic Therapy
Founding member
North American Lymphedema Education Association
  (NALEA)
Jamesburg, New Jersey, United States

Judith Nudelman, MD
Clinical Associate Professor of Family Medicine
Alpert Medical School
Brown University
Providence Community Health Centers
Providence, Rhode Island, United States

Pamela Lynne Ostby, PhD, RN, OCN, CLT
Research Specialist
Sinclair School of Nursing
University of Missouri
Columbia, Missouri, United States

Nicolle Samuels, MSPT, CLT-LANA, CWS, CKTP
Director of Rehabilitation and Wellness Services
Certified Lymphedema Therapist (Instructor)
Certified Wound Specialist
Certified Kinesiotaping Practitioner
Academy of Lymphatic Studies
Adjunct Professor
University of South Dakota
Briar Cliff University
Director of Rehabilitation and Wellness Services
Hegg Memorial Health Center
Rock Valley, Iowa, United States

Brad G. Smith, MS, CCC-SLP, CLT
Speech Language Pathologist
Certified Lymphedema Therapist
Specialist Instructor
Norton School of Lymphatic Therapy
Sammons Cancer Center-Dallas
Baylor University Medical Center
Dallas, Texas, United States

Julie M. Soderberg, MPT, ATC, CLT-LANA
Lymphedema Program Coordinator
Providence Little Company of Mary
National Lymphedema Center
Torrance, California, United States

Rebecca Spigel, PT, DPT, CLT-LANA, STAR/C
University of Chicago Medicine
Chicago, Illinois, United States

Sarah A. Stolker, MSPT, CLT-LANA
Primary Instructor
Norton School of Lymphatic Therapy
Physical Therapist
Certified Lymphedema Therapist
David C Pratt Cancer Center
Mercy Hospital
Creve Coeur, Missouri, United States

Nicole L. Stout, DPT, CLT-LANA, FAPTA
Partner
3e Services, LLC
Sarasota, Florida, United States

Joachim E. Zuther, CDT Clinical Instructor, CLT-LANA
Founder, Director
Academy of Lymphatic Studies
Founding member
North American Lymphedema Education Association
  (NALEA)
Sebastian, Florida, United States

Chapter 1

Anatomy

1 Anatomy

1.1 Circulatory System

The circulatory or cardiovascular system involves the combined functioning of the heart, blood, and blood vessels to supply oxygen and nutrients to organs and tissues throughout the body and to carry away waste products. Among its vital functions, the circulatory system increases blood flow to meet increased energy demands during exercise, and it regulates body temperature. When foreign substances or organisms invade the body, the circulatory system transports disease-fighting elements of the immune system, such as white blood cells and antibodies, to the regions under attack. Also, in the case of injury or bleeding, the circulatory system sends clotting cells and proteins to the affected site, which stop bleeding and promote healing.

1.1.1 Components

The heart, blood, and blood vessels are the three structural elements that form the circulatory system, with the heart as its motor.

Heart

The heart is divided into four chambers—the right atrium, the right ventricle, the left atrium, and the left ventricle. The walls of these chambers consist of muscle tissue called myocardium, which contracts continuously and rhythmically to pump blood. The pumping action of the heart occurs in two stages for each heartbeat—the diastole, when the heart is at rest, and the systole, when the heart contracts to pump deoxygenated blood toward the lungs (pulmonary circulation) and oxygenated blood to the body (systemic circulation). During each heartbeat, typically about 60 to 90 mL of blood is pumped out of the heart.

Blood

Blood is made up of three types of cells: red blood cells, which carry oxygen; white blood cells, which fight disease; and blood-clotting platelets. All of these cells are carried through blood vessels in a liquid called plasma. Plasma is yellowish in color and consists of water, salts, proteins, vitamins, minerals, hormones, dissolved gases, and fats.

Blood Vessels

Three types of blood vessel can be differentiated, forming a complex network of tubes throughout the body. The arteries carry blood away from the heart, and the veins carry blood toward the heart. Capillaries are the smallest links between the arteries and veins, where oxygen and nutrients diffuse into body tissues. The inner layer (intima) of blood vessels is lined with endothelial cells that create a smooth passage for the transit of blood. This inner layer is surrounded by connective tissue (media) and smooth muscle, which enable the blood vessel to expand or contract.

Arteries have thicker walls than veins, to withstand the pressure of blood being pumped from the heart. Arteries also have a much better-developed system of smooth muscles in their walls. Blood in the veins is at lower pressure, and the smooth musculature is not as well developed as it is in the arteries. Veins therefore have one-way valves, which allow blood to flow only toward the heart and prevent it from pooling. Capillaries, the smallest blood vessels, are only visible under the microscope. Ten capillaries lying side by side are barely as thick as a human hair.

The systemic circulation carries oxygenated blood from the heart (leaving the left ventricle) via the aorta to all the tissues in the body except the lungs, and returns deoxygenated blood, carrying waste products such as carbon dioxide, back to the heart (right atrium). The pulmonary circulation carries this spent blood via the pulmonary artery from the heart (leaving the right ventricle) to the lungs. In the lungs, the blood releases its carbon dioxide and absorbs oxygen. The oxygenated blood then returns to the heart (in the left atrium) via the pulmonary vein before transferring to the systemic circulation.

1.1.2 Systemic Circulation

Smaller arteries branch off from the aorta, leading to various parts of the body. These smaller arteries in turn branch out into even smaller arteries, called arterioles. Branches of arterioles become progressively smaller in diameter, eventually forming the capillaries. Once blood has reached the capillary level, blood pressure is greatly reduced.

The thin walls of the capillaries allow dissolved oxygen and nutrients from the blood to diffuse

1

across to a fluid known as interstitial fluid, which fills the gaps between the cells of tissues or organs. The dissolved oxygen and nutrients then enter the cells from the interstitial fluid by diffusion across the cell membranes. Meanwhile, carbon dioxide and other waste products leave the cells diffuse through the interstitial fluid, cross the capillary walls, and enter the blood. In this way, the blood delivers nutrients and removes waste without leaving the capillary tube.

Blood capillaries merge at their venous ends to form tiny veins, called venules. These veins in turn join together to form progressively larger veins. Ultimately, the veins converge into two large veins: the inferior vena cava, bringing blood from the lower half of the body; and the superior vena cava, bringing blood from the upper half. These two large veins join at the right atrium of the heart.

Because the pressure is dissipated in the arterioles and capillaries, blood in the veins flows back to the heart at very low pressure, often running uphill when a person is standing. Flow against gravity is made possible by the one-way valves, located several centimeters apart, in the veins. When surrounding muscles contract—for example, in the calf or arm—the muscles squeeze blood back toward the heart. If the one-way valves are working properly, blood travels only toward the heart and cannot lapse backward. Veins with defective valves that allow the blood to flow backward become enlarged or dilated to form varicosities.

The lymphatic system represents an accessory route by which lymph fluid can flow from the tissue spaces into the bloodstream. En route to the venous circulation, lymph travels through successive lymph nodes, thereby filtering the impurities from the lymph fluid (▶ Fig. 1.1).

The cardiovascular system is closely associated with the lymphatic system. The commonalities between the two systems include
- Superficial, deep, and organ systems.
- Similar vessel structure.
- Leukocytes (both systems contain monocytes and lymphocytes).
- Blood plasma (the lymphatic system returns percolated or filtered blood plasma to the bloodstream).
- Serum proteins (lower concentration in the lymphatic system).
- Common pathways to the heart.
- Protection of the body from infection and disease.

The main differences between the two systems include:
- The lymphatic system is not a closed circulatory system. It is therefore more appropriate to speak of lymph transport rather than of lymph circulation.
- There is no central pump in the lymphatic system.
- The lymph transport is interrupted by lymph nodes.

1.2 Lymphatic System

1.2.1 Function

The lymphatic system is part of the circulatory system and consists of a network of lymphatic vessels that carry a clear fluid called lymph (from Latin lympha = water). The lymphatic system has multiple interrelated functions. The main function is to collect and transport tissue fluids from the intercellular spaces in all the tissues of the body back to the venous system (fluid homeostasis). It absorbs and transports fatty acids as chyle from the digestive system, and plays a crucial role in the immune response. Lymph nodes and other lymphatic organs filter the lymph to remove microorganisms and other foreign particles.

1.2.2 Components of the Lymphatic System

The lymphatic system consists of lymphoid organs, a conducting network of lymphatic vessels, and the circulating lymph fluid.

Lymphoid organs can be divided into two categories: primary lymphoid organs and secondary lymphoid organs.

Primary lymphoid organs (bone marrow and thymus) are responsible for the production of T and B lymphocytes. Bone marrow is responsible for both the production of T lymphocytes and the creation and maturation of B lymphocytes, which will colonize the secondary lymphoid organs. B lymphocytes immediately join the circulatory system and travel to secondary lymphoid organs, whereas T lymphocytes travel from the bone marrow to the thymus, where they develop further.

Secondary lymphoid organs include the thymus, lymph nodes, spleen, tonsils, Peyer's patches, and mucosa-associated lymphoid tissue (MALT). These peripheral organs are arranged as a series of filters monitoring the contents of the lymph fluid, tissue fluid, and blood. The lymphoid tissue filtering these fluids is arranged in different ways. Secondary lymphoid tissues are also the location where mature lymphocytes are activated by antigens, thus initiating adaptive immune response (see also 1.3.4 later in this chapter).

1.2.3 Embryology and Development of the Lymphatic System

The lymphatic system begins to develop by the end of the fifth gestational week. The lymphatic vessels, lymph nodes, and spleen develop from the mesoderm.

The mesoderm is the middle layer of the three primary germ cell layers. The other two layers are the ectoderm and endoderm. The mesoderm differentiates to give rise to several tissues and structures, including connective tissue, muscle, bone, and the urogenital and circulatory systems.

The lymphatic system develops independently in close association with veins and begins with a more or less regular series of small and blind-ending outgrowths (lymph sacs) in close proximity to some of the embryonic veins. These lymph sacs are developed by the confluence of numerous venous capillaries, which initially lose their connections with the venous system, but later, on the formation of the sacs, regain them. The lymphatic system is therefore developmentally an offshoot of the venous system, and the lining walls of its vessels are endothelial.

Lymph sacs develop from fusion and dilation of mesenchymal spaces. Adjacent spaces fuse into a network of dilated lymphatic capillaries that establish a primitive lymphatic system by the end of the second month. In the human embryo, there are six lymph sacs from which the lymphatic vessels are derived: two paired, the jugular and the posterior lymph sacs; and two unpaired, the retroperitoneal and the cisterna chyli. Lymph sacs develop in a craniocaudal direction, from the jugular to the pelvic region. All of the lymph sacs except the cisterna chyli are, at a later stage, divided up by slender connective tissue bridges and transformed into groups of lymph nodes. The lower portion of the cisterna chyli is similarly converted, but its upper portion remains as the adult cisterna.

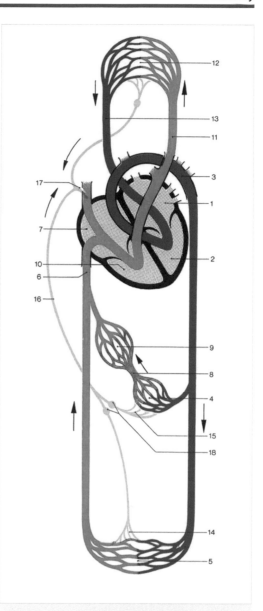

Fig. 1.1 Organs of circulation. 1, left atrium; 2, left ventricle; 3, aorta; 4, blood capillary network of the intestines; 5, blood capillary network of other organs; 6, inferior vena cava; 7, right atrium; 8, portal vein; 9, blood capillary network of the liver; 10, right ventricle; 11, pulmonary artery; 12, blood capillary network of the lungs; 13, pulmonary vein; 14, vessels of the superficial and deep lymphatic system; 15, lymphatic vessels draining the intestinal system; 16, lymphatic trunks; 17, venous angles; 18, lymph nodes. (From Kahle W, Leonhardt H, Platzer W. Color Atlas/Text of Human Anatomy, Vol. 2: Internal Organs. 4th ed. Stuttgart/New York: Thieme; 1993.)

1.3 Topography of the Lymphatic System

The lymphatic system is divided into the superficial and deep layers and is separated by the fascia (connecting the skin to the underlying tissue). The superficial (suprafascial) layer is responsible for the drainage of skin and subcutaneous tissue, whereas the deep (subfascial) lymphatic system drains the lymph from muscle tissue, tendon sheaths, nervous tissues, the periosteum, and joint structures (some distal joints on the extremities drain via the superficial layer). The transport vessels of the superficial system are embedded in the subcutaneous fatty tissue; deep transport vessels generally accompany blood vessels and are grouped together with them in the same membrane. Perforating vessels connect the deep system with the superficial system.

The lymphatic system of the internal organs represents a subcategory of the deep system.

1.3.1 Lymph Fluid

Once the interstitial fluid enters the lymphatic system, it is called *lymph*. Lymph fluid is a clear and transparent semifluid medium, with the exception of the cloudy chylous fluid found in lymph vessels draining the intestinal system (fatty acids absorbed by intestinal lymphatics produce a cloudy or milky appearance of the lymph fluid).

Lymph fluid is composed of *lymphatic loads*. This term was coined by Földi and summarizes all those substances that leave the interstitial areas via the lymphatic system.

1.3.2 Lymphatic Loads

Lymphatic loads include protein, water, cellular components and particles, and fat.

Protein

In the course of a day, at least half of the proteins circulating in the blood will leave the blood capillaries (and the postcapillary venules) and travel into the interstitial spaces. Given this fact, the protein concentration in the interstitium continues to remain lower than that of the blood. Proteins in the interstitium perform such important tasks as cell nutrition, immune defense, and blood coagulation (fibrinogen). They are also responsible for the transport of fats, minerals, hormones, and waste products. Proteins play a vital role in fluid balance;

for example, maintenance of the colloid-osmotic pressure difference (see also Chapter 2, Filtration and Reabsorption).

Proteins are unable to reenter the bloodstream via the blood capillaries.

> The return of the proteins circulating in the interstitium back into the bloodstream is facilitated by the lymphatic system. Intercellular openings (▶ Fig. 1.2 and ▶ Fig. 1.3) in the lymph capillary level allow the large protein molecules to be absorbed.

Foreign proteins such as those resulting from the breakdown of bacteria also constitute a lymphatic load.

The implications resulting from insufficient protein return in case of lymphedema will be discussed in Chapter 3.

Water

Approximately 10 to 20% of the water leaving the blood capillary system by way of filtration comprises the lymphatic load of water. This remaining fraction of filtrate is returned to the blood circulation via the thoracic duct, the right lymphatic duct, and the venous angles, and amounts to approximately 2 to 3 liters per day. However, considerably larger volumes of lymphatic load of water than the roughly 3 liters returned by the thoracic duct and the right lymphatic duct are produced throughout the body during the course of a day. The blood capillaries in the lymph node level reabsorb most of the remaining filtrate (see Lymph Nodes later in this chapter).

The lymphatic load of water plays an essential role in the body's fluid management and serves as a solvent for other lymphatic loads.

Cells and Particles

White blood cells (as well as some red blood cells) leave the blood capillaries continuously and are absorbed by the lymphatics. The circulation of lymphocytes back into the bloodstream plays an essential role in the immune response of the body.

Cell fractions resulting from trauma or tissue neoformation as well as bacteria and cancer cells are also transported by the lymphatic system. Cancer cells use the lymphatic system to form metastases in lymph nodes and other tissues.

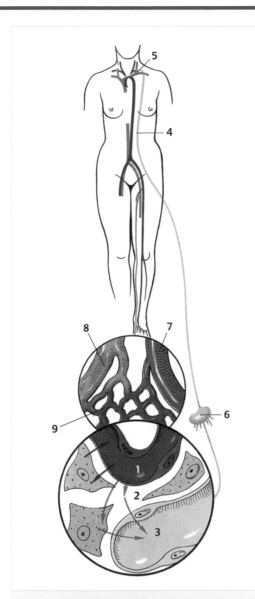

Fig. 1.2 Lymphatic return. 1, blood capillary; 2, interstitial tissues; 3, lymph capillary; 4, larger lymph vessels (collectors and trunks); 5, venous angle; 6, lymph nodes; 7, precapillary artery; 8, postcapillary vein; 9, blood capillaries. (From Kahle W, Leonhardt H, Platzer W. Color Atlas/Text of Human Anatomy, Vol. 2: Internal Organs. 4th ed. Stuttgart/New York: Thieme; 1993.)

Other particles entering the body by way of inhalation, digestion, or injury (dust of various sources, dirt, fungal spores, and other cellular components) are also absorbed by the lymphatic vessels and transported to the lymph nodes, where immune response mechanisms are activated.

Fatty Acids

Certain fat compounds cannot be reabsorbed by the blood vessels of the small intestines and are absorbed by the intestinal lymph vessels, also referred to in the literature as chylous vessels. In addition to the lymphatic loads described previously, chylous vessels return fatty acids and fat compounds back to the bloodstream. If fat is part of the lymph, the normally transparent lymph fluid takes on a milky color.

1.3.3 Lymphatic Vessels

Lymphatic vessels, also referred to as lymphatics, are found in all areas with a blood supply. Until recently, the central nervous system (CNS) was an exception to this rule. The brain, which is supplied by blood vessels and is part of the CNS, has been thought to be deficient of lymphatic vessels, as they have gone undiscovered due to their hidden location. In 2015, independent from each other, two different groups of researchers[1,2] discovered the existence of a functional lymphatic vessel system surrounding the blood vessels in the brain's meninges, the membranes enveloping the brain and spinal cord.

The system is managed by the brain's glial cells and was named the glymphatic system in recognition of its dependence on these cells. Lining the dural sinuses, the glymphatic system moves immune cells and fluid from the cerebrospinal fluid, a clear liquid surrounding the brain and spinal cord, and is connected to the deep lymph nodes of the neck.

The discovery of the lymphatic system in the CNS may change the traditional thought of the brain being an immune privileged organ. Research indicates that lymphatic clearance of the brain may play an important role in neuroimmunological diseases, and disruption of this lymphatic pathway may be involved in neurological disorders associated with immune system dysfunction, such as Alzheimer's disease, Parkinson's disease, multiple sclerosis, and meningitis, which affect tens of millions of individuals worldwide.[3]

Lymphatic vessels can be differentiated between lymph capillaries, precollectors, lymph collectors, and lymphatic trunks. The following section discusses the different characteristics of each vessel.

Lymph Capillaries

Lymph capillaries are also referred to in the literature as initial lymph vessels and represent the

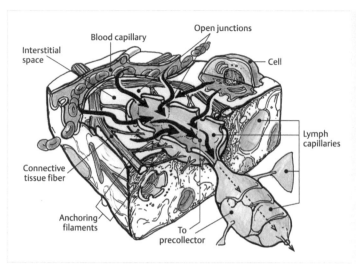

Fig. 1.3 Lymph capillary and anchoring filaments.

beginning of the lymphatic drainage system. They originate in close proximity to blood capillaries as closed or dead-end tubes in the interstitial spaces of the subendothelial layers of the skin and in mucous membranes (▶ Fig. 1.2 and ▶ Fig. 1.3). The lymph capillaries of the superficial lymphatic system are connected to each other and form a unit covering the entire surface of the body like a network, also known as the *initial lymph vessel plexus*. The meshes of this plexus are finer in the areas of the fingers (flexor aspect), palms, and soles of the feet.

Lymph capillaries resemble blood capillaries but have distinct differences. The lymph capillaries are slightly larger, have a more irregular lumen, and are more permeable than blood capillaries. Because of their unique structure, lymph capillaries are able to absorb macromolecules (e.g., proteins). The flat endothelial cells of lymph capillaries are arranged in a single layer. Cell junctions may have a continuous connection (*tight junction*), lay adjacent to each other, or overlap each other. The overlapping structures of the endothelial cells create inlet valves (*open junctions*). This structural adaptation ensures the return of protein, water, and other macromolecular substances to the cardiovascular system.

Semi-elastic fibers, also referred to in the literature as *anchoring filaments*, connect the microfiber network located in the subendothelial layer of the lymph capillaries with the surrounding connective tissue (▶ Fig. 1.3). This enables the lymph capillaries to stay open even under high tissue pressure.

The main purpose of lymph capillaries is *lymph formation*, that is, the absorption of lymphatic loads into the lymphatic system.

As discussed earlier, approximately 20% of the blood capillary filtrate remains in the interstitium, causing an increase in the volume and pressure of interstitial fluid. The more fluid accumulates, the more the connective tissue fibers are stretched away from each other, subsequently causing a pull on the anchoring filaments that connect the lymph capillaries with the surrounding fiber network.

The anchoring filaments transfer this force to the lymph capillary, which in turn will dilate and cause the open junctions of the endothelial cells to open like inlet valves. The difference in pressure between the inner lumen of the lymph capillary (lower pressure) and the surrounding tissue (higher pressure) creates a suction effect, facilitating the movement of tissue fluid and other components from the interstitial space into the lymphatic system.

This directional flow of lymphatic loads ends when the lymph capillary is filled to capacity. In this phase, the pressure inside the lymph capillary is actually greater than the pressure in the surrounding interstitial tissues. This pressure difference causes the open junctions (or inlet valves) to close. The opening and closing mechanism of the lymph capillaries adapts to the volume of fluid in the interstitial spaces. This repetitive process will continue in those areas with blood supply and ultrafiltration of fluid from the blood capillaries.

Mobilization of connective tissue from the outside (see also Chapter 4, Manual Lymph Drainage) can also manipulate anchoring filaments with subsequent opening of lymph capillaries, thereby increasing the uptake of lymphatic loads into the lymphatic system.

Lymph capillaries do not contain valves; thus, lymph fluid is able to move freely in all directions throughout the initial lymph vessel plexus. Under physiological conditions, lymph fluid moves from the capillaries into the precollectors because the resistance in the slightly bigger precollectors is lower than in the lymph capillaries.

Precollectors

Precollectors represent the connection between lymph capillaries and collectors. Precollectors of the superficial lymphatic system generally connect the lymph capillaries with the superficial collectors embedded in the subcutaneous fatty layer of the tissue. Some of these precollectors perforate the fascia and create a connection between the superficial and deep lymphatic system (*perforating precollectors*).

The wall structure of precollectors varies. Endothelial cells have predominantly tight junctions, and smooth musculature is present in some areas in the wall. There are also areas with open junctions between endothelial cells as in lymph capillaries. Precollectors may also contain valves, although in fewer numbers than those found in collectors.

It is postulated that the main purpose of precollectors is the transport of lymph fluid from the capillaries to lymph collectors. Due to the capillary-like wall structure in some areas, precollectors are able to absorb lymphatic loads. This is why these vessels are also referred to in some of the literature as part of the initial lymphatics.

Lymph Collectors

Lymph collectors transport lymph fluid to the lymph nodes and the lymphatic trunks. The diameter of collectors varies between 0.1 and 0.6 mm; their walls are structured similarly to those of

veins and consist of three distinct layers. The inner layer (intima) consists of endothelial cells and a basal membrane, the medium layer (media) contains a network of smooth musculature, and collagen tissue is present in the outer layer (adventitia).

Collectors contain valves, which, as in venous vessels, allow the flow of fluid in one direction only (proximal). The interval between the valves is irregular and varies between 6 and 20 mm (up to 10 cm in larger trunks). The segment of a collector located between a proximal and a distal pair of valves is called a *lymph angion* (▶ Fig. 1.4). The media in valvular areas of lymph collectors contain less smooth musculature than the angion area. Lymph angions have an autonomic contraction frequency of about 10 to 12 contractions per minute at rest (*lymphangiomotoricity*).

In healthy lymph collectors, the proximal valve is open during the systole, whereas the distal valve is closed; in the diastole, the opposite is the case. This permits directional flow of lymph fluid from distal to proximal angions. In lymphangiectasia (dilation) with valvular insufficiency, the lymph flow may reverse into distal lymph angions (*lymphatic reflux*).

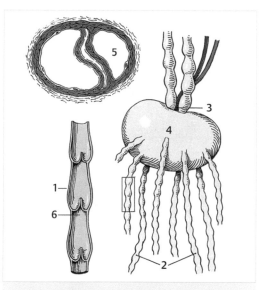

Fig. 1.4 Lymph collectors. 1, lymph collector; 2, afferent lymph collector to lymph node; 3, efferent lymph collector from lymph node; 4, lymph node; 5, cross section through a lymph collector in the area of the valves; 6, lymph angion. (From Kahle W, Leonhardt H, Platzer W. Color Atlas/Text of Human Anatomy, Vol. 2: Internal Organs. 4th ed. Stuttgart/New York: Thieme; 1993.)

Lymph collectors have the ability to react to an increase in lymph formation with an increase in contraction frequency. The increase in lymph fluid entering the lymph angion will cause a stretch on the wall of the angion, which in turn results in an increase in lymphangiomotoricity (*lymphatic safety factor*; see also Chapter 2, Safety Factor of the Lymphatic System).

Other factors that may influence lymphangio-motoricity are external stretch on the lymph angion wall (e.g., manual lymph drainage), temperature, activity of muscle and joint pumps, diaphragmatic breathing, pulsation of adjacent arteries, and certain tissue hormones. Stimulation of the local sympathetic tone may also increase the pulsation frequency of lymph collectors.

As stated earlier, the superficial and deep lymph collectors can be differentiated. The transport vessels of the superficial lymphatic system are embedded in the subcutaneous fatty layer of the skin and follow a fairly straight path within their drainage areas toward the lymph nodes, whereas the collectors belonging to the deep and organ systems follow the anatomy of larger blood vessels and organ vessels, respectively.

> Lymph collectors are responsible for draining lymphatic loads from certain body areas, known as *tributary or drainage areas*. Most drainage areas of the superficial lymphatic system are subdivided into *lymphatic territories*.

Lymphatic territories consist of several collectors that are responsible for the drainage of the same body area. All collectors in a lymphatic territory transport lymph fluid into the same group of lymph nodes (regional lymph nodes). Lymphatic territories are separated by *lymphatic watersheds* (see discussion later in this chapter). Traversing toward the lymph nodes, collectors on the extremities parallel the watersheds, whereas collectors on the trunk tend to originate at the watersheds.

Connections between lymph collectors belonging to the same territory (*intraterritorial lympho-lymphatic anastomoses*) are frequent

and important to ensure sufficient return of the lymph fluid from peripheral areas. Connections between lymph collectors of adjacent territories are much less frequent. These interterritorial anastomoses vary depending on location (see also later in this chapter).

Lymphatic Trunks

These vessels show the same wall structure as lymph collectors, but generally they contain a more developed muscle structure in the media. Lymphatic trunks, like lymph collectors, are innervated by the sympathetic nervous system. Intralymphatic valves have the same structure and passive function as in collectors.

> Lymph collectors transport the lymph fluid from the superficial, deep, and organ systems to the lymphatic trunks, which then forward the lymph to the venous angles (▶ Fig. 1.5).

Lumbar Trunks

The left and right lumbar trunks are responsible for the drainage of the lower extremities, the lower body quadrants, and the external genitalia (▶ Fig. 1.6 and ▶ Fig. 1.7). Both lumbar trunks, together with the gastrointestinal trunk (which brings lymph fluid from the stomach and digestive system, the liver, and the pancreas), form the *cisterna chyli* (▶ Fig. 1.6 and ▶ Fig. 1.7). Chylous lymph fluid from the digestive system is mixed with the transparent lymph fluid from various other tissues (described in Superficial Layer and in Deep Layer, later) in the cisterna chyli. The location of this saclike reservoir varies but is usually between the vertebral levels T11 and L2 (anterior); it is between 3 and 8 cm long, and its width varies between 0.5 and 1.5 cm.

Thoracic Duct

The thoracic duct originates together with the cisterna chyli and represents the largest lymph trunk in the body. The length varies between 36 and 45 cm, and its width between 1 and 5 mm. Its

Lymph capillaries → Precollectors → Collectors → Lymph nodes → Trunks → Venous angles

Fig. 1.5 The pattern of lymphatic return to the venous system.

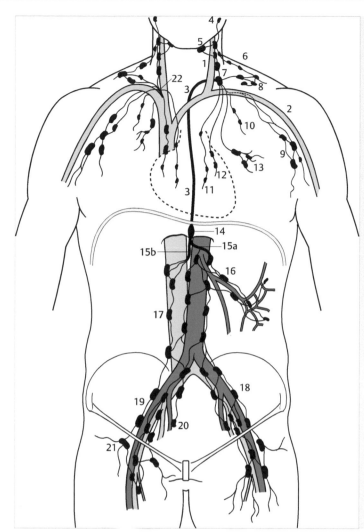

Fig. 1.6 The most important lymphatic trunks and lymph node groups of the body. 1, internal jugular vein (left); 2, subclavian vein (left); 3, thoracic duct; 4, parotid nodes; 5, submandibular nodes; 6, concomitant nodes of the accessory nerve; 7, internal jugular nodes with (left) jugular trunk; 8, supraclavicular nodes with (left) supraclavicular trunk; 9, axillary nodes with (left) subclavian trunk; 10, intercostal nodes with (left) intercostal trunk; 11, parasternal nodes with (left) parasternal trunk; 12, anterior mediastinal nodes with (left) anterior mediastinal trunk; 13, tracheobronchial nodes with (left) tracheobronchial trunk; 14, cisterna chyli; 15a, left lumbar trunk; 15b, right lumbar trunk; 16, mesenteric nodes; 17, lumbar nodes; 18, iliac nodes; 19, iliac nodes; 20, iliac nodes; 21, inguinal nodes; 22, right lymphatic duct. (From Wittlinger H, Wittlinger D, Wittlinger A, Wittlinger M. Dr. Vodder's Manual Lymph Drainage. Stuttgart/New York: Thieme; 2001.)

origin is located between the peritoneum and the vertebral column and varies, as with the cisterna chyli, between T11 and L2 (▶ Fig. 1.6 and ▶ Fig. 1.7). On its way to the venous angle, the thoracic duct perforates the diaphragm together with the aorta at the aortic hiatus and runs in the posterior mediastinum in the cranial direction. In the majority of cases, the thoracic duct empties the lymph fluid (average 3 liters per day, representing approximately three-quarters of the total body lymph fluid) into the left venous angle. The left venous angle is composed of the left internal jugular and left subclavian vein (▶ Fig. 1.7). Valves at the junction between the venous angle and the thoracic duct prevent reflux of venous blood into the lymphatic system.

Right Lymphatic Duct

This 1- to 1.5-cm-long trunk is generally formed by the confluence of the right jugular, supraclavicular, subclavian, and parasternal trunks and connects with the venous system in the area of the right venous angle (formed by the right internal jugular and subclavian veins). Approximately one-quarter of the lymph fluid passing through the body in the course of a day returns to the venous system via the right lymphatic duct (▶ Fig. 1.6 and ▶ Fig. 1.7).

The jugular, supraclavicular, subclavian, and parasternal trunks are bilateral and located in the upper half of the body. They connect either separately or together with the thoracic duct or the right lymphatic duct with the respective venous

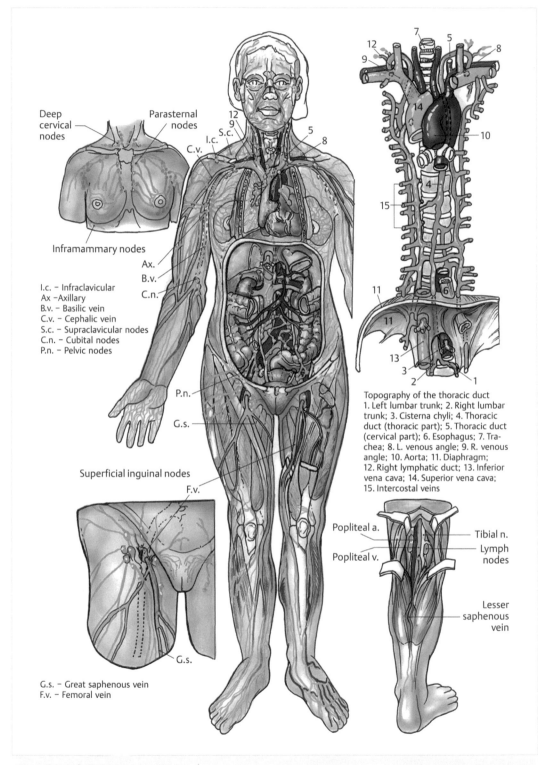

Deep cervical nodes

Parasternal nodes

12
9
S.c.
I.c.
C.v.

5
8

Inframammary nodes

Ax.
B.v.
C.n.

I.c. – Infraclavicular
Ax –Axillary
B.v. – Basilic vein
C.v. – Cephalic vein
S.c. – Supraclavicular nodes
C.n. – Cubital nodes
P.n. – Pelvic nodes

P.n.

G.s.

Superficial inguinal nodes

F.v.

G.s.

G.s. – Great saphenous vein
F.v. – Femoral vein

12
9
7
5
8
14
10
4
15
11
11
6
13
3
2
1

Topography of the thoracic duct
1. Left lumbar trunk; 2. Right lumbar trunk; 3. Cisterna chyli; 4. Thoracic duct (thoracic part); 5. Thoracic duct (cervical part); 6. Esophagus; 7. Trachea; 8. L. venous angle; 9. R. venous angle; 10. Aorta; 11. Diaphragm; 12. Right lymphatic duct; 13. Inferior vena cava; 14. Superior vena cava; 15. Intercostal veins

Popliteal a.
Popliteal v.

Tibial n.
Lymph nodes

Lesser saphenous vein

Fig. 1.7 Lymphatic system: overview.

angle (additional trunks in that area, which are not primarily relevant to the management of lymphedema, are omitted).

Jugular Trunk

The jugular trunk is formed by the confluence of the efferent lymph vessels coming from the internal jugular lymph nodes, which filter the lymph originating in the head and neck (▶ Fig. 1.6 and ▶ Fig. 1.8).

Supraclavicular Trunk

The supraclavicular trunk is formed by efferent lymph vessels of the supraclavicular lymph nodes, which filter the lymph coming from the head and neck areas, the shoulder region, and parts of the mammary gland (▶ Fig. 1.8).

Subclavian Trunk

This trunk (approximately 3 cm long) drains the lymph originating from the axillary lymph nodes, which are responsible for filtering lymph from the upper extremities, the upper quadrants (anterior and posterior), the majority of the mammary gland, and the shoulder region (▶ Fig. 1.6 and ▶ Fig. 1.8).

Parasternal Trunk

Coming from the parasternal lymph nodes, this trunk drains part of the mammary gland as well as parts of the pleura, diaphragm, liver, pericardium, and striated musculature in the chest and abdominal areas (see Drainage of the Mammary Gland later in this chapter).

1.3.4 Lymphatic Tissues

Lymphatic tissue is made up of a framework of reticular fibers, which are produced by reticular cells. Lymphatic tissue may be found either as scattered foci of cells, or as dense nodules within connective tissue (especially in the intestines as tonsils or Peyer's patches), or as aggregations of lymphoid cells enclosed within a capsule such as the lymph nodes, spleen, and thymus (▶ Fig. 1.9). Generally, it can be said that lymphatic tissues are dedicated to produce and distribute lymphocytes.

Lymph Nodes

Lymph nodes have three main functions.

Protective Function

Lymph nodes serve as filters for harmful material (e.g., cancer cells, pathogens, dust, and dirt) in the lymph fluid.

Immune Function

Lymph nodes are responsible for the production of antigen-stimulated lymphocytes (antibodies). Lymphocytes are white blood cells, which circulate in the blood and the lymphatic system. They harbor in the lymph nodes and spleen and are part of the immune system responsible for both directly (T cells and macrophages) and indirectly (B cells producing antibodies) attacking foreign invaders. The antibodies produced in the lymph nodes leave via efferent lymph collectors and travel within the lymph fluid to the blood for distribution throughout the body. The number of lymphocytes in efferent lymph vessels is greater than in afferent vessels.

Thickening of the Lymph Fluid

Blood capillaries inside the lymph nodes reabsorb a large portion of the water content in the lymph fluid, thereby reducing the amount of lymph returning via the thoracic duct (and the right lymphatic duct) into the venous system.

> The number of these round, kidney-shaped, or bean-shaped encapsulated lymphatic organs in an average human varies between 600 and 700, with most of the nodes located strategically in the intestines and the head–neck areas (place of entry for pathogens).

Their size in adults varies between 0.2 and 0.3 cm. The shape, number, and size of lymph nodes depend on factors such as age, sex, and constitution. A set number of lymph nodes are present at birth; although lymph nodes increase and decrease in size during the course of life, they do not regenerate or vanish.

Most lymph nodes are embedded in fatty tissue and are arranged in either groups or chains. Their capsular area consists of dense connective tissue.

Lymph fluid enters the lymph nodes via afferent lymph collectors, which perforate the capsular area, and leaves the nodes at the hilus area

The Lymphatic System
Superficial and deep layers of lymph nodes of the neck, pericervical lymphatic circle

1. Occipital lymph nodes
2. Deep occipital lymph nodes
3. Retroauricular lymph nodes
4. Preauricular lymph nodes
5. Infraauricular lymph nodes
6. Deep parotid lymph nodes
7. Zygomatic lymph node
8. Nasolabial lymph node
9. Buccinator lymph node
10. Submandibular lymph nodes
11. Submental lymph nodes
12. Anterior jugular lymph nodes
13. Lateral jugular lymph nodes (deep)
14. Substernocleidomastoid lymph nodes
15. External jugular lymph nodes
16. Accessory lymph nodes
17. Subtrapezoid cervical lymph nodes
18. Supraclavicular lymph nodes
19. Scalenus lymph node
20. Cephalic lymph node
21. Central axillary lymph nodes
22. Infraclavicular lymph nodes
23. Subclavian trunk
24. Jugular trunk
25. Supraclavicular trunk
26. Right lymphatic duct
27. Tracheobronchial trunk
28. Lacrimal gland
29. Mammary gland

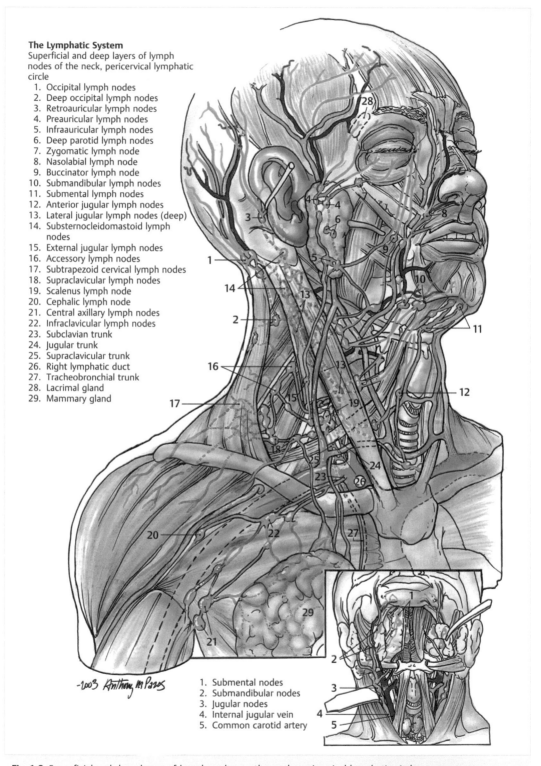

1. Submental nodes
2. Submandibular nodes
3. Jugular nodes
4. Internal jugular vein
5. Common carotid artery

Fig. 1.8 Superficial and deep layers of lymph nodes on the neck; pericervical lymphatic circle.

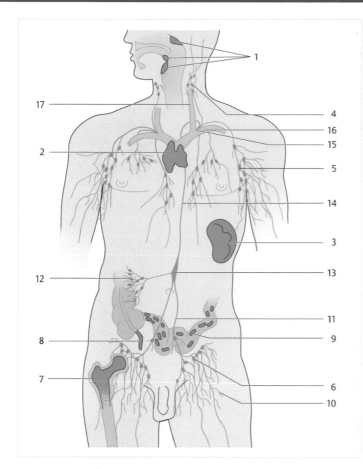

Fig. 1.9 Lymphatic tissue, lymph vessels, and regional lymph nodes. 1, tonsils; 2, thymus; 3, spleen; 4, cervical nodes; 5, axillary nodes; 6, inguinal nodes; 7, bone marrow; 8, appendix; 9, Peyer's patches in the intestinal system; 10, afferent lymph collectors to the inguinal nodes; 11, lumbar trunks; 12, intestinal nodes; 13, cisterna chyli; 14, thoracic duct; 15, left venous angle; 16, subclavian vein; 17, internal jugular vein. (From Faller A, Schuenke M. The Human Body. Stuttgart/New York: Thieme; 2004.)

via efferent lymph collectors (▶ Fig. 1.10). Collectors also interconnect lymph nodes; for example, an efferent lymph collector of one node may also represent an afferent lymph collector for the node situated further proximally (secondary node). To ensure sufficient filter function, lymph fluid will pass in most cases through more than one lymph node before it reenters the blood circulation.

The inside of lymph nodes consists of trabeculae, which compartmentalize the lymph node lumen. Those trabeculae originating at the hilus area contain the intranodal blood vessels. A large number of lymphocytes and macrophages are located between the trabeculae and are connected by a loose net of fibers.

The lymph fluid circulates within the sinus system, which is located between the capsular area, the trabeculae, and the clusters of defense cells. Upon entering the intranodal sinus system via afferent lymph collectors, the lymph flow is considerably slower than in collectors, which enables

macrophages to better identify and phagocytose harmful substances.

In many cases, regional lymph nodes represent the first line of defense in the lymph transport. The drainage or tributary area of a group of regional lymph nodes may include several lymphatic territories. For example, the tributary area for the lymph nodes located in the groin (inguinal lymph nodes) consists of the lower extremities, gluteal area, external genitalia (skin), perineum, and lower body quadrants (abdominal and lumbar areas).

1.4 Lymphatic Watersheds

Watersheds represent linear areas on the skin that separate territories from each other and contain relatively few lymph collectors (▶ Fig. 1.11 and ▶ Fig. 1.12). Although collectors within the same territory anastomose frequently, connections between collectors of adjacent territories are much less frequent.

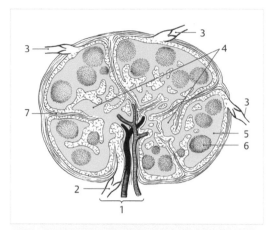

Fig. 1.10 Cross section of a lymph node. 1, hilus area (blood vessels enter and blood and lymph vessels leave the lymph node); 2, efferent lymph collector from lymph node; 3, afferent lymph collector to lymph node perforating the capsular area; 4, lymphoreticular tissue between the outer layer of the lymph node and the hilus; 5, sinus system; 6, lymphatic follicles; 7, trabeculae. (From Feneis H, Dauber W. Pocket Atlas of Human Anatomy. Stuttgart/New York: Thieme; 2000.)

Watersheds located on the trunk and between the trunk and extremities are discussed in the following section.

1.4.1 Sagittal Watershed

The sagittal watershed, also referred to as the median watershed, connects the vertex with the perineum (anterior and posterior). It divides the lymphatic drainage of the head, neck, trunk, and external genitalia into equal halves.

1.4.2 Horizontal Watershed

The upper horizontal watershed separates the neck and shoulder territory from the territories of the arm and thorax. It forms a line from the jugular notch (manubrium), running laterally to the acromion, and continues posterior to the vertebral levels between C7 and T2.

The lower horizontal (or transverse) watershed starts at the umbilicus and follows the caudal limitation of the rib cage to the vertebral column. This

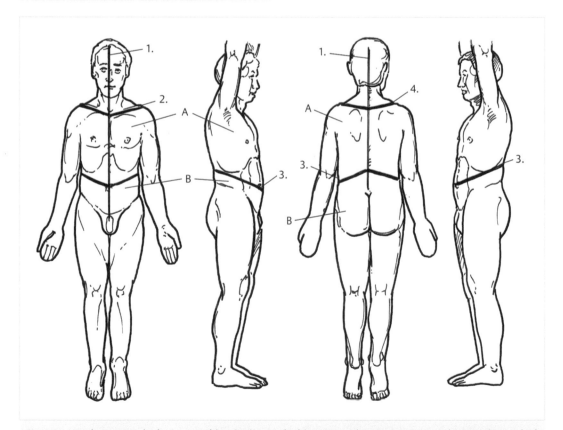

Fig. 1.11 Lymphatic watersheds. 1, sagittal (median) watershed (anterior and posterior); 2, upper horizontal watershed (anterior); 3, horizontal (transverse) watershed (anterior and posterior); 4, upper horizontal watershed (posterior); A, upper quadrants (anterior and posterior); B, lower quadrants (anterior and posterior).

The lymphatic system

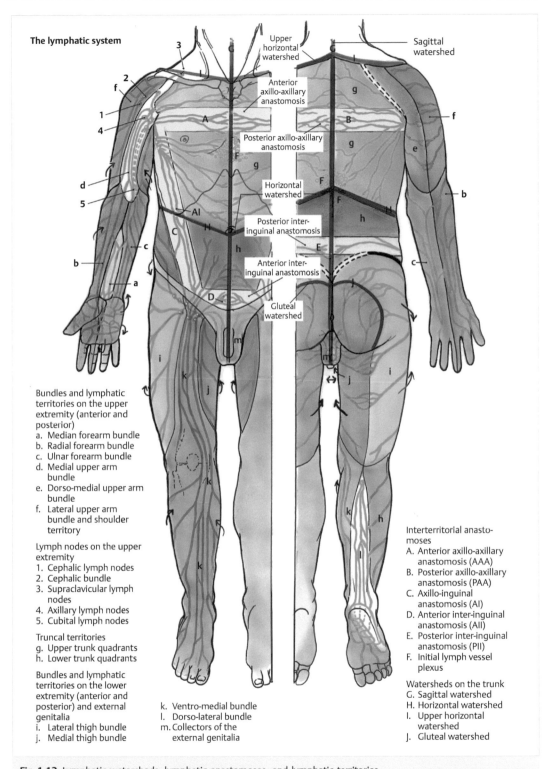

Upper horizontal watershed

Sagittal watershed

Anterior axillo-axillary anastomosis

Posterior axillo-axillary anastomosis

Horizontal watershed

Posterior inter-inguinal anastomosis

Anterior inter-inguinal anastomosis

Gluteal watershed

Bundles and lymphatic territories on the upper extremity (anterior and posterior)
a. Median forearm bundle
b. Radial forearm bundle
c. Ulnar forearm bundle
d. Medial upper arm bundle
e. Dorso-medial upper arm bundle
f. Lateral upper arm bundle and shoulder territory

Lymph nodes on the upper extremity
1. Cephalic lymph nodes
2. Cephalic bundle
3. Supraclavicular lymph nodes
4. Axillary lymph nodes
5. Cubital lymph nodes

Truncal territories
g. Upper trunk quadrants
h. Lower trunk quadrants

Bundles and lymphatic territories on the lower extremity (anterior and posterior) and external genitalia
i. Lateral thigh bundle
j. Medial thigh bundle

k. Ventro-medial bundle
l. Dorso-lateral bundle
m. Collectors of the external genitalia

Interterritorial anastomoses
A. Anterior axillo-axillary anastomosis (AAA)
B. Posterior axillo-axillary anastomosis (PAA)
C. Axillo-inguinal anastomosis (AI)
D. Anterior inter-inguinal anastomosis (AII)
E. Posterior inter-inguinal anastomosis (PII)
F. Initial lymph vessel plexus

Watersheds on the trunk
G. Sagittal watershed
H. Horizontal watershed
I. Upper horizontal watershed
J. Gluteal watershed

Fig. 1.12 Lymphatic watersheds, lymphatic anastomoses, and lymphatic territories.

watershed separates the upper from the lower territories on the trunk.

The sagittal and horizontal watersheds create four territories on the trunk; these territories are also known as quadrants (see also 1.6.3 Lymphatic Drainage of the Trunk later in this chapter).

1.4.3 Watersheds between the Trunk and the Extremities

The watershed separating the lower extremities from the trunk (inguinal watershed) starts at the pubic symphysis and follows the iliac crest to the apex of the sacrum. A line starting at the coracoid process, traveling along the axillary fold, and then continuing posterior to roughly the midpoint of the spine of the scapula separates the arm from the trunk (axillary watershed).

The location and direction of the valves inside lymph collectors inhibit the flow of lymph between adjacent territories under normal conditions. Some lymph fluid may cross the watershed via lymph capillaries (initial lymphatic plexus).

In case of lymph stasis, lymph fluid is able to move against the normal flow, over the watershed, and through alternative routes:

- Dilated capillaries of the initial lymph vessel plexus (▶ Fig. 1.12). Congested lymph fluid causes the lymphatics in the affected area to dilate. The subsequent greater resistance in these dilated collectors and precollectors forces the lymph back into the lymph capillaries (dermal backflow) and across the watershed.
- Abnormal dilation of lymph collectors may eventually result in valvular insufficiency. The valvular insufficiency leads to a retrograde flow of lymph from the congested territory to an adjacent territory free from edema. These pathways are known as *interterritorial anastomoses* (▶ Fig. 1.12 and ▶ Fig. 1.13).

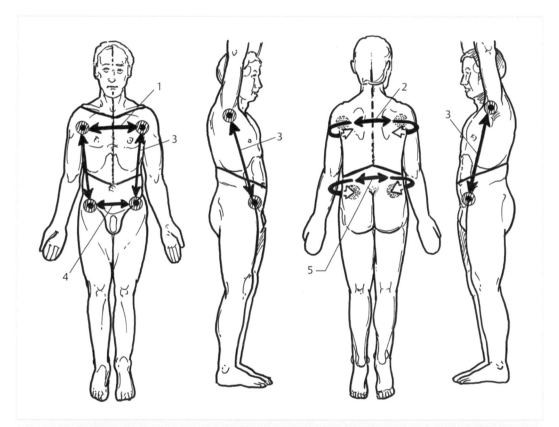

Fig. 1.13 Lymphatic anastomoses. 1, anterior axillo-axillary (AAA) anastomosis; 2, posterior axillo-axillary (PAA) anastomosis; 3, axillo-inguinal (AI) anastomosis, also known as inguinal-axillary (IA) anastomosis; 4, anterior interinguinal (AII) anastomosis; 5, posterior interinguinal (PII) anastomosis.

1.5 Interterritorial Anastomoses

If normal lymph flow within a territory is interrupted, activation of interterritorial anastomoses may prevent the onset of swelling as part of the body's own avoidance mechanisms to lymph stasis (see also Chapter 3, Avoidance Mechanisms). If swelling is present, accumulated lymph fluid can be rerouted manually by use of these anastomoses. For example, if lymphedema is present in the right upper extremity, the axillo-axillary anastomoses on the anterior and posterior thorax as well as the axillo-inguinal anastomosis on the right side can be utilized to reroute lymph fluid into adjacent tributary areas. (Refer to Chapter 5 for a more in-depth discussion of anastomoses in the treatment of lymphedema.)

Lymph collectors on the trunk generally originate at the watersheds and run in a straight line toward their regional lymph nodes. Some of these collectors originate "in line" or horizontal to the collectors of an adjacent territory. These collectors seem to anastomose more frequently than others in the same territory.

1.5.1 Anterior Axillo-axillary (AAA) Anastomosis

This connection is found between the right and left upper quadrants. Collectors of this anastomosis create a connection between the contralateral axillary lymph node groups on the anterior side of the trunk.

1.5.2 Posterior Axillo-axillary (PAA) Anastomosis

This is the connection between the contralateral axillary lymph nodes on the posterior side of the upper quadrants.

1.5.3 Axillo-inguinal (AI) Anastomosis

In axillo-inguinal anastomosis, also known as inguinal axillary (IA) anastomosis, collectors of the ipsilateral upper and lower quadrants connect and form a connection between the axillary and inguinal lymph node groups of the same sides.

1.5.4 Anterior Interinguinal (AII) Anastomosis

This anastomosis is located over the mons pubis area and connects the contralateral inguinal lymph nodes on the anterior lower body quadrants.

1.5.5 Posterior Interinguinal (PII) Anastomosis

Collectors forming this anastomosis are found on the sacrum and connect the contralateral inguinal lymph node groups on the posterior lower body quadrants.

1.6 Lymphatic Drainage and Regional Lymph Node Groups of Different Body Parts

Lymphedema manifests itself almost exclusively in the skin and subcutis. This section concentrates on the superficial lymphatic system in different body sections and will only occasionally remark on the lymphatic drainage of the deep lymphatic and organ systems (▶ Table 1.1). In the discussion that follows, the number of lymph nodes is noted in parentheses.

1.6.1 Lymphatic Drainage of the Scalp and Face

Most of the collectors in this area drain toward lymph nodes that are arranged in a circular pattern along the head–neck border. Most of the efferent collectors of the circle pass to the deep cervical lymph nodes (see Lateral Group later in this chapter). The following regional lymph nodes are collectively referred to as the *pericervical lymphatic circle.*

Submental Lymph Nodes (Two to Three)

Location

Beneath the platysma, embedded in fatty tissue between the anterior bellies of the digastric muscles (▶ Fig. 1.8, ▶ Fig. 1.14, and ▶ Fig. 1.15).

Tributaries

Central portion of the lower lip and the chin.

Table 1.1 Tributaries and efferent drainage of regional lymph nodes

	Lymph nodes	Superficial tributaries (skin)	Efferent vessels
1	Submental	Central portion of the lower lip; chin and cheek	To 6 → VA
2	Submandibular	Medial portion the lower eyelid; cheek; nose; upper and lower lip; lateral chin	To 6 → VA
3	Parotid	Temporoparietal of scalp; forehead; upper eyelid; lateral part of lower eyelid; anterior auricle	To 6 → VA
4	Posterior auricular	Parietal portion of scalp; posterior auricle	To 6 and 7 → VA
5	Occipital	Occipital portion of scalp, upper part of neck	To 7 → VA
6	Internal jugular	Receives lymph fluid from 1 to 5	Jugular trunk → VA
7	Accessory	Receives lymph fluid from 4 and 5	8 → VA
8	Supraclavicular	Receives lymph fluid from 7 and intercostal lymph nodes; skin of anterolateral neck; portions of lateral upper arm; portions of mammary gland	Supraclavicular trunk → VA
9	Parasternal	Mammary gland (~25%)	Parasternal trunk → VA
10	Axillary	Upper extremity; mammary gland (~75%); upper quadrants (anterior/posterior)	Subclavian trunk → VA
11	Inguinal	Skin of penis and scrotum; lower vagina; perineum; anus; buttocks; lower quadrants (anterior/posterior)	Pelvic lymph nodes → Lumbar lymph nodes → Lumbar trunk → Cisterna chyli → Thoracic duct → VA

Abbreviation: VA, venous angle.

Submandibular Lymph Nodes (Three to Six)

Location

The superficial surface of the submandibular saliva gland behind the mandible (► Fig. 1.8, ► Fig. 1.14, and ► Fig. 1.15).

Tributaries

Medial portion of the lower eyelid, cheek, nose, upper eyelid, and lateral part of the lower lip and chin.

Parotid Lymph Nodes

(About eight in the deep and nine nodes in the superficial group; number varies greatly in the literature.)

Location

The superficial group is embedded in the subcutaneous fatty tissue around the parotid gland and directly anterior to the ear; the deep group is embedded in the parotid gland (► Fig. 1.8 and ► Fig. 1.14).

Tributaries

Temporoparietal scalp, forehead, upper eyelid, lateral portion of the lower eyelid, and skin of the anterior auricle.

Posterior Auricular Lymph Nodes (Two to Three)

Location

At the mastoid insertion of the sternocleidomastoid muscle, beneath the auricularis posterior muscle (► Fig. 1.8 and ► Fig. 1.14).

Tributaries

Parietal portion of the scalp and posterior auricle.

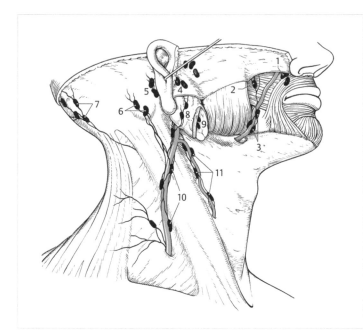

Fig. 1.14 Superficial lymph nodes of the neck and head. 1, nasolabial node (below the nasolabial fold); 2, buccinator node (deep within the buccinator muscle); 3, mandibular nodes (located on the mandible); 4, parotid nodes (preauricular); 5, infra-auricular nodes (posterior auricular); 6, mastoid nodes (posterior auricular); 7, occipital nodes; 8, deep parotid nodes (beneath the parotid fascia); 9, intraglandular nodes (embedded within the parotid gland); 10, lateral superficial nodes (external jugular lymph nodes); 11, anterior superficial nodes (anterior jugular lymph nodes). (From Feneis H, Dauber W. Pocket Atlas of Human Anatomy. Stuttgart/New York: Thieme; 2000.)

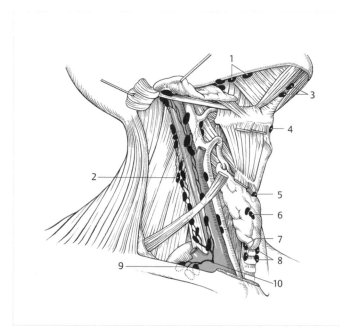

Fig. 1.15 Deep lymph nodes of the neck and head. 1, submandibular nodes; 2, internal jugular nodes; 3, submental nodes; 4, infrahyoid nodes; 5, prelaryngeal nodes; 6, thyroid nodes; 7, paratracheal nodes; 8, pretracheal nodes; 9, supraclavicular nodes; 10, right venous angle. (From Feneis H, Dauber W. Pocket Atlas of Human Anatomy. Stuttgart/New York: Thieme; 2000.)

Occipital Lymph Nodes (One to Three)

Location

Insertion of the semispinalis capitis muscle (▶ Fig. 1.8 and ▶ Fig. 1.14).

Tributaries

Occipital portion of the scalp and the upper part of the skin on the neck.

1.6.2 Lymphatic Drainage of the Neck

An anterior and lateral group of lymph nodes can be differentiated in the neck region. These groups are further divided into deep and superficial nodes.

Anterior Group

The nodes belonging to this group are irregular and inconsistent. The superficial nodes (anterior jugular lymph nodes) are grouped around the anterior jugular vein; its tributary areas include portions of the skin and musculature of the anterior neck (▶ Fig. 1.14).

The deep nodes of this group are arranged anterior and lateral to the larynx, the trachea, and the thyroid gland. This deeper set drains the lower part of the larynx, the thyroid gland, and the upper part of the trachea. The efferent collectors of the superficial and deep group drain into the deep cervical lymph nodes, which are part of the lateral group (▶ Fig. 1.8 and ▶ Fig. 1.15).

Lateral Group

The nodes belonging to the superficial portion (external jugular lymph nodes) are grouped along the exterior jugular vein between the parotid gland and the supraclavicular lymph nodes. The deep portion of this group is embedded in fatty tissue, which extends from the base of the skull to the venous angle area. The nodes form chains and follow the borders of the lateral neck triangle, which is outlined by the sternocleidomastoid (anterior), the upper trapezius (posterior) muscles, and the clavicle (inferior). Numerous connections are present between the deep lateral lymph node chains (▶ Fig. 1.8 and ▶ Fig. 1.15).

Internal Jugular Lymph Nodes (10–20)

Location

Posterior to the sternocleidomastoid muscle and along the internal jugular vein

Tributaries

Scalp and face (pericervical lymphatic circle), nasal cavities, palate (hard and soft), tongue, tonsils, auris media, pharynx, and larynx (including vocal cords).

The efferent vessels converge into the jugular trunk (see Lymphatic Trunks previously in this chapter), which connects to the venous angle either directly or via the thoracic duct, or to the right lymphatic duct, respectively (▶ Fig. 1.8 and ▶ Fig. 1.15).

Accessory Lymph Nodes (5–20)

Location

Along the upper trapezius and anterior to the accessory nerve.

Tributaries

Receive lymph fluid from the occipital and posterior auricular lymph nodes.

Additional Tributaries

Occipital portion of the scalp, skin of the lateral neck, and portions of the neck musculature.

The efferent vessels from the accessory lymph nodes connect with the supraclavicular lymph nodes (▶ Fig. 1.8).

Supraclavicular Lymph Nodes (4–12)

Location

Between the inferior belly of the omohyoid muscle and the sternohyoid muscle (venous angle area), behind the clavicle.

Tributaries

Transport lymph coming from the accessory lymph nodes.

Additional Tributaries

Skin of the anterolateral neck, intercostal lymph nodes, lateral upper arm, and portions of the glandular tissue of the breast.

Efferent vessels from the supraclavicular nodes converge into the supraclavicular trunk (see Lymphatic Trunks previously in this chapter), which connects to the venous angle either directly or via the thoracic duct or right lymphatic duct, respectively (▶ Fig. 1.8).

The proximity and possible connections of the supraclavicular trunk with the thoracic duct and other trunks terminating in the venous angle area explain why metastatic tumors from the mammary gland, lung, and esophagus, as well as from reproductive and intestinal organs, can be found in the supraclavicular lymph nodes.

1.6.3 Lymphatic Drainage of the Trunk

Four territories or quadrants can be differentiated on the trunk (▶ Fig. 1.11 and ▶ Fig. 1.12). The upper territories (anterior and posterior) are located between the upper and lower horizontal watersheds (see discussion earlier in this chapter) and the axillary watershed, which separates the trunk from the upper extremity (see 1.4.3 previously in this chapter). Regional lymph nodes for the upper territories are the axillary lymph nodes. The lower horizontal watershed and the watershed separating the lower extremity from the trunk outline the lower territories (anterior and posterior); regional nodes are the inguinal lymph nodes. Upper and lower territories are separated by the sagittal watershed (see discussion earlier in this chapter) into right and left upper and lower quadrants.

The collectors of all four quadrants are arranged like spokes on a wheel, with the origin emanating from the watersheds and the center in the regional lymph node groups (▶ Fig. 1.12 and ▶ Fig. 1.16). Some of the collectors form connections with collectors of adjacent territories, allowing interterritorial lymph flow (see 1.5 previously in this chapter).

The structure of the initial lymphatic system corresponds with the conditions described in Lymph Capillaries previously in this chapter. The initial lymph vessel plexus covers the entire surface of the anterior and posterior trunk, including the watershed areas (▶ Fig. 1.12).

Lymph fluid may use the plexus vessels to move from the extremities to the trunk, bypassing the regional lymph nodes, or to move between quadrants.

Drainage of the Mammary Gland

Regional Lymph Nodes

Axillary (and indirectly supraclavicular) and parasternal nodes.

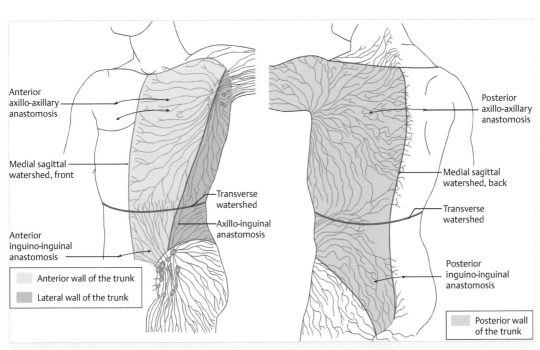

Anterior axillo-axillary anastomosis

Medial sagittal watershed, front

Anterior inguino-inguinal anastomosis

Transverse watershed

Axillo-inguinal anastomosis

Posterior axillo-axillary anastomosis

Medial sagittal watershed, back

Transverse watershed

Posterior inguino-inguinal anastomosis

Anterior wall of the trunk

Lateral wall of the trunk

Posterior wall of the trunk

Fig. 1.16 Superficial lymphatic system of the trunk with watersheds and anastomosis. (From Wittlinger H, Wittlinger D, Wittlinger A, Wittlinger M. Dr. Vodder's Manual Lymph Drainage. Stuttgart/New York: Thieme; 2001.)

1

Axillary Lymph Nodes (10–24)

Location

Consistency in a triangular outline, where the apex is the axilla, the anterior border is the pectoralis minor, and the posterior border the subscapularis muscle. Most nodes are embedded in fatty tissue; others are arranged around blood vessels (lateral thoracic and subscapular arteries, axillary vein) and nerves (subscapular nerve). Axillary nodes can be found in the epifascial and subfascial systems and are divided into five groups (▶ Fig. 1.7, ▶ Fig. 1.16, and ▶ Fig. 1.17):

- Anterior (pectoral) group.
- Posterior (subscapular) group.
- Central group.
- Lateral (infraclavicular) group.
- Apical group.

Tributaries

Axillary lymph nodes receive lymph from the ipsilateral upper quadrant (anterior and posterior), the ipsilateral mammary gland (about 75%), and the ipsilateral upper extremity.

The efferent vessels from the axillary lymph nodes converge into the subclavian trunk (see Lymphatic Trunks previously in this chapter), which connects to the venous angle area either directly or via the thoracic duct or right lymphatic duct, respectively.

Parasternal (Internal Mammary) Lymph Nodes (Four to Six)

Location

At the anterior border of the intercostal spaces and parallel to the internal mammary artery (▶ Fig. 1.17 and ▶ Fig. 1.18).

Tributaries

Mammary gland (about 25%), parts of the liver and pleura, diaphragm, pericardium, and striated musculature in the chest and abdominal areas. The efferent vessels pass via the parasternal trunk to the venous angle area.

The lymphatic vessels of the mammary gland originate in a plexus in the interlobular spaces and on the walls of the lactiferous ducts. Those vessels from the central part of the glandular tissue pass to an intricate plexus situated beneath the areola. This plexus also receives the lymphatics from the skin over the central part of the mammary gland and those from the areola and nipple. About four efferent vessels leave this area and drain roughly three-quarters (preferably the lateral quadrants) of the breast to the axillary nodes. The vessels draining the medial part of the mammary gland originate in the same intraglandular plexus and pierce the thoracic wall to connect with the parasternal lymph nodes, which drain approximately one-third (preferably the medial quadrants) of the glandular tissue.

The intraglandular plexus interconnects all drainage areas of the breast. With this connection, the lateral quadrants may also drain into the parasternal nodes and the medial quadrants into the axillary lymph nodes.

Metastases in breast cancer are most often found in the central axillary lymph nodes.

1.6.4 Lymphatic Drainage of the Upper Extremity

Lymph vessels of the upper extremity are divided into a superficial and a deep layer. Connections between the two layers are found in both

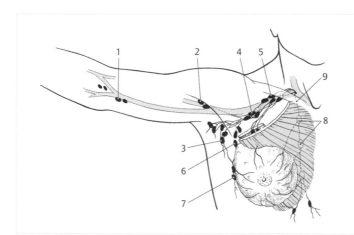

Fig. 1.17 Drainage of the mammary gland. 1, cubital nodes; 2, lateral (infraclavicular) group of axillary nodes; 3, posterior (subscapular) group of axillary nodes; 4, central axillary nodes; 5, apical axillary nodes; 6, anterior (pectoral) group of axillary nodes; 7, paramammary nodes (on the lateral margin of the mammary gland); 8, parasternal nodes; 9, parasternal trunk. (From Feneis H, Dauber W. Pocket Atlas of Human Anatomy. Stuttgart/New York: Thieme; 2000.)

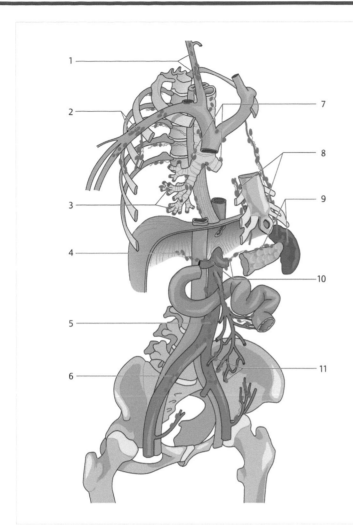

Fig. 1.18 Regional lymph nodes of the trunk. 1, deep cervical nodes; 2, axillary nodes; 3, bronchopulmonary nodes; 4, hepatic nodes; 5, common pelvic nodes; 6, pelvic nodes; 7, tracheobronchial nodes; 8, parasternal nodes; 9, nodes of the spleen and pancreas; 10, colic (abdominal) nodes; 11, mesenteric nodes (100–150). (From Faller A, Schuenke M. The Human Body. Stuttgart/New York: Thieme; 2004.)

directions. In the area of the hand, the connection from deep to superficial dominates. Perforating precollectors (see earlier discussion in this chapter) create connections from superficial to deep in other areas of the arm.

The regional lymph nodes for both layers are the axillary lymph nodes.

Superficial Layer

The meshes of the initial lymph vessel plexus, which pervades the skin everywhere, are finer in the palm and the flexor aspects of the fingers. Territories on the upper extremity (and the lower extremity) are also referred to as *bundles* (▶ Fig. 1.12 and ▶ Fig. 1.19).

Collectors on the Hand

A pair of collectors, which run on the sides of each digit (originating on the second digit) and incline backward to reach the dorsum of the hand, drains the digital plexuses.

From the dense plexus of the palm, collectors traverse in different directions. Collectors belonging to the *mesothenar territory* drain the central palmar plexus and run on the volar side between the thenar and hypothenar eminence upward to form the medial forearm territory. The *radial hand territory* drains the radial border of the palm, the web space between the index and the thumb, and the thenar eminence. The *ulnar hand territory* drains the ulnar border of the palm, the hand, and the hypothenar eminence. Collectors belonging to

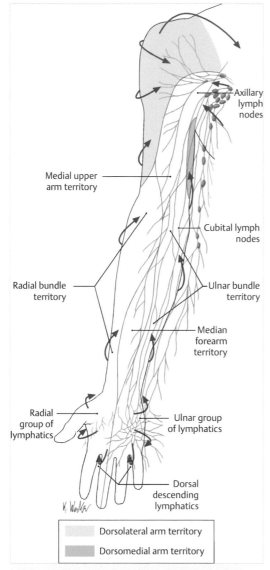

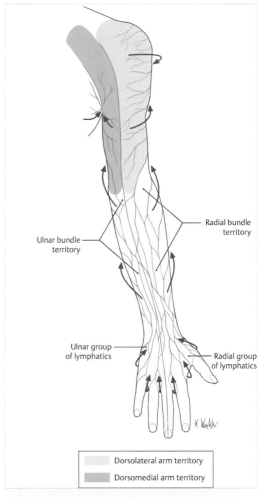

Fig. 1.19 (a,b) Superficial lymphatic system of the upper extremities, (a) front (palmar) and

(b) back (dorsal) (From Wittlinger H, Wittlinger D, Wittlinger A, Wittlinger M. Dr Vodder's Manual Lymph Drainage. Stuttgart/New York: Thieme; 2001)

the *descending hand territory* are responsible for the drainage of the web spaces as well as the adjacent skin covering the palmar metacarpophalangeal joints. The collectors belonging to the radial, ulnar, and descending territories pass around the hand to join the collectors on the dorsum of the hand, which are also responsible for the drainage of lymphatic loads coming from the interphalangeal joints. From the dorsum of the hand, the lymph vessels pass the wrist to join the collectors of the forearm.

Collectors on the Forearm

The 20 to 30 collectors in this area are subdivided into the radial, ulnar, and median territories. The *median forearm territory* represents a continuation of the mesothenar hand territory and is located on the anterior surface of the forearm. Collectors coming from the dorsum of the hand continue on the forearm with the *radial and ulnar forearm territories*, which accompany the cephalic and basilic veins, respectively. The collectors of both bundles pass around the forearm to converge together with the median territory in the antecubital area, where they decrease in number.

Antecubital lymph nodes, located adjacent to the basilic vein, may provide additional filter stations for the collectors of the ulnar territory. Antecubital lymph nodes vary in number.

Vessels belonging to the radial forearm territory occasionally ascend with the cephalic vein to the axillary or supraclavicular lymph node groups. Kubik described this drainage pathway as the *long upper arm type* (present in 16% of the population), which may have an important function in the case of axillary lymph node dissection (e.g., individuals with long upper arm type may not develop secondary upper extremity lymphedema).

Collectors on the Upper Arm

The collectors coming from the forearm continue to travel to the axillary lymph node group along the *medial upper arm territory*, which is located between the biceps and the triceps muscles on the medial upper arm. Collectors of this territory also drain the skin on the dorsomedial upper arm and shoulder.

The lateral upper arm territory is responsible for the drainage of the skin on the dorsolateral upper arm and shoulder. Its collectors drain partly into axillary and supraclavicular lymph nodes. The vessels passing to the supraclavicular nodes generally accompany the cephalic vein along the infraclavicular fossa. This pathway is also described as the *cephalic bundle*, which may contain a varying number of lymph nodes (deltoideopectoral nodes).

Deep Layer

Subfascial tissues (except metacarpophalangeal and interdigital joints) drain via the deep lymphatic system; its vessels accompany the deep blood vessels. In the forearm, they consist of four sets, corresponding with the radial, ulnar, volar, and dorsal interosseous arteries. On the upper arm, the collectors generally follow the brachial artery and transport the lymph fluid toward the axillary lymph nodes.

1.6.5 Lymphatic Drainage of the Lower Extremity

As with the arm, the lymph vessels on the lower extremity are divided into a superficial and deep layer with the exception of the toes. The fascia between the subcutis and the muscle layer is absent in toes; a distinction between the two layers is therefore not possible.

Both layers communicate via perforating precollectors. There are also connections between the superficial and deep layers of the inguinal lymph nodes (▶ Fig. 1.7 and ▶ Fig. 1.20).

Superficial Layer

Superficial Inguinal Lymph Nodes (6–12)

Location

Grouped around the great saphenous vein and embedded in fatty tissue, these nodes are found in the upper part of the medial femoral triangle (outlined by the inguinal ligament, sartorius muscle, and adductors) and can be divided into two groups. The nodes belonging to the horizontal group are arranged as a chain situated immediately below the inguinal ligament. The nodes arranged around the saphenous perforation belong to the vertical group (▶ Fig. 1.7 and ▶ Fig. 1.20).

Tributaries

The horizontal group receives lymph fluid from the integument of the penis, scrotum, lower part of the vagina, perineum, anus, buttock, and anterior and posterior truncal wall below the level of the umbilicus (lower quadrant). The vertical group is chiefly responsible for the superficial lymphatic vessels of the lower extremity; they also receive

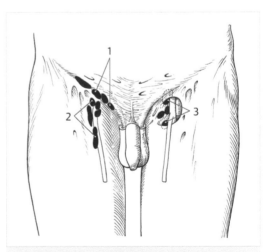

Fig. 1.20 Inguinal lymph nodes. 1, inguinal nodes, horizontal group (superficial); 2, inguinal nodes, vertical group (superficial); 3, deep inguinal nodes. (From Feneis H, Dauber W. Pocket Atlas of Human Anatomy. Stuttgart/New York: Thieme; 2000.)

some of the vessels that drain the integument of the penis, scrotum, vagina, perineum, and buttock.

The efferent vessels perforate the fascia below the inguinal ligament, and most of the collectors follow the pelvic artery to connect with the pelvic lymph nodes (▶ Fig. 1.7 and ▶ Fig. 1.21). From there, the lymph fluid continues to pass through the lumbar lymph nodes (located along the vertebral levels L5–L1) and the lumbar trunks to reach the cisterna chyli and the thoracic duct (▶ Fig. 1.7 and ▶ Fig. 1.22).

Collectors on the Foot

The meshes of the initial lymph vessel plexus, which pervades the skin everywhere, are finer on the sole of the foot and the flexor aspects of the toes. Collectors on the dorsum of the foot drain the majority of the sole, the toes, and the medial malleolus area and pass the ankle on the anterior and medial side to continue as part of the ventromedial territory on the lower leg. Collectors draining the lateral malleolus and the lateral and posterior border of the foot (including portions of the lateral sole) continue as collectors belonging to the dorsolateral territory on the leg in the proximal direction (▶ Fig. 1.12 and ▶ Fig. 1.23).

Collectors of the Lower Leg and Knee

Two territories can be distinguished on the lower leg. The *ventromedial territory* drains the majority of the foot (continuation of the collectors coming from the dorsum of the foot and the medial mal-

leolus) as well as the skin of the lower leg, except an area of skin in the middle of the calf. Collectors of the ventromedial group are larger and more numerous than those belonging to the *dorsolateral territory*. Collectors of the dorsolateral group commence on the lateral and posterior border of the foot, drain the portion of skin located in the middle of the calf, and follow the small saphenous vein to the superficial popliteal lymph nodes. From the superficial popliteal lymph nodes, the lymph continues to the deep popliteal lymph nodes and from there, following subfascial collectors, to the deep inguinal lymph nodes (▶ Fig. 1.7, ▶ Fig. 1.12, and ▶ Fig. 1.24).

Collectors of the ventromedial territory run up the leg with the great saphenous vein and pass with it behind the medial condyle of the femur to the thigh (▶ Fig. 1.12, ▶ Fig. 1.23, ▶ Fig. 1.25, and ▶ Fig. 1.26). The vessels decrease in number below the medial knee to an average of 4 to 6 collectors (from 5–10 on the lower leg). Surgical interventions on the knee, especially incisions on the medial aspect of the knee, may lead to more serious postoperative swelling involving tissues distal to this joint.

Collectors on the Thigh

The vessels belonging to the ventromedial territory continue to follow the great saphenous vein to the superficial inguinal lymph nodes. The lateral thigh territory drains the skin of the lateral thigh and the lateral buttock. The medial thigh territory is responsible for the medial thigh, the medial

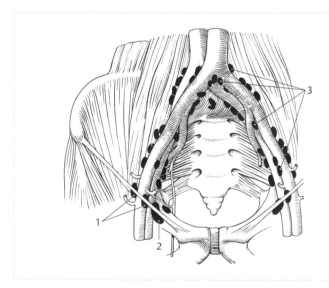

Fig. 1.21 Pelvic lymph nodes. 1, lacunar nodes; 2, lymph node of Cloquet or Rosenmüller; 3, pelvic nodes. (From Feneis H, Dauber W. Pocket Atlas of Human Anatomy. Stuttgart/New York: Thieme; 2000.)

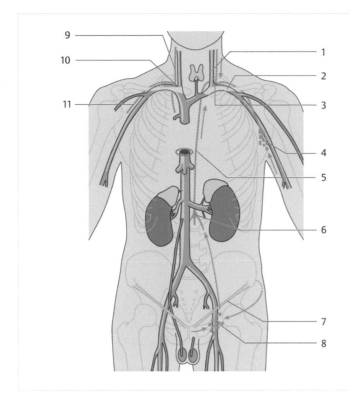

Fig. 1.22 Lymphatic pathways. 1, internal jugular vein; 2, subclavian vein; 3, left venous angle; 4, axillary nodes; 5, thoracic duct; 6, cisterna chyli; 7, inguinal ligament; 8, inguinal nodes; 9, jugular trunk; 10, right venous angle; 11, subclavian trunk. (From Faller A, Schuenke M. The Human Body. Stuttgart/New York: Thieme; 2004.)

buttock, and the perineum. A watershed running through the middle of the buttocks and the posterior thigh to the popliteal fossa separates both territories (gluteal watershed; ▶ Fig. 1.12).

Deep Layer

The deep lymphatic system in the lower extremities drains musculature, tendons, ligaments, and joint structures. The deep vessels below the knee consist of three sets, the anterior and posterior tibial and the peroneal, which accompany the corresponding blood vessels. All three transport the lymph to the deep popliteal lymph nodes.

The deep collectors on the thigh tend to follow the deep femoral artery and run toward the deep inguinal lymph nodes. Collectors in the gluteal area follow the gluteal artery and transport the lymph fluid to the pelvic lymph nodes.

Deep Popliteal Lymph Nodes (Four to Six)

Location

Embedded in the fat contained in the popliteal fossa (▶ Fig. 1.7 and ▶ Fig. 1.24).

Tributaries

Portions of the skin drained by collectors belonging to the dorsolateral bundle (superficial popliteal nodes drain into the deep popliteal lymph nodes); muscle and tendon tissue of the feet, lower legs, and distal part of posterior thigh; posterior portions of the ankle and knee joints.

The efferent vessels of the deep popliteal lymph nodes pass through the adductor hiatus and follow the femoral artery to the deep inguinal lymph nodes.

1

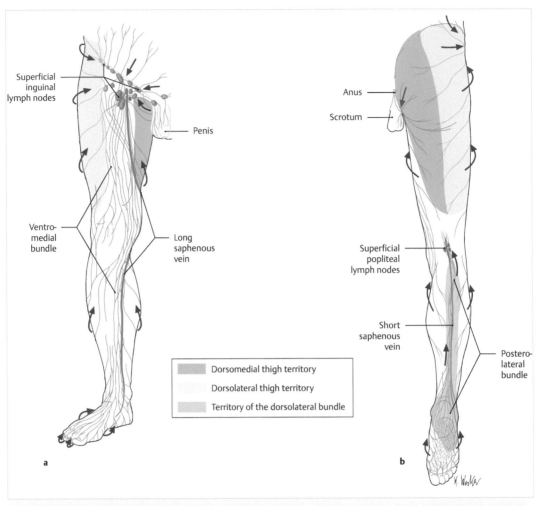

Superficial inguinal lymph nodes

Penis

Ventro-medial bundle

Long saphenous vein

Anus

Scrotum

Superficial popliteal lymph nodes

Short saphenous vein

Postero-lateral bundle

Dorsomedial thigh territory

Dorsolateral thigh territory

Territory of the dorsolateral bundle

a

b

Fig. 1.23 (a, b) Superficial drainage territories of the lower extremities and the adjacent trunk. The arrows indicate the main directions of lymphatic drainage (a) front (anterior) and (b) back (posterior). (From Wittlinger H, Wittlinger D, Wittlinger A, Wittlinger M. Dr Vodder's Manual Lymph Drainage. Stuttgart/New York: Thieme; 2001.)

Deep Inguinal Lymph Nodes (One to Three)

Location

Below the fascia on the medial side of the femoral vein. If three nodes are present, the most inferior node is situated below the junction of the great saphenous and femoral veins, the middle in the femoral canal, and the superior node in the lateral part of the femoral ring. The upper lymph node is also known as the lymph node of Cloquet or Rosenmüller (▶ Fig. 1.20 and ▶ Fig. 1.21).

Tributaries

Deep inguinal nodes receive the lymph transported by the deep lymph collectors accompanying the femoral artery, lymph fluid from the glans and corpus penis, and the outer layer of the clitoris. Lymph fluid previously filtered by the superficial inguinal lymph nodes also passes through the deep group.

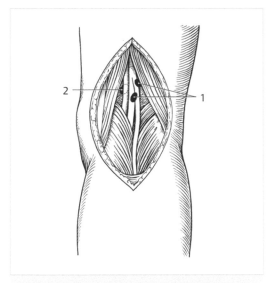

Fig. 1.24 Popliteal nodes. 1, superficial popliteal nodes; 2, deep popliteal nodes. (From Feneis H, Dauber W. Pocket Atlas of Human Anatomy. Stuttgart/New York: Thieme; 2000.)

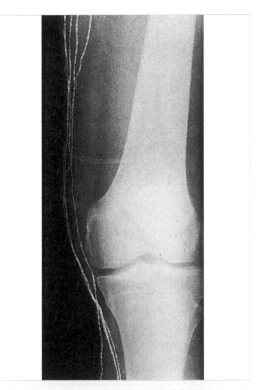

Fig. 1.26 Radiograph of the ventromedial territory.

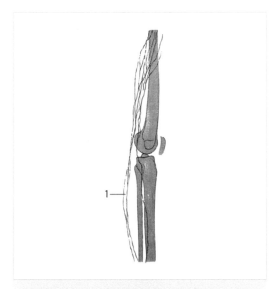

Fig. 1.25 Ventromedial territory on the lower extremity. 1, collectors of the ventromedial territory passing the knee behind the medial femur condyle. (From Kahle W, Leonhardt H, Platzer W. Color Atlas/Text of Human Anatomy, Vol. 2: Internal Organs. 4th ed. Stuttgart/New York: Thieme; 1993.)

References

[1] Louveau A, Smirnov I, Keyes TJ, et al. Structural and functional features of central nervous system lymphatic vessels. Nature. 2015; 523(7560):337–341

[2] Aspelund A, Antila S, Proulx ST, et al. A dural lymphatic vascular system that drains brain interstitial fluid and macromolecules. J Exp Med. 2015; 212(7):991–999

[3] Dissing-Olesen L, Hong S, Stevens B. New Brain Lymphatic Vessels Drain Old Concepts. EBioMedicine. 2015; 2 (8):776–777

Recommended Reading

Bates DO, Levick JR, Mortimer PS. Change in macromolecular composition of interstitial fluid from swollen arms after breast cancer treatment, and its implications. Clin Sci (Lond). 1993; 85(6):737–746

Clodius L, Foeldi M. Therapy for lymphedema today. Inter Angio 1984:3

Földi E, Földi M, Clodius L. The lymphedema chaos: a lancet. Ann Plast Surg. 1989; 22(6):505–515

Földi M, Földi E. Das Lymphoedem. Stuttgart: Gustav Fischer Verlag; 1991

Földi M, Kubik S. Lehrbuch der Lymphologie. Stuttgart: Gustav Fischer Verlag; 1999

Guyton AC. The lymphatic system, interstitial fluid dynamics, edema, and pulmonary fluid. In: Guyton AC, ed. Textbook of Medical Physiology. 7th ed. Philadelphia, PA: WB Saunders; 1986:361–373

Olszewski W. Peripheral Lymph: Formation and Immune Function. Boca Raton, FL: CRC Press; 1985

Tortora GJ. Grabowski SR. Principles of Anatomy and Physiology. 7th ed. New York, NY: HarperCollins College; 1993

Weissleder H, Schuchardt C. Lymphedema, Diagnosis and Therapy. 3rd ed. Köln: Viavital-Verlag; 2001

Zöltzer H, Castenholz A. The composition of lymph [in German]. Z Lymphol. 1985; 9(1):3–13

Chapter 2

Physiology

2 Physiology

2.1 Introduction

One of the main functions of the lymphatic system is to facilitate fluid movement from the tissues back to the blood circulation. A basic understanding of the complexities of fluid transfer between the blood capillaries, the tissues, and the lymph capillaries helps understand the lymphatic system and its role in fluid homeostasis.

2.2 Heart and Circulation

The cardiovascular system is an elaborate network designed to deliver oxygen and nutrients to body organs and to remove waste products of metabolism from the tissues. Its main components are the heart and a system of vessels that transport blood throughout the body. The part of the circulatory system that delivers blood to and from the lungs is called the pulmonary circulation, and the flow of blood throughout the rest of the body is administered by the systemic circulation (high-pressure system) (▶ Fig. 2.1).

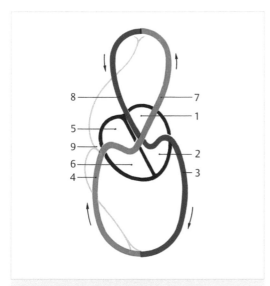

Fig. 2.1 Pulmonary and systemic circulation. 1, left atrium; 2, left ventricle; 3, aorta; 4, inferior vena cava; 5, right atrium; 6, right ventricle; 7, pulmonary artery; 8, pulmonary vein; 9, return of the lymphatic system to the low pressure system. (From Kahle W, Leonhardt H, Platzer W. Color Atlas and Textbook of Human Anatomy, Vol. 2: Internal Organs. 4th ed. Stuttgart-New York: Thieme; 1993.)

Blood that has been oxygenated in the lungs is pumped out of the left ventricle of the heart through the aorta, the largest artery in the body. The aorta arches upward from the left ventricle of the heart to the upper chest and then travels down toward the abdomen, forming the main trunk of the arterial circulation. It then branches off into numerous smaller arteries, which deliver oxygen-rich blood to the various body systems. These arteries further subdivide into smaller vessels, the precapillary arterioles. Precapillary arterioles in turn branch off into even smaller tubes, the blood capillaries, which are so thin that blood cells can only pass through them in single file. Blood capillaries consist of an arterial and a venous loop.

The walls of the larger arteries and arterioles are made up of an outer layer consisting of connective tissue (adventitia), smooth musculature in the middle layer (media), and an inner layer of endothelial cells (intima). The walls of the small capillaries do not contain any muscle fibers; they consist only of a single layer of endothelial cells (▶ Fig. 2.2). This wall structure enables an exchange of certain substances between the blood capillaries and the surrounding tissues (wall permeability). The endothelial cells, which form the capillary wall, control its permeability. Across their walls, exchanges occur between blood and tissue fluids, oxygen (O_2), carbon dioxide (CO_2), nutrients, water, inorganic ions, vitamins, hormones, immune substances, and metabolic waste. A large part of the waste products are extracted from the blood as it flows through the kidneys.

The average blood capillary is approximately 1 mm long, and the lumen diameter is approximately 8 μm. The flow velocity within a capillary amounts to about 0.2 mm per second, and the number or density of blood capillaries in a given tissue is proportional to its metabolic activity. Estimates indicate that if all capillaries of the body were placed end to end, they would reach 60,000 miles (about 96,500 kilometers). If split in half, they would cover an area equal to 1.5 football fields.

The blood leaving the blood capillaries through the postcapillary venules has a lower oxygen content. On its way back to the heart, the venous blood passes through progressively larger veins and connects with the right atrium via the superior and inferior vena cava. The pressure inside the thin-walled venous vessels is considerably lower

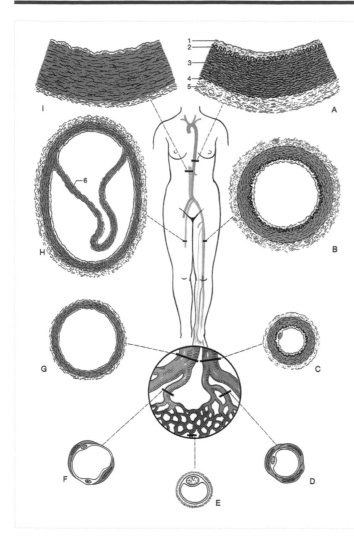

Fig. 2.2 Layers in the walls of blood vessels in various parts of the systemic circulation. A, aorta: 1, intima; 2, internal elastic membrane; 3, media (with fenestrated elastic membranes) containing smooth musculature; 4, external elastic membranes; 5, adventitia. B, larger peripheral arteries. C, smaller peripheral arteries. D, precapillary arterioles (their media are formed by one or two circular layers of smooth musculature (precapillary sphincter). E, blood capillaries (their walls do not contain smooth musculature). F, postcapilary veins (their walls contain irregularly distributed muscle cells). G, smaller peripheral veins (their walls consist of endothelium and a thin layer of spirally arranged smooth musculature, but most do not have a distinct three-layered structure). H, larger peripheral veins (same wall structure as G; smaller and larger veins have numerous valves (semilunar pockets), which open in the direction of the heart. Valves are absent in the superior and inferior vena cava and the veins of the portal circulation, kidneys, and brain; 6, cross section of a venous valve. I, inferior vena cava (the wall has a well-developed intima; the longitudinal muscle strands in the media are arranged in small bundles). (From Kahle W, Leonhardt H, Platzer W. Color Atlas and Textbook of Human Anatomy, Vol. 2: Internal Organs. 4th ed. Stuttgart-New York: Thieme; 1993.)

than in the arterial system (▶ Fig. 2.3). A system of valves inside the larger veins prevents pooling of venous blood in the lower extremities. In fact, the pressure in the venous system is so low that a sufficient return of blood to the heart would not be possible without the help of the muscle and joint pumps, diaphragmatic breathing, and the suction effect of the heart during the relaxation phase, or diastole. Together with a functioning valvular system, these supporting mechanisms propel the venous blood back to the heart.

The blood leaves the right ventricle to reach the pulmonary circulation via the pulmonary artery, which carries blood with a low oxygen content to the lungs. There, it branches off into two arteries, one for each lung, to reach the thin-walled pulmonary capillaries, where CO_2 leaves and exits the body through the mouth and nose. Oxygen reenters the blood through the pulmonary capillaries, and the freshly oxygenated blood returns to the left atrium via the pulmonary vein. In pulmonary circulation, the roles of arteries and veins are the opposite of those in the systemic circulation (▶ Fig. 2.1).

2.3 Blood Pressure

Blood pressure is the force of blood pushing against the walls of blood vessels. It is measured in millimeters of mercury (mm Hg) and reaches its highest value in the left ventricle and aorta during the systole, in which the blood is pumped from the heart into the systemic circulation. Its lowest value occurs during the diastole of the heart muscle.

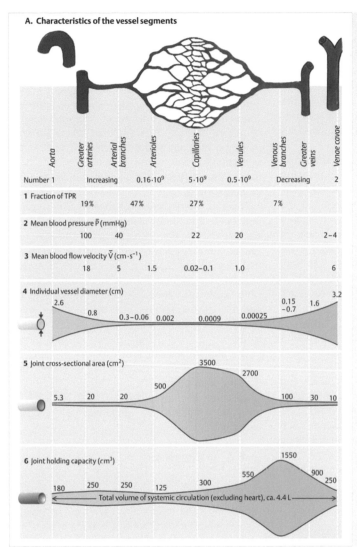

A. Characteristics of the vessel segments

	Aorta	Greater arteries	Arterial branches	Arterioles	Capillaries	Venules	Venous branches	Greater veins	Venae cavae
Number	1	Increasing		$0.16 \cdot 10^9$	$5 \cdot 10^9$	$0.5 \cdot 10^9$	Decreasing		2
1 Fraction of TPR		19%		47%		27%		7%	
2 Mean blood pressure $\bar{P}$ (mmHg)		100	40			22	20		2–4
3 Mean blood flow velocity $\bar{V}$ (cm·s⁻¹)		18	5	1.5	0.02–0.1	1.0			6

4 Individual vessel diameter (cm)

2.6   0.8   0.3–0.06   0.002   0.0009   0.00025   0.15 –0.7   1.6   3.2

5 Joint cross-sectional area (cm²)

5.3   20   20   500   3500   2700   100   30   10

6 Joint holding capacity (cm³)

180   250   250   125   300   550   1550   900   250

Total volume of systemic circulation (excluding heart), ca. 4.4 L

Fig. 2.3 Mean blood pressure values in different blood vessel segments and other characteristics. TPR, total peripheral flow resistance. (From Despopoulos A, Silbernagl S. Color Atlas of Physiology. 5th ed. Stuttgart-New York: Thieme; 2003.)

The blood pressure inside blood vessels is in inverse proportion to their distance from the heart; for example, it decreases as the distance increases and is lower in capillaries than in arteries.

Blood pressure varies with age, sex, and constitution of the individual. A rough rule of thumb for normal systolic pressure in adults is 100 plus the age of the individual. The diastolic pressure should be around two-thirds of the value of the systolic pressure.

The mean blood pressure is a value half of the sum of systolic and diastolic values and should be around 100 mm Hg for a normal individual in good health. Its value decreases continuously between the arterial and the venous end of the systemic circulation. In the veins near the heart, the pressure amounts to only 1.5 to 4 mm Hg (► Fig. 2.3). Sufficient venous return to the heart depends on supporting mechanisms described earlier.

The pulmonary circulation also belongs to the low-pressure system; its systolic value in the pulmonary artery amounts to about 25 mm Hg.

2.3.1 Blood Capillary Pressure

The diameter of blood vessels in the arterial system decreases the farther they branch out; the resistance within these vessels is in inverse proportion to their diameter (i.e., the smaller the vessel, the greater the resistance). If the resistance within a vessel increases, the blood capillary pressure (BCP) will decrease (▶ Fig. 2.3; see also 2.4.4 later in this chapter).

Because of the large diameter of the aorta and the larger arteries, the mean blood pressure in these vessels decreases only minimally. The resistance in the precapillary arterioles and the blood capillaries is notably higher (smaller diameter), causing a considerable decrease in pressure within these vessels. The mean pressure in the arterial end of the blood capillary amounts to approximately 29 mm Hg (BCP_{art}) and that on the venous end to approximately 14 mm Hg (BCP_{ven}).

Contraction or dilation of the ringlike smooth muscles in the media of precapillary arterioles (*precapillary sphincters*) also has an effect on BCP. In the contraction phase of these sphincters, the lumen of the precapillary arterioles decreases, and the blood will be rerouted directly into postcapillary venules via arteriovenous anastomoses. Less blood reaches the blood capillaries, and the BCP will decrease. If the sphincter dilates, more blood enters the blood capillaries, and the pressure inside the capillaries will subsequently increase (*vasodilation*).

The sympathetic branch of the autonomic nervous system controls the precapillary sphincter. It can regulate the flow of blood through the capillaries according to the metabolic needs of the tissue (e.g., hypoxia in the tissues supplied by the capillaries), external factors (temperature), or hormones.

The BCP may also increase due to insufficient venous return (venous or cardiac insufficiency, pregnancy). Venous stasis causes the thin-walled veins to dilate, resulting in venous pooling and a subsequent increase in venous pressure. The venous stasis will also affect the blood capillaries in that the blood volume inside the capillaries increases, thus leading to an increased BCP (*passive vasodilation*). Variations in BCP may have significant effects on lymphedema and swellings of other geneses due to increased filtration values (see also 2.6.3 later in this chapter).

2.4 Capillary Exchange

The body can be viewed as being composed of two basic fluid volume compartments: intravascular and extravascular. The intravascular compartment is composed of cardiac chambers and blood vessels and contains blood; the extravascular system represents everything outside of the intravascular compartment. The extravascular compartment is made up of many subcompartments, such as the interstitial, cellular, and lymphatic subcompartments, and a specialized system containing cerebrospinal fluid.

There is a constant exchange of fluids, gases, nutrients, and other substances between these compartments. The primary sites of this exchange are the blood capillaries within the blood capillary bed; the blood capillary bed consists of several capillaries supplied by the same precapillary arteriole. Some substances are transported across the endothelial membrane, but material (especially water) also leaves through pores in the capillary walls.

The clinical relevance of capillary exchange to lymphedema is discussed later in section "Filtration and Reabsorption."

Diffusion, osmosis, filtration, and reabsorption are the mechanisms involved in capillary exchange.

2.4.1 Diffusion

> Diffusion is the equilibrating movement of molecules and other particles in solution from an area of higher to an area of lower concentration (concentration gradient).

When areas of higher and lower concentrations are connected, more particles diffuse from the place of high concentration to the place of lower concentration than in the opposite direction (net diffusion). Substances undergoing net diffusion are said to move down their concentration gradient; for example, from higher to lower concentration. After a certain time, these substances become evenly distributed: they reach *diffusional equilibrium*. In this state, there is no further net diffusion. The exchange of substances in diffusion is independent of energy (passive process) and influenced by the following factors.

Temperature

Diffusion occurs more rapidly if temperature increases.

Concentration Gradient

The larger the difference in concentration, the faster the diffusion.

Size of the Molecules

Smaller molecules (e.g., O_2) diffuse more rapidly than larger ones (e.g., protein).

Surface Area

The larger the area, the faster the diffusion.

Diffusion Distance

The shorter the distance, the more effective (and faster) the diffusion.

Diffusion can be differentiated between simple and slow. In simple diffusion, the migration of molecules from a place of higher to lower concentration (or temperature) occurs without any separation along the concentration gradient. In the body, this form of diffusion would occur within the interstitial spaces or the cells. In case of slow diffusion, a membrane separates the involved mediums (▶ Fig. 2.4).

To better understand the movement of molecules through blood capillary walls or cell membranes, the following example is helpful. A container of water is separated by a membrane into two compartments. Sugar molecules are placed in one of the compartments but not in the other. The membrane is completely permeable for both the sugar and the water molecules. Although the sugar molecules will move in all directions, more of them will move (or diffuse) from the side of the container where they are in greater concentration to the other compartment of the container. At the same time, the water molecules will diffuse from the compartment where they are in greater concentration through the pores of the membrane to the side where they are in lesser concentration. Equilibrium (no more movement) will be reached with equal concentrations of sugar and water in both compartments (▶ Fig. 2.5).

It is important to understand that diffusion is exclusively responsible for the exchange of O_2 and CO_2 in all the tissues in the body. The majority of the nutrients and other substances obtained by the body, as well as the removal of waste products, are supplied by diffusion as well. To ensure sufficient gas exchange and metabolism, a short diffusion distance is imperative. In healthy conditions, every tissue cell is usually within 2 to 3 cell diameters of the supplying blood capillary.

Clinical relevance: In cases of swelling, the distance between the blood capillaries and the cells supplied by these capillaries increases. This increase in diffusion distance will result in a drastic decrease in the supply of oxygen and nutrients to the cells. Waste products and CO_2 will accumulate in the cells and interstitial tissues. This situation results in an environment extremely susceptible to infection, skin breakdown, cell damage, and delayed healing. It is imperative to initiate therapeutic decongestive measures in the very early stages of tissue swelling to avoid these complications or to promote healing in already damaged tissue.

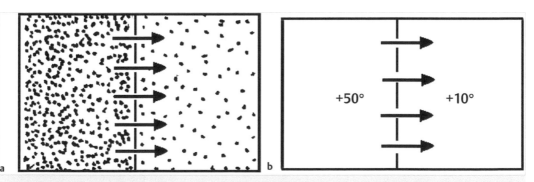

Fig. 2.4 (a,b) Diffusion. **(a)** Slow diffusion (a membrane separating the two media is slowing down the migration of molecules from a place of higher to a place of lower concentration). **(b)** Temperature diffusion (temperature moves down the pressure gradient from high to low).

2

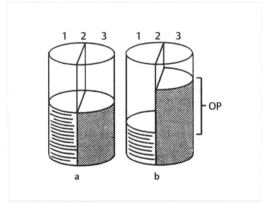

Fig. 2.5 (a,b) Osmosis. 1, a chamber containing water; 2, membrane; 3, a chamber containing a solution of sugar and water. (a) The membrane is permeable to water and sugar (slow diffusion). (b) The selective membrane is impermeable to sugar but permeable to water. OP, osmotic pressure (measured in mm Hg). The increased water level in chamber 3 causes an elevation in hydrostatic pressure.

2.4.2 Osmosis and Osmotic Pressure

Osmosis is the movement or diffusion of water molecules from a place of higher water concentration to a place of lower water concentration across a selectively permeable (or semipermeable) membrane, which is permeable only to water molecules and impermeable to other molecules.

Cell membranes in the body are generally permeable to water; water equilibrates throughout the body by osmosis.

To better understand the process of water moving through cell membranes, the example of the water container will be used again. A container of water is separated by a membrane into two compartments. Sugar molecules are placed in one of the compartments but not in the other. The membrane is permeable only to the water molecules but impermeable to the sugar molecules. In the sugar solution, the concentration of water is lower; sugar molecules take up space that water molecules would otherwise occupy. The water molecules will diffuse from the side of the container where they are in larger concentration across the

selective membrane to the other compartment of the container. The sugar molecules are unable to cross the membrane; osmosis occurs only toward one side of the container (toward the side with the sugar solution), leading to a rise of the water level on this side of the container. The hydrostatic pressure in this side of the container will increase, leading to a pressure difference between the two sides of the membrane. This is called the osmotic pressure and is measured in mm Hg (▶ Fig. 2.5).

To move the water back into the other side of the container (the compartment with the larger concentration of water molecules), a pressure equal to the osmotic pressure needs to be applied to the increased water level on one side of the container. This pressure is needed to overcome the hydrophilic effect of the sugar molecules.

The most abundant substance to diffuse through cell membranes is water. Enough water moves in each direction through the cell membranes per second to equal an amount about 100 times the volume of the cell itself.

Clinical relevance: Because the volume of water moving into and out of the cells is the same, the volume of the cells remains constant. However, under certain conditions a concentration difference for water may develop across a membrane. In the case of lymphedema and an impaired lymphatic system, the protein concentration within the interstitial tissue fluid will increase (high-protein edema) in that area. The hydrophilia of these proteins and the higher solute concentration in the interstitium will cause the water molecules to move toward the interstitial space, causing an increase in volume of the affected area. To overcome this osmotic pressure—that is, to force the water molecules back into the cells and blood capillaries—it is necessary to apply an appropriate pressure to the edematous area.

2.4.3 Colloid Osmosis and Colloid Osmotic Pressure

The concentration of proteins in the plasma amounts to approximately 75 g per liter of plasma. Proteins are the only dissolved substances in the plasma that do not diffuse readily through the blood capillary membranes. Those proteins leaving the blood capillaries into the interstitial fluid are soon removed from the interstitial spaces by the lymphatic system. Therefore, the concentration of the proteins in the plasma averages about three times more than the protein concentration in most interstitial fluids. Proteins in the plasma cause a higher colloid osmotic pressure (COP_{PL}; also known as oncotic pressure) than proteins in the interstitial fluid (interstitial fluid colloid osmotic pressure; COP_{IP}). Normal values for the COP_{PL} average about 25 mm Hg.

Clinical relevance: The effects of increased protein concentration in lymphedema and the subsequent increase of the COP_{IP} of the interstitial fluid have already been discussed in section "Osmosis and Osmotic Pressure." Patients and therapists should be cautious using external compression pumps in the treatment of lymphedema. These devices may temporarily remove water from the interstitial tissues, mechanically leaving the proteins behind. The result will be an increased COP_{IP} (i.e., the protein molecules will attract more water out of the blood capillaries). Diuretics may have the same effect (see Chapter 3, Therapeutic Approach to Lymphedema).

In case of a decrease in the amount of protein in the blood (hypoproteinemia), the oncotic pressure of the plasma proteins (COP_{PL}) will decrease. This will result in more water leaving the blood capillaries and accumulating in the tissues. The swelling resulting from hypoproteinemia affects the entire body surface (generalized edema) and should not be confused with lymphedema.

2.4.4 Filtration and Reabsorption

Another example for passive exchange of water across a membrane is filtration.

This process depends on a pressure gradient between both sides of the membrane and always moves from the area of higher to the area of lower pressure.

As discussed earlier, the blood capillary membrane is permeable to water (solvent) containing micromolecules (solutes) but impermeable to larger molecules such as plasma proteins.

The pressure gradient is produced by the blood pressure; the pressure inside blood capillaries is greater than the pressure in the interstitial fluid. Another force affecting filtration is the colloid osmotic pressure of the plasma proteins.

Ernest Henry Starling (1866–1927) discovered that under normal conditions the average BCP and the colloid osmotic pressure of the plasma proteins are approximately identical (Starling's equilibrium). But because the BCP in the arterial end of the capillary (29 mm Hg) is higher than the COP (25 mm Hg), water is filtered through the capillary

membrane into the interstitium → filtration ($BCP_{art} > COP_{PL}$).

At the venous end of the capillary, the BCP (14 mm Hg) is lower than the colloid osmotic pressure of the plasma proteins (25 mm Hg); water is reabsorbed back into the blood capillaries → reabsorption ($BCP_{vm} < COP_{pL}$) (▶ Fig. 2.6, ▶ Fig. 2.7).

The water leaving the blood via filtration washes over the tissue cells carrying nutrients and other solutes with it. Fluid returning through reabsorption

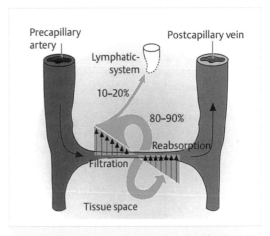

Fig. 2.6 Filtration and reabsorption on the blood capillary level. (From Faller A, Schwenke M. The Human Body. Stuttgart-New York: Thieme; 2004.)

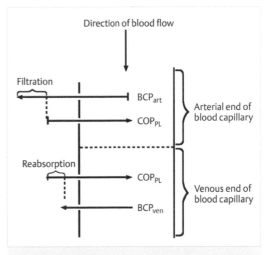

Fig. 2.7 The effects of blood capillary pressure (BCP_{art} and BCP_{ven}) and colloid osmotic pressure of the plasma proteins (COP_{PL}) on filtration and reabsorption.

2

deposits waste products from the cells back into the venous system. This "balance" in filtration and reabsorption changes frequently by contraction or dilation of the precapillary sphincter (see 2.3.1 previously in this chapter). In the dilation phase of the sphincter, the BCP may increase to a value allowing only filtration to occur. If the sphincter contracts, the BCP may decrease so much that only reabsorption takes place over the entire length of the capillary (▸ Fig. 2.8).

In the course of a day, approximately 20 L of fluid (representing 0.5% of the plasma in the flowing blood) is filtered by the nonrenal blood capillaries into the interstitial space. About 80 to 90% of this filtrate is reabsorbed back into the blood capillaries. The remaining fraction of about 10 to 20% is also known as the net filtrate and accounts for the roughly 3 L that are returned to the blood circulation via the lymphatic system.

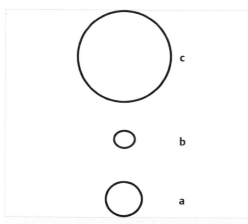

Fig. 2.8 (a–c) The effect of the precapillary sphincter musculature on blood capillary pressure and blood pressure in the precapillary arterioles. (a) Lumen diameter of the precapillary arterioles in normal muscle tone. (b) Contraction of the precapillary sphincter muscles causes a decrease in lumen diameter of the precapillary arterioles. Less blood reaches the blood capillaries, causing a decrease in blood capillary pressure. The blood pressure proximal to the precapillary arterioles increases. (c) Dilation of the precapillary sphincter muscles causes an increase in the lumen diameter of the precapillary arterioles. More blood reaches the blood capillaries, causing an increase in blood capillary pressure. The blood pressure proximal to the precapillary arterioles decreases.

Additional factors affecting filtration and reabsorption are the interstitial fluid colloid osmotic pressure (COP_{IP}) and the interstitial fluid pressure (IP).

Interstitial fluid colloid osmotic pressure (COP_{Ip}): Although the blood capillary membrane is usually impermeable toward the protein molecules, approximately half of the proteins circulating in the blood manage to leave the blood capillaries and the postcapillary venules in the course of a day. The permeability toward protein varies between the different tissues and depends on the individual microstructure. As outlined previously, the presence of proteins in the perivascular space results in colloid osmotic pressure in the interstitium (COP_{Ip}), which averages about 8 mm Hg. COP_{Ip} will cause the water molecules to move toward the interstitial space and thus "works against" the effort of the proteins in the blood to reabsorb the fluid.

Interstitial fluid pressure (IP): This is the pressure located in the interstitial fluid. For reasons not further elaborated in this book, it is extremely difficult to measure the value of this pressure. Some authors report negative (subatmospheric) values, while others report positive values. If the value is positive, it represents a force working against filtration and supporting reabsorption; if it is negative, it supports filtration and works against reabsorption.

Net Filtration Pressure

To determine this value at the arterial end of the blood capillary, it is necessary to subtract all the inward forces from the outward forces on the capillary.

Outward Forces

BCP_{art}, COP_{IP}, IP (if negative).

Inward Forces

COP_{PL}, IP (if positive).

Under normal conditions, the outward forces are greater than the inward forces on the arterial end of the capillary.

Net Reabsorption Pressure

To determine the net reabsorption value on the venous end of the blood capillary, the outward forces have to be subtracted from the inward forces.

Inward Forces

COP_{PL}, IP (if positive).

Outward Forces

BCP_{ven}, COP_{IP}, IP (if negative).

> Under normal conditions, inward forces outweigh outward forces on the venous end of the blood capillaries.

Clinical relevance: Almost all therapeutic measures and activities (as well as pathologies) will have an effect on net filtration and net reabsorption. Knowing about the relationship and interactions between filtration and reabsorption, it is easy to understand why some therapeutic measures or activities help and support the lymphatic system, whereas others work against it.

Increased net filtration: An increase in BCP results in more water leaving the blood capillaries. BCP increases if the blood volume entering the capillary increases (vasodilation). Possible causes are massage, changes in temperature (ice, heat, sauna, sunburn), passive vasodilation (insufficient venous return), strenuous exercise, infection, and other factors (▶ Fig. 2.9).

More water leaving the blood capillaries results in an increase in lymphatic load of water. In most cases, this will not present a problem for healthy individuals with a functioning lymphatic system. The lymphatic system is capable of coping with an increase of lymphatic load by activating its safety factor (see 2.5.2 later in this chapter).

However, if the lymphatic system is impaired or already overloaded, such as in edema and lymphedema, the lymphatic system in many cases is unable to respond to a local increase in net filtrate. To avoid additional problems and setbacks in treatment progress, it is necessary to avoid causes responsible for a significant increase in net filtration (heat, infection, strenuous exercise, impaired venous return).

Increased net reabsorption: Supporting the reabsorption of water from the interstitial areas back into the blood capillaries is a therapeutic goal in the management of edema and lymphedema. Increasing the tissue pressure by the skillful application of compression, with either special bandage materials or compression garments, will help achieve that goal (see Chapter 4, Compression Therapy). Simultaneous to increasing the net reabsorption, the net filtration will be decreased.

2.5 Physiology of the Lymphatic System

Now that the different factors affecting the movement of fluid through the capillary membranes have been covered, it becomes necessary to discuss the physiological capabilities of the lymphatic system to understand one of its most vital functions: the removal of proteins and other substances, along with active edema protection by the removal of interstitial fluid.

2.5.1 Lymph Time Volume and Transport Capacity of the Lymphatic System

The lymph time volume (LTV) is the amount of lymph fluid the lymphatic system is able to transport in a unit of time. LTV is lower at rest and higher during activity.

The transport capacity (TC) of the lymph vascular system represents the amount of lymph fluid transported by the lymphatic system utilizing its maximum amplitude and frequency. It is equal to the maximum lymph time volume (TC = LTV_{max}).

Under physiological conditions, the LTV at rest is equal to about 10% of the TC of the lymphatic system. The difference between LTV and TC represents the *functional reserve* (FR) of the lymphatic system (▶ Fig. 2.10).

To clarify the relationship between normal LTV, the TC, and the FR of the lymphatic system, the example of the thoracic duct will be used. As discussed in Chapter 1, the normal volume of lymph fluid returned to the blood circulation by the thoracic duct equals 2 to 3 L in 24 hours. In certain pathologies, volumes of more than 20 L of lymph fluid per day are measured. The FR enables the lymphatic system to respond to a volume increase in lymph fluid and proteins in the tissue with an increase in LTV.

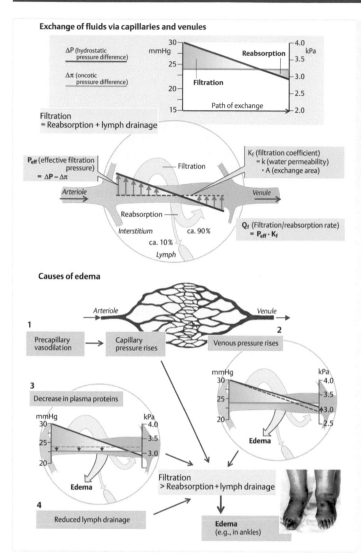

Exchange of fluids via capillaries and venules

Filtration
= Reabsorption + lymph drainage

P_{eff} (effective filtration pressure)
$= \Delta P - \Delta \pi$

K_f (filtration coefficient)
= k (water permeability)
· A (exchange area)

Q_f (Filtration/reabsorption rate)
$= P_{eff} \cdot K_f$

Causes of edema

1 Precapillary vasodilation → Capillary pressure rises

2 Venous pressure rises

3 Decrease in plasma proteins

4 Reduced lymph drainage

Filtration
> Reabsorption + lymph drainage

Edema
(e.g., in ankles)

Fig. 2.9 Causes of edema. 1, vasodilation (heat, massage, infection, strenuous exercise); 2, passive vasodilation due to insufficient venous return (venous or cardiac insufficiency, pregnancy); 3, hypoproteinemia (malnutrition, kidney, and liver diseases); 4, reduced transport capacity of the lymphatic system. (From Despopoulos A, Silbernagl S. Color Atlas of Physiology. 5th ed. Stuttgart-New York: Thieme; 2003.)

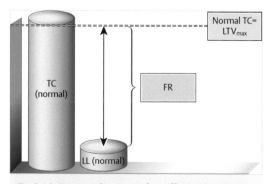

Fig. 2.10 Functional reserve of a sufficient lymphatic system. FR, functional reserve of the lymphatic system; LL, lymphatic loads or lymph volume; LTV, lymph time volume ($TC = LTV_{max}$); TC, transport capacity of the lymphatic system.

2.5.2 Safety Factor of the Lymphatic System

The body's ability to respond to an increase in the lymphatic load of water (increase in net filtrate) and protein consists of active and passive edema protective measures.

Passive edema protection: An increase in the volume of water leaving the blood capillaries results in an elevated volume of fluid accumulating in the interstitial tissue; the interstitial fluid pressure will subsequently increase. Referring to the earlier discussions in the sections "Net Filtration Pressure" and "Net Reabsorption Pressure," it is clear that an increase in IP will decrease net filtration and increase net reabsorption pressures, thus enhancing edema protection. The additional water in the interstitium will lower the concentration gradient of the interstitial proteins, thus lowering COP_{IP}. These passive measures allow more fluid to be reabsorbed back into the blood capillaries.

Active edema protection: The lymphatic system activates its safety factor; that is, it responds to an increase in lymphatic load of water and protein with an increase in lymph formation on the lymph capillary level, as well as an elevated contraction frequency in lymph collectors and trunks (increase in LTV) (▶ Fig. 2.11).

The effects of fluid accumulation in the interstitial tissues on lymph capillaries and anchoring filaments are discussed in Chapter 1, Lymph Capillaries. The increased intralymphatic pressure in collectors and trunks stimulates the smooth musculature inside the wall of the lymph angions, which leads to an increase in contraction frequency and amplitude in these vessels.

An increase in the amount of protein in the tissue (inflammation) will also activate the safety factor. Protein accumulation causes COP_{IP} to increase, which in turn results in more water leaving the capillaries. The resulting elevated water load has the same effect on the lymphatic system as previously outlined.

The lymphatic system is said to be sufficient if the TC is greater than the lymphatic load of water and protein.

2.6 Insufficiency of the Lymphatic System

Insufficiency occurs if the TC of the lymphatic system is smaller than the lymphatic load (TC < LL); lymphatic insufficiency will induce edema (local or generalized) in the interstitial area.

There are three forms of insufficiency that can result in either edema or lymphedema: dynamic, mechanical, or combined insufficiency.

2.6.1 Dynamic Insufficiency

Dynamic is the most common insufficiency and is also known as *high-volume insufficiency*. In this case, the lymphatic load (of water or of protein and water) exceeds the TC of the anatomically and functionally intact lymphatic system (LL > TC); as discussed earlier, the limit of the FR of the lymphatic system is its TC (▶ Fig. 2.12).

Dynamic insufficiency occurs if active and passive edema protective measures are exhausted, and results in edema.

Edema is a swelling caused by the accumulation of abnormally large amounts of fluid in the

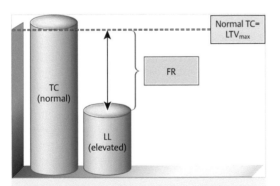

Fig. 2.11 Lymphatic safety factor. The sufficient lymphatic system reacts to an increase of lymph volume with an increase in lymph angiomotoricity. FR, functional reserve of the lymphatic system; LL, lymphatic loads or lymph volume; LTV, lymph time volume (TC = LTV_{max}); TC, transport capacity of the lymphatic system.

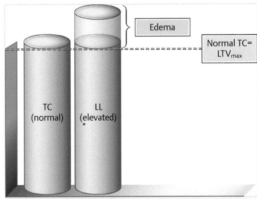

Fig. 2.12 Dynamic insufficiency. The lymph volume exceeds the transport capacity of the healthy lymphatic system, resulting in the onset of edema. LL, lymphatic loads or lymph volume; LTV, lymph time volume (TC = LTV_{max}); TC, transport capacity of the lymphatic system.

2

intercellular tissue spaces of the body, which is visible and/or palpable (pitting). It is a symptom rather than a disease or disorder and may be caused by cardiac insufficiency, immobility, chronic venous insufficiency (stage I and II), hypoproteinemia, pregnancy, and other factors.

Clinical relevance: If dynamic insufficiency is present over long periods of time (e.g., months; the duration varies depending on the condition and severity), secondary damage to the lymphatic system is imminent. The intralymphatic pressure increases in lymph collectors working at their TC over extended time periods, resulting in possible damage to the collector walls and their valvular system. Secondary damage to the lymph collectors could cause a reduction in their TC, which would exacerbate the situation.

To avoid secondary damage to the lymphatic system and the tissues, it is imperative to reduce the lymphatic load of water (or protein and water in the case of inflammation) as soon as possible. In localized edema, this is usually achieved by elevation, compression, and exercise. Manual lymph drainage (MLD) is not the therapy of choice in cases of dynamic insufficiency. MLD increases a reduced TC of the lymphatic system; it is not possible to elevate the normal TC of an overloaded but otherwise healthy lymphatic system by use of MLD.

Compression therapy and MLD are strictly contraindicated in edema caused by cardiac insufficiency (*hemodynamic insufficiency*) due to the elevated fluid volumes returning to the heart, which may cause cardiac overload or additional damage.

2.6.2 Mechanical Insufficiency

Typical for mechanical insufficiency, also known as *low-volume insufficiency*, is a reduction in the TC of the lymphatic system due to functional or organic causes (▶ Fig. 2.13).

The impairment is so severe that the lymphatic system is unable to manage a normal lymphatic load (TC < LL [normal]) or to respond to an increase in the lymphatic load of water and protein.

Surgery, radiation, trauma, or inflammation (organic causes) involving the lymphatic system

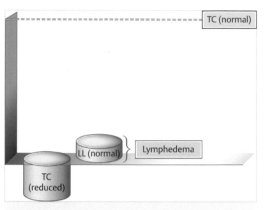

Fig. 2.13 Mechanical insufficiency. The transport capacity falls below the normal lymph volume. LL, lymphatic loads or lymph volume; TC, transport capacity of the lymphatic system.

can result in mechanical insufficiency. Functional causes may involve paralysis of the lymph vessels as a response to certain drugs or toxins (filariasis), as well as valvular insufficiency as a result of lymph vessel dilation. The walls of the lymph angions may become fibrotic due to high intralymphatic pressure and subsequent seepage of proteins into the wall structure (mural insufficiency).

The inability of the lymphatic system to perform one of its basic functions, for example, the removal of water and protein from the tissues, will result in high-protein edema or lymphedema.

Clinical relevance: Lymphedema, if left untreated, will lead to serious consequences. The stagnation of water, protein, and other waste products in the interstitium may cause tissue damage. The protein-rich swelling elongates the diffusion distance and thus reduces the ability of the body's defense mechanisms as a result of the impaired circulation of macrophages and lymphocytes. This leads to a high susceptibility to infections (cellulitis).

To reduce lymphedema and to avoid further damage, it is imperative to treat this condition by means of complete decongestive therapy (CDT; see Chapter 4) and to avoid conditions that may lead to excessive vasodilation (increased net filtrate) and infections. CDT has few or no side effects and shows excellent long-term results.

2.6.3 Combined Insufficiency

In combined insufficiency, the TC of the lymphatic system is reduced, and the volume of the lymphatic loads is simultaneously elevated (▶ Fig. 2.14).

The maximum degree of this insufficiency is reached if the TC is reduced below the level of normal lymphatic loads (mechanical insufficiency), and the volume of lymphatic loads is greater than the TC of a healthy lymphatic system (dynamic insufficiency). The combination of these insufficiencies may lead to severe tissue damage (necrosis) and chronic inflammation in the affected areas.

The presence of either dynamic or mechanical insufficiency may lead to combined insufficiency. As discussed earlier in this chapter, if dynamic insufficiency presents over long periods of time, the walls and valves of lymph collectors may experience damage. The resulting reduction of its TC will lead to combined insufficiency.

If mechanical insufficiency is present and the lymphatic load of water or protein and water increases, combined insufficiency will be the result.

Clinical relevance: To avoid further complications in the presence of dynamic insufficiency, the primary goal is to reduce the lymphatic loads. The clinical goal in lymphedema (mechanical insufficiency) is to reduce the interstitial swelling as soon as possible. It is also important to understand that infection, trauma, and certain forms of exercise result in an increase in lymphatic loads, which may lead to combined insufficiency with further complications. To avoid this situation and to further compliance, it is necessary to provide patients suffering from lymphedema with as much information as possible (see Chapter 5, Patient Education, Precautions).

2.7 Edema and Lymphedema at a Glance

The term "swelling" can be interchangeably used with edema; in some cases, the swelling must be considered as lymphedema. While the initial causes for the formation of the swelling are different, all involve the accumulation of fluid in the soft tissues of the skin due to a dynamic or mechanical insufficiency of the lymphatic system.

To understand the differences between edema and lymphedema, it is important to consider that a large portion of the human body consists of water. According to Guyton's *Textbook of Medical Physiology*, the water content of an average-weight male is approximately 60%, and in a female approximately 55%. In a male weighing 160 pounds, this amounts to about 40 L of water. About two-thirds of the water resides inside the body's cells in the intracellular fluid compartment, and one-third is located outside the cells in the extracellular compartment. Of the fluid residing outside the cells, one-fifth is located inside blood vessels as intravascular fluid. The remaining fluid (~10.5 L) is distributed in the interstitial tissue between the cells (interstitial fluid).

Fluids, gases (oxygen and carbon dioxide), nutrients, and waste products are constantly exchanged between the blood and the interstitial tissue. The primary sites of this exchange are the blood capillaries, which are the smallest blood vessels and part of the body's microcirculation. Blood capillaries have very thin walls, consisting of only a single layer of cells. Gaps between these cells enable the exchange of substances from the blood capillaries into the tissues and back. The water located in the interstitial tissue spaces is fluid that has leaked out of blood capillaries (see also 2.4.4 in this chapter).

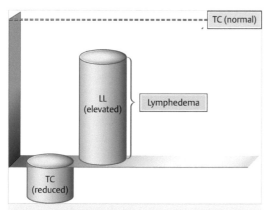

Fig. 2.14 Combined mechanical/dynamic insufficiency. LL, lymphatic loads or lymph volume; TC, transport capacity of the lymphatic system.

> Edema takes place when excess levels of interstitial fluid accumulate; this can occur if too much water leaves the blood capillaries, or if the water located in the tissues is not being reabsorbed efficiently back into the blood capillaries. Edema may affect the entire body (anasarca, or generalized edema) or only certain parts of the body (localized edema).

2

Under normal conditions, the body strives to maintain a balance of fluid in the tissues by ensuring that about the same amount of water entering the body also leaves it. However, several factors can upset the fluid balance in the body, which may cause the onset of edema.

2.7.1 Edema

As outlined earlier in this chapter, edema is a symptom rather than a disease in itself that can be caused by several conditions, including
- Congestive heart failure.
- Chronic venous insufficiency.
- Immobility (prolonged standing or sitting, paralysis).
- Pregnancy.
- Pressure from tight jewelry, tight bandages, or compression garments.

In all these cases, the accumulation of fluid in the interstitial tissues is caused by insufficient return of venous blood, also known as venous pooling. The high volume of blood and the consequent increase in hydrostatic pressure inside the veins and blood capillaries make it difficult for fluid to move from the tissues back into the vessels. While the lymphatic system tries to correct this imbalance by working harder, the elevated levels of tissue fluid are too high for the lymph vessels to compensate.

Edema may also be caused by a change in the concentration of serum proteins (hypoproteinemia). Proteins in the blood have the ability to retain some water and salts within the blood, and a lower level of proteins may affect the movement of fluid in and out of blood capillaries, causing excess levels of water to accumulate in the tissues. A loss of serum proteins may be caused by kidney, liver, or thyroid diseases, malnutrition, excessive bleeding, chronic draining wounds, and excessive burns. Inflammatory reactions caused by traumatic events and arthritis are also a common cause of the onset of edema.

Edema is a visible and palpable accumulation of excess levels of fluid within the tissues. Gentle, steady pressure with a thumb on the edematous tissues produces a temporary indentation (pitting edema). Edema can be a transitory or permanent symptom, and its treatment focuses on the correction of the underlying condition; if this condition can be resolved, the edema dissipates. If the underlying cause cannot be corrected, edema may be treated by elevation of the affected body part, wearing compression garments, diuretics, or dietary changes focusing on a low salt intake.

2.7.2 Lymphedema

Lymphedema results from the inability of the lymphatic system to perform one of its basic functions: the removal of water and protein from the tissues of a certain portion of the body. This insufficiency can be caused by developmental abnormalities of the lymphatic system (primary lymphedema) or damage to the lymphatic system such as the removal or radiation of lymph nodes in cancer surgery or infection of the lymphatic system (secondary lymphedema). Lymphedema can present in the extremities, head and neck, trunk, or external genitalia. The accumulation of protein and water in the tissues may be gradual in some patients and sudden in others; the result is always a high-protein edema. The high-protein content in lymphedema can lead to secondary complications, such as hardening of the tissues over time, infections, and increase in volume, especially in untreated or mistreated lymphedema.

> Contrary to edema, which is a low-protein swelling, lymphedema is a disease rather than a symptom and its underlying cause, the insufficiency of parts of the lymphatic system, cannot be reversed. Lymphedema does not dissipate by itself and continues to progress without adequate treatment.

The goal of lymphedema management is to reduce the lymphedematous swelling to a normal or near-normal size utilizing remaining healthy lymph vessels and other lymphatic pathways. Once the lymphedema is decongested, the secondary goal is to maintain the reduction and to prevent the reaccumulation of lymph fluid. These goals can be achieved with the internationally recognized "gold standard" of lymphedema treatment known as complete decongestive therapy (CDT). CDT is recognized as the therapy of choice for lymphedema by many international and national societies and associations concerned with lymphedema.

The pathophysiology of lymphedema is discussed in Chapter 3. Chapters 4 and 5 cover the various intervention techniques for this condition.

2.8 Understanding Starling's Equilibrium

It can sometimes be helpful to seek tangible, commonplace examples of biological, physical, chemical, or physiological processes to reinforce comprehension. In this example of "dehydrated beans," many of the processes at work in the microcirculation are represented and can be studied.

2.8.1 Process 1

For instance, if one were to prepare a soup requiring the addition of beans, these beans would most likely come in a dehydrated form requiring rehydration. To rehydrate the beans, the cook would need to soak the beans for many hours in a bowl of water. After a suitable amount of time has passed, the cook is likely to see the following results.

Expected findings (▶ Fig. 2.15):
- Wet beans (swollen with water).
- Little water remaining in the bowl.
- The skin of the beans may be ruptured.

Unexpected findings:
- A completely homogenized mixture of beans and water (mush/soup).

Principles at Work: Physiological Comparison

As such, what "physical principles" are at work to support our expected findings?
- Hindered diffusion: Why? The skin of the bean is a semi-permeable membrane. It holds back substances (proteins) that are too large to pass through its pores but allows water to pass unimpeded. Protein is retained, water moves in freely. Blood capillary walls act to retain large molecules and cells but allow water to pass freely.
- Colloid osmosis: Why? Because beans are nearly all protein and the diffusion is unidirectional. (Only water moves inward.)
- Colloid osmotic pressure (COP): Why? Because many of the beans (proteins) required more space in which to store the water causing pressure, "rupturing" the skins. Blood plasma retains pressure (because of proteins) against the vessel wall, which does not rupture but accommodates and can be measured (▶ Fig. 2.16).

2.8.2 Process 2

Now supposing we wrap the beans in cheesecloth and lift them out of the bowl. Do the beans leak water back into the bowl? No.
- Expected finding: The beans hold the water and remain saturated. Gravity has no effect.

Why is this? The colloid osmotic pressure generated between the beans (proteins) and water is greater than the atmospheric pressure plus that created by the skin around them, including the pressure of the cheesecloth covering.

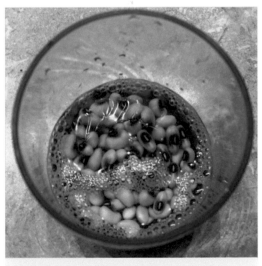

Fig. 2.16 Hindered diffusion. Water moves freely through semipermeable membrane. Proteins are retained.

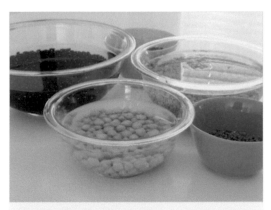

Fig. 2.15 Colloid osmosis. Unidirectional flow of water into the beans.

Principles at Work: Physiological Comparison

- COP_{PL} exceeds BCP = absorption. Colloid osmotic pressure of the plasma (COP_{PL}) is greater than BCP, which is represented by the low external (inward) pressure of the container.
- No ultrafiltration (UF). Blood (protein-rich beans) will not spontaneously leak water without a mechanical force "tearing" water away.

2.8.3 Process 3

So how can water be liberated from the swollen beans (plasma proteins)? What would need to occur?

The way to liberate the water from the beans is to gently squeeze them "mechanically" in the cloth. This external pressure causes a force greater than the beans' ability to retain water and the water is pulled away from the proteins. Only water leaks back into the bowl, while proteins are held back by the semipermeable membrane (skins).

Principles at Work: Physiological Comparison

- BCP exceeds COP_{PL} = Ultrafiltration. In the arterial limb of the capillary, BCP exceeds colloid osmotic pressure (of plasma); this process is called ultrafiltration (UF). Water leaves the blood's microcirculation (or beans) and proteins are retained. Following this ultrafiltration process, a measure of water has "filtered" back into the bowl (interstitium).

2.8.4 Process 4

What happens if the beans are dipped or immersed back into the bowl and pressure around them is released? Reabsorption (R) will occur as the proteins again generate an attraction for water to resaturate, regaining full osmotic pressure.

Principle at Work: Physiological Comparison

- COP_{PL} exceeds BCP = reabsorption. In the venous limb of the capillary, blood is dehydrated,

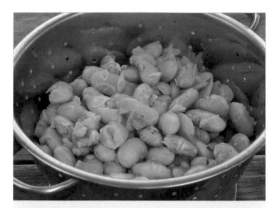

Fig. 2.17 Ultrafiltration. Swollen beans retain water. Liberation requires mechanical force.

therefore BCP is low and COP of the plasma proteins overwhelms BCP creating a migration of water toward the proteins.

2.8.5 Process 5

Now what if the bowl (which before contained only water) actually contained partially saturated beans?

When we dip the cheesecloth with beans into the water, some of the water travels through the cheesecloth and some soaks into the beans in the bowl (interstitium). So it could be said that the free beans in the bowl reduced the amount of water that could return to the beans in the cloth (▶ Fig. 2.17).

Principle at Work: Physiological Comparison

- COP_{IP} increases UF, decreases reabsorption.

Like a magnet for water, interstitial proteins generating colloid osmotic pressure (COP_{IP}) hold water outside of the blood vessel that would otherwise return to the blood. This force assists the "leaking" (ultrafiltration) of water from the capillary (beans) into the interstitium (bowl) while simultaneously reducing water volume that would return to the venous limb (bean) via reabsorption.

Recommended Reading

Földi M, Kubik S. Lehrbuch der Lymphologie. Germany: Gustav Fischer Verlag; 1999

Guyton AC, Hall JE. Textbook of Medical Physiology. 9th ed. Philadelphia, PA: WB Saunders; 1996

Kügler C, Strunk M, Rudofsky G. Venous pressure dynamics of the healthy human leg. Role of muscle activity, joint mobility and anthropometric factors. J Vasc Res. 2001; 38(1):20–29

Kuhnke E. Die Physiologischen Grundlagen der Manuellen Lymphdrainage. Physiotherapie. 1975; 66:723–730

Silbernagl S, Despopoulos A. Color Atlas of Physiology. 6th ed. New York, NY: Thieme Medical Publishers; 2009

Weissleder H, Schuchardt C. Erkrankungen des Lymphge-faes-systems. Köln: Viavital Verlag; 2000

2

Chapter 3

Pathology

3 Pathology

3.1 Lymphedema

3.1.1 Definition

Lymphedema is a very common and serious condition, affecting at least 3 million Americans. It occurs if the transport capacity (TC) of the lymphatic system has fallen below the normal lymphatic load (LL; see Chapter 2, Mechanical Insufficiency), resulting in an abnormal accumulation of water and proteins principally in the subcutaneous tissues.

Lymphedema may be present in the extremities, trunk, abdomen, head and neck, external genitalia, and internal organs; its onset is gradual in some patients and sudden in others. Most patients in the western hemisphere develop lymphedema after surgery and/or radiation therapy for various cancers (breast, uterus, prostate, bladder, lymphoma, melanoma), in which case it is referred to as secondary lymphedema. Other patients develop it without obvious cause at different stages in life (primary lymphedema), and still others develop it after trauma or deep vein thrombosis. In developing countries, parasites (filariasis) account for millions of cases.

Lymphedema is serious because of its long-term physical and psychosocial consequences for patients; it continues to progress if left untreated. If lymphedema combines with other pathologies (cardiac and venous insufficiency, chronic arthritic conditions, etc.), the pathophysiological effects are further exacerbated due to the additional stress placed on the already compromised lymphatic system (see Chapter 2, Combined Insufficiency). Its cosmetic deformities are difficult to hide, and complications do occur frequently (fibrosis, cellulitis, lymphangitis, lymphorrhea, etc.). Lymphedema is also serious because of the pervasive lack of medical expertise in the diagnosis and treatment of this condition and the tendency of clinicians to trivialize lymphedema in patients who have been treated for cancer.

3.1.2 Incidence and Prevalence of Lymphedema

There is no consistency in the data on the general incidence and prevalence of lymphedema. Incidence rates vary greatly, which results from the variety of measurement techniques and definitions used in studies that evaluate the rates of lymphedema, as well as a general lack of literature on the incidence of primary and secondary lymphedema.

Worldwide, 140 to 250 million cases of lymphedema are estimated to exist, with filariasis, a parasitic infestation (see Secondary Lymphedema later in this chapter), being the most common cause.

> In the United States, the highest incidence of lymphedema is observed following breast cancer surgery, particularly among those who undergo radiation therapy following axillary lymph node dissection (ALND).

Besides skin cancer, breast cancer is the most common type of cancer among women in the United States. The incidence of breast cancer (treatment) related lymphedema (BCRL) is generally poorly documented due to delayed onset of symptoms and the lack of standardized diagnostic criteria. Up to 40% of the 3 million cancer survivors in the United States will develop BCRL.[1,2] All women are at risk for developing breast cancer and a woman's chance of developing breast cancer increases with age. The majority of breast cancer cases occur in women older than 50 years. Although breast cancer is less common at a young age, younger women tend to have more aggressive types of breast cancer than older women, which may explain why survival rates are lower among younger women. Incidence also varies within ethnic groups and geographical location within the United States (▶ Table 3.1).

Table 3.1 Incidence of breast cancer by age

By age 30 y	1 out of 2,212
By age 40 y	1 out of 235
By age 50 y	1 out of 54
By age 60 y	1 out of 23
By age 70 y	1 out of 14
By age 80 y	1 out of 10
Ever	1 out of 8

Source: Adapted from National Cancer Institute, 1999.

Other cancer survivors at risk for lymphedema include those who have undergone surgery and/or radiation treatment for malignant melanoma of the upper or lower extremities; prostate cancer; gynecologic cancers; ovarian and testicular cancers; and colorectal, pancreatic, or liver cancers.

The incidence of secondary lower extremity lymphedema is even less well documented than that for secondary upper extremity lymphedema. Lymph node dissection for malignant melanoma has been shown to have an incidence risk of lymphedema of up to 80%, although other studies suggest an incidence between 6 and 29%.[3] Treatment for cervical, endometrial, and vulvar malignancies has been shown to have an incidence risk of lymphedema between 5 and 49%; incidence rates increase if treatment involves radiation therapy.[3] In prostate cancer, the incidence of lymphedema has been observed at 3 to 8%, which has been shown to increase with the use of radiation therapy by three- to fourfold.[3]

It is generally thought that the more lymph nodes are removed during any surgical procedure, the higher the incidence of lymphedema. The true numbers of patients suffering from any form of lymphedema are unknown.

In general, studies with longer follow-up show a higher incidence and more severe swelling. Some authors feel that with more conservative surgical procedures (modified radical mastectomy), and the use of sentinel node procedure (see discussion in Secondary Lymphedema later in this chapter), the incidence has decreased. Presently, there is not enough follow-up information available to state this with certainty.

Prevalence rates for primary lymphedema (see Primary Lymphedema later in this chapter) have been reported to be 1.15 in 100,000 individuals under the age of 20 years. Congenital lymphedema is clinically evident at birth and accounts for 10 to 25%; lymphedema praecox accounts for 70 to 80% of all primary lymphedema cases.[4]

Based on the numbers above and other statistics, it is estimated that 2 to 3 million secondary and 1 to 2 million primary lymphedema cases are currently in existence in the United States.

> Lymphedema may develop anytime during the course of a lifetime in primary cases. Secondary cases may occur immediately postoperative, within a few months, a couple of years, or 20 years or more after surgery.

3.1.3 Lymphedema Incidence among Non–Breast Cancer Patients

Lymphedema is recognized as a significant breast cancer survivorship issue; however, this chronic, progressive condition can also occur after the treatment of other solid tumors, particularly those requiring lymph node dissections. While there have been several studies examining the incidence and risk factors for lymphedema following the treatment of breast cancer,[5] less is known about lymphedema following the treatment of other tumors.

Our research group performed a systematic review and meta-analysis of the oncology-related medical literature to determine the reported incidence of and risk factors for lymphedema after treatment of cancers other than breast carcinoma.[6] We searched three major medical indices (MEDLINE, Cochrane Library databases, and Scopus) to identify all prospective studies of posttreatment lymphedema published from 1972 to 2010. These studies were identified and categorized according to the type of malignancy. Detailed information related to the surgical procedure, radiation therapy, follow-up interval, lymphedema measurement criteria, and lymphedema incidence was extracted from each article. The Quality Assessment Tool for Diagnostic Accuracy Studies[7] was used to score individual study quality, with scores ranging from 0 (worst quality) to 14 (best quality). Overall estimates of lymphedema incidence were calculated using weighted averages, on the basis of study size, for each type of malignancy.

Forty-seven eligible studies were identified that evaluated secondary lymphedema in patients with melanoma ($n = 19$ studies), gynecologic cancer ($n = 25$), genitourinary cancer ($n = 8$), head and neck cancer ($n = 1$), and sarcoma ($n = 1$). The median (range) study quality scores were as follows: melanoma, 7 (4–10); gynecologic cancer, 7 (4–10); genitourinary cancer, 5 (3–9); head and neck cancer, 5 (4–10); and sarcoma, 7. Of the 8,341 patients included in these reports, 16% had been diagnosed with lymphedema, with a reported incidence of 0 to 73%. This variability in the reported incidence can be attributed to the significant heterogeneity among the studies' clinical lymphedema definitions, lymphedema measurement methods, and follow-up durations.

Patients with sarcoma had the highest pooled incidence of lymphedema (30%), followed by patients with gynecologic cancer (20%), melanoma (16%), genitourinary cancer (10%), and head and neck cancer (4%) (▶ Table 3.2). Among patients with melanoma, those undergoing ALND had a much lower incidence of lymphedema (5%) than did those undergoing inguinofemoral lymph node dissection (28%). Overall, 2,837 patients in 22 studies underwent pelvic lymph node dissection for various malignancies; their incidence of lymphedema was 22%. The incidence of lymphedema among 1,716 patients in 18 studies treated with radiation was 31%.

The results of our meta-analysis led us to conclude that the incidence of lymphedema varies widely according to primary tumor type, treatment, and anatomic region. Currently, no gold standard exists for defining or measuring lymphedema in the clinical setting, and lymphedema after cancer treatment is often overlooked and underdiagnosed. All patients who undergo lymph node dissection for the treatment of solid tumors should be considered to be at lifetime risk for developing lymphedema. Increased awareness is needed among health care providers, and postoperative surveillance is critical. At a minimum, surveillance should include observation for signs of swelling and assessment of lymphedema-associated symptoms, such as limb heaviness and tightness, because early detection and treatment of this condition is imperative.

3.2 Lymphedema Genetics

3.2.1 Hereditary Lymphedema

In western countries, the predominant presentation of lymphedema is secondary as a result of cancer treatment. However, there are forms of primary lymphedema, which run in families (hereditary) that have been recognized as early as 1892 by Milroy.[8] Despite this long history, it was only in the last 10 to 15 years that, with the explosion of molecular lymphology, advances in genetics have taken place.[9,10] The true incidence is not clear because there does not exist standardized evaluation protocols, few centers are equipped to focus on patients with genetic-linked lymphatic abnormalities, and testing options are limited. In

Table 3.2 Incidence of lymphedema among non–breast cancer patients

Type of malignancy	No. of patients	No. of studies	Lymphedema assessment	Pooled, weighted incidence (%)	Incidence, range (%)
Genitourinary	1,060	8	Subjective: extremity circumference	11	3–9
Bladder	267			16	3–9
Penile	244			21	4–5
Prostate	549			4	4–6
Gynecologic	2,829	25	Subjective: extremity circumference, water displacement, common toxicity criteria[5]	25	0–73
Cervical	1,657			27	2–49
Endometrial	168			1	1[a]
Vulvar	1,004			30	0–73
Head and neck	139	1	Subjective: extremity circumference	4	5–8
Sarcoma	54	1	Subjective	30	30[a]
Melanoma	4,259	19	Subjective: extremity circumference, volume	9	1–66
Upper extremity				3	1–39
Lower extremity				18	6–66

[a]No range in incidence as there was only one study for each of these disease sites.

patients with primary lymphedema, it is reasonable to estimate that 5 to 10% are hereditary based on our current knowledge and testing ability. There is a slightly higher incidence in females, with males generally presenting at birth and females at puberty; however, this is not diagnostic. Examination of the lymphatic system defects in these patients has demonstrated developmental aplasia, hypoplasia, and hyperplasia of the lymphatic vessels and nodes which leads to lymphedema. The majority of patients described so far have autosomal dominant mutations, meaning a single mutated gene passed on to the next generation is sufficient to cause disease. Others are autosomal recessive requiring a mutated gene from each parent. Some of these genes have reduced penetrance, meaning that even though the gene may be present, its effect may not be seen. There are also genes that have varied levels of presentation. These features understandably require careful evaluation by the clinical team.

The Online Mendelian Inheritance in Man (OMIM) catalog focuses mainly on inherited genetic diseases.[11] This catalog is frequently updated and easily searchable. Focusing on lymphedema or lymphangiectasia, there are almost 40 syndromes that have lymphedema as a component and many of these have multiple phenotypic abnormalities involving the lymphatic system.[11] There are also additional syndromes that do not yet have entries in OMIM.[12]

The Known Genes

There are 11 genes implicated so far in syndromes with lymphedema either as a primary phenotype or as a consistent feature, more genes without a solid associated lymphedema syndrome, and 6 syndromes with chromosomal abnormalities (▶ Table 3.3). These mutations and chromosomal abnormalities are spread across the human genome and it appears unlikely that genes yet to

Table 3.3 Lymphedema-related syndromes with identified genes, genes without syndromes, and chromosomal aneuploidy associated with lymphedema

Syndrome	Gene	Main manifestations	OMIM	IP	Candidate locus
Syndromes with genes					
Hereditary lymphedema 1A (Milroy)	FLT4 (VEGFR3)	Congenital lymphedema[13]	153100	AD	5q35
Hereditary lymphedema 1C	GJC2	Lymphedema of limbs, onset 1–15 y[14]	613480	AD	1q41
Lymphedema-distichiasis syndrome	FOXC2	Leg lymphedema and distichiasis[15]	153400	AD	16q24
Hennekam lymphangiectasia-lymphedema syndrome	CCBE1	Lymphedema of limbs, intestinal lymphangiectasia, mental retardation[16]	235510	AR	18q21
Hypotrichosis-lymphedema-telangiectasia syndrome	SOX18	Lymphedema, alopecia, telangiectasia[17]	607823	AD	20q13
Lymphedema-choanal etresia syndrome	PTPN14	Leg lymphedema, blockage of nasal airways (choana)[18]	608911	AR	1q32
Emberger's syndrome	GATA2	Leg lymphedema, immune dysfunction, deafness[19]	614038	AD	3q21
Microencephaly-lymphedema-chorioretinopathy	KIF11	Microencephaly[20]	152950	AD	10q23
Milroylike lymphede-	VEGFC	Lymphedema[21]	615907	AD	4q23

(Continued)

Table 3.3 continued

Syndrome	Gene	Main manifestations	OMIM	IP	Candidate locus
ma					
Oculodentaldigital lymphedema	GJA1	Lymphedema, face, eyes[22]	164200	AD	6q22
Sotos	NSD1	Lymphedema, over-growth[23]	117550	AD	5q35
Noonan (subset)	PTPN11	Lymphedema, chy-lous reflux[24]	163950	AD	12q24
Cholestasis-lymphe-dema (Aagenaes)	?		214900	AR	15q1
Mutations without syndromes					
? Lymphedema lym-phangiectasia	HGF	Various lymphedema (15)	–		7q21
?	MET	Various lymphedema (15)	–		7q31
Chromosome abnor-malities					
Klinefelter's syndro-me	?	Associated lymphe-dema	–	–	XXY
Turner's syndrome	?	Associated lymphe-dema	–	–	XO
Trisomy 13	?	Associated lymphe-dema	–	–	13
Trisomy 18	?	Associated lymphe-dema	–	–	18
Trisomy 21	?	Associated lymphe-dema	–	–	21
Trisomy 22	?	Associated lymphe-dema	–	–	22

Abbreviations: AD, autosomal dominant; AR, autosomal recessive; IP, inheritance pattern; OMIM, Online Mendelian Inheritance in Man.

be discovered will be segregated to more focused areas. It is interesting to note that all the mutations so far have been found on the q or long arm of the chromosomes. Whether this will hold true for new genes will have to be seen.

What This Means to Patients in the Clinic

Although major advances in understanding genetic development of the lymphatic system and lymphedema-related syndromes have occurred recently, defining the link between the clinical phenotype and the genotype is still far from adequate. The first step is detailed evaluation by the clinical team to obtain a good history and physical exam which is paramount to phenotyping the patient. This phenotyping should also include imaging of the lymphatic system to define more clearly the defects seen in the system. Without clear distinctions between patients within and outside of specific syndromes, the sophisticated genetic techniques will not be as powerful.

The second step is to obtain genotype information. This will largely fall to the geneticist or knowledgeable physician on the team. After obtaining consent from the patient, a requirement due to the type of information which can be obtained by analysis of genetic material regardless of whether the patient is in a study or not, a sample is collected to isolate DNA. This sample can be blood, scrapings of cheek cells, mouthwash following vigorous rinsing, or a small piece of tissue if an operative procedure has taken place. Standardized protocols are used to isolate DNA from these samples. The number of family members who are available and whether the search will be for a particular gene(s) or for a new gene will determine what type of analysis will be employed. Sophisticated linkage analysis may take place, whole genome, specific gene, or exome sequencing may be utilized, or newer gene-chip technology could be employed.[10,20,25,26] Centers have varying levels of expertise with these techniques and some specific gene testing is commercially available and associated costs must be considered.

The Future

We know from studies in mice that there are many more genes that can impact the lymphatic system which do not yet have a corresponding gene in man or the corresponding mutations have yet to be discovered. There are also many human syndromes which as of yet have no gene defect associated with them. These areas are clearly where future advances will need to be made. In addition, improvements in availability and sophistication of genetic testing and more comprehensive and careful phenotyping of the physical and lymphatic system by clinicians should push the field forward.

The goal of investigating the genetics of lymphedema-related syndromes is to be able to bring these discoveries back into the clinic and impact patient lives. If we can identify genes that are paramount to the growth and development of the lymphatic system, then we may be able to harness this knowledge to grow (or inhibit) the lymphatic system when and where it is not functioning correctly. In addition, by carefully defining the syndromes that exhibit lymphedema, we may be able to devise specific genetic treatment plans and timing to correct or ameliorate the defects. Unfortunately, the recent history of genetic treatment has yet to yield success and we are still lacking in our understanding of the specific genes, interactions, and milieu needed for future treatment.

3.2.2 Etiology of Lymphedema

Lymphedema can be classified as primary or secondary, based on underlying etiology. However, this classification usually has little significance in determining the method of treatment (▶ Table 3.4).

Primary Lymphedema

> Primary lymphedema represents a developmental abnormality (dysplasia) of the lymphatic system, which is either congenital or hereditary. It can present as a variety of abnormalities.

Hypoplasia

This most common form of dysplasia refers to the incomplete development of lymph vessels; that is, the number of lymph collectors is reduced, and the diameter of existing lymph vessels is smaller than normal.

Hyperplasia

The diameter of lymph collectors is larger than normal in this dysplasia (*lymphangiectasia* or *megalymphatics*). The dilation of the lymph collectors results in a malfunction of the valvular system within the collectors, which often leads to lymphatic reflux.

Table 3.4 Etiology of lymphedema

Primary lymphedema	Secondary lymphedema
Aplasia	Dissection of lymph nodes
Hypoplasia	
Hyperplasia (lymphangiectasia/megalymphatics)	Radiation
	Trauma
Fibrosis of lymph nodes	Surgery
Agenesis of lymph nodes	Infection
Congenital	Malignancies
<35 years of age: lymphedema praecox	Chronic venous insufficiency
>35 years of age: lymphedema tarda	Immobility Self-induced

Aplasia

The absence of single lymph collectors, capillaries, or lymph nodes associated with this abnormality may be a cause for the development of primary lymphedema.

Fibrosis of the inguinal lymph nodes (Kinmonth's syndrome) presents an additional cause for the onset of primary lymphedema. The fibrotic changes primarily affect the capsular and trabecular area of the involved lymph nodes. This may affect lymph transport in the afferent lymph collectors.

With the understanding of basic lymphatic system physiology, it becomes evident that the TC of the lymphatic system in all the above-mentioned abnormalities is reduced (▶ Fig. 3.1). As discussed in Chapter 2, lymphedema occurs if the TC of the lymphatic system falls below the normal LL.

Although the developmental abnormalities are present at birth, lymphedema may develop at some point later in life. It may not develop at all as long as the (reduced) TC of the lymphatic system is sufficient to manage the LLs. Primary lymphedema is often classified by the age of the patient at the onset of swelling.

Congenital lymphedema is clinically evident at birth or within the first 2 years of life. A subgroup of patients with congenital lymphedema has a familial pattern of inheritance, which is termed Milroy's disease. If primary lymphedema presents after birth but before the age of 35 years, it is called *lymphedema praecox*, which is the most common form of primary lymphedema and most often arises during puberty or pregnancy. *Lymphedema tarda* is relatively rare and develops after the age of 35 years.

Primary lymphedema almost exclusively affects the lower extremity (unilateral and bilateral) and involves mostly females. The swelling usually starts at the foot and ankle and gradually involves the remainder of the extremity. It may occur without any known impetus or may develop after minor trauma (insect bites, injections, sprains, strains, burns, cuts), infections, or immobility. These triggering factors produce additional stress to the already impaired lymphatic system, resulting in mechanical insufficiency (▶ Fig. 3.2).

Secondary Lymphedema

The mechanical insufficiency present in secondary lymphedema is caused by a known insult to the lymphatic system.

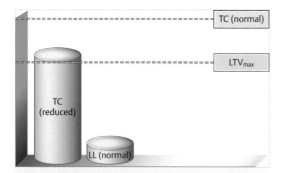

Fig. 3.1 Reduced transport capacity in the subclinical stage of lymphedema. LL, lymphatic loads or lymph volume; LTV, lymph time volume (TC = LTV_{max}); TC, transport capacity of the lymphatic system.

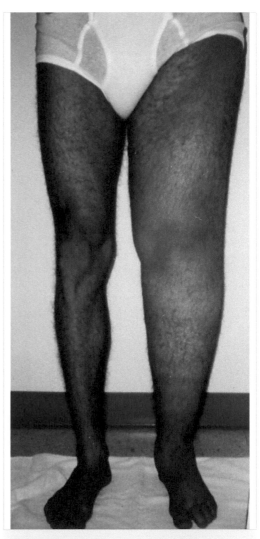

Fig. 3.2 Primary lymphedema of the left lower extremity.

Most common causes for secondary lymphedema include surgery and radiation, trauma, infection, malignant tumors, immobility, and chronic venous insufficiency (CVI).

Lymphedema may also be self-induced.

Surgery and radiation: As outlined earlier, this is by far the most common cause for secondary lymphedema in the United States. Surgical procedures in cancer therapy commonly include the removal (dissection) of lymph nodes. The goal of these procedures is to eliminate the cancer cells and to save the patient's life.

A side effect in lymph node dissection is the disruption in the lymph transport. If the remaining lymphatics are unable to manage the LL, secondary lymphedema will develop.

In the early years of breast cancer surgery, *radical mastectomy* was the only option available for patients. Radical mastectomy includes the removal of the entire mammary gland, the axillary lymph nodes, and the pectoralis muscles under the breast. Although common in the past, radical mastectomy is now rarely performed and is recommended only if the cancer cells have spread to the muscles under the mammary gland. *Modified radical mastectomy* is now more commonly performed. This procedure includes the removal of the breast and part of the axillary lymph nodes. In certain forms of breast cancer, a *simple* or *total mastectomy* is performed, in which only the mammary gland, but not the axillary lymph nodes, is removed.

Today, many women with breast cancer are given the choice between mastectomy and *lumpectomy*. In lumpectomy, also referred to as breast-conserving surgery, only the part of the mammary gland containing the malignant tumor and some of the normal surrounding tissue are removed. Most women after breast surgery, especially after lumpectomy, receive radiation treatment (▶ Fig. 3.3).

Sentinel lymph node biopsy (SLNB), a relatively new technique, was developed to determine if cancer cells have spread to the axillary nodes and trunks, without having to perform a traditional ALND during which, on average, about 10 to 15 axillary lymph nodes are removed. An SLNB requires the removal of only those lymph nodes to which the mammary gland drains first (sentinel

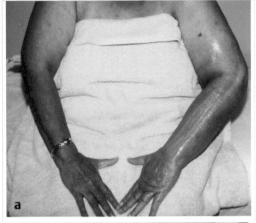

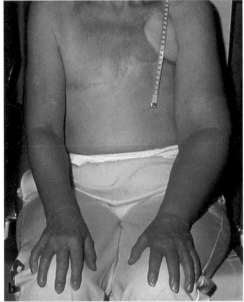

Fig. 3.3 (a) Secondary lymphedema of the left upper extremity. (b) Secondary lymphedema of the left upper extremity following bilateral mastectomy.

nodes) before reaching the rest of the axillary lymph nodes. A pathologist then closely reviews one to three lymph nodes. If they do not contain malignant cells, the chance that the remaining axillary nodes are cancer free is approximately 95%, and removal of additional axillary nodes may be avoided.

Radiation (or radiotherapy) is the treatment of cancer and other diseases with ionizing radiation. The goal of this therapy is to destroy cancer cells that may linger after surgery. It uses either precisely aimed, high-energy, external beam radiation or radioactive seeds that are implanted in the tumor area. Malignant cells often grow at a faster rate than normal cells; this makes many cancers very sensitive, that is, vulnerable to radiation.

Although radiation damages both cancer cells and normal cells, the normal cells are able to repair themselves and continue to function properly. Radiation is usually administered 5 days a week for several weeks and may also contribute to the onset of lymphedema. Rays can cause fibrosis in the tissues, leading to an impaired lymph transport, and hinder the regeneration of lymph vessels. Radiation may also affect nervous tissue, which can result in numerous problems affecting either the lymphedema itself or the patient's ability and compliance during the treatment of the lymphedema (radiation plexopathy; see 3.2.7 later in this chapter).

Trauma: Traumatic insults involving the lymphatic system may cause a significant reduction in lymph flow, resulting in secondary lymphedema (burns, larger skin abrasions). Scar tissue hinders regeneration (lympholymphatic anastomosis) of lymph collectors, further exacerbating the problem. Posttraumatic secondary lymphedema develops from a mechanical insufficiency of the lymphatic system as a result of tissue lesions and should not be confused with posttraumatic edema. Posttraumatic edema is a local result due to trauma, which usually recedes after a few days (see 3.14 later in this chapter).

Infection: Recurrent acute or chronic inflammatory processes affecting the lymphatic system may result in mechanical insufficiency. If inflammation involves lymph nodes (lymphadenitis) or collectors (lymphangitis), the walls tend to become fibrotic and the lymph fluid coagulates and obliterates the lymphatics, thus creating blockage to the lymph flow. In addition to the existing mechanical insufficiency, there is an increase in the volume of LL, resulting in combined insufficiency.

Lymph node and lymph vessel infections can be caused by bacteria (especially *Streptococcus*) and fungal infections. The inflammatory process affecting intra- and periarticular tissues in rheumatoid arthritis may spread to the lymphatics, presenting another cause for mechanical insufficiency (see 3.18 later in this chapter).

The most common cause for inflammation of the lymphatic system and lymphedema in general is filariasis.

Lymphatic Filariasis

Lymphatic filariasis is the primary cause of lymphedema worldwide and is a painful and extremely disfiguring disease, which has been identified by the World Health Organization (WHO) as the second leading cause for permanent and long-term disability in the world. It is a tropical disease, endemic in more than 80 countries in Africa, India, Southeast Asia, and South America, as well as in the Pacific Islands and the Caribbean. Lymphatic filariasis is rare in the United States, and it is likely that those who contract it will have visited endemic regions.

According to the WHO, 1.3 billion individuals are at risk from the disease and over 120 million people are currently affected, with approximately 40 million being disfigured by lymphedema and suffering from recurrent infections and other secondary conditions.

Filariasis is caused by three types of round parasitic filarial worms, with *Wuchereria bancrofti* being the most common type. The other types, *Brugia malayi* and *Brugia timori*, are endemic to Southeast Asia.

Lymphatic filariasis is transmitted to humans by different types of mosquitos that bite while carrying infective-stage larvae. At the time of the bite, the larvae enter the wound and are deposited in the victim's skin; from there, the parasitic larvae migrate to the lymphatic system, where, over a period of 6 to 12 months, they develop into adult worms and mate. Male and female worms live together and form "nests" in the nodes and vessels of the lymphatic system. Adult worms live for a period of approximately 4 to 6 years; male worms can grow to 3 to 4 cm in length, whereas females can reach 8 to 10 cm.

The females produce millions of microscopic worms (microfilariae) during their lifetime, which circulate in the host's bloodstream and are then again ingested by biting mosquitos. Once inside the mosquito, the microfilariae develop into infective-stage larvae, which then again are transmitted to other individuals, thus completing the transmission cycle (▶ Fig. 3.4**a**).

During their lifetime inside the host's lymphatic system, the worms cause dilation of and damage to the lymphatics, restricting the normal flow of lymph, and cause swelling, fibrosis, and infections to lymph vessels and nodes (lymphangitis, lymphadenitis).

While infection by larvae generally occurs in childhood in individuals living in endemic

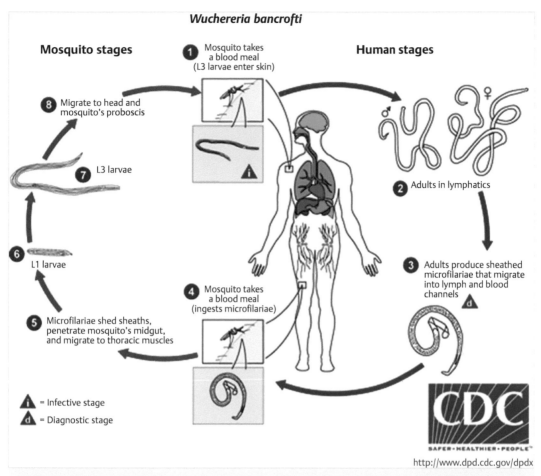

Fig. 3.4 (a) Lifecycle of *Wuchereria bancrofti*. (Reproduced with permission from the Centers for Disease Control and Prevention.) *(continued)*

countries, the painful and disfiguring symptoms of this condition typically manifest themselves later in life.

Lymphatic filariasis may present asymptomatically with no external signs of disfigurement or infection but with acute (infections, fever, swelling) or chronic subclinical lymphatic damage. The chronic stage includes lymphedema, which can grow to monstrous proportions and may affect the extremities (most often the legs), breasts, and the external genitalia (labia, scrotum, and penis) causing pain, disability, and sexual dysfunction (▶ Fig. 3.4**b**).

Lymphatic filariasis is typically diagnosed through blood tests that detect the presence of microfilariae in the blood as well as through antigen detection tests.

The primary treatment approach for individuals affected by lymphatic filariasis is pharmaceutical (diethylcarbamazine [DEC], albendazole, and ivermectin) and aims to eliminate adult worms and circulating microfilariae, thus interrupting the transmission cycle. Another important goal is to eliminate lymphatic filariasis as a public health problem by preventive measures involving mass drug administration covering the entire at-risk population of a country.

The goal of the Global Alliance to Eliminate Lymphatic Filariasis (GAELF) is to stop the spread of filarial infection and to eradicate this disease through distribution of free medication. To interrupt the transmission of infection, mass drug administration should be implemented in endemic regions for a period of 4 to 6 years.

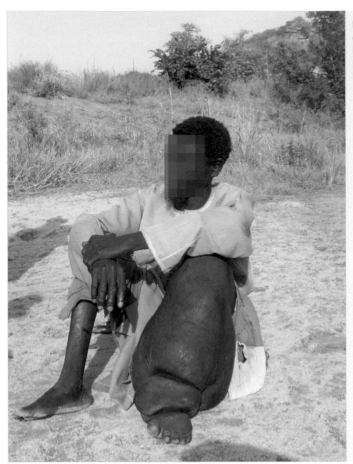

Fig. 3.4 *(cont.)* **(b)** A Nigerian man with elephantiasis, the most extreme form of lymphatic filariasis. (Reproduced with permission from The Carter Center/ Emily Staub.)

Foreigners visiting endemic countries are rarely infected; however, as a preventive measure, mosquito bites should be avoided by sleeping under a mosquito net, using insect repellents, wearing long-sleeved shirts and long pants, and refraining from being outside between dusk and dawn, when mosquitos are most active.

Lymphedema caused by lymphatic filariasis can be treated effectively with complete decongestive therapy (CDT), if available. Other measures to improve lymphedema and infections are patient education in self-care, including hygiene, skin care, compression therapy, exercises, and elevation of the affected extremity.

Malignant Tumors

Malignant tumors may mechanically block the lymph flow by pressing against lymphatic structures from the outside (see 3.2.7 later in this chapter). Malignant cells may also infiltrate the lymphatic system and proliferate in either lymph vessels (malignant lymphangiosis) or lymph nodes, thus blocking the flow of lymph (▶ Fig. 3.5). Modified CDT protocols may be applied to address the symptoms associated with malignancies (▶ Fig. 3.6).

Chronic Venous Insufficiency

Insufficient venous return results in an increase in venous blood pressure. The subsequent elevation in blood capillary pressure causes an increase in net filtrate (see 3.12 later in this chapter). In its primary function to actively prevent edema, the lymphatic system tries to compensate for the higher volume of the LL of water by the activation of its safety factor (see Chapter 2, Safety Factor of the Lymphatic System). Without initiation of adequate therapy for the venous problem, the lymphatic system may develop a mechanical insufficiency (combined insufficiency) over time, due to the constant strain (▶ Fig. 3.7).

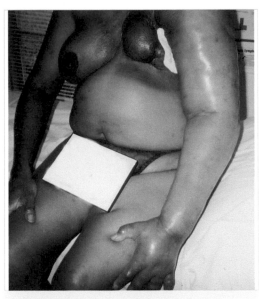

Fig. 3.5 Malignant lymphedema of the left upper extremity.

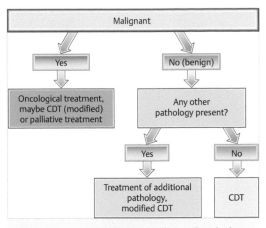

Fig. 3.6 Therapeutic approach in malignant lymphedema.

Immobility

If left without proper care, immobility caused by injuries to the spinal cord, stroke, or cerebral hemorrhage may eventually result in similar problems as discussed earlier (e.g., insufficient venous return with subsequent lymphatic overload).

Self-Induced Lymphedema

By use of a tourniquet (bandages, rubber band), some individuals produce a combination of venous and lymphatic obstruction on an extremity that produces the signs and symptoms of lymphedema. The ligature mark is usually easily identifiable just proximal to the swelling. This condition is extremely rare. If a therapist suspects self-induced lymphedema (also known as artificial lymphedema), it is recommended that he or she contact the referring physician following the evaluation (▶ Fig. 3.8).

3.2.3 Stages of Lymphedema

Currently, there is no cure or permanent remedy for lymphedema. The TC in the damaged lymph vessels cannot be restored to its original level (see Chapter 2, **Fig. 2.13**).

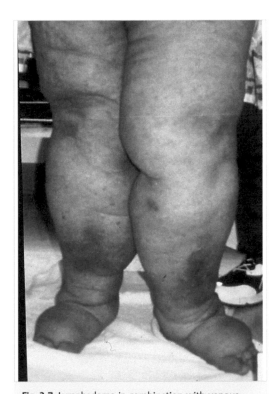

Fig. 3.7 Lymphedema in combination with venous insufficiency (stage 2) on both lower extremities.

If lymphedema is present, the lymphatic system is mechanically insufficient, that is, the TC has fallen below the normal LL.

3

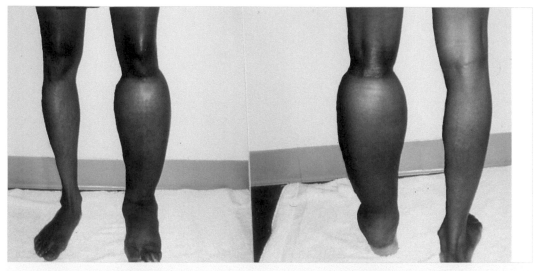

Fig. 3.8 Self-induced lymphedema of the left lower extremity (note the ligature mark on the left knee).

Although the swelling may recede somewhat during the night in some early-stage cases, lymphedema is a progressive condition. Regardless of genesis, lymphedema, in most cases, will gradually progress through its stages if left untreated (▶ Table 3.5).

There is no specific period of time for a patient to remain in a particular stage. For example, a patient will not necessarily be in stage 1 for 4 months and then progress to stage 2 for 6 months before moving to stage 3.

Stage 0

This stage is also known as the subclinical stage, or prestage, of lymphedema. In this stage, the TC of the lymphatic system is subnormal, yet remains sufficient to manage the (normal) LL (▶ Fig. 3.1). This situation results in a limited functional reserve (FR) of the lymphatic system (see Chapter 2, Lymph Time Volume and Transport Capacity of the Lymphatic System).

Patients who have undergone surgery (or had trauma) involving the lymphatic system and do not experience the onset of lymphedema are said to be in a *latency stage*, which is a subcategory of stage 0. For example, those women who have had surgery for breast cancer (with or without lymph node dissection and radiation) and do not present with postmastectomy/lumpectomy lymphedema are considered to be in a latency stage. Again, in

these cases, the TC is subnormal but still sufficient to drain the normal LL.

Table 3.5 Stages of lymphedema with typical symptoms

Stages of lymphe-dema	Characteristics
• Latency stage	• No swelling
• Lymphangiopathy (also stage 0/pre-stage/subclinical stage)	• Reduced transport capacity (TC) • "Normal" tissue consistency
Stage 1 (reversible stage)	• Edema is soft (pitting)
	• No secondary tissue changes
	• Elevation reduces swelling
Stage 2 (spontaneously irreversible stage)	• Lymphostatic fibrosis • Hardening of the tissue (no pitting)
	• Stemmer's sign positive
	• Frequent infections
Stage 3 (lympho-static elephantiasis)	• Extreme increase in volume and tissue texture with typical skin changes (papillomas, deep skin-folds, etc.)
	• Stemmer's sign positive

A condition known as *lymphangiopathy* presents if the TC is reduced by congenital malformations (dysplasia) of the lymphatic system. As long as the subnormal TC can manage the LL, lymphedema is not clinically present.

Patients in a prestage are "at risk" of developing lymphedema. The reduction in FR results in a fragile balance between the subnormal TC and the LL. The onset of lymphedema correlates to the ability of the lymphatic system to compensate for any added stress to the system or the frequency of certain occurrences that may cause an increase in LL of water (or water and protein) in the limb at risk.

Patient information and education, especially following surgical procedures, can dramatically reduce the risk of developing lymphedema (see Chapter 5, Precautions and Traveling with Lymphedema).

Stage 1

This stage, also known as the *reversible stage*, is characterized by soft-tissue pliability without any fibrotic alterations. Pitting is easily induced, and the swelling retains the indentation produced by the (thumb) pressure for some time (▶ Fig. 3.9). In early stage 1, it is possible for the swelling to recede overnight.

With proper management in this early stage, it is possible for the patient to expect reduction of the extremity to a normal size (compared with the uninvolved limb). Without proper care, progression into stage 2 in the vast majority of cases is inevitable.

It is difficult to distinguish stage 1 lymphedema from edemas of other geneses. The clinician needs to take into account the patient's history and whether the swelling resolves with conventional management (compression, elevation) or not (refer to 3.6 and 3.7 later in this chapter).

Stage 2

Stage 2, also known as *spontaneously irreversible lymphedema*, is primarily identified by tissue proliferation and subsequent fibrosis (lymphostatic fibrosis). Over time, the tissue becomes more indurated, and pitting is difficult to induce. In stage 2, the Stemmer's sign is positive (▶ Fig. 3.10). A Stemmer's sign is positive if the skin from the dorsum of the fingers and toes cannot be lifted, or lifted only with difficulty (compared with the uninvolved side). A positive Stemmer's sign is considered accurate to diagnose lymphedema of the extremities; the absence of a Stemmer's sign, however, does not exclude the presence of lymphedema (false-negative Stemmer's sign).

In many cases, the volume of the swelling increases, which exacerbates the already compromised local immune defense (increased diffusion distance). Because of this, infections (cellulitis) in this stage are common.

Volume reduction can be expected if proper treatment is initiated in this stage of lymphedema. In most cases, the indurated tissue will not completely recede in the intensive phase of CDT (see Chapter 4). Reduction of fibrotic tissue is achieved mainly in the second phase of CDT with compression and good patient compliance (▶ Fig. 3.11).

Lymphedema often stabilizes in stage 2. In those patients suffering from recurrent infections, the lymphedema may develop into stage 3, lymphostatic elephantiasis.

Stage 3 (Lymphostatic Elephantiasis)

Typical for this stage are an increase in volume of the lymphostatic edema and further progression of the tissue changes. Lymphostatic fibrosis

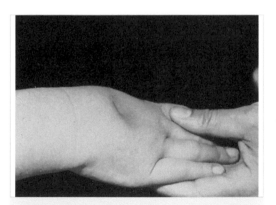

Fig. 3.9 Pitting lymphedema (stage 1) on the right hand.

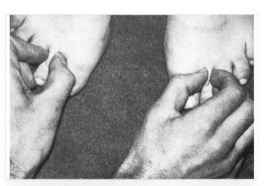

Fig. 3.10 Positive Stemmer's sign on the second toe of the right foot in lower extremity lymphedema.

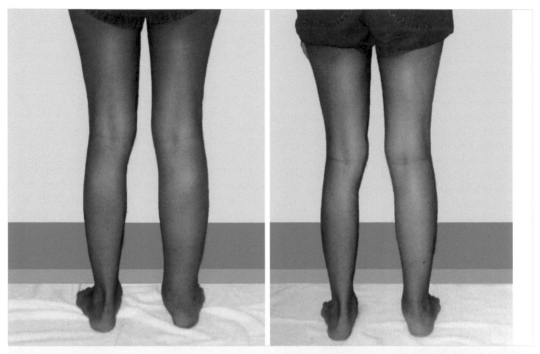

Fig. 3.11 Primary lymphedema of the right lower extremity **(a)** before and **(b)** after complete decongestive therapy.

increases in firmness, and other skin alterations, such as papillomas, cysts and fistulas, hyperkeratosis, mycotic infections of the nails and skin, and ulcerations, develop frequently. Pitting may or may not be present. The natural skinfolds, especially on the dorsum of the wrist and ankle, deepen, and the Stemmer's sign becomes more prominent. In many cases, cellulitis is recurrent (▶ Fig. 3.12).

If lymphedema management starts in this stage, reduction can still be expected. To achieve good results, it is necessary to extend the duration of the intensive phase of CDT. In many cases, the intensive phase has to be repeated several times. Even extreme cases of lymphostatic elephantiasis can be reduced to a normal or near-normal size with proper care and patient compliance (see 3.11 later in this chapter).

Tissue changes or the progression of fibrosis remains the clinical trait to distinguish between the stages of lymphedema.

Tissue changes commonly seen in the progression of lymphedema are proliferation of connective tissue cells, production of collagen fibers, and an increase in fatty deposits and fibrotic changes (lymphostatic fibrosis). The fibrotic tissue tends to become sclerotic over time, increasing in firmness.

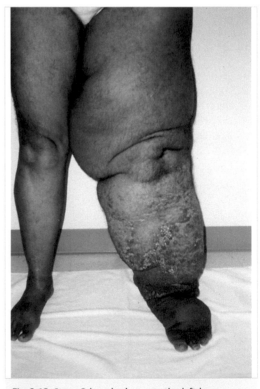

Fig. 3.12 Stage 3 lymphedema on the left lower extremity.

3

Lymphostatic fibrosis is initially noticed at the distal end of the extremities, fingers, and toes (► Fig. 3.13).

Pitting is generally more pronounced in the early stages of lymphedema and occurs if pressure is applied with the examiner's thumb on the edematous tissue. Pitting is usually tested on the distal extremity (preferably over bony prominences) and occurs because of the displacement of fluid in the tissue caused by pressure with the flat thumb. The pitting response (indentation produced by pressure) can remain on the tested area for some time if there are minimal fibrotic skin changes present.

Angiosarcoma (Stewart–Treves syndrome; see also 3.2.7 later in this chapter) may develop in long-lasting lymphedema, particularly in patients with stage 3 lymphedema. This type of angiosarcoma may develop in primary or secondary lymphedema and is characterized by extensive malignancy; it is highly lethal. Reliable data on the incidence of angiosarcoma in lymphedema are not available at this time.

3.2.4 Grading of Lymphedema Based on Severity

Extremity volume is not considered within the different stages of lymphedema. The severity of unilateral lymphedema in relation to volume can be assessed within each stage as minimal (less than 20% increase), moderate (20–40% increase), or

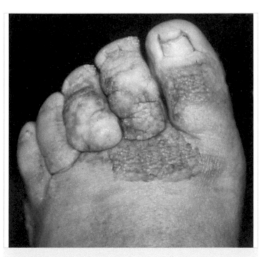

Fig. 3.13 Lymphostatic fibrosis, papillomas, and fungal infections of the left foot.

severe (more than 40%) increase in limb volume (► Table 3.6).

3.2.5 Precipitating Factors for Lymphedema

For a patient "at risk," the possible development of lymphedema depends on many factors (see 3.2.6 later in this chapter). Some patients are able to effectively compensate for a decrease in TC and FR by the regeneration of lymph vessels, utilizing alternative collateral circulation routes and lymphovenous anastomoses, and increasing the lymph time volume of remaining collectors. These patients may not exhibit signs or symptoms of lymphedema as long as the lymphatic system has found a way to compensate.

As discussed earlier, lymphedema may develop anytime during the course of a lifetime in primary cases. In secondary cases, the swelling may occur immediately postoperative, within a few months or a couple of years, or 20 years or more after surgery.

Based on the pathology and pathophysiology, as well as patient reports, certain triggers that cause the onset of lymphedema can be identified (for a more detailed review of precipitating factors and prevention of lymphedema, refer to Chapter 5, Precautions).

Lymphedema Risk Reduction (Venipuncture and Blood Pressure)

The surgical procedures used for individuals affected by breast cancer may be mastectomy, partial mastectomy, or lumpectomy. Along with the actual breast surgery for cancer, axillary lymph nodes are removed and/or radiated. As a result of axillary lymph node clearance, the normal lymphatic drainage from the extremity is impaired, and some patients experience the onset of lymphedema. Accumulated lymph in the edematous arm provides a rich culture medium for bacteria, which makes lymphedematous tissues extremely

Table 3.6 Grading of lymphedema based on severity

Severity of lymphedema	Volume increase
Minimal	<20%
Moderate	20–40%
Severe	>40%

susceptible to infections. Simple injuries and puncture wounds can develop into local or generalized infections that may produce further lymphatic destruction and blockage. To reduce the risk of these postoperative complications, most patients are advised to not have blood pressure readings taken on, intravenous infusions in, or blood samples taken from the arm on the operated side.

Very few published data are available to document the exact risk of lymphedema from performing blood pressure readings, blood draws, and injections on the affected extremity. Lack of research and normal variations in an individual's lymphatic system (numbers or sizes of lymph nodes) make it difficult to quantify personal risk from each triggering factor.

While further research is needed, health care professionals are encouraged to minimize the risk of lymphedema by taking blood pressure readings and blood draws from and giving injections to the nonaffected limb whenever possible. In patients with breast cancer on both sides, these procedures should be performed on the leg or the foot. If this is not possible, the procedure should be carried out on the nondominant arm. If one side has had no lymph node removal, the arm on that side should be used, regardless of whether it is the dominant arm. In an emergency, however (such as a car accident), and if an intravenous line must be started, medical professionals must be allowed to do what they need to do to start the intravenous line as soon as possible.

If a port is present, blood draws should be taken directly from there. In patients with "bad" veins, good hydration and some form of heat (heat pads, warm water) help dilate the veins prior to cannulation.

To avoid the onset of lymphedema, or infections in lymphedema, health care professionals should follow expert consensus regarding best practice to avoid lymphedema and inform patients with breast cancer about their risk for lymphedema. Until further research is available, the National Lymphedema Network's Position Statement on risk reduction practices should be used to deliver information to patients.

Not all medical professionals are familiar with the precautions for avoiding lymphedema, so patients have to be particularly watchful advocates for themselves. Lymphedema alert bracelets are available from the National Lymphedema Network. Wearing this bracelet increases the odds of remaining lymphedema-free and at the same time educates the medical community.

Increase in Blood Capillary Pressure

Active hyperemia (vasodilation) that results from a local or systemic application causes an increase in blood flow, which ultimately will increase the LL of water and stress a compromised lymphatic system (see Chapter 2, **Fig. 2.9**). Examples of active hyperemia include local hot pack, other thermal modalities (diathermy, electrical stimulation, ultrasound), massage, vigorous exercise, and infection of the limb "at risk." Hot tubs and saunas, hot weather, and high humidity, as well as injuries, are additional triggering factors.

Passive vasodilation as a result of the obstruction of the venous return will also result in increased net filtrate and place additional stress on the compromised lymphatic system. Examples include CVI, cardiac insufficiency, and immobility, as well as the examples listed under the next category.

Fluctuation in Weight Gain and Fluid Volumes

Pregnancy and obesity, excessive weight gains during the menstrual cycle (cyclic idiopathic edema), and certain medications are known to trigger the onset of lymphedema by causing additional stress (LL) on the compromised lymphatic system.

Injury

Even in subclinical stages of lymphedema, the immune response is reduced as a result of edematous saturation of the tissues on a microscopic level. Any insult to the integrity of the skin may cause infection, thus triggering the onset of lymphedema. Examples include insect bites, pet scratches, injections, intravenous cannulation, blood pressure measurements on the involved extremity, cuts, and abrasions.

Changes in Pressure

The change in cabin pressure during an airline flight, coupled with inactivity, may trigger the onset of lymphedema. The reduced cabin pressure may allow more fluid into the tissue spaces. Additional inactivity allows for venous pooling, which will eventually cause an increased pressure at the blood capillary level, thereby increasing filtration and the LLs (see Chapter 5, Traveling with Lymphedema).

3.2.6 Avoidance Mechanisms

In an effort to maintain fluid homeostasis, the body has the ability to respond to lymphostasis, which may prevent the manifestation of lymphedema. The following discussion will focus on the body's compensatory mechanisms.

Safety Factor

Lymph collectors not affected by either blockage (surgery, radiation, trauma) or malformation will increase their contraction frequency and amplitude (lymphangiomotoricity) in an effort to compensate for those collectors affected by mechanical insufficiency. These compensating collectors are located in the same tributary area. The mechanisms involving the lymphatic safety factor are described in Chapter 2, Safety Factor of the Lymphatic System.

Collateral Circulation

Lymph collectors circumnavigating blocked areas may be able to avoid the onset of lymphedema by redirecting lymph fluid into areas with sufficient lymph drainage. Lymph collectors of the lateral upper arm, for example, may drain into the supraclavicular lymph nodes. This may be significant in case of ALND because part of the lymph fluid may be rerouted around the axillary area into the supraclavicular nodes. The chance to avoid the manifestation of lymphedema, in this case, of the arm, is even greater if the individual's collectors of the lateral upper arm communicate with those located in the radial forearm territory (long upper arm type; see Chapter 1, Superficial Layer). If this connection exists, lymph fluid from the forearm and upper arm would be able to bypass the blocked axillary area into the supraclavicular nodes.

Interterritorial anastomoses present another possible bypass for lymph fluid. If the normal flow of lymph within a truncal territory is interrupted by lymph node dissection, the interterritorial anastomoses may prevent the onset of swelling in those quadrants that would normally drain into the dissected lymph node groups. The higher the number of anastomoses, as described in Chapter 1, Interterritorial Anastomoses, the better the chance of avoiding lymphedema.

Lympho-Lymphatic Anastomosis

Severed lymph collectors tend to reconnect after a relatively short time (2–3 weeks). Newly formed lymph vessels reconnect the distal with the proximal lymph vessels' stump (▶ Fig. 3.14). Scar tissue may prevent lympho-lymphatic anastomoses. Lymph collectors separated due to blunt trauma (no skin breakage) will regenerate more effectively than collectors disconnected by incisional trauma.

Lymphovenous Anastomosis

The distal end of a severed lymph collector may connect with an adjacent vein, creating a natural shunt. Lymph fluid then directly voids into venous blood.

Lymph Vessels in the Adventitia of Blood Vessels

Larger blood vessels have their own nutrient blood vessels (vasa vasorum vessels), which supply the wall of the larger arteries and veins with oxygen and nutrients.

There are also lymph vessels in the adventitia of larger blood vessels (lymph vasa vasorum). With lymphedema present, LLs may reach these lymph vasa vasorum vessels via tissue channels. Lymph

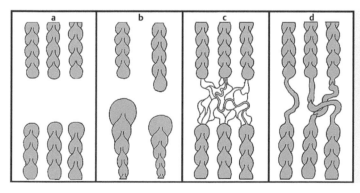

Fig. 3.14 Reconnection of lymph collectors following blunt trauma. **(a)** Severed lymph collectors. **(b)** Intralymphatic pressure in the distal lymph collector stump increases. **(c)** Newly formed lymph vessels connecting the distal and proximal lymph vessel stumps. **(d)** Lympho-lymphatic regeneration.

vessels in the adventitia of blood vessels have the ability to increase their activity, thus providing an additional drainage pathway for stagnant lymph fluid.

Macrophages

If protein-rich fluid accumulates in the tissues, monocytes leave the blood capillaries in large numbers. Once in the tissues, they are macrophages (phagocytes) and will digest accumulated protein molecules. The subsequent decrease in tissue protein concentration will result in an increased reabsorption and a decrease in net filtrate, which will help reduce the LLs. The digested protein molecules are broken down into amino acids, which do not present a LL, and are removed by the blood circulatory system.

3.2.7 Complications in Lymphedema

Lymphedema is often combined with other pathologies and conditions, which either aggravate the existing symptoms or present additional complicating factors in the treatment of lymphedema.

The following is a list of the most common complications.

Reflux

It is defined as retrograde flow of lymph fluid caused by valvular insufficiency of lymph collectors. Valvular insufficiency is the result of hyperplasia, dilation of collectors due to constant strain or blockage of lymph flow, or organic changes in the walls of lymph collectors (mural insufficiency; see Chapter 2, Mechanical Insufficiency).

If valvular insufficiency is present, lymph fluid is propelled not only to proximal but also to distal (retrograde flow) during the contraction of lymph angions. Reflux presents as blisterlike formations (*lymphatic cysts*) on the surface of the skin, commonly in the axillary (▶ Fig. 3.15), cubital, genital (see Chapter 5, **Fig. 5.25**), and popliteal areas. Lymphatic cysts contain lymph fluid, which may be clear or chylous. If chylous, the reflux originates from the intestinal lymph system.

Clinical Relevance

Lymphatic cysts may easily break open, presenting an entryway for pathogens, which can cause

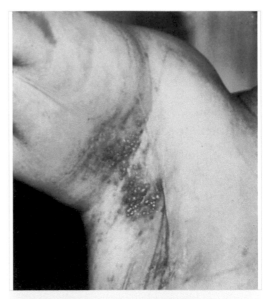

Fig. 3.15 Lymphatic cysts in the right axilla.

infection. Burst cysts associated with leaking of lymph fluid (lymphorrhea) are termed *lymphatic fistulas*.

To avoid damage to cysts and to prevent infection, it is recommended to cover the cyst with sterile gauze during treatment (local antibiotics should be applied around the fistulas) and not manually work on or around the cysts and fistulas. Cysts should be padded with soft foam material (donut or **U**-shaped padding) to avoid direct contact with the bandage materials while the patient wears the bandages.

Radiation Fibrosis

Radiation fibrosis is reaction of the skin to irradiation, leaving visible and/or palpable changes in the skin and subcutaneous tissue. The skin in radiation fibrosis appears reddish brown (▶ Fig. 3.16), and superficial blood vessels may be dilated in the irradiated area (telangiectasia) (▶ Fig. 3.17). The newly formed scar tissue may be soft or hard, and the skin may adhere to the underlying fascia.

Clinical Relevance

The tissue changes in radiation fibrosis tend to get worse over time, possibly resulting in compression of venous blood vessels and subsequent dilation of superficial veins.

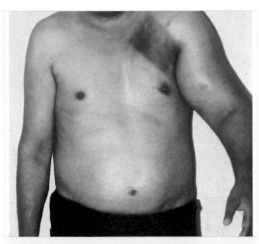

Fig. 3.16 Radiation fibrosis in a patient with secondary lymphedema on the left upper extremity.

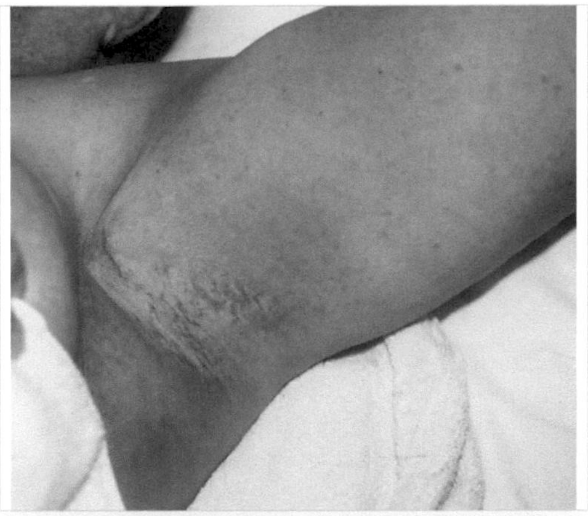

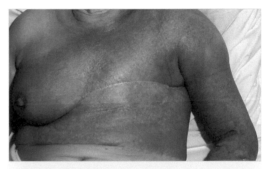

Fig. 3.17 Telangiectasia in the left axilla.

> Radiation fibrosis may cause pain, limitations in range of motion (ROM) if near a joint, paresthesia, pareses, and paralysis, which can occur even years after the radiation therapy was administered.

The skin in radiation fibrosis may also be more fragile. To avoid mechanical damage to the irradiated skin, CDT presents a local contraindication in radiation fibrosis if there is adhesion to the fascia or if the radiated area is painful. Movements designed to mildly stretch the affected skin area should be incorporated into the exercise program. CDT techniques may be applied with lighter pressures if skin discoloration or telangiectasia and/or dilated superficial veins are present and the skin is pliable.

Infection

Bacterial (especially *Streptococcus*) and fungal infections are common in patients with lymphedema (especially stages 2 and 3). Clinical symptoms of cellulitis are fever and tenderness; the skin is red with indistinct margins (▶ Fig. 3.18).

Fungal infections may involve the skin and/or nails and most often affect the lower extremities (▶ Fig. 3.19). Nails generally take on a yellow color, split, flake, and grow too thick. Symptoms in

Fig. 3.18 Cellulitis in a patient with secondary lymphedema of the left upper extremity.

fungal infections of the skin include itching, crusting, scaling, and maceration between the toes. The skin may be moist or dry and may show a grayish-white film. A sweet odor is often associated with fungal infections.

Clinical Relevance

Episodes of cellulitis (or erysipelas) usually require a course of systemic antibiotics. CDT is generally contraindicated until the infection has cleared. Therapy for the fungal infection with local or systemic antifungal medication precedes lymphedema treatment.

Hyperkeratosis

Hyperkeratosis is defined as hypertrophy of the corneous layer of the skin. This condition is often associated with lymphedema, especially on the

3

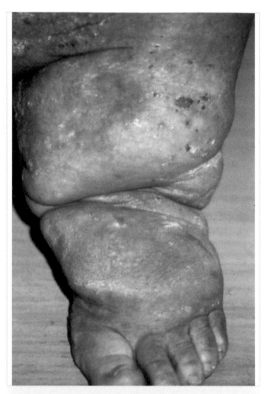

Fig. 3.19 Fungal infections and lymphorrhea on lymphedema of the left lower extremity.

lower extremity. Wartlike papillomas are generally observed on the feet and toes. Skinfolds may be deepened.

Clinical Relevance

Good skin hygiene is necessary to avoid possible infections in the moist skinfolds. Hyperkeratosis may be treated with over-the-counter medication or, in extreme cases, may be surgically removed (after decongestion), especially if papillomas interfere with the donning of compression garments. Because papillomas are elevated nodules, care must be taken to not tear the papillomas while donning the garments.

Scars

Scars located perpendicular to lymph collectors may present a blockage to lymph drainage, especially if the scar tissue adheres to the underlying tissues and/or exceeds 3 mm in width.

Clinical Relevance

The treatment of fresh scars is covered later in this chapter under Traumatic Edema. Older scars causing discomfort, blocking lymph flow, or hindering exercise protocols may be treated with techniques and materials designed to soften the indurated tissue (foam, manual techniques, nonthermal ultrasound).

Malignancies

Blockage of the lymphatic return may be caused by malignant tumors, in which case the swelling would be categorized as malignant lymphedema. As described previously in this chapter, a rare form of malignancy may develop as a result of long-standing lymphedema (angiosarcoma or Stewart–Treves syndrome). Malignant cells may also infiltrate the lymphatic system, causing blockage to the lymph flow (malignant lymphangiosis) (▶ Fig. 3.20).

Signs and symptoms of malignancies include sudden onset and fast progression of the swelling, pain (especially in the swollen extremity), paresthesia, paresis and paralysis, enlarged lymph nodes, ulcerations on the skin, varicose veins on the thorax, and elevated shoulder due to pain on the involved side in upper extremity involvement (▶ Fig. 3.21).

Changes in the color and integrity of the skin may also indicate malignancies: cellulitislike redness is often associated with malignant lymphangiosis (▶ Fig. 3.20) (the redness does

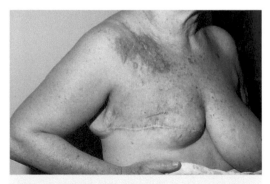

Fig. 3.20 Malignant lymphangiosis.

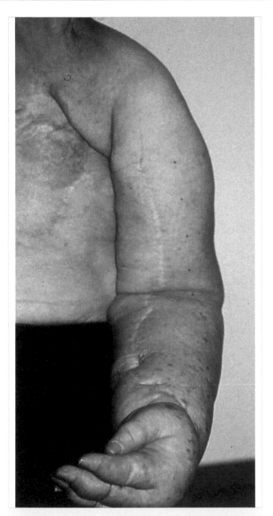

Fig. 3.21 Malignant lymphedema of the left upper extremity.

Paresis and Paralysis

Partial or complete loss of motor function may be caused by injuries to peripheral nerves, the spinal cord, stroke or cerebral hemorrhage, infiltration of nervous tissue by malignant tumors, or radiation (radiation plexopathy).

Clinical Relevance

Immobility is detrimental to the lymphatic return. Modifications to the exercise program are necessary to address impaired motor function. Patients may need assistive devices to enhance mobility.

Genital Swelling

It is frequently present in combination with lower extremity lymphedema. In 40 to 60% of the male lymphedema population, the external genitalia (scrotum and/or penis) may also present with significant swelling, in addition to the lower extremity involvement. Females are affected less frequently.

Clinical Relevance

These patients should be thoroughly instructed in self-management issues (e.g., hygiene, the application of bandages or pads to the swollen area, appropriate clothing, etc.). It is important that compression garments incorporate the genital swelling (pantyhose, compressive body parts; refer to the appropriate sections in Chapters 4 and 5).

Other Pathologies Combined with Lymphedema

Lymphedema is often combined with other conditions and pathologies that may worsen the symptoms associated with lymphedema or complicate the treatment protocol with additional obstacles.

Clinical Relevance

It is necessary to incorporate modifications in the treatment protocol for lymphedema to appropriately address signs and symptoms associated with any additional pathologies.

Examples

Lymphedema and Cardiac Insufficiency

Abdominal techniques are contraindicated; the affected extremity (especially in leg lymphedema)

not appear suddenly as in cellulitis but develops slowly over the course of weeks and months). Hematomalike discolorations on the skin may indicate the presence of angiosarcoma.

Clinical Relevance

If any of the above symptoms are present, if lymphedema is therapy-resistant, or if there is a sudden relapse in swelling in previously treated lymphedema, a physician must be consulted immediately. Modified CDT protocols may be applied to reduce and alleviate the symptoms associated with malignancies (palliative care).

should be treated only in sections to avoid too much venous blood and lymph fluid returning to the heart during the treatment. Lighter compression is necessary for the same reason.

Lymphedema and Obesity

Obesity contributes to the onset of lymphedema and often worsens the symptoms of existing lymphedema (see 5.18). In a 2008 study conducted by researchers at the University of Missouri, Columbia, it was suggested that the risk of developing upper extremity lymphedema following breast cancer surgery was 40 to 60% higher in women with a body mass index (BMI) classified as overweight or obese, compared with women of normal weight. In their study, which included 193 breast cancer survivors, the researchers also reported that the risk of lymphedema is especially high in overweight or obese women who undergo cancer treatment involving the dominant side or who experience postoperative swelling.

Excessive weight and obesity may also contribute to the onset of primary and secondary lymphedema involving the lower extremities. Excessive weight, especially morbid obesity, can have a negative impact on the return of lymphatic fluid from the legs; additional fluid volumes associated with obesity may overwhelm an already impaired lymphatic system. Direct pressure on lymphatic vessels by excess fatty tissue, impaired diaphragmatic breathing, and decreased muscular function can also be factors contributing to the manifestation of lymphedema. CVI is often associated with obesity. The increased burden on the lymphatic system in CVI can play a significant role in the manifestation of lower extremity lymphedema.

The progress of treatment of existing lymphedema may be seriously hampered in patients with a high BMI. With obese patients it is often difficult to apply bandages, especially in cases of lymphedema affecting the lower extremities. Furthermore, the compressive materials (bandages, garments) applied to the affected extremities have a tendency to slide in obese patients. Compression garments may have to be custom made, creating an additional financial burden on the patient.

Exercise—a very important aspect of the management of lymphedema—may be made difficult as well. Mobility problems associated with a high BMI can affect the patient's participation in

treatment, and exercise protocols used in lymphedema therapy for the upper and lower extremities may have to be modified accordingly.

Weight management and proper nutrition are essential for successful long-term lymphedema management (see also 3.11.7 later in this chapter).

Lymphedema and Orthopaedic Problems

Symptoms associated with lymphedema and orthopaedic pathologies will magnify each other and may even exacerbate the current presentation of either or both pathologies. Relevant combinations are "frozen" shoulder and upper extremity lymphedema or hip/knee problems associated with lymphedema of the leg. To interrupt the vicious cycle, it is necessary to address all involved pathologies. It is often advised to prioritize treatment according to the more limiting factors found during the assessment.

Lymphedema and Venous Insufficiency

Venous insufficiency contributes to the onset of lymphedema and worsens symptoms of existing lower extremity lymphedema (see 3.12 later in this chapter). The additional presence of venous ulcerations necessitates proper wound care (▶ Fig. 3.22; see also 3.13 and 3.13.6 later in this chapter). It is recommended that the lymphedema therapist incorporate the materials prescribed by the physician into the compression bandage.

Although venous insufficiency will benefit from CDT for lower extremity lymphedema, it is imperative to observe possible complications associated with venous insufficiency (thrombophlebitis). These complications may present a contraindication for the treatment of lymphedema.

Lymphedema and Diabetes

Diabetes is often associated with dry skin, frequent infections, neuropathy, slow-healing wounds, and high blood pressure. To address these problems, the treatment protocol for lymphedema may be modified accordingly, with more emphasis on skin hygiene. If ulcerations are present, the incorporation of wound care into the protocol becomes necessary. As with venous ulcers, it is recommended that the lymphedema therapist use and incorporate the materials prescribed by the physician into the compression bandage.

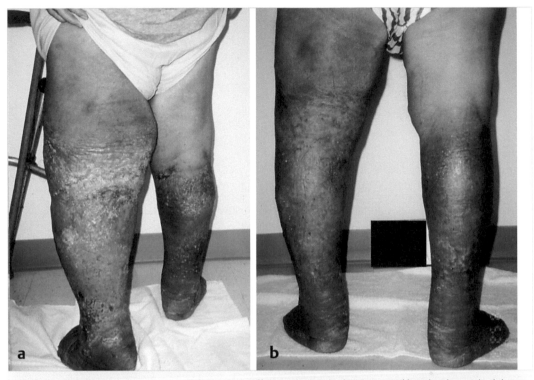

Fig. 3.22 Lymphedema in combination with venous insufficiency (stage 3), ulcerations, and lymphorrhea on both lower extremities (a) before and (b) after complete decongestive therapy.

3.3 Axillary Web Syndrome

3.3.1 Definition

Axillary web syndrome (AWS) is a condition that may develop after interruption to the axillary lymphatics such as ALND, sentinel lymph node dissection (SLND), trauma, or an obstruction from cancer. It is a visible and palpable web of tissue that becomes taut with shoulder abduction. It is located in the axilla region and often extends distally along the anterior, medial upper arm toward the antecubital space and may extend as far as the base of the thumb. In patients with a thin body type, it may also extend proximally along the lateral chest wall (▶ Fig. 3.23a). In a few cases, subcutaneous nodules have also been reported along the cord. It has the appearance of a tight cord of tissue being stretched underneath the skin (▶ Fig. 3.23b) and is sometimes referred to as "cording." Other terms used to describe AWS include Mondor's disease, lymphatic cording, subcutaneous fibrous banding, fiddle-string phenomenon, lymph vessel fibrosis, lymphangiofibrosis thrombotica occlusiva, and lymph thrombosis. AWS is painful and can limit ROM of the shoulder, elbow, wrist, and trunk. The cord tends to be more extensive in patients who have had ALND compared with those who have had SLND. AWS should not be analogous with soft-tissue tightness, because many patients have soft-tissue tightness following ALND but do not have AWS.

3.3.2 Risk Factors

Risk factors for developing AWS include ALND, lower BMI, younger age, radical mastectomy, numbness due to intercostobrachial nerve injury, positive lymph node status, and hematoma. AWS appears more often in patients with a thin body type for reasons unknown. It is suggested the cord may be more difficult to detect in heavier-set patients because the thick layer of subcutaneous tissue may cover the cord. The subcutaneous fat tissue may also make it more difficult for the skin

3

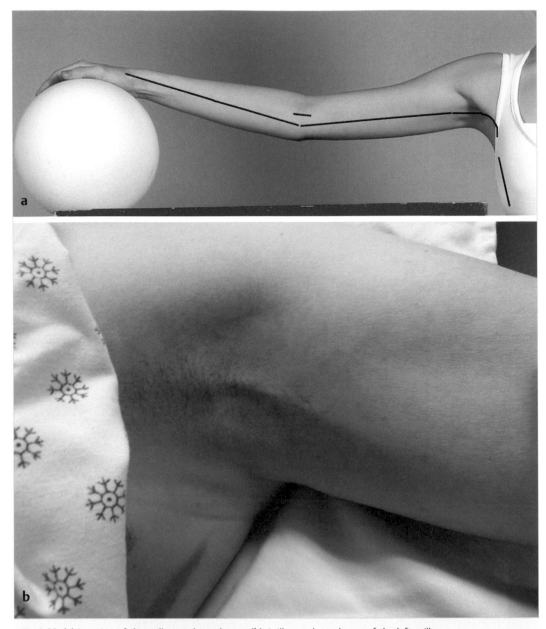

Fig. 3.23 (a) Location of the axillary web syndrome. (b) Axillary web syndrome of the left axilla.

to adhere to the underlying tissue caused by the cord.

3.3.3 Physiology/Pathophysiology

It has been indicated that AWS is a variant of Mondor's syndrome. Mondor's syndrome is caused by a thrombosed superficial vein and presents as a cord on the chest wall, which is painful, tender, and causes skin retraction and pulling. AWS development is thought to be caused by an injury to the axillary lymphatics following ALND, trauma, or an obstruction from cancer. An interruption of the lymphovenous channels causes a thrombosis and stagnation of the lymphovenous fluid, resulting in inflammation, fibrosis, and shortening of the tissue. Tissue biopsies of the cord taken from a small number of patients have indicated dilated lymphatics, a fibrin clot in the lymphatics, and venous thrombosis.

Imaging studies on AWS demonstrated the cords were not compatible with a vein, nerve, or fascia, suggesting the cords were lymphatic in origin. These imaging studies determined that AWS is likely not a result of a venous thrombosis.

3.3.4 Incidence, Onset, and Duration of AWS

The reported incidence of AWS is variable, ranging from 6 to 72%. The incidence is higher with ALND (range: 6–72%) compared to SLND (0.9–41%). AWS most often occurs in the early postoperative period beginning approximately 1 to 5 weeks following surgery. Later onset of AWS coming on months to years later has also been described, though less common. Previous studies suggested AWS resolves on its own within 2 to 3 months, but more current studies have determined AWS can linger for months to years later. Cords will also resolve and then return days to years later for reasons unknown. The variation in the onset and duration makes it difficult to determine the actual incidence of AWS; therefore, the reported incidences may be higher.

3.3.5 Assessment and Documentation

Evaluation for the presence of AWS can be performed by fully abducting the arm with the elbow extended. The axilla, medial arm, elbow, forearm, wrist, hand, and trunk should be assessed through observation and palpation. Not all cords are visible, so palpation of the affected areas is necessary to fully evaluate the extent of the cords.

All patients following ALND from breast cancer or melanoma should be standardly assessed for AWS. A recent study demonstrated shoulder abduction ROM was significantly lower in women with AWS compared to those without in the early time period following surgical breast cancer. Typically, there is a postoperative delay in the development of AWS, with patients having fairly normal ROM within the first few weeks. Within a few weeks, the patient starts to experience tightening and pain in the arm, which begins to limit ROM. The patient may come to the clinic with the affected arm in a protected position of shoulder protraction, internal rotation, and elbow flexion, with wrist flexed and supinated because it is painful to let the arm rest by the side. Shoulder abduction is the most limited movement in most cases, but elbow extension can also be limited especially with arm abduction. The cord is taut and painful with palpation.

With a severe cord that extends to the elbow or base of the thumb, the cord will be easily detected by the attempt to position the arm at the side with elbow extended. The patient will not be able to extend the elbow or wrist fully and a cord can be visible and palpable in the forearm. If the cord is located in the axilla, the cord will become visible or palpable when the arm is abducted and a stretch is applied to the cord. In thin patients, a cord may be visible on the lateral chest wall at the end range of shoulder abduction and trunk side-bending. Some patients will report tension in the lateral chest wall similar to the cording symptoms felt in the arm and axilla even though a cord may not be observed. The reason the cord may not be visible in this area may be due to the presence of subcutaneous fatty tissue. A thorough assessment of all affected areas is indicated so that fragments of the cord are not missed.

Some cords may be hidden under subcutaneous tissue and may not become immediately apparent. AWS has been found in patients who appear to have full ROM following a standard shoulder assessment. Patients describe their shoulder as feeling "different" or experience pulling or twinges with specific movements or activities. Patients can often replicate the symptoms by positioning themselves in the position of discomfort. Once in this position, a cord often becomes apparent in the affected area. Treatment for the cord should be performed with the patient in this selected position.

Documentation of AWS is necessary to demonstrate severity of the condition, effectiveness of treatment, and patient progress. Suggested documentation includes

- Medical history.
- Patient function, pain level, and awareness of cording.
- Location of the cords (i.e., axilla, upper arm, elbow, forearm, wrist, hand, chest/trunk).
- Number of cords, length of cords, and if the cords are visible and/or palpable.
- Active and passive ROM of the extremity and trunk.
- Posture assessment.
- Lymphedema measures.
- Photos.

3

3.3.6 Therapeutic Approach

From a therapist's perspective, any indication of AWS should not be ignored. Evidence supports that physical therapy involving stretching and strengthening exercises, ROM, and manual techniques improves shoulder function, pain, and quality of life in breast cancer patients with AWS. Manual lymphatic drainage (MLD) has added benefit of reducing arm lymphedema. Treatment of AWS can rapidly reduce the pain caused by the tension of the cord and dramatically improve ROM and function. Without treatment, AWS could cause prolonged shoulder immobility which could lead to secondary problems such as altered movement patterns, poor posture, malalignment, muscle imbalance, impingement, frozen shoulder, soft-tissue tightness, and chronic pain.

An effective manual technique used to treat AWS is skin traction starting at the most distal portion of the cord and working proximally. It involves a gentle stretch on the superficial tissue over the cord. Using the palmar surface of the fingers, both hands are placed approximately 2 to 10 cm apart along the cord and a stretch is applied along the direction of the cord in the opposite direction (▶ Fig. 3.24). Once the patient no longer feels tension in the area, the arm is repositioned into further abduction to apply more tension on the cord. Feedback from the patient is imperative throughout treatment as the cord may become tight in another area as one area is relieved. Work the area of the cord where the patient indicates tightness. The elbow should stay extended throughout the progression into abduction. Wrist extension can also be applied to achieve tension on the cord.

Cord bending is another manual technique used to treat AWS. While the cord is tensed when the patient is positioned in a stretch, a perpendicular pressure is applied on the cord with the thumbs while bending the tissue in the opposite direction with the other fingers. Cord bending should be applied to the area of the cord where the patient indicates tightness. This technique can also be used in the pectoral region to stretch the tissue (▶ Fig. 3.25).

The cords may break or release during treatment and a palpable and sometimes audible pop can be experienced. No adverse effects have been reported following the breaking of the cords though it is important to be cautious and avoid being overly aggressive in trying to break the cords until further research is obtained on the exact mechanics of the cord breaking. It is not known whether the noise is due to the actual cord or the supporting fibrous tissue around the cord breaking, or to another cause. If a cord does break, an immediate increase in ROM is experienced. To reduce anxiety, it is beneficial to explain to the patient that the cord may break and that he or she may hear and feel the cord release during treatment and to reassure him or her that this is a normal response. Gentle manual techniques are quite effective in helping resolve the cords without being overly aggressive.

If the cord extends into the arm, a gentle but effective approach to the rapid resolution of the cord is the short-term use of gradient compression bandaging. Low-stretch compression bandages achieving a gradient compression can be used for 1 to 3 days. Less compression is needed compared

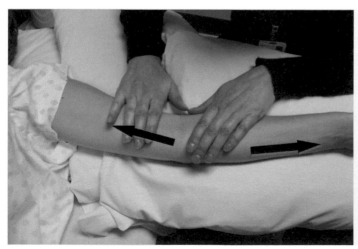

Fig. 3.24 Skin traction.

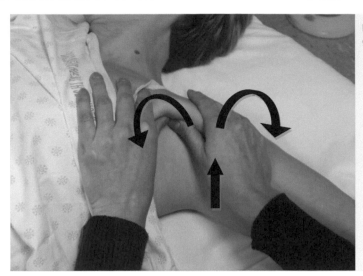

Fig. 3.25 Bending of the pectoral region (cord bending technique).

with regular lymphedema compression bandaging; therefore, two to three compression bandages with appropriate padding are usually sufficient. If there is lymphedema involvement, the appropriate compression to treat the lymphedema is indicated. Like all bandaging, close monitoring and patient education are necessary to avoid complications. A compression garment is not as effective in resolving the cord.

Instruction in a home exercise program is dependent on the location and severity of the cord. Gentle ROM exercises should be initiated at the most distal portion of the cord first. A cord that extends to the base of the thumb can be quite painful; therefore, thumb and wrist extension in addition to elbow extension may be all the patient can tolerate initially. Proximal ROM exercises (such as pendulum exercises and/or the finger walk on the wall) can be added as the cord resolves distally. The patient can be instructed in a self-skin stretch, similar to a nerve stretch, by placing the affected hand on the wall with the wrist extended, forearm supinated, elbow extended, arm abducted below 90 degrees, and scapula depressed. The palmar surface of the unaffected hand can be used to apply a gentle proximal stretch on the cord (▶ Fig. 3.26). This self-skin stretch of the cord can also be applied with more advanced stretches such as pectoralis and latissimus dorsi stretches or other exercises indicated by therapist. A caregiver can also be instructed in manual techniques to stretch the cord to help increase the ROM.

It is important to focus on postural education throughout treatment. Myofascial release,

craniosacral techniques, scar mobilization, joint mobilization, nerve glides, and strengthening can also be incorporated into the treatment as indicated by the therapist. Nonsteroid anti-inflammatory drugs and opioids may also be beneficial for pain management related to AWS. Anecdotally, adjunct modalities, such as low-level laser therapy (LLLT), have also been utilized to treat AWS, but there is no scientific evidence to support the use.

3.4 Impact of Lymphedema on Quality of Life

Lymphedema affects psychological well-being and quality of life of people of all ages,[4] cultures,[27,28,29,30] and genders.[31] Although the majority of research has been done in the area of BCRL,[32] and the highest proportion of patients living with lymphedema in the developed world may be survivors of breast cancer,[33] studies show that patients suffering from either primary or secondary lymphedema experience a negative impact on their quality of life from this chronic disease.[4,32,34,35,36,37]

The association of quality of life and lymphedema has long been a concern, with research dating back over three decades.[4,38,39,40] Primary lymphedema is reported to affect 1.15/100,000 people under 20 years of age.[4] As far back as 1985, Smeltzer et al reported findings from a longitudinal study at the Mayo Clinic of children and adolescents with primary lymphedema that led to recommendations that adolescents, in particular, be referred for psychological counseling.

3

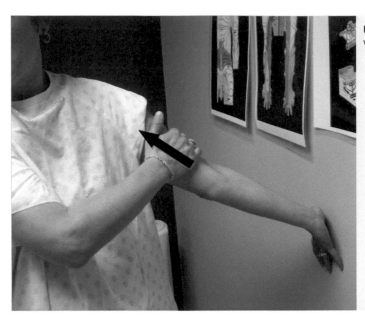

Fig. 3.26 Self-stretching of the cord with proximal skin stretch.

A decade later, noting the absence of a validated tool for assessing quality of life among patients living with lymphedema, despite the general clinical awareness of such a problem, Augustin et al[41] developed and validated a tool for assessment of quality of life in lymphedema. They found that patients with primary and secondary lymphedema showed marked impairment in quality of life in all areas assessed (e.g., physical status, everyday life, social life, emotional well-being, treatment, satisfaction, and profession/household), compared with patients with early-stage venous insufficiency, and comparable reductions in quality of life compared with patients with venous leg ulcers.

In an area of greater investigation, researchers reporting quality-of-life outcomes among breast cancer survivors with lymphedema detail impairments in both physical and psychological aspects of life.[42,43] For example, in a systematic review of the psychosocial impact of lymphedema, 19 of 23 studies related to BCRL summarized the effect of lymphedema and treatment on individuals in the psychological and psychosocial domains.[32] The impact of lymphedema was reported to include negative self-identity, emotional disturbance, and psychological distress. Social impact included feelings of marginalization and perceived public insensitivity, financial burden, social isolation, and perceived diminished sexuality.[32] In addition, among 11 quantitative studies, poorer social well-being was statistically significant in persons with lymphedema. All 12 of the reviewed qualitative studies reported negative psychological and social impact related to lymphedema.[32] In addition, studies and subsequent instrument development using cognitive and emotional parameters have identified the concepts of self-efficacy and self-regulation as influential predictors of successful coping and adherence in at-risk populations for the development of BCRL.[43] Self-efficacy is one's belief that he/she can affect a situation or condition and self-regulation is the ability to control emotion, behavior, and distractions that may interfere with preset goals to control any given health threat.[44] An understanding of lymphedema lends itself to positive coping and increased feelings of self-empowerment, thus advancing one's health literacy and the ability to evaluate current coping and management strategies.[2,42] Studies of individuals with primary lymphedema are needed to correlate decreased self-efficacy and self-regulation to adherence.

It is important to continuously develop item content that represents new research findings as related to contributing factors that impact quality of life, such as psychological and psychosocial parameters (e.g., perceptions of self-efficacy and self-regulation).[43] In addition to the LYMQOL (a quality of life measure for limb lymphedema),[45] Klernäs et al[46] introduced a shortened version of the quality-of-life inventory for lymphedema (LyQLI). The LyQLI is a 45-item inventory demonstrating good internal consistency, reliability, face validity, and concurrent validity that encompass three domains: physical, psychosocial, and practical. Although further research is needed to assess sensitivity, it has the potential for use in the clinical setting and cross-sectional studies that are specific to individuals with both primary and secondary lymphedema.[46] Planning care for individuals with lymphedema should include education, access to ongoing interactive support and medical treatment with health care providers, and evaluation of psychological and psychosocial parameters, all of which contribute to improved patient outcomes and, subsequently, may lead improved quality of life.[2,42,47,48,49]

Physiological symptoms may compromise normal activities of *daily* living (e.g., sleeping, driving, carrying items, household chores, occupational responsibilities, dressing, or gardening and other leisure activities),[50,51,52,53] domestic role,[54] and family responsibilities.[52] Survivors with lymphedema experience more symptoms (increase in arm and shoulder size; tighter fitting clothing, sleeve cuff, and jewelry; limited elbow function; arm/hand weakness; loss of sleep secondary to arm discomfort; tenderness; swelling; pitting; blistering; firmness/tightness; heaviness; stiffness; aching; breast swelling) than those survivors without lymphedema.[34,54,55,56,57] In a study by Fu et al[58] (data from 250 women. $n = 60$ healthy women; $n = 42$ women with BCRL; and $n = 148$ women at risk for LE), updated evidence was reported that breast cancer survivors with LE continue suffering from multiple lymphedema symptoms in the upper extremity on the side affected by breast cancer. Arm swelling was reported by all survivors with LE, with others also reporting arm tightness, arm heaviness, arm firmness, arm aching, tingling, limited arm movement, stiffness, seroma formation, limited finger movement, increased arm temperature, and limited elbow movement. There were no reports of blistering in either the LE or at-risk group.[58] In addition, a cut-off was established between the three groups of participants. A diagnostic cut-off of three symptoms was made between the breast cancer survivors with lymphedema and the healthy adult group (sensitivity = 94%; specificity = 97%) and a cut-off of nine symptoms was made between the lymphedema group and the at-risk groups (sensitivity = 64%; specificity = 80%).[58]

While breast cancer survivors report that they are most fearful of a cancer recurrence, it is noted that their second greatest fear is that they will develop lymphedema.[59] The majority of breast cancer survivors are 65 years of age or older,[60] and although chronological age alone is not the only factor to consider when classifying older adults, Nazarko[61] reported that they are three times more likely to develop BCRL than younger people and are at risk for delayed diagnosis due to the coexistence of other forms of edema and comorbidities.[62] Konecne and Perdomo[63] reported that lymphedema can lead to functional limitations for elderly individuals (e.g., decreased ability to reach, lift, push, pull, twist, carry, shove, and grasp), which in turn could affect their quality of life. As people living with primary and secondary lymphedema grow older, the impact on quality of life may burgeon.[62]

This chapter focuses on the personal impact on quality of life when living with lymphedema based on qualitative studies of individuals and families and the objective impact on quality of life in areas such as function and finances. Personal quotations (Armer, unpublished data) and studies that are selected for review reveal the universal and widespread impact of this chronic condition.

3.4.1 Personal Views of Lymphedema across the Globe

It's like giving birth. Everybody can tell you it feels like this and this, but until you experience it yourself, you don't know …
If you've got children and you've got a husband, you've got to be up. There's no time to be sick … It does influence relationships, especially with your husband … My husband likes a good-looking woman with breasts and a nice body and everything. So it has been hard work for me to, to survive this whole thing …
I think at first … you try to have a lot of hope that this thing … is a temporary sort of situation. And I think that, um, the disappointment, with time and as you realize it's not going to go away, something that you have to cope with for the rest of your life, so it is a disappointment.
V, breast cancer survivor and professional business woman, living with lymphedema, South Africa

Since going through breast cancer five years ago and developing a swollen arm my doctor says [it] will only get bigger … caring for my family has been very difficult …

3

I fight cancer, through my weakness and through my struggle ... I struggle ...
Sacrifice ... I am a humble person. I am grateful for everything, every day. I am grateful ...
There are other times when I think about my thick arm because of the weight of the arm. But then I have to put it out of my head ... there are other things to worry about, a decent place to live, running water ...

E, breast cancer survivor and hourly domestic worker, living with lymphedema, South Africa

Going through treatment for breast cancer (41 years ago) was nothing compared to all these (39) years with lymphedema.

R, breast cancer survivor and retired secretary, living with lymphedema, Midwestern United States

These quotations reveal the personal dimensions of living with lymphedema following breast cancer treatment in two very disparate parts of the world, with comments resonating with the impact on quality of life among individuals of vastly different ages and cultures. It is important that health professionals hear the voices of the individuals they treat who are living with the challenges of lymphedema.

3.4.2 Impact of Minimal Limb Volume Change on Quality of Life among Survivors with Lymphedema

A recently published prospective cohort study[55] assessed symptoms, quality of life, and health status among women undergoing surgery for breast cancer. Serial upper extremity circumference,

perometry (Juzo, Cuyahoga Falls, OH) volume, and symptom reports were assessed every 3 months for 1 year and then every 6 months for the next 18 months. A model adapted from Wilson and Cleary[64] and Ware and Sherbourne[65] guided the analysis suggesting that health-related quality of life, such as specific health measures (symptoms and limb volume change [LVC]) and generic health measures (function and quality of life), is among the best predictors of future health outcomes (such as expenditures, response to treatment, work productivity and disability, and mortality). Analysis revealed that although functional status tended to decrease slightly, but not significantly, with increase in volume change from 5 to $\geq 15\%$, symptoms increased significantly with volume increase and quality of life decreased significantly even with mild limb volume increase[51] (▶ Fig. 3.27).

These findings underscore the importance of assessing symptoms, limb volume, function, and quality of life among individuals living with lymphedema. They reveal the association of even mild increase in limb volume with decreased quality of life and support the imperative for early, effective, evidence-based interventions for those meeting the diagnostic criterion for lymphedema.[55]

Economic Impact of Lymphedema for Survivors

A retrospective cohort study[66] using inpatient databases for five states through the Agency for Healthcare Research and Quality's (AHRQ) Healthcare Cost and Utilization Project (HCUP) was conducted for women aged at least 18 years who underwent lumpectomy or mastectomy for breast cancer with a concurrent axillary lymph node

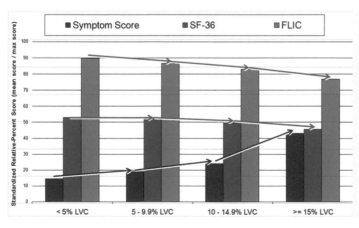

Fig. 3.27 Graph of symptom score, function (36-Item Short Form Health Survey [SF-36]), and quality of life (Functional Living Index-Cancer [FLIC]) by categories of limb volume change. (Reproduced with permission from Cormier et al.[55])

procedure. ICD-9 classification codes were used to identify cases between January 1, 2007, and December 31, 2009. The purpose of the study was to calculate hospital costs associated with complicated lymphedema incidence after breast cancer surgery.[66] Of 56,075 women, 1,279 (2.3%) were admitted with complicated lymphedema at least once within 2 years of surgery and experience fivefold more all-cause hospitals admissions compared to women without lymphedema. Substantially higher hospital costs were associated in the lymphedema group than the nonlymphedema group of patients: $58,088 versus $31,819 per patient ($p < 0.001$).[66]

Another team, headed by a health-economist researcher, conducted a study to estimate costs associated with lymphedema by comparing the total cost of insurance claims for survivors with breast cancer lymphedema with that of a matched cohort of breast cancer patients without lymphedema.[67] Claims data from a national employment-based database of 1,877 individuals with an average age of 48.8 years and a 9.6% lymphedema occurrence rate were used. There was a 3:1 match of breast cancer controls to breast cancer–lymphedema patients, matched by breast cancer treatment characteristics (mastectomy, lumpectomy, node dissection; chemotherapy; radiation therapy). A regression model was performed to compare the risk of cellulitis or other infections in survivors with and without lymphedema and to estimate costs associated with lymphedema.[67]

The research findings of Shih et al revealed that those with lymphedema had a statistically greater risk of submitting health claims because of cellulitis or lymphangitis and other complications.[67] Furthermore, 2-year estimated health claims costs were more than $22,000 greater for those survivors with BCRL than for those without lymphedema, with approximately $13,500 of these excess claims not being related to cancer treatment.[67] As related specifically to quality of life, breast cancer survivors with lymphedema utilized more psychological counseling services than breast cancer survivors without lymphedema.[67]

It is important to note that these data are drawn from a database of employed adult women with health insurance, and so these data reflect the more well-represented, higher-insured, less-vulnerable population with and at risk for lymphedema; other uninsured or underinsured groups may have greater complications and health costs, and subsequently greater impact on their quality of life.

Impact of Lymphedema on Family Life

Findings from a series of ethnographic studies by Radina and Armer[68,69] revealed information on coping with chronic illness and the impact of lymphedema on women's family roles; resiliency among women with post–breast cancer lymphedema and their families; and the survivor's transition from caregiver to care-receiver.

Coping with Chronic Illness: Impact of Lymphedema on Women's Family Roles

The first study investigated the effect of lymphedema on women and their families regarding task completion and family functioning using the Family Adjustment and Adaptation Response Model.[52] For example, following the development of lymphedema, women may no longer be able to move furniture, carry in groceries, and care for children or aging parents as they used to. Families who were more flexible in modifying daily tasks and who had preexisting resources for coping with stressors were found to have more positive outcomes than did those families who were rigid and coped poorly with stressors.

Resiliency among Women with Lymphedema and Their Families

The second study was guided by the Resiliency Model of Family Stress, Adjustment, and Adaptation.[68] This investigation into how lymphedema onset and its related stressors impact women and their families found three particular stressors: (1) required modification of daily tasks; (2) lymphedema as a reminder of breast cancer; and (3) frustration with medical professionals.

Transition from Caregiver to Care-Receiver: Functionally Autonomous Survivors with Lymphedema

The third study explored women's experiences of off-time life course transitions from being the caregiver to becoming a care-recipient as a result of post–breast cancer lymphedema.[69] Women in the prime productive years of work and family unexpectedly making the transition to the role of receiver of care is often an abrupt change which was out of step with age and developmental peers.

Two dominant themes were revealed: (1) not wanting to be a burden and (2) desiring to live an independent lifestyle. Even in the presence of family and friends willing to help, women wanted to continue to live autonomously as they had done before.

These qualitative studies provide insight into the impact of lymphedema for survivors and their families. Together, they provide evidence which corroborates and further illuminates the findings of Shigaki et al[70] and others[50,51,52,53] about the impact of lymphedema on both the individual and the family in compromising the domestic role and activities of daily living. Radina and Armer[52] found that families were in large part responsible for the individual's adaptation and adjustment to living with lymphedema. These studies suggest that interventions within the family could increase the resiliency of patients with chronic illnesses. Therefore, health professionals should be concerned with the entire family, or even community, rather than just the individual.

Coping with Lymphedema

A qualitative study by Heppner et al[27] examined the stressors associated with lymphedema following breast cancer and the roles of coping and social support in response to the stress. This study used intensive semi-structured interviews and consensual qualitative research methods. Survivors with lymphedema experienced a broader array of stressors than previously reported in the literature. These findings included the following themes: (1) lymphedema impact is pervasive; and (2) approach coping rather than avoidant coping is reported to be beneficial.

Stressors associated with lymphedema included (with scale of frequency of reports; number representing cases supporting the theme; and the most frequently reported are in bold)
- **Concerns about (and excessive time demands related to) maintenance of daily activities (10).**
- **Physical symptoms and pain associated with lymphedema (10).**
- Negative emotional and cognitive reactions (9).
- Lack of concerns and caring of health care providers (9).
- Concerns regarding their prognosis (7).
- Attractiveness and sexual issues (6).
- Negative social support (6).
- Lack of adequate health insurance coverage (6).
- Stress and anxiety in partners/children (5).
- Absence of social support (2).

- Cultural-related stressors (1).

Coping strategies to manage lymphedema-related stressors were reported as
- **Actively sought information or treatment options (10).**
- **Learned physical strategies to manage lymphedema symptoms (10).**
- **Accepted the limitations associated with lymphedema symptoms (10).**
- **Focused on the positive aspects of life (10).**
- Used spiritual/religious methods (9).
- Openly talked and educated about lymphedema (9).
- Maintained leisure and recreational activities (6).
- Used ineffective coping methods (5).
- Impact of their racial and socioeconomic backgrounds on coping (1).

Among social support and social resources for coping with lymphedema-related stressors were
- **Opportunity to nurture others (10).**
- Reliable alliance of others besides partners (9).
- Reliable alliance of partners (8).
- Concern and support from health care providers (7).
- Spiritual support from others (5).
- Maintaining the status quo (3).

This qualitative study examining coping strategies and stressors reported by breast cancer survivors provides guidance for health professionals in assessing coping and stresses experienced by those living with lymphedema. Together, these qualitative studies lay the foundation for research designed to develop and evaluate interventions to strengthen family function, enhance coping, and lessen the stresses associated with this chronic condition.

Reframing the Situation

The literature furthers the understanding of the impact of lymphedema on quality of life among those living with this chronic condition.[39,52,55,70] A final quote captures the essence of the possibility of reframing what may have proved to have been both an unexpected and devastating life event, whether the emergence of primary or secondary lymphedema.

It [lymphedema] isn't minor, but the gratitude is that I have learned so much about my body. Because out of negative experiences can come positive, and I suppose that's one of the ways I cope. I try to look for what positive can come from this. And if you can see positives, you can cope a little better. It doesn't become so dramatic.

U, participant in urban setting in Midwestern US, data from Heppner et al[27]

The effect of lymphedema is indeed both qualitative, with personal and family impact, and quantitative, with quality of life, functional, and financial impact, and with universal and widespread reach. Around the globe, lymphedema impacts the quality of life of those it affects.

Research studies such as those reviewed here provide insight into the personal nature and challenges of living with lymphedema and the foundation for evidence-based interventions to enhance quality of life for individuals and families living with lymphedema.

3.5 Early Identification and Conservative Treatment: Clinical Implications and Interventions

3.5.1 Introduction

The natural course of lymphedema is a relatively slow onset and progression over time. With regard to secondary lymphedema, there is often a known incident that damages the lymphatic system and escalates an individual's risk for developing the condition. In such a circumstance, monitoring and screening the at-risk individual for the onset of lymphedema should be implemented to facilitate early identification and enable early intervention.

Early identification and management of lymphedema requires a standardized approach for screening and monitoring for symptoms associated with early swelling in the limb or body region. In order to successfully identify lymphedema early, it is important for the clinical provider to have an understanding of the early-onset presentation, recognize patient-reported symptoms consistent with the onset, incorporate clinical measurement tools that provide a reliable assessment of tissue changes, and utilize a diagnostic threshold that is sensitive enough to promote early intervention.

When lymphedema is identified at an early, even subclinical, stage, the treatment intervention is altered from traditional CDT. The components of CDT are still recognized as foundational for treating early lymphedema, but modifications are

appropriate to reduce the intensity of intervention.

This chapter will review the requisite knowledge to enable early identification and to understand the protocols for early intervention as well as provide an evidence-based clinical model that promotes early detection and treatment of lymphedema.

3.5.2 Pathophysiology and Presentation of Early Lymphedema

It is well documented that the lymphatic system does not function as a linear system of fluid flow. Variation exists in vessel anatomy across regions and segments of the body, which introduces wide variability in the trajectory of lymphatic fluid movement.[71] Within different body regions, there is further variation in lymphatic vessel density and fluid flow patterns. Due to these nuanced differences in lymphatic vessel patterns and function among body regions, the onset of lymphedema can be variable.

Lymphatic Watersheds

Anatomic variation in the lymphatic system is partly described by the theory of lymphatic watersheds. Watersheds are areas within a body region that delineate a pattern of fluid flow. Early work in mapping the lymphatic system identified these nuanced vessel trajectories within the system. More recent work has demonstrated that these watersheds and their systemic variation contribute an important consideration for early identification of the onset of lymphedema. Lymphatic congestion does not happen ubiquitously along a limb or throughout the entirety of a body region. The onset is gradual, starting in one area of the limb and progressing. Stanton and colleagues identified that this onset begins within certain regions of a limb and progresses to adjacent areas if the condition is untreated and becomes more chronic.[72]

3.5.3 Regional Swelling

The concept of regional edema accumulation prior to the onset of chronic lymphedema was established by Stanton and colleagues and clinically validated in the breast cancer population by Stout et al. These findings suggest that fluid begins to accumulate in particular areas of a body region prior to the onset of broader regional swelling.

3

This is attributed to segmental lymphatic drainage patterns that differ between the superficial and subfascial compartments of the limb.[72] When lymphatic disruption occurs, there is an increase in the lymphatic pressure in the subfascial muscle compartments due to these tissues having little compliance. This results in poor lymphatic drainage from the superficial tissue into the deeper compartments, a requisite mechanism for fluid drainage. The result is superficial lymphatic vessel overload and congestion of fluid in the interstitial tissues. This supports the contention that the initial clinical presentation of lymphedema may be segmental in nature and may be distributed, initially, in tissue superficial to the muscle compartments. When exploring this mechanism in a cohort of breast cancer patients with subclinical lymphedema, segments of the limb associated with larger muscle groups were identified as the first regions of the limb to demonstrate clinically meaningful swelling. Further, volumetric changes in these segments predicted the onset of lymphedema.[73]

The demonstration of regional swelling prior to full limb or body region has important implications for early identification of lymphedema. Evidence suggests that segments of the limb or body region may initially present with fluid congestion and swelling symptoms that can be identified using standardized measurement methodology. When consistent measures are utilized to monitor tissue changes over time, early identification of tissue congestion and subclinical lymphedema can be achieved.

3.5.4 Early Identification

Early identification is an important concept for lymphedema management. As lymphedema becomes more chronic, the condition worsens through progressively more severe grades of tissue pathology and swelling. Early-stage lymphedema typically presents with mild swelling and little to no soft-tissue fibrosis. Treatment intervention in an early stage requires less resources from the health care delivery team and lessens the burden on the individual. Evidence supports that early intervention may prevent the condition from progressing to a more chronic, severe stage.[74] The progression of lymphedema to chronic stages is debilitating both physically and psychologically. Therefore, identification at an early stage is also optimal for an individual's quality of life.

The most obvious clinical sign of lymphedema is visible swelling in the tissue; however, fluid congestion begins to occur and causes tissue changes prior to obvious visible clinical signs of swelling. In order to identify lymphedema at the earliest presentation, the population at risk should be monitored for early self-reported symptoms of lymphedema, clinically assessed by a health care provider with appropriate test and measurements, and encouraged to participate in risk reduction behaviors. Using a standardized clinical intervention that proactively monitors for early symptoms enables identification of the earliest changes in tissue congestion and promotes early management.

Subclinical fluid congestion in interstitial tissue results in sensory symptoms that patients often describe as numbness, aching, tingling, or feelings of fullness or heaviness in the limb or body region.[54] Individuals will often report an intermittent bout of swelling that reportedly dissipates and may "come and go" from time to time. These subjective symptoms are frequently predictive of the onset of lymphedema in the at-risk population and should be proactively monitored for and acted upon when reported.[54]

A number of clinical measurement tools are available for assisting in the diagnosis and monitoring of lymphedema. These tools and their clinical validity and relevance are highlighted elsewhere in this text. While it is important for health care providers to choose clinically valid measurement tools for early identification of lymphedema, it is far more vital that tissue assessment with these tools is conducted in a proactive manner using consistent measurement methodology. Optimally, in the population at risk for secondary lymphedema, a baseline measure of the limb volume or tissue fluid is established prior to the inception of cancer treatments known to damage the lymphatic system. Measures are then repeated at routine intervals using consistent methodology to assess change over time. When monitoring the limb, it is prudent practice to use the contralateral, unaffected limb as a control for changes that may be attributed to weight fluctuations or systemic fluid retention. A prospective surveillance model enables the early identification and treatment of subclinical lymphedema.

Prospective Surveillance Model

The Prospective Surveillance Model (PSM) was originally described by Stout and colleagues as a standardized model for proactive assessment and monitoring for the onset of lymphedema in an at-risk population.[74] Using this standardized model, lymphedema was detected at a subclinical level and managed using conservative intervention. The model is an effective approach to identify early lymphedema and mitigate the progression of the condition. It has good clinical utility and feasibility.

The PSM begins with an assessment of an individual's level of mobility, function, weight, and limb volume ideally taken at the point of cancer diagnosis and prior to the onset of any cancer-mitigating treatments. These clinical measures establish a baseline and enable comparison measures over time. The framework of the PSM requires proactive reassessment of these clinical tests at intervals over time during and after cancer treatment, in the absence of overt symptoms, to identify changes from baseline and to determine if the changes are clinically meaningful.[75] When clinically meaningful changes are identified, treatment is initiated. Used in this standardized approach, the PSM serves as a screening mechanism that aids in the early identification of lymphedema.

The decision to intervene for early lymphedema is made based on a clinically meaningful limb volume or fluid change from baseline, with consideration for the contralateral limb. This diagnostic threshold is identified as > 3 to 5% LVC from baseline. Subjective sensory symptoms may or may not be present but should be assessed. Intervention should be conservative at this point in order to manage the swelling congestion in the tissue. At this stage, lymphedema is considered subclinical as there may not be overt visible swelling and no obvious tissue changes likely to be visible or palpable.

3.5.5 Early Intervention

The most relevant outcome of early detection is to enable early intervention of lymphedema when the condition is in a reversible, early stage. When lymphedema is identified early, conservative treatment interventions can be implemented that are less intense and less costly. Early intervention is supported by a large and growing body of literature that has evolved since the seminal research regarding subclinical lymphedema early detection in the late 2000s.[76] Early intervention takes the form of both proactive/preventive interventions and condition management interventions once the subclinical threshold for lymphedema is identified.

Preventive Early Intervention

The original PSM as described by Stout and colleagues did not prescribe any intervention prior to the development of lymphedema. The model demonstrated strong evidence for a screening and monitoring framework to promote early identification of lymphedema. The model was expanded in further research to include preventive interventions along with the interval monitoring and screening recommendations. A recent systematic review highlights that the integration of exercise and self-MLD techniques, taught to the at-risk individual at baseline, and reinforced with the interval reassessment interventions, results in reduced rates of lymphedema as compared to controls who received no education or intervention for prevention.[77]

These findings suggest that the standardized methodology offered by the PSM is further augmented when accompanied by interventions designed to enhance lymphatic function, mainly through exercises, skin care, and lymphatic system stimulation. The PSM model is an effective framework to promote early identification of lymphedema and, with these additional aspects, it also serves a potentially preventive role in condition development.

Early Intervention for Lymphedema Management

The PSM offers a framework to promote early identification of lymphedema. Early identification of lymphedema is only meaningful if intervention is provided to reduce the initial presentation of fluid congestion so as to alter the trajectory of the condition and prevent progression to a more advanced stage. Optimally, this intervention is a conservative approach to alleviate the fluid congestion in the tissues without introducing a burdensome plan of care for the patient. The early intervention should consist of compression therapy, self-lymphatic decongestion techniques, exercise, and education.

Compression

Compression therapy is a well-established modality, used in standard lymphedema treatment protocols. Compression garments increase the interstitial pressure of tissue offering a counter-pressure that prevents the accumulation of fluid in the tissues and enables fluid re-uptake into the

3

venous circulation. Compression garments are used in traditional CDT during the maintenance phase, after limb volume has been maximally reduced by intensive therapy. The goal of compression garments is to maintain limb volumes and prevent the reaccumulation of lymphedema after intensive decongestive therapy.

The role of compression therapy in early lymphedema, however, is different. Early detection enables identification of fluid congestion in the tissue prior to the condition having caused significant soft-tissue changes. Therefore, the fluid is more dynamic as the lymphatic system is not yet unduly strained or incapable of evacuating fluid from the tissue. Compression therapy in the early stages of swelling can be utilized at a reduced level of pressure and over lesser duration than in traditional CDT.

In early lymphedema, compression garment pressure is recommended at lower levels: 20 to 30 mm Hg for the arm and hand piece and 30 to 40 mm Hg for the leg. These lower levels of compression enable a meaningful shift in fluid dynamics at the tissue level, but provide gentler supportive compression to the limb. A short trial of compression garments in early lymphedema is an effective intervention to overcome the initial fluid congestion and reduce limb volume to near-normal states.

Early trials studying the PSM utilized compression therapy in the presence of subclinical lymphedema as a daily application over a 4 to 6 week time period. No night compression was indicated. Following reassessment and when fluid congestion was determined to have abated, the garment wear was further reduced to only include times of excess activity or strain on the limb, including exercise, heavy lifting activities, or if the limb became symptomatic.

Lymphatic Decongestion

Several studies support the use of self-MLD education as a mechanism to improve the lymphatic function and diminish fluid congestion in early stages. Evidence suggests that the use of self-MLD techniques as a part of a preventive protocol can reduce the onset of lymphedema. These reports vary in their recommendations as to the timing of self-MLD, locations of the body where self-MLD should be conducted, and frequency with which it should be carried out. It is reasonable to deduce, based on existing research, that a routine of, at least, daily self-MLD should be incorporated into an early preventive intervention.

Exercise

Movement of large muscle groups is known to facilitate improved lymphatic fluid flow. Muscle pumping action, with or without compression therapy, enhances lymphatic vessel activity and perpetuates lymphatic fluid flow. Movement-based exercise programs have been suggested as a component of preventive intervention protocols. Early evidence suggests that there may be a protective benefit from resistive exercise; however, more research is needed to better articulate these interventions to assure safety in the at-risk population.

Education

Education is a hallmark of lymphedema management and is especially important in the at-risk population as a part of the prospective surveillance protocol. The rationale for initiating intervention through assessment and education at baseline is to enable optimal timing for individuals to develop an understanding of their risk and to familiarize themselves with symptoms that should be attended to.

3.5.6 Summary

The PSM provides a framework for assessment and intervention that enables the early identification and treatment of lymphedema. The model has been expanded to include additional functional measures as well as intervention components that are known to reduce the risk of developing lymphedema. ▶ Fig. 3.28 outlines the components of the PSM that could be implemented into clinical practice to enable ongoing assessment of the at-risk individual in

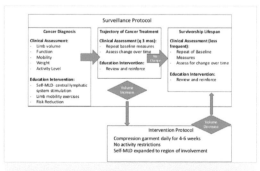

Fig. 3.28 Prospective surveillance protocol for early identification and early intervention for lymphedema.

an effort to identify lymphedema onset at the earliest presentation, thereby facilitating early, conservative intervention.

3.6 Diagnosis of Lymphedema

Lymphedema is a disease without a "gold standard" or single unifying diagnostic criterion that is reproducible, universally accepted, and generalizable. Despite the fact that the disease is dynamic, the current diagnostic criteria are based almost solely on physical exam findings. Due to the lack of a universally accepted diagnostic standard, the incidence of lymphedema will inevitably vary with the method used to define its presence.

Lymphedema is a disease which can only be diagnosed clinically. As there is no universal criteria, any objective measurement criteria to diagnose it will be inherently arbitrary. As Cheville has written: "There is no one value or standard you can use to say, 'OK, if you meet that you have lymphedema, and if you don't, well then you don't have it'."[78] Therefore, the diagnosis will rely on clinical evaluation, symptom evaluation, and objective measurements.

The Agency for Healthcare Research and Quality (AHRQ) Technology Review of Lymphedema stated: "Is there any 'gold standard' method to formally grade or measure the severity of lymphedema?"

Based on the evidence in the extracted studies, there does not appear to be a gold standard to formally "This stage may exist for monthsgrade or measure the severity of lymphedema."[79]

Most studies have focused on secondary lymphedema, primarily BCRL, and there is relatively little literature on lower extremity, truncal/breast, genital, abdominal, head and neck, and primary lymphedema.

In an effort to create an objective measurement guideline to diagnose lymphedema, various measurement standards have been used: volume measurements, bioimpedance to measure fluid in the tissues, and symptoms surveys. Again, as it is a clinical diagnosis and one that may vary over time, it is essential that the clinician utilizes all modalities and recognizes that lymphedema can be subtle and variable and "patient-reported signs and symptoms are often the first indications of clinically relevant lymphedema."[80]

3.6.1 Diagnosis of Lymphedema— Various Approaches

- "The 2-cm rule": This applies to a circumferential measurement discrepancy between two limbs, and its sensitivity and specificity are directly related to the number of measurements obtained and whether they are used to create a limb volume. Armer et al found that using a single-point discrepancy, on women followed up for 5 years, resulted in a 91% incidence of lymphedema.[81] The NLN position paper on Early Detection of Breast Cancer Related Lymphedema has stated that a single 1 cm increase from baseline should result in a 1-month follow-up and a 2 cm increase should result in treatment referral. Clearly, this interlimb discrepancy diagnosis cannot be generalized to nonlimb lymphedema.[82]
- Limb volume measurement: This can be obtained from circumferential measurements, perometry, or volume displacement measurement. Circumferential measurements can be used to calculate arm volumes with either a two-point system: frustum sign method (volume of a truncated cone) or disk model method (summed truncated cones). The significant limb volume discrepancy to diagnose lymphedema has not been clarified; 5% volume increase has been found to have a 91% sensitivity rate and a 10% increase corresponded to a 49% sensitivity.[82,83] One study measured accuracy of limb volume calculated by incremental measurements, and concluded that while 4-cm measurements were accurate for arm volumes, leg volumes could be obtained with 4-, 8-, or 12-cm incremental measurements.[84]
- Physical examination: Stanton et al used perometry and physical examination[85] and found that for breast cancer patients whose volume measurements were within normal limits examination discovered early signs of lymphedema: decreased visibility of veins, smoothing of the contours of the medial elbow region, increased skin and subcutis thickness on palpation, and pitting edema. Limitation of edema to focal regions was noted, for example, hand and wrist only or upper arm. Stemmer's sign, fixation of digital skin, is a time-honored sign of lymphedema. Thickening of the skin and skin elasticity has been correlated with successful treatment of lymphedema, and another objective measurement that can be utilized.[86,87]
- Symptoms: Patients will report symptoms of swelling, warmth, heaviness, tingling,

3

tightness, and/or skin changes. Armer et al have developed the University of Missouri Lymphedema and Breast Cancer Questionnaire (LBCQ) survey to assess BCRL. Symptoms can precede overt swelling and latency stage lymphedema may only present with symptoms or subtle physical findings as mentioned earlier. Yost et al have developed a validated questionnaire for lower extremity lymphedema, and this can be accessed from their article.[80] There are other validated survey tools which are available for a fee.

- Newer technologies: Bioimpedance spectroscopy (BIS) has been marketed specifically to diagnose latent lymphedema, stage 0—prior to physical changes. The device measures extracellular fluid, but requires accurate use and sequential measurements and is not useful in patients with fibrosis. As early diagnosis and prospective monitoring of lymphedema have been proved to minimize BCRL,[88] bioimpedance is a measurement modality, which, combined with a full assessment of the patient, can aid in detecting early lymphedema. The device's literature states that it is not intended to diagnose or predict lymphedema, yet it has been proposed to be utilized in this manner. Clinically, it is a useful adjunct to a full clinical evaluation, and can have a role in perspective survelliance.[88,89]
- Imaging: Per the AHQR review: "The validity of ultrasound, lymphoscintigraphy (LAS), computed tomography (CT) scan, or magnetic resonance imaging (MRI) was evaluated in four studies. There is little evidence for the validity of these tests owing to the limited number of studies, small sample sizes, a questionable reference standard in one study, and questionable means of scoring LAS in two studies."[79]
- Nonextremity lymphedema: the NLN position paper on BCRL suggests that for truncal and breast lymphedema, patients be examined for "objective" evidence/visualization of swelling in the chest or trunk and symptoms referable to the area. Williams stated, "there is no fully validated method to assess these areas," despite the possible incidence of truncal/breast lymphedema in up to 70% of treated patients.[84,90,91]
- Skin elasticity is impacted by lymphedema. Studies are just emerging to create objective measurement devices.[86,87] Additionally, clinical exam will identify changes in skin elasticity.

- Head and neck lymphedema: Patients treated for head and neck cancer have been assessed externally using the Földi scale and internally with endoscopy, and found to have a high incidence of lymphedema—up to 50%.[92]
- Lymphedema rating scales: The Földi scale, the Common Toxicity Criteria v3 lymphedema, the LVF Location, Volume, Fibrosis Scale by Kasseroller, RG, and International Society of Lymphology Staging (below). Most scales rely exclusively on volume, which is of little value in bilateral or nonlimb lymphedema.

3.6.2 International Society of Lymphology (ISL) Lymphedema Staging

ISL Stage 0

It is a subclinical state where swelling is not evident despite impaired lymph transport.

This stage may exist for months or years before edema becomes evident.

ISL Stage 1

This represents early onset of the condition where there is accumulation of tissue

fluid that subsides with limb elevation. The edema may be pitting at this stage.

ISL Stage II

Limb elevation alone rarely reduces swelling and pitting is manifest.

ISL Late Stage II

There may or may not be pitting as tissue fibrosis is more evident.

ISL Stage III

The tissue is hard (fibrotic) and pitting is absent. Skin changes such as thickening, hyperpigmentation, increased skin folds, fat deposits, and warty overgrowths are present.

Yet, with any evaluation, a thorough patient history is vital to making the diagnosis, and often before lymphedema manifests with physical symptoms, there are subtle symptoms and history that aid in making the diagnosis.

3.6.3 History

The history should be taken to assess both primary and secondary lymphedema and other medical conditions that cause swelling.

There are the classic cardinal signs for history of present illness: location, quality, radiation, intensity/severity, onset, aggravating factors, alleviating factors, and associated symptoms.

The pattern of illness/symptoms should be obtained. Lymphedema is a dynamic process. The nature of the onset should be documented: sudden, insidious, a provoking incident such as trauma, or infection. The nature of the symptoms: wax and wane, progressive, and again provoking behaviors such as exercise, heat, prolonged standing.

The pattern of swelling gives important clues as to the diagnosis. In primary lymphedema, the swelling typically begins distally—usually in the toes, although rarely hands may be involved, and progresses proximally. Lipedema is a disorder of subcutaneous fatty tissue, tends to affect women, and disproportionably involves the lower half of the body while sparing the area below the ankles. In lipedema, the affected areas are typically hypersensitive to touch and pressure. Secondary lymphedema occurs in the quadrant at risk after disruption of the regional lymphatics due to surgery, radiation, injury, and/or infection. The swelling of secondary lymphedema can start in any portion of the quadrant. In lymphedema secondary to venous insufficiency, there will be a history of varicose veins, venous stasis changes, and/or deep vein thrombosis, and the swelling usually begins distally and initially resolves with elevation.

Patients should be asked if there is a family history of swelling and limbs that do not reduce despite weight loss and/or elevation. Body habitus and familial body habitus give important clues as to lipedema and primary lymphedema.

Foreign travel history is important to assess filariasis.[93]

Disruption to the lymphatic system should be assessed: history of trauma, surgery, radiation, chemotherapy, venous thrombosis, immobility, and history of skin infections.

Secondary causes of swelling should be assessed, such as congestive heart failure (CHF), renal failure, venous insufficiency, varicosities, hepatic insufficiency, hypothyroidism, neuropathies, reflex sympathetic dystrophy, and any paralysis.

Additionally, medications can cause peripheral edema, so a thorough medication history, both prescribed and over the counter, should be obtained.

History of symptoms that are associated with swelling should be obtained: heaviness, achiness, tight clothing or jewelry, noticeable swelling, changes in contours of the body, obscuring of bony or tendon landmarks, marks left by clothing or other pressure, warmth, color changes of the skin, numbness, paresthesia, and the temporal pattern of these symptoms. A validated questionnaire for breast cancer patients, the LBCQ questionnaire, has been developed by Armer.[81] Cheville and coworkers have developed a questionnaire for lower extremity lymphedema.[80]

As with any patient, a full history of present illness, past medical history, and social history—with attention to occupation, functionality, exercise, family history, and review of systems—including screening for mood disorders, should be performed. Additional special questionnaires for assessment of function, pain, and symptoms should be utilized.

Directed by the area where lymphedema is suspected, a thorough review of systems should be obtained.

As always, symptoms of pain should be documented and scored.

3.6.4 Physical Examination

General

Vital signs, including BMI should be obtained; weight should be obtained at every visit. General observation of gait, balance, and use of limbs should be noted.

A general physical examination should be performed, within the health care provider's area of expertise—clearly, this will vary with training, but ideally the most complete physical examination that the practitioner had been trained and expertise to perform should be obtained. For example: for head and neck lymphedema, endoscopic evaluation is preferred, as well as a functional swallowing evaluation.

Assessment of cardiac, pulmonary, hepatic, dermatologic, neurologic, and musculoskeletal systems should be performed.

Specific for Lymphedema

The patient should be examined in all four quadrants of the body, with attention to noticeable swelling, obscuring of tendon and bony landmarks, skin exam, surgical scars, musculoskeletal function, and neurologic examination. The skin examination should focus on changes in the cutis, thickening, fibrosis, color changes, skin lesions, a full nail examination, varicosities, venous stasis changes, and evaluation of all wounds. Presence of Stemmer's sign should be documented.

The skin changes associated with progressive lymphedema should be assessed: thickening, papillomatosis, hyperkeratosis, lymph vesicles, and/or fistulas.

In the breast, skin thickening can present as a "peau d'orange" pattern.

As described earlier, a quantitative measurement of the patient should be obtained, if possible: interlimb volume for limb edema obtained as calculated volumes, perometry measurements, and/or water displacement measurements.

Additionally, to assess general extracellular fluid, serial BIS measurements can be obtained —with awareness that the L-dex is not intended to diagnose or predict lymphedema (see manufacturer's information 10)—using consistent guidelines that involve an empty bladder, avoidance of caffeine and alcohol, and lying prone for adequate period. BIS measures extracellular fluid and can assist in the diagnosis of lymphedema. The device is not reliable once there is skin fibrosis (ImpediMed correspondence).

For suspected nonlimb lymphedema, the patient should be examined for overt swelling—pitting or nonpitting, changes of the skin and subcutis, and use of photography may be helpful to document external physical examination abnormalities, as in breast/truncal, genital, abdominal, and head and neck edema.

Lymphedema is edema just composed of lymphatic fluid. Patients will present with edema that is due to CHF, nephrotic syndrome, hepatic insufficiency, and vascular insufficiency. They can have coexisting lymphedema as well if the lymphatic system is damaged. Additionally, morbid edema can cause lymphedema due to obstruction.

Reassessment

As lymphedema is a chronic condition, reassessment is crucial.

A focused history of symptoms and modalities used to treat the condition should be obtained.

Weight, height, and BMI should be obtained, as well as current medications and interval medical conditions should be documented.

Symptoms and pain, as well as body function, should be assessed.

Quantitative measurements should be documented, if applicable. For limb volumes, a 3% increase from a "normal" baseline is considered indicative of subclinical lymphedema and a 5% increase is considered both sensitive and specific for lymphedema. As Stanton has documented, observation of subtle changes may indicate clinically significant disease, even in the absence of volume increases. If bioimpedance is used as an adjunctive measurement, serial measurements with close attention to accuracy should be obtained: the manufacturer states that "L-dex values of above +10 or increase of 10 may indicate lymphedema."[89]

The concept of a treated chronic disease should be employed: a patient who has responded to CDT and compression may subsequently present with reduced limb or body volume and reduced symptoms, but as lymphedema is chronic, this documents a reduction in the severity of their disease and possibly a regression of their ISL stage, and is not an end point, but merely an excellent response to treatment.

3.6.5 Medical Education about Lymphedema

Unfortunately, the extent to which the lymphatic system is studied in medical school is typically observation during gross anatomy and discussion of enlarged lymph nodes in pathophysiology. The topic of lymphedema is rarely, if ever, discussed. The majority of medical school graduates will not have sufficient medical education to possibly even be aware of the disease, and they will likely have insufficient education to diagnose it.

Postgraduate medical education tends to ignore lymphedema as well, as there are virtually no questions on it in board exams, nor is it featured in continuing medical education.

Even in specialties relating to areas where secondary lymphedema can be a side effect of treatment, medical oncologists, surgeons, and radiation oncologists do not routinely receive education on the disease, diagnosis, or treatment of lymphedema.

A recent study by Kaiser Permanente, of practicing physicians in a staff model HMO setting, documented that medical oncologists and surgeons, and female physicians in general, were better informed about BCRL, yet only 44% of physicians who treated women with breast cancer had ever made a lymphedema treatment referral.[94]

A personal observation: attending a survivorship conference, sponsored by Harvard Medical School, at a major cancer center, I spoke to the medical director of the Livestrong Clinic, whose mission statement included treatment of lymphedema, and this director was unaware of how to treat lymphedema. When contacted, their physical therapy department had hired lymphedema therapists, but did not know their level of training, and proposed making lymphedema a "sentinel event" which is synonymous with significant medical error. Additionally, the published information on this illustrious institution's website on lymphedema contained many factual errors. Despite contacting the medical director of the institution, the website has never been updated, and subsequent survivorship conferences by this institution have not addressed lymphedema.

Additionally, one of their closely affiliated hospitals has consistently measured women with perometers to diagnose lymphedema and for surveillance, but has consistently published articles to "debunk" lymphedema risk reduction behaviors and to reassure surgeons that the risk of lymphedema with sentinel node biopsy is so low that doing the procedure during a prophylactic mastectomy, where it is likely to not be necessary for staging, should be considered without concern for risk of causing lymphedema.[95,96] As they "define" lymphedema as a 10% volume increase in the at-risk arm, they will be inherently missing many cases of lymphedema, as simple volume increase, at 10%, without evaluation of skin elasticity or symptoms, will inherently miss many women with BCRL. One study showed that the vast majority of women with BCRL in their assessment group were missed by simple volume measurement.[97] A full clinical examination and symptom assessment is imperative.

The medical profession has ignored lymphedema, and as there is no standard for diagnosis, all studies will inherently be inconsistent. As there are no uniform objective criteria for diagnosis, clinicians cannot be given a simple test, and must perform a full assessment of the patient and make a clinical judgment. This requires knowledge and understanding of the condition.

Case Study

A 58-year-old woman was treated for breast cancer with breast conservation and radiation. It has been 5 years since her cancer diagnosis and she has completed 5 years of tamoxifen therapy. Approximately 3 years ago, she underwent a course of CDT for lymphedema of the left, treated, arm and wears compression garments. She works in a clerical position and notes that she has tingling and aching in the arm, which is worse at night and often wakes her from sleep.

On examination, her arm has focal swelling at the proximal portion with thickening of the skin and obscuring of veins, and the skin is lighter in appearance. This area of thickening measures 2 to 3 cm wider than her untreated arm, but the other parts of her arms are equal in size, and there is no visible swelling in the dorsum of her hand, nor obscuring of tendons.

On examination of her treated breast, the skin is thickened, with prominent pores, and still has residual radiation tanning.

The "red flags" in this case are the history of lymphedema because the greatest predictor of progressive lymphedema is a history of mild lymphedema,[98] the history of axillary surgery and radiation, and the symptoms of aching and tingling.

This patient most likely does not have a 10% volume increase in the affected arm, but clinically she has breast and truncal lymphedema and limb lymphedema with fibrosis and would benefit from treatment of her breast and trunk with MLD and compression garments as well as treatment of her focal area of fibrosis; and as her symptoms are worse at night, showing her how to apply bandages and advising her to wear different night garments might help toward reducing the swelling, fibrosis, and symptoms in her arm. She was discharged from lymphedema therapy without follow-up, and at over 5 years out from breast cancer treatment, she has most likely been discharged from many of her physicians. Yet her risk of lymphedema and progression of lymphedema is lifelong.

3.6.6 Summary

There is no single, unifying diagnostic criteria for lymphedema. Current diagnostic criteria tend to focus on limb lymphedema.

It should be realized that without unifying diagnostic criteria for lymphedema, there will be inherent variations in diagnosis, reported incidence, and prevalence of the disease.

Lymphedema is a dynamic process and reliance solely on physical diagnosis could result in disease being missed.

3

A thorough history is crucial, as is obtaining some form of objective measurement that is consistent to the health care professionals' practice. Lymphedema can exist in the absence of 2-cm limb circumference discrepancy. Symptoms can precede and coexist with clinically apparent lymphedema. Physical examination can fluctuate with treatment, provoking conditions, and comorbidities.

Lymphedema can coexist with lipedema, venous insufficiency, CHF, and other medical comorbidities.

Reliance on a single modality to diagnose lymphedema could result in disease being missed: patients should be assessed by symptoms, history, physical examination, and objective measurements.

Medical education is often lacking in lymphedema, at all levels of medical providers and at all stages of their clinical careers.

3.7 Evaluation of Lymphedema

Accurate and timely diagnosis of lymphedema is essential so that the appropriate amount of treatment can be applied in a prompt, cost-effective, and minimally intensive fashion. Despite the growing body of evidence regarding the evaluation, treatment, and early intervention/prevention of lymphedema, many controversies and knowledge gaps exist. This translates into continued delays in the diagnosis and access to treatment for many patients. Once diagnosed, patients want timely treatment but the current treatment paradigm often requires that patients get on long waiting lists until an appointment is available.

Lymphedema is a dynamic condition regardless of the stage. Managing a latency stage is vastly different from managing a severe stage III lymphedema; yet, both are chronic and require lifelong care. Different levels of intervention are required according to the stage, severity, and complexity of lymphedema.[99] Certified lymphedema therapists and lymphedema clinics must embrace this more evolved approach toward managing lymphedema and change the strategy used in scheduling initial evaluations and triaging patients for the actual treatment.

Lymphedema and other swelling disorders exist along a vast spectrum of presentations encountered during the initial evaluation. These presentations can be divided into three distinct categories: (1) patients presenting with clear objective signs and/or chronic history of lymphedema with or without possible infection, (2) patients without clear objective signs who complain of subjective complaints and subtle sensory changes in the affected area, and (3) patients who present for a prehabilitation visit to establish a baseline measurement prior to any surgery, radiotherapy, or treatment that will remove lymph nodes and/or will put the patient at risk of developing lymphedema (▶ Table 3.7).

Clinics may want to develop a simple preevaluation questionnaire to assist their staff with triaging and setting up lymphedema evaluations based on these categories versus a "first-come, first-served" model. The probable stage, severity, and complexity of lymphedema need to be factored in when scheduling. Clinics must also ensure that staff screen patients for possible infections that require urgent medical care and give recommendations for patients to seek medical treatment immediately.

It is important to note the time since onset, current symptoms, and known risk factors. Many clinics have long waiting lists to see patients with advanced stage chronic lymphedema for full intensive phase CDT treatment. A patient with stage 0/I lymphedema who is having sensory changes or subclinical symptoms of lymphedema cannot wait 1 to 2 months to be evaluated. There must be a mechanism in place to trigger the early intervention evaluation in a time-sensitive fashion, so prompt treatment of early-stage 0/I lymphedema can be initiated. Studies have demonstrated that upward of 80% of lymphedema is not diagnosed until stage II.[1] Studies have also shown that mild BCRL is a predictor of more severe lymphedema, and if left untreated, approximately 50% of cases will progress to more severe lymphedema in 5 years.[99] Similarly, a study found almost 80% of women mentioned symptoms of lymphedema to their health care provider, yet only 47% received treatment. The majority of patients receiving treatment were already in late stage, having moderate to severe symptoms.[1]

A comprehensive evaluation process requires adequate time to perform a complete systems' review, yet it should be focused toward the presenting symptoms and/or diagnosis. The evaluation will provide the necessary data for differential diagnosis, to quantify and/or stage the condition, and to determine if CDT or parts of CDT are indicated for treatment. It is often the first time a patient has met a health care provider who is a specialist in the field of lymphedema, and the

Table 3.7 Framework for triaging and scheduling patients, setting time frames, and scope of treatment based on presentation of lymphedema symptoms

Presentation of lymphedema symptoms	Time from scheduling to evaluation	Scope of evaluation and treatment	Frequency and duration of treatment
Prehabilitation of patients who will be at risk for developing lymphedema (pretreatment or preoperative)	• May need expedited evaluation due to planned surgical date • Must be prior to scheduled surgery or treatment	• Pretreatment baseline • Focus on any current impairments • Plan for potential issues throughout treatment	• Initial visit and further pre-tx visits if significant issues that will affect surgery • Post-op visit(s) • Surveillance visits
Patients with subclinical, subjective complaints	• Need to be seen as soon as possible • Within 7 days	• Compare to pretreatment baseline if possible • Educate on exercise, skin care, and use of compression	• Depends on other treatments they are receiving • See at least one to three visits over 4–6 weeks • Ensure compliance and no progression of symptoms
Patients with objective signs of edema, chronic symptoms, previous treatment, no current signs and symptoms of wounds or infection	• Can be put on wait list • Schedule at the patient's convenience	• Full evaluation geared to successful CDT treatment • Assess any barriers to care prior to initiating treatment	Full CDT; 5 days per week × 3–4 + weeks depending on severity Once measured for garments can reduce to 3 × week if needed until garment fitting
Patients with objective signs of edema, chronic symptoms, previous treatment with current signs and symptoms of wounds or infection	• Need to be prescreened for possible infection prior to being placed on wait list • If needed must be sent to MD • Coordinate transition from acute care to outpatient	• Prescreen for urgent medical issues • If possible, infection must be referred to definitive medical treatment • Otherwise full evaluation geared to successful CDT treatment • Assess any barriers to care prior to initiating treatment	• Full CDT; 5 days per week × 3–4 + weeks depending on severity • Coordinate with wound care if needed • Begin bandaging once infection properly treated to prevent progression of lymphedema

patient often lacks basic information about the condition. Patients may not realize the relevance of their entire medical and/or surgical history, which, along with their personal history, often reveals the subtle and progressive onset of their lymphedema or the potential to acquire lymphedema. In all cases, a thorough evaluation performed by the therapist can clarify the medical diagnosis and establish the rehabilitation diagnosis as a basis for skilled therapy services. Patients may be cleared for therapy, but many referring physicians may not realize the systemic effects that CDT and its component parts have on the human body. The evaluation can also prevent unnecessary or unsafe treatment, by recognizing contraindications and/or precautions for treatment. Patients will occasionally present to the lymphedema clinic with an inaccurate diagnosis on the referral, as any swelling or edema that looks severe is dubiously termed lymphedema. To be accurately diagnosed

as lymphedema, there must be an abnormality of the lymphatic system, whether acquired or developmental, that ultimately results in a mechanical insufficiency. When no clear cause for edema can be established after a thorough evaluation process, it is incumbent on the therapist to contact the referring physician for further medical work-up and consultation.

Thorough evaluation allows the therapist to identify the patient's goals and impairments in function, determine the rehabilitation diagnosis, determine the prognosis for treatment, and develop a comprehensive plan of care. It will also assess education style, barriers to care, and the need for other medical treatments for concomitant conditions. The plan of care will include setting short-term and long-term patient-centered goals, selecting all appropriate interventions (such as bandaging, MLD, compression garments, remedial exercise, and self-care), and developing a

3

comprehensive discharge plan. It is imperative during the initial evaluation that the therapist determines the need for skilled care and confirms that the patient will have the ability to independently perform their self-care management. Otherwise, treatment may not proceed until the necessary caregiver(s) or assistance is in place. Similar attention must be given to the patient's ability to obtain the necessary supplies and garments. If no clear source of insurance or self-pay option exists at the time of evaluation, then this needs to be arranged prior to initiating treatment. A therapist should not get midway through the intensive phase of decongestion, only to discover that the patient is not able to obtain the necessary garments because this would render the treatment useless. Many patients have significant financial restrictions that limit their ability to get appropriate compression garments. A plan must be in place prior to initiating treatment.

Prior to the actual evaluation, it is important for the therapist to get as much information as possible about the patient's condition. This will help focus the evaluation as the therapist will have a better understanding of the extent of the lymphedema and the impact on the patient's life. This can be accomplished by having all new patients fill out a pretreatment lymphedema questionnaire similar to one used by the National Lymphedema Network.[100] At the least, a simple form assessing functional status, work status, caregiver status, available social support, living situation, and transportation status will offer the therapist significant insight into the patient's abilities and resources. Once the evaluation is completed, the therapist can select appropriate functional outcome and/or quality-of-life measures for the patient to fill out. Oftentimes, a patient may have multiple functional issues and more than one tool will be needed to adequately gauge their progress and outcomes. These include such tools as the recently validated Lymphedema Life Impact Scale (LLIS),[101] LYM-QOL,[45] the Lymph-ICF,[102] the Lymphedema and Breast Cancer Questionnaire (LBCQ),[54] the ULL-27[103] for upper limb lymphedema, or the FLQA-I[41] for arm or leg lymphedema. The use of such disease-specific tools may benefit the clinician by providing outcome measures to assess the effectiveness of treatment and will aid in the clinical assessment.[45] As mentioned, these tools can be used in conjunction with other common measures of functional status such as the Disabilities of the Arm, Shoulder, and Hand Questionnaire (DASH), the Lower Extremity Function Scales (LEFS), and

Timed Up and Go (TUG), to name a few. This is particularly important when patients have preexisting comorbid conditions.

The patient evaluation includes both subjective and objective components that will be combined to form a comprehensive assessment of the patient's condition. Földi stated, "Medical histories, inspection, palpation, and percussion are increasingly neglected, and diagnoses are based on laboratory data. What is lost is an understanding of the interconnections."[104] The advantage of having a thorough lymphedema evaluation by a specially trained clinician is that he or she has the capacity to make the interconnections and ensure that proper treatment is provided based on a full understanding of the patient's condition. The first few minutes of the evaluation yields critical information about the patient's situation. How did the patient ambulate into the room? Is the patient demonstrating any signs of physical exertion? Is he or she sitting on the chair or on the treatment table with appropriate posture? Is someone with the patient for support? Do they appear anxious or upset? Observation starts the moment one sees the patient for the first time.

It is often helpful to begin the evaluation when the patient is still dressed by asking him or her about the history of the onset and development of the edema. The patient should be thoroughly questioned about the course of the swelling, going as far back into his or her history as required. Did the swelling develop slowly or rapidly? Was the presentation distal or proximal? Is there pain or discomfort? Does the patient have a known cause or causes for the edema that could result in secondary lymphedema. How old was he or she when any symptoms started? Is there a family history of swelling? Did the patient ever have an infection related to the swelling? If so, how many infections has he or she been treated for? Where was the infection located? What treatment(s) did the patient receive? Was he or she hospitalized for the infection? Is the patient currently under any prophylactic care for infections?

Allowing some time to establish a clinical relationship is important, as it allows the therapist time to educate the patient on how the lymphatic system works as they progress through the evaluation process. This will help the patient understand why the therapist must evaluate the entire body and why the patient needs to put on a gown for both evaluation and treatment. A thorough review of the patient's past medical and surgical history is required at this time, along with rectifying the patient's medication list, as this must be assessed for common medications that may cause edema, such as calcium channel blockers. What the patient reported should match their recorded health history, as patients often forget about very important medical conditions and/or surgical history. Recent diagnostic tests, laboratory work, and medical treatments should be noted. Any prior treatment, including self-care for their edema, should also be noted. Patients who have had previous treatment elsewhere should try to have their medical records from that treatment available during their initial evaluation. Patients should also have a list or bring any compression garments (day and night), bandages, and the specific name/model of any pneumatic compression devices (PCD they may be using or have used in the past.

Pain must be assessed and documented along with all other important baseline vital signs. The onset, location, duration, and description of pain should be noted along with factors that change the level of pain. Many patients will try to differentiate between pain and discomfort, or they will neglect to mention the pain in other areas of their body. Encourage patients to report any pain because it may affect their ability to tolerate treatment or participate in their self-management. Therapists should not challenge the patient on whether lymphedema is or is not painful, as many patients have varying degrees of pain. When there is no clear reason for the pain, further medical evaluation may be needed, particularly in the patient with a history of cancer treatment. Patients with lymphedema may have other underlying conditions that contribute to their symptoms, but have been overlooked due to the presence of edema.

The initial evaluation also serves to educate patients on general treatment protocols within the lymphedema clinic. Patients should be shown how to put on the gown and drape their body with a sheet if required. Patients need to be educated on meticulous hand hygiene and why they should keep their shoes off the treatment table and their bare feet off the floor. The therapist must also assess functional activities such as the ability to don and doff clothing and shoes, general mobility, toileting/incontinence issues, and overall self-care. Timing how long it takes patients to change into a gown can give a general indication as to their self-care status, as can their ability to accomplish this alone or with assistance. At this time, patients should be offered a chaperone, if institutional policy requires that one be present. This is particularly important in the case of genital lymphedema assessment. If the patient is a minor, then the parent or legal guardian must be in the room for the entire evaluation regardless of diagnosis.

The upper extremity patient should be in a patient gown that leaves the entire thorax above the waist/transverse watershed visible. Having the gown open toward the back allows for more discrete examination to begin on the posterior thorax. Similarly, the lower extremity patient must be in a gown that leaves the entire region below the transverse watershed visible. Patient education occurs throughout the evaluation as the therapist explains many concepts to the patient, such as why the contralateral limb must be assessed, and why unaffected tissue needs to be inspected. Education with anatomic depictions of the different superficial lymphatic territories, watersheds, and anastomoses is very important so that the patient has adequate understanding of how treating unaffected tissue influences affected tissue.

The appearance of the involved limb(s), body part, and/or quadrants along with observations on the unaffected areas should be noted first, gaining an appreciation for the symmetry or asymmetry of the body region involved and the general condition of the skin. What observable areas of lymph drainage are affected? Document any observable skin changes such as scars, wounds, fibrosis, discoloration, peau d'orange, hyperkeratosis, papillomas, and lymph cysts. Note the presence of collateral veins, abnormal skinfolds, radiation markers, and implanted devices visible under the skin, along with any possible areas of infection. Are there areas with excessive dryness, moisture, or contracture of the skin? Are there areas of lipodermatosclerosis or hemosiderin staining? Examine any notable areas more closely to assess their impact on lymphatic transport at the surface level. Will the direction and location of a scar impede normal surface drainage? Do observable surface radiation changes possibly represent deeper radiation fibrosis? Are there skin fragility issues that will have an impact on treatment? Does the observation of this tissue warrant palpation for further assessment?

Careful observation allows for safe and effective palpation of relevant tissue. Palpation will allow the therapist to gain a better sense of the affected tissue. It is important to explain what you are expecting to feel during palpation as you check the various tissues and parts of the body. Is the edema pitting or nonpitting? Is there tenderness with palpation using light touch or deeper pressure? What is the texture and temperature of the skin in the affected regions versus the unaffected regions? Is there a Stemmer's sign on the fingers or toes? Are there subtle tissue changes or loss of usual anatomic architecture or is the limb fibrotic and dense? Does the affected region feel heavier on one side compared to the other? This is often the case with truncal, breast lymphedema, and with lobules of tissue on the medial thighs, back, and upper arms. The quality and location of any abnormal palpation should be documented. A body diagram may be helpful to accurately locate areas of concern. Photographs are also important, but must only be taken once written consent has been obtained and is documented in the patient's record. Photographic technique needs to be operationally defined so that patient photographs are taken in a consistent manner. Keep the distance between the subject and the camera consistent and take photographs with similar lighting. Also ensure the patient's privacy is protected as much as possible, keeping identifiable features out of the photo when able.

Next, measurements should be taken for limb volume, girth, or other appropriate measures of the area involved (such as head, neck, breast, and genital lymphedema). It is important that anthropometric measurements are taken for comparison to a baseline height, weight, and calculated BMI. Patients going through cancer treatment often have significant changes in weight that must be accounted for throughout treatment. Circumferential measurements taken with a tape measure are standard and can be used for simple girth measurements or the numbers can be placed in volumetric programs that convert the circumferential measurements to limb volume. Commercially available volumetric programs are available for limb volumes. These programs automatically calculate the percentage reduction achieved during treatment and compare limbs, generating reports that can be part of the patient record. Other testing methods such as BIS and infrared perometry are possible measurement tools. Specific protocols should be followed to ensure standardization of any of these techniques.

ROM, muscle-strength testing, flexibility, and sensation are assessed to make sure any possible deficiencies will not inhibit participation in lymphedema treatment. Posture, balance, and gait must be assessed for similar reasons. If the patient will have to negotiate stairs while bandaged, this will also need to be assessed. Any deficiencies that will affect treatment outcome for the lymphedema must be addressed. Specific functional tasks should be assessed if there is any question as to the patient's ability to perform a specific task. The clinician must anticipate the effect of any type of bandaging on the patient's function. If bandaging creates an unsafe environment, action must be taken to remediate the situation. Patients should never be sent home with a bandage that puts them at unnecessary risk of falls or other injuries.

Patients should be given further education prior to leaving the initial evaluation. At the very least, they need disease-specific information on the treatment of lymphedema. Patients should be informed about the components of CDT, the daily requirements for treatment, any costs associated with treatment (such as bandages and garments), special clothing, and appropriate shoes (required for lower extremity treatment). Meticulous skin and nail care along with risk-reduction education should be covered. The subject of garments and durable medical equipment (DME) needs to be discussed. Depending on the location, many clinics use outside vendors to provide DME services. Consent forms are required to release protected health information to companies that provide these services. The patient will need to work with these companies to ascertain his or her DME benefits for compression garments. Treatment cannot start until a clear payment source is identified for the garments and bandages. Other situations the patient should deal with because they might prevent treatment being started immediately include obtaining further medical clearance; arranging work schedules according to the Family and Medical Leave Act (FMLA); arranging for assistance at home; obtaining reliable transportation; and obtaining necessary insurance authorizations for treatment (▶ Table 3.8).

The evaluation process may not be fully complete by the time the patient leaves the clinic, especially if there are concerns regarding medical clearance. The therapist may need additional time to collect appropriate medical records to adequately synthesize and formulate the assessment of the patient's condition. Regardless, the patient will need clear follow-up instructions due to the complexity of the requirements for initiating treatment. It is vital that the therapist provides a written checklist or plan for the patient. This acts as a guide for upcoming treatment and continued education.

The final steps of the evaluation are to establish the prognosis with both the expected improvement and amount of time needed to obtain the improvement. A plan of care should also be

Table 3.8 Common examples of barriers to care for successful CDT treatment

Types of barriers to care	Examples
Medical/physiological	• Requires further medical clearance • Comorbid medical conditions • Symptoms of lymphedema • Pain
Psychological/psychosocial	• Lack of support • Social isolation • Public insensitivity • Anxiety/depression
Self-management	• Complexity of self-treatment • Inability to perform self-care for hygiene • Unable to perform basic ADLS • Inadequate home support
Financial	• Limited insurance coverage • Limited or no coverage for DME/garments • Limited financial resources
Occupational	• Limited time off from work to attend treatment • Needs to arrange FMLA/work schedule • Unable to work while in bandages • Occupational role changes
Geographical	• Geographical disparities • Clinics too far away for regular care
Transportation	• Inadequate or lack of transportation • Mobility issues affecting type of transportation • Complicated traffic issues

determined with functional goals that have objective criteria and a temporal basis. The direct interventions include the components of CDT and any other interventions that are needed to reach the goals. A discharge plan also needs to be formulated that clearly defines when a patient will be ready for discharge to his or her self-maintenance phase of care. It is important to remember that the evaluation will often be used by insurance companies and DME companies to determine if services will be provided. The evaluation is an opportunity to advocate for the patient to ensure he or she gets the proper care and treatment for lymphedema. The therapist must not feel pressure to start treatment until the conditions have been met that will allow treatment to be successful. Quite often, once the patient realizes what is involved with CDT, he or she needs to make further plans prior to starting intensive treatment. With chronic lymphedema, there is time to plan for treatment. Early intervention and surveillance require a different set of standards, and treatment must be timely.

3.7.1 Surveillance and Early Intervention

The management of cancer-related secondary lymphedema has the potential to be significantly different with the advent of prehabilitation baseline assessment and early intervention management, along with newer diagnostic modalities that have high sensitivity and specificity to detect early changes.[105] Patients scheduled to have cancer surgeries, chemotherapy, or radiotherapy treatments that will subject the lymphatic system to damage should be sent for pretreatment baseline assessment. Prehabilitation assessments are most commonly performed prior to breast cancer surgeries, but are becoming increasingly common for melanoma, gynecological, prostate, head, neck, and certain other cancers, such as sarcomas.

The prehabilitation baseline evaluation establishes a reference point prior to any treatment intervention. The evaluation assesses ROM, strength, sensation, limb volume/girth, functional activity, work status, and exercise habits. The evaluation assesses for any preexisting deficits or impairments. It also provides patient education, activity modification, and exercises as part of a postoperative or posttreatment plan of care.

The early-intervention model is based on knowledge of the anatomy, physiology, and pathophysiology of the lymphatic system. The concept of a mechanical insufficiency, as outlined by Földi, is central to understanding how and why lymphedema can develop.[104] This concept can be put into clear and concise patient-focused language and visualizations, so the patient understands the importance of early detection. A simple drawing of Transport Capacity, Lymphatic Load and Functional Reserve, similar to the diagrams in this text, can show a patient the potential change in capacity after surgery. Other techniques include using analogies of different size cups or vehicles that carry the LLs, or even showing a small container with the amount of fluid that could represent an early change. For BCRL, this change can be quite small, as was demonstrated by the Bethesda group work in 2008, where a significant volume change of 83 mL from the baseline assessments was detected (▶ Fig. 3.29).[74]

The patient gains a visual representation of the physiological process that could put him or her at risk of developing lymphedema and the small amounts of fluid that represent a clinically significant change. This serves as a basis for risk-reduction education. Therapists can review the different components of risk reduction to show the patient how many triggers for lymphedema affect the LL, causing it to surpass the TC. This information may seem too detailed, as patients are often overwhelmed at the time of cancer diagnosis. But research has demonstrated positive effects for patients receiving preoperative information and education about lymphedema.[106]

Simple anatomic drawings showing superficial lymph vessels draining to their respective regional lymph nodes also help patients conceptualize the area(s) that will be at risk. Similarly, anatomic drawings of a lymph node with its many afferent vessels and few efferent vessels can be useful for a patient undergoing SLNB. The concept that a single lymph node may have respective uptake from more than one anatomic region can be challenging for a patient. Once shown how a lymph node functions, patients gain perspective on their situation. Clear definitions and descriptions of the areas at risk are vital for the patient to have full understanding of where to look for symptoms. Previous risk-reduction and patient education for BCRL focused on arm lymphedema. However, we are well aware of the issues with truncal, chest, and breast lymphedema in this population. Similarly, for other types of cancer, patients must be told from where the lymph nodes will be removed and how many will be removed. They should be shown what territories drain to those nodes and the areas at risk should be acknowledged.

The surveillance model should standardize the intervals for regular postoperative follow-up. Suggested intervals begin as early as 1 month after surgery, followed by surveillance assessments at 3-month intervals, at least during the first year.[105] Patients should know not to delay reporting any symptoms of heaviness or tightness in the at-risk territory. It is no longer appropriate to wait until their symptoms progress. The goal of surveillance and early intervention is to preempt the progression symptoms that may not be reversible. The therapist needs to give the patient permission to ask questions and report symptoms that were historically disregarded. The patient with subjective complaints of heaviness and fullness needs a timely lymphedema evaluation, even if he or she is not at one of the standardized surveillance points. Based on newer understandings of risk factors associated with development of BCRL, the onset of mild edema should never be minimized. Since most research on early intervention and surveillance is from the BCRL domain, we should not directly apply it to other cancers. To date, multiple studies have been published with preliminary data on other types of cancer-related lymphedema. In 2015, the American Cancer Society published an excellent overview of the progress made in the treatment and prevention of cancer-related lymphedema, which summarizes the current body of knowledge.[107]

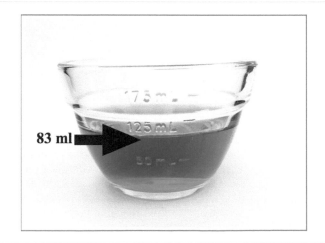

Fig. 3.29 Visual model of subclinical lymphedema volume to help patients understand early symptoms of breast cancer–related lymphedema concept based on CANCER study by Stout et al.[74]

Lymphedema is dynamic in nature, especially in its early stages. Patients may be having confounding symptoms from other treatments such as chemotherapy, additional surgeries, and radiotherapy. Treatment should not be withheld during this time, especially if the patient is reporting subjective complaints of heaviness and fullness. We must not let symptoms progress to a stage where they need full decongestive treatment. These early symptoms have been shown in the literature to naturally progress to more severe symptoms without treatment.[74] Treating these early symptoms requires much less intensity. Full CDT is not required and individual components of treatment can be applied as needed with much less cost. Patients are able to learn skills that will help them manage the condition over a lifetime. They may have similar symptoms in the future and will gain confidence in understanding their body and their reaction to certain activities, treatments, exercises, and compression garments.

The surveillance and early-intervention/prehabilitation model must acknowledge deficiencies in the insurance/reimbursement system. Many countries utilize treatment only when impairment diagnoses are made.[105] This is too late for the majority of patients who have known risk factors. If their insurance will only pay for garments and/or treatment once markedly visible edema is present, then we are subjecting them to a more intensive treatment model from the beginning. Using the prospective surveillance and screening model, patients and providers will need to bridge the time-sensitive gap for obtaining treatment and acquiring properly fitted garments. This will require current lymphedema programs to revamp the waiting-list concept of treating chronic lymphedema. Evidence from BCRL has shown most patients are likely to develop lymphedema in the first 3 years after treatment.[1] The 6- to 9-month point is regarded to be a critical time for early symptoms to occur. Patients with any type of initial symptom need to see a certified lymphedema therapist in a timely fashion. Researchers have recently published various cost-analysis models that show the increased costs of treating late-stage BCRL.[108,109] These studies have not included the patient-related costs for lost wages, lost leisure time, pain, psychological distress, or added self-care time.[105]

Efforts should continue toward the active promotion of the early-intervention model, even though it has not been studied exhaustively, as it is based on the strong body of evidence compiled so far in the age of modern lymphedema treatment. The shift in perspective from impairment-based care to that of secondary prevention, which utilizes a prospective surveillance model to prevent common chronic disease-related sequelae,[105] is vital to the advancement of the therapist role in the treatment and management of lymphedema. In 2011, the NLN Medical Advisory Committee (MAC) issued a position paper on "Screening and Measurement for Early Detection of Breast Cancer-Related Lymphedema."[82] In 2012, researchers introduced a prospective model for rehabilitation and early-intervention for breast cancer survivors.[75] These documents give both patients with breast cancer diagnosis and those specific health care providers who treat them the guidelines for setting the prospective surveillance model as the standard of care. The strength of this document was further acknowledged when the National Accreditation Program for Breast Centers (NAPBC) issued updated guidelines in 2011 that referenced this National Lymphedema Network position paper.[110]

Researchers are currently evaluating genetic polymorphisms associated with the possible development of secondary lymphedema related to cancer. They are establishing the models that may use skin biopsies or serum biomarker proteins to establish further early identification and risk stratification of patients who may be more likely to develop lymphedema. This could lead to future targeted molecular of pharmacological treatments.

3.8 Research in Lymphedema: Issues of Measurement and Assessment of Occurrence

Quantifying and diagnosing lymphedema (LE) has been problematic to date, despite the fact that researchers have used various methods to measure the limb with LE.[50,84,109,111] Perhaps, the most common criterion for diagnosis has been a finding of 2 cm or more difference in arm circumference (or 200-mL difference in LV) between affected and nonaffected limbs.[50,109] In part because of difficulties in measurement and diagnosis and delayed onset, the reported incidence of LE varies greatly among women treated with surgery and radiation for breast cancer.[112,113] Research involving careful measures and an extended follow-up period is an important step in supplying the reliable incidence and prevalence figures needed to study and treat LE.[47,50,105,111,114] Reviews of the literature have

3

estimated the overall incidence of lymphedema as 15.5% which varied by malignancy (p < 0.001).[6] Other studies have reported LE up to 40%,[115] from 6 to 30%,[113] 6.7 to 6.25%,[116] and from 43 to 94%.[111] Petrek and Heelan[113] noted that the study with the shortest follow-up (12 months) reported the lowest incidence (6%); likewise, one of the studies with the longest follow-up (11 years) reported the highest incidence (24%). This broad statistical range of findings probably reflects major breakthroughs in breast cancer treatment, including progress in breast conservation and therapeutic combinations that have led to increased survivorship[117,118]; inconsistent criteria for defining LE[50]; and small samples, retrospective analyses, and the psychometric difficulties (e.g., reliability) in assessing LE.[50,119] The Missouri 60-month data from a single prospectively followed sample reflect a range of 7 to 46% (6 months), 38 to 82% (24 months), and 43 to 94% (60 months) LE occurrence, depending upon LE definition and time point (▶ Fig. 3.30).[111]

There is a common misconception that LE is not a problem of the present or future due to modern procedures such as SLNB and breast conservation surgical approaches. However, the latest published data reveal LE occurrence to be at a significant level of concern in spite of these improved techniques.[120] Clinicians and researchers report modest estimates of LE following breast cancer surgery even for SLNB-only patients.[120] The latest American College of Surgeons Oncology Group (ACOSOG) data reveal LE incidence of 7% after SLNB only at a short follow-up at 6 months; those receiving further nodal dissection were not included in this analysis.[117,118] Because this SLNB-only group with node-negative disease represents the group at lesser risk for LE and because this LE occurrence is

commonly reported by clinical observation rather than objective limb measurement, there is a high probability that the condition is under-represented.

Breast conservation surgery and radiation therapy are standard options for breast cancer treatment, depending on stage. In addition, Giuliano et al conducted a randomized clinical trial ($N = 891$), and reported that patients with limited sentinel lymph node metastatic breast cancer treated with breast conservation and systemic therapy who received an SLND alone compared with ALND did not result in inferior survival.[118] Since radiation exposure is associated with trauma to the lymphatic system, risk for LE is likely to continue in women treated with state-of-the-art treatment modalities,[121] and although SLND has decreased the incidence of LE,[122] ALND remains the standard of care for those cases with more nodal involvement, thereby creating a cohort of breast cancer survivors at continuing lifetime risk of LE.[119] Increased measurement accuracy and long-term follow-up will result in a better understanding of the incidence and prevalence of LE following current therapeutic approaches for breast cancer treatment and will enable more informed decisions to be made regarding early- and late-onset LE risk factors, interventions, and management.[119] In addition, appropriate sampling decisions can be made for the next stage of risk reduction and management-intervention research.

In a 3-year follow-up study in Britain of breast cancer patients ($N = 188$ retained of 251 enrolled, with 25.1% attrition due to death [7.5%], lost to follow-up [7.1%], declining to continue [7.1%], and unable to continue due to illness [3.2%]), 20.7% developed LE, with risk factors identified as hospital skin puncture, mastectomy, and BMI > 26.[123] Of

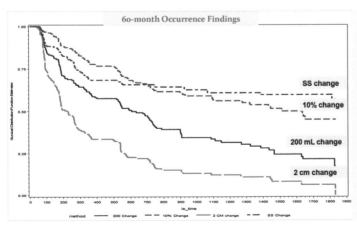

Fig. 3.30 Comparison of four methods for estimating lymphedema using observations from baseline to 60 months postsurgery and survival analysis. (Reproduced with permission from Armer and Stewart.[111])

the 39 with LE, 20 (51.3%) were diagnosed prior to the 3-year follow-up. These 20 included 9 (45%) diagnosed by 6 months and 16 (80%) by 12 months. Beyond these 20 who were diagnosed prior to the 3-year follow-up, 19 more (48.7%) were found to have LE at the 3-year follow-up.[123] This finding suggests a bimodal distribution of early- and late-onset LE which needs to be further explored over time. As noted earlier, data from the original Missouri R01 study (▶ Fig. 3.30) reveal LE occurrence at 43 to 94% at 60 months across all treatment groups, dependent upon LE definition.[111] Early survivor analysis projections at 12 months were confirmed at 24 months for early-onset LE, and the research team continued to examine these trends at 36 to 60 months through 84 months to document occurrence of late-onset LE.[111] Based on even the lowest estimates for the United States alone, LE affects hundreds of thousands of women and represents a major societal problem.[124,125]

Early detection and intervention hold the greatest promise of reducing this widespread condition.[73,74,105,123] Additional identification of epidemiological and clinical factors associated with risk and incidence will provide the necessary foundation for risk-reduction intervention. However, personal and historical characteristics such as age, weight, infection, radiation therapy, and axillary dissection are generally believed to affect women's risk for LE onset[123,124] and research has found that patient adherence to self-management is the most important factor in treating LE.[2,115,126] A contributing factor to successful adherence is having knowledge about the condition. In a study of 166 women with BCRL, Alcorso et al[127] reported a significant correlation between higher adherence and greater knowledge of lymphedema. Further research studies with rigorous design and larger sample sizes are needed to learn more about factors influencing patient adherence and effective self-management strategies for LE symptoms. For example, many of the most promising LE management techniques are time-consuming, very difficult for patients to accomplish themselves, and may be vulnerable to incomplete patient adherence without strong support and practical assistance from family or friends.[52,128] Such support and practical assistance may diminish over time, changes which need to be followed in survivors as they age.[62,81,129,130,131] Unfortunately, support groups and training in practical problem-solving are not always available to patients; therefore, health care providers need to offer evidence-based alternatives.

As limited as the physiological interventions that have proved to be effective in LE management may be, evaluation of psychosocial interventions has been even more limited. Preliminary research suggests that the lack of social support and avoidant coping are related to psychosocial and functional morbidity in LE patients.[32,70,127,129] As survivors age, avoidant coping may be more prevalent, thus leading to long-term problems. A qualitative study by Heppner et al[27] revealed that helpful coping strategies included approach-coping actions rather than avoidant actions, and that social support was a significant component of coping. Thus, psychosocial factors such as social support and applied problem-solving capacity may serve as personal and environmental resources. If available, these resources may allow women to successfully manage their chronic condition and its emotional and psychological impact; but a lack of these resources may exacerbate the functional impact of LE. These early findings suggest that further study is needed to better understand psychosocial factors, especially applied problem-solving capacity and social support, in relation to the progression of LE over an extended time period.[27,130] The addition of an educative-supportive program that continues throughout survivorship is a necessary component of prospective surveillance for physiological changes.[48,132]

To further develop programs of research on intervention directed at LE risk reduction, early detection, treatment, and symptom management, it is crucial that researchers and clinicians conduct investigations with increased precision in LE measurement to establish its current incidence and prevalence among breast cancer survivors and identify protective mechanisms over an extended time period. Before the outcomes of available treatments for the management of LE and its complications can be examined scientifically, it is necessary to carry out the following five steps: (1) the establishment of standardized operational definitions for lymphedema assessment, diagnosis, and treatment; (2) the establishment of accurate and reliable methods of measuring LV both at diagnosis and for the purpose of evaluating response to treatment; (3) the determination of LE incidence, prevalence, and associated symptoms across time; (4) the examination across time of the frequency and impact on daily living of LE symptoms and, concomitantly, the level of perceived coping effectiveness and the effectiveness of self-management strategies to manage the symptoms; and (5) the identification of protective mechanisms that reduce the severity and progression of LE, increase the effectiveness of self-management strategies, and enhance posttreatment psychosocial adjustment and functional health status.[111]

3.8.1 Measurement Issues in Lymphedema

The ideal volumetric measurement for LE would be easy to use, accessible, quick, noninvasive, hygienic, inexpensive, reliable, quantifiable, suitable for any portion of the limb, and able to provide information on shape.[50,109] Existing measures that are easy to use and inexpensive have limited reliability and do not address the functional impact of LE.[133] Limb volume measurements need to be performed routinely, preoperatively as well as at follow-up. Currently, no "gold standard" clinical protocol exists that is easy to use, noninvasive, and reliable for measuring the affected limb in the clinical setting. The Missouri study compares the currently accepted clinical LE assessment measures, examining how these methods converge and diverge in identifying early- and late-onset LE occurrence trends over time.[111] Such work will help establish a measurement standard that is both rigorous and clinically feasible, a key development that will help the fields of lymphology and LE move forward substantially and efficiently.

Although **water displacement** has been regarded as the sensitive and accurate "gold standard" for volume measurement in the laboratory setting, it is little used clinically because it is cumbersome and messy, requiring sanitation between patients and access to both a water source and drain. It is usually applied to a certain part of the limb and does not provide data about localization of the edema or the shape of the extremity (▶ Fig. 3.31).[50,107,109] A standard deviation of 2 mL for repeated measures of the arm has been reported by Swedborg.[134] One quandary is that water displacement is contraindicated in patients with open skin lesions.

Circumference measurements taken at various points of a body part are used most frequently to quantify LE (▶ Fig. 3.32), but several problems exist.[108] Limits for acceptable difference between repeated circumferential measurements of the normal adult arm, forearm, and wrist are 0.2 cm,[135] a standard rarely met clinically. Although circumferences may appear to be simple measures, control of intra- and intermeasurer reliability is difficult. Volume calculations assume a

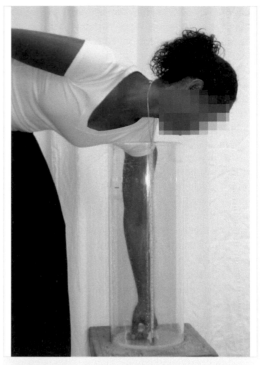

Fig. 3.31 Water displacement with use of a volumeter. (Photo courtesy of J. Cormier.)

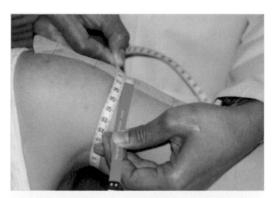

Fig. 3.32 Circumferences for limb girth. (Photo courtesy of J. Armer.)

circular circumference, which is seldom the case. This systematic methodological error gives a slightly higher volume than the true value. Studies report correlations with water displacement ranging from 0.70 to 0.98.[109,136] Because of the irregular shape of the hand, circumference measurements are inaccurate for determining volume of the hand. Severe limitations exist for this method, as well, when skin damage exists. Handling the extremity and contacting equipment raise hygienic concerns.[50] The circumferential method is considered time-consuming and requires considerable experience, although it is inexpensive in terms of equipment resources.

The **Perometer 400T/350S** (Juzo, Cuyahoga Falls, OH) is an optoelectronic volumetry (OEV) device developed to meet the need for a quick, hygienic, and accurate method of limb volume calculation (► Fig. 3.33). It works similarly to computer-assisted tomography, but uses infrared light instead of X-rays.[109] The light sources (two arrays of infrared-emitting diodes at right angles to each other) are set along two sides of a 46×46 cm frame with corresponding light sensors (two arrays of infrared-detecting diodes) opposite the light sources.[74,109,136] Where the path of the array of 360 infrared light beams is interrupted by the limb, the receivers in the limb's shadow are not lit, allowing the OEV to calculate a precise transection. Dimensions along the x and y axes are measured to an accuracy of 10^{-4} m.[109] Transections are measured every 3 mm and the volume is calculated by a computer.[109] The Perometer 400T/350S has a standard deviation with repeated measures of 8.9 mL, which is less than 0.5% of the arm volume.[109,136] This device can measure the volume and transection of any part of

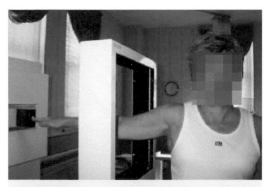

Fig. 3.33 Perometer (Juzo, Cuyahoga Falls, OH). (Photo courtesy of J. Armer.)

the limb, display the shape of the limb or limb segment, and make accurate calculations of change in volume in seconds. Given the observed precision of the perometer, the Missouri research team has conceptualized LE as a continuous (rather than dichotomous) variable, supporting a more robust test of the link between severity of LE (measured in percent of LV difference between affected and nonaffected limbs and LVC over time) and selected psychosocial processes and functional health.

Bioelectrical Impedance

Single-frequency bioelectrical impedance has become more frequently used in clinical and research settings to measure upper limb extracellular fluid.[137] Proponents report ease of use and low risk of user error, suggesting this measurement method may have advantages for use in community-based settings, as compared with some other measurement methods. The feasibility of using single-frequency bioelectrical impedance to detect upper limb LE in nonlaboratory settings was examined by a team at Vanderbilt University. Ridner et al[138] used a standardized protocol to assess impedance ratios among healthy normal women, breast cancer survivors with LE, and breast cancer survivors without LE with participants seated in an upright position (rather than the usual protocol of supine position; see ► Fig. 3.34). Ratios of healthy normal controls and breast cancer survivors without LE were very similar, while those values were markedly different from the values assessed in the survivor group with LE ($p < 0.001$). The authors suggest these findings support the conclusion that impedance ratios determined by single-frequency bioelectrical impedance can be used as markers for LE in nonlaboratory (community) settings when a standardized protocol is used. Single and multifrequency impedance were highly correlated in an earlier study by Ridner et al.[138] In another study, Fu et al collected bioelectrical impedance data from healthy women, women with BCRL, and women at-risk for LE ($N = 250$).[58] Reliability, sensitivity, and specificity of bioelectrical

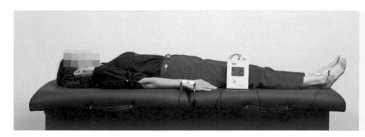

Fig. 3.34 Bioelectrical impedance. (Courtesy of ImpediMed, Inc.)

3

impedance were reported as acceptable in all three groups. However, it was reported that using a diagnostic cutoff of L-Dex ratio > +7.1 discriminated between at-risk breast cancer survivors and those with lymphedema with 80% sensitivity and 90% specificity; therefore, other assessment methods should be integrated to identify 20% of missed lymphedema cases.[139]

Tissue Dielectric Constant (Linda Koehler)

Water displacement, girth circumference, perometry, and BIS are suitable measuring devices for the extremities, but they do not have the ability to measure localized edema. Tissue dielectric constant (TDC) has the potential of identifying and quantifying edema in localized areas of the body that the other measures cannot adequately measure such as swelling of the trunk or head and neck region. TDC is dependent on the amount of water in the tissue. A probe is placed on the skin and a low electromagnetic wave is emitted into the tissue. A portion of the electromagnetic wave is reflected back to the probe indicating the amount of local tissue water under the area of the probe. The local tissue water measure displays as a dimensionless number, TDC, ranging from 1 to 80. A higher number signifies a higher amount of water in the localized area. Pure water has a value of around 80. Different size probes are available to measure different depths under the skin ranging from 0.5 to 5 mm (▶ Fig. 3.35). The 2.5-mm probe depth is the proposed effective depth for lymphedema. In unilateral breast cancer involvement, literature suggests taking TDC measures bilaterally and comparing the at-risk/affected side to the unaffected side by calculating an interarm TDC ratio. To calculate the interarm TDC ratio, the at-risk/affected side TDC measure is divided by the unaffected TDC measure (i.e., $\frac{TDC_{affected}}{TDC_{unaffected}}$). Standardized thresholds have yet to be determined, but current literature suggests a TDC ratio ≥ 1.30 for the anterior forearm and 1.45 for the anterior biceps may be indicative of preclinical latent lymphedema in individuals following breast cancer treatment. Other literature suggests a threshold of 1.2 to 1.26 to be indicative mainly of chronic lymphedema. Further research is needed to substantiate a suitable TDC threshold for the breast cancer population and provide guidelines and interpretation of TDC measures for other areas of the body and patient populations.

3.8.2 Issues in Psychosocial Factors Influencing Adaptation to Breast Cancer Lymphedema

LE is a serious problem. Beyond the physical symptoms and risks noted earlier, challenges associated with LE may also lead to posttreatment

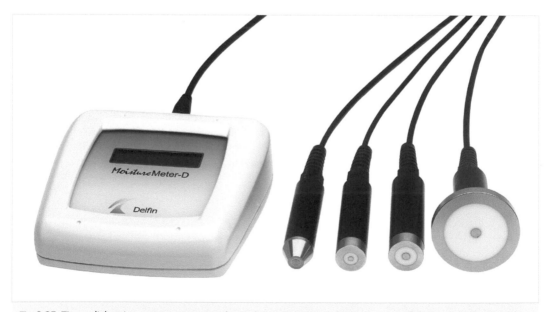

Fig. 3.35 Tissue dielectric constant measuring device (MoistureMeter-D device courtesy of Delfin Technologies Ltd.)

psychological and psychosocial distress. Tobin et al[140] were among the first researchers to examine the psychological morbidity of LE. They observed that breast cancer patients who did not experience arm swelling seemed more successful in assimilating the experience of breast cancer and moving on. Patients with arm swelling reported more difficulty in several domains of psychosocial adjustment. One patient aptly described the difficulty: "The breast is not so bad. At least it is hidden, but everybody keeps asking about my arm."[140] A qualitative analysis of three focus groups of women breast cancer survivors diagnosed with lymphedema was conducted by Ridner et al[141] to examine perceptions of support and a variety of issues that were identified as critical in managing LE.[141] Three central themes emerged from the data: lack of social support; lack of resources for LE self-care; and imposed self-advocacy. Participants voiced the need for more help with self-management of LE, including education for patients and health care providers, social and instrumental support, and overall recognition that lymphedema is a chronic condition. Minimizing the condition and feelings of marginalization contribute to psychological and psychosocial symptoms that negatively affect successful LE management.[141]

As is often the case, the initial studies investigating a particular problem are not theory-driven, but descriptive. Although descriptive studies can be informative, the lack of theory-driven research can inhibit more complete understanding of an area. Moreover, the initial studies examining the link between LE and psychosocial adjustment are limited by measurement problems of both LE and psychosocial adjustment, as well as by several research-design issues that limit experimental rigor. After reviewing the LE literature, Petrek and Heelan[113] noted that the scanty evaluation of LE may be attributed to several factors, including a history of relative neglect of women's health problems and, perhaps most importantly, the traditional view that quality of life is less important than the eradication of cancer and detection of recurrence. Unfortunately, neglect of LE has not only meant that many women go undiagnosed and fail to receive basic preventive information (see Fu et al),[106] but also inhibited the development of effective psychosocial interventions. Treatment of LE has been, and continues to be, a major challenge for health care professionals.[27,119,127,129]

There is a need for more rigorous, prospective studies examining the role of psychosocial factors in the development and progression of LE. Longitudinal studies will have clearer implications for interventions for women at risk for LE. Researchers and clinicians need to continue collecting and analyzing data during the years of survivorship because a substantial amount of LE develops more than 1 to 3 years after cancer diagnosis,[111] because causes of delayed-onset LE differ,[119,123] and because long-term physical and psychosocial ramifications of living with LE are unknown.[116]

Summary

Of 3 million women with breast cancer in the United States (and nearly 14.5 million cancer survivors of all types),[33] at least one in four is likely to have LE within 11 years[33,113] and to experience a wide range of potentially debilitating outcomes as a result. At this point, much remains unknown about LE measurement, incidence, and correlates, including effective and ineffective self-management strategies. There is a dearth of evidence about how psychosocial factors such as problem-solving and social support might reduce LE onset, severity, and progression. Very little is known about the full impact of early- and late-onset LE on psychosocial health and functional health. Lack of research on these topics inhibits understanding of LE, its impact, and the development of effective intervention strategies to reduce the debilitating outcomes that make LE a major health risk. Studies with prospective design and long-term follow-up are essential to address the gaps in the field. Rigorous extended follow-up will increase our understanding of factors related to late-onset LE and long-term management of both early- and late-onset LE.

3.8.3 Theoretic Framework for Research

The Missouri team's examination of LE takes as its guide a biobehavioral model of cancer, stress, and disease progression proposed by Andersen et al,[142] as well as emerging models of stress and coping.[143] Research clearly indicates that both minor and major stressors can substantially affect a person's psychological and physiological well-being.[144] Early evidence suggests that these effects continue over the long term.[27] Moreover, in the past 15 years, growing empirical evidence suggests that psychosocial factors, such as problem-solving and social support, play key roles in adaptive responses to stress.[145] In particular, individual characteristics, such as problem-solving and environmental systems, including social support, can be protective mechanisms that reduce the risks associated with life crises and transitions.[143] Thus, we conceptualize problem-solving and social support as potential protective mechanisms that could reduce the progression of LE[27]; these factors are on the left side of ▶ Fig. 3.36. The center of ▶ Fig. 3.36 reflects our conceptualization of LE in terms of both objective and subjective indicators—specifically LVC and associated LE symptoms—and coping effectiveness and symptom management, respectively. Because the measurement of LVC has been problematic in the past, we include two measurement methods, the traditional circumferential measurement and infrared perometry. Likewise, because very little is known about coping with LE, we examine coping through measurement of LE coping efficacy, as well as ways of managing LE symptoms. Objective and subjective assessments describe different dimensions of LE, which may help further our understanding of not only the physical aspects of LE, but also the cognitive and affective components associated with coping with this disease. Finally, the right side of ▶ Fig. 3.36 depicts multiple dimensions of treatment outcomes, namely psychosocial adjustment, specifically psychosocial distress, cancer-related quality of life, family functioning, and adjustment to chronic illness, as well

as functional health status. Overall quality of life is conceptualized as encompassing and being impacted by psychosocial adjustment and functional health status. The outcome of overall quality of life should be a key focus of future intervention research.

Because both effective problem-solving and high social support have been implicated as protective mechanisms in the progression of LE,[27] and because social support and problem-solving capacity may be critical personal and environmental resources in coping with and managing the disease course,[27,131] we use instruments designed to provide a fine-grained assessment of problem-solving and six different types of social support to assess these variables. In addition, since patient adherence has been suggested as an important variable in LE progression over the long term,[146,147] we examine the association of LE coping efficacy and symptom management in predicting LVC, LE-associated symptoms, and outcomes of psychosocial adjustment and functional health status. Preliminary analysis reveals that the identified psychosocial variables account for considerable variance in long-term psychosocial adjustment following cancer treatment.[27,131] It appears that attachment social support is the most beneficial single factor predicting global psychological symptoms of distress immediately after surgery,

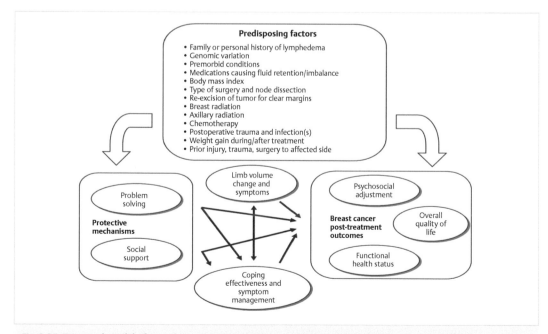

Fig. 3.36 Structural model of post–breast cancer treatment outcomes. (Adapted from Armer et al.[131])

whereas problem-solving control emerges as a stronger predictor of psychological adjustment 1 year later. Further, problem-solving perceptions of personal control, followed by attachment support, were the best predictors of functional adjustment both immediately after surgery and 1 year later. Additionally, it appears that both immediately after surgery and 1 year later, poor social support appears to have a somewhat stronger association with psychological distress than a relative abundance of support. This suggests there may be a critical threshold of support that can be investigated with additional longitudinal data. Initial work suggests these tools provide precise data relevant to identifying such a threshold. These relationships will be further explored in longer-term follow-up, both over time and between those with LE and without LE. By tracking changes in these variables over time, along with changes in functional health status and psychosocial adjustment, researchers are able to investigate predisposing variables (e.g., problem-solving ability, social support), and posttreatment coping effectiveness and symptom management as predictors of LVC, psychosocial adjustment outcomes, and functional health status over time. The goal is to identify variables that influence LE risk reduction, disease progression, and psychosocial adjustment and functional health over an extended period of time, which can inform subsequent interventions and provide a foundation for a future focus on both patient compliance and overall quality of life.

The application of a rigorous LV measurement protocol makes possible the accurate future comparisons of LE occurrence and treatment effectiveness across multiple sites, therapeutic modalities, and patient characteristics. Some studies have relied on measuring LE as a dichotomous variable (e.g., ≥ 2 cm limb difference) using often imprecise and unreliable measurement tools such as circumferences alone without baseline measures; this approach has not allowed examination of LVC and other symptoms that may begin immediately after surgery and/or radiation, that may evolve over the following years and decades, and that are not easily detected with current measurement strategies. The added measurement precision of a continuous variable (rather than a dichotomous variable), preoperative baseline measurements, and the addition of a second assessment (such as symptoms and/or perometer) provides a more stringent examination of the relationships among protective mechanisms (problem-solving and social support), LV, LE-related symptoms, LE

coping effectiveness, and post–breast cancer treatment psychosocial adjustment and functional health status. Moreover, the prospective longitudinal design with repeated measures allows researchers to rigorously examine these relationships over time.

In addition to employing state-of-the-art detection and measurement of LVC, researchers need to employ multidimensional measures of perceived social support and problem-solving. Use of validated instruments in LE research will allow researchers to identify the particular forms of social support and approaches to problem-solving that are associated with successfully managing both early- and late-onset LE. The results of such studies will provide important information about what kind of problem-solving and social support interventions might be most helpful in dealing with LE. Identifying these coping assets and deficits in social support and problem-solving is an essential foundational step toward developing psychosocial interventions to administer and evaluate as part of ongoing programs of research in this area. Ultimately, these research programs have great potential to influence clinical practice guidelines and patient compliance for those living with and at risk for LE.

As noted earlier, it is conservatively estimated that 20 to 40 out of every 100 women treated for breast cancer with contemporary treatment modalities will experience LE in their lifetimes. Indeed, in the Missouri preliminary work, 39% of 103 women returning for follow-up after breast cancer treatment (mean time since diagnosis = 36 months) had ≥ 2 cm difference in circumference between the limbs at one or more points.[81,111] Using the most conservative LE definitions, LE occurrence was 38% (based on 10% volume change) and 39% (based on symptom report) at 24 months.[81,111] The Missouri team continues to follow these trends over time as late-onset LE occurs and continues to compare occurrence, progression, management, and impact among early- and late-onset LE. Over the past decade, breast conservation techniques, most often coupled with radiotherapy, have been used widely in an effort to diminish unpleasant, lasting side effects (such as LE) long associated with more radical treatments.[6] Similar medical optimism regarding reduction in LE has been associated in recent years with the advent of SLNB procedures that spare the breast cancer patient the more invasive and traumatic ALND.[6] However, preliminary observations indicate that the incidence of LE following surgical methods of breast conservation, such as lumpectomy and partial mastectomy combined with radiotherapy, may be equal to or in fact not statistically different from the incidence following traditional surgical treatment (mastectomy with or without radiation).[6,121,123] Further national cooperative group clinical trials are under way to more fully examine these questions of comparative treatment outcomes.

The findings from the Missouri,[81,111] Bethesda,[73,74] Massachusetts General,[148] and MD Anderson Cancer Center[55,149,150] programs of study will have potentially widespread clinical applications in developing and testing protocols for consistent, accurate, noninvasive, and labor- and cost-effective measurement of the limb with LE. Potential application is considerable for both upper and lower extremity LE attributable to surgery, radiation, and other adjunct treatment for malignancies, including breast, melanoma, prostate, ovarian, and other cancers involving lymph node dissection and irradiation. Moreover, examining the link between protective mechanisms, LVC, coping effectiveness, and outcomes of psychosocial adjustment and functional health status repeatedly over time will lead to a more complete understanding of the pathophysiology and consequences of early- and late-onset LE, and subsequently to more appropriate care. Also, identifying potential protective mechanisms could greatly inform clinical treatment and risk-reduction interventions. Accurate and consistent anthropometric measurements are essential to scientific evaluation of the effectiveness of LE treatments, as well as to sound clinical assessment of disease management and progression.[50] The protocols applied in the reviewed research provide such accuracy.

The ongoing Missouri program of study[81,111] is an example of an epidemiological study of the natural occurrence of LE following cancer treatment, as are the MD Anderson Cancer Center,[55,149,150] Massachusetts General,[148] and Bethesda studies.[73,74] For example, from the Missouri study's inception, the researchers have followed two cohorts, one of which developed LE following breast cancer treatment and an at-risk group that did not. By applying survival analysis theory, all the researchers know about the at-risk group is that its members do not yet meet the criteria for LE; it is not known whether they will eventually meet such criteria.[81] At-risk individuals have altered lymphatic function that may impede the body's ability to take up excess lymph that escapes into the extracellular spaces; some experts consider this to

be stage 0 or latent lymphedema.[104,112,113] The findings from data collected with this approach over time from pre-op to several years postdiagnosis will do much to inform our understanding of individual and collective risk factors in the development of early- and late-onset LE. Such data will subsequently inform the development and implementation of risk-reducing interventions for patients treated for breast cancer and other cancers in which lymph nodes are sampled, removed, and irradiated.

As a further example of research to come, researchers are just beginning to understand that women treated for breast cancer develop a unique sarcopenic obesity—weight gain without concurrent gains in lean body mass.[151] The condition of having compromised lymph vessels predisposes women to weight gain in those areas,[152,153] and weight gain itself is a risk factor for late-onset LE. The problem is particularly troublesome in this case because of the biological mechanism leading to the weight gain—compromised lymph vessels that leak lymph into surrounding fat cells, which causes them to enlarge. This is not a problem that can be controlled by eating less and exercising more. Thus, we need to study how women cope with this long-term problem that can present itself years after breast cancer treatment.[151,152,153] Future longitudinal study has the potential to aid our understanding of factors influencing late-onset LE and how patients cope with the risk factors and LE itself.

3.8.4 Looking to the Future: Imperatives for Research to Support Guidelines for Secondary LE

It is now time that earlier findings from cross-sectional, retrospective, and self-report studies be examined in the context of today's advances in surgical, radiation, and hormonal therapies with cohorts of survivors followed with rigorous anthropometric and self-report methodology from pre-op over time. The Missouri, Massachusetts General, MD Anderson Cancer Center, and Bethesda datasets have the potential to become landmark prospective studies in cancer-related LE: the focus of these cross-disciplinary longitudinal prospective studies examining more precise LV measurement, other treatment-related symptoms, and psychosocial adjustment and functional health correlates is promising. The combination of subjective and objective assessment of LE is revealing of the complexity of the LE diagnosis and the fact that subjective symptoms may occur before objective volume changes.[73,81,104] Until recently, no reliable and valid method of assessing LVC has been available in the United States other than water displacement, which is not clinically practical and thus not used routinely for LE diagnosis. Circumferences were frequently seen as too time-consuming and unreliable without proper training and monitoring. The result has been that LE in breast cancer survivors is underdiagnosed and undertreated, leaving a large number of women with poor outcomes and compromised quality of life and functional health. More sophisticated continuous measurement of LVC with the perometer (and potentially electrical impedance) and its correlation with coping effectiveness, psychosocial adjustment, and functional health provide a more robust test of this association, and greatly increase our understanding of the impact of LE over the long term. This could be accomplished with prospective surveillance program that includes a holistic approach to monitoring at-risk individuals for physiological changes with interval measurements and psychological assessment. An assessment of perceptions of self-efficacy and self-regulation should be included for evaluation of successful adherence to risk-minimizing behaviors.[47] In addition, multidisciplinary studies such as the Missouri study are among the first to attempt to rigorously identify protective mechanisms that could inform risk reduction and management interventions.

Although not addressed since 2009, the Medicare Evidence Development & Advisory Committee (MEDCAC) panel presented a charge for researchers and clinicians to discuss the means by which evidenced-based medicine can best be pursued to determine the appropriate diagnostic and treatment methods for lymphedema to inform public policy.[154,155] Recognizing that 1.4 million individuals are conservatively estimated to be affected with LE and millions more are at risk of developing secondary LE and that lymphedema has a major societal impact on health, quality of life, functional status, family, and finances, we believe that surveillance is needed to capture the true significance of this distressing condition.

This field has a variety of effective assessment modalities: circumferences, symptom self-report, water displacement, perometry, and electrical impedance spectroscopy, among others. Valid and reliable methods must be applied systematically in the at-risk population to assess emergence to lymphedema for risk reduction, detection, and early intervention. These measures must be applied in the affected population to assess progression and response to treatment for prevention and early management of complications.

Evidence at the highest level supports CDT (and its five component parts) for the treatment of lymphedema (Chapter 5).[156,157] There is increasing evidence for the use of the individual components of CDT under the guidance of a specialty-trained therapist for mild to moderate lymphedema and, recently, in subclinical lymphedema.[156,157,158] Promising studies are under way to evaluate adjunct therapies under selected circumstances.

The challenge is great, but the potential rewards are equally great. We need more well-designed studies with precise measurements, larger well-defined study cohorts, followed over longer time periods, with stand-alone and bundled interventions incorporating standard-of-care versus optimal-care guidelines.[156,157] Further, the compilation of multiple large datasets, as is under way in the American Lymphedema Framework Project (ALFP) minimum dataset, provides new opportunities to ask more sophisticated questions of the existing and future datasets in lymphedema.[159] Together, these will lead to more definitive evidence-based recommendations for the optimal management of lymphedema.

3.9 Radiation-Induced Brachial Plexopathy and Lymphedema

Radiation-induced brachial plexopathy (RIBP) is caused by radiation damage to the brachial plexus, a network bundle of nerves located near the neck and shoulder. The nerves forming the brachial plexus originate at the spinal cord in the neck and are responsible for the sensory and muscular innervation of the entire upper extremity (▶ Fig. 3.37).

The beneficial effects of radiation therapy in breast cancer and other malignant diseases are well known and documented. However, this life-saving therapy has potentially adverse effects on several body systems, which are exposed to the rays during treatment, such as skin, nerves, and internal organs.

In breast cancer, radiation treatment is administered to the axillary area, chest, or neck. Radiation damage to this network of nerves can result in sensory and/or motor damage, with or without

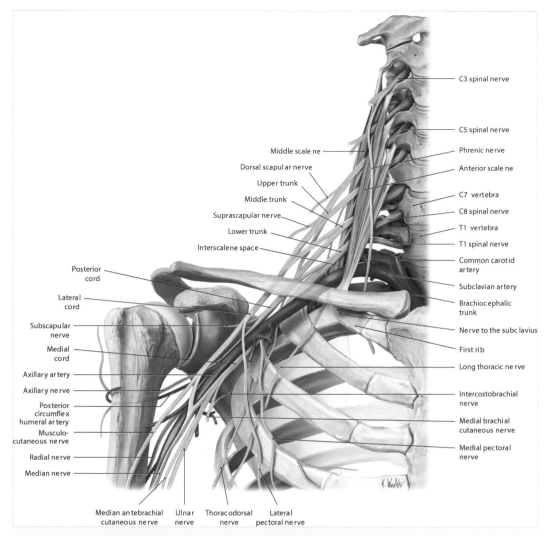

Fig. 3.37 Course of the brachial plexus, right side, anterior view. (From Thieme Atlas of Anatomy, General Anatomy and Musculoskeletal System. © Thieme 2005, Illustration by Karl Wesker.)

accompanying pain in the brachial plexus distribution in the arm. Symptoms may include paresthesia (tingling, pricking, numbness), dysesthesia (abnormal sense of touch, such as burning, itching, feeling of an electric current, "pins and needles," pain), decreased sensitivity, partial loss of movement (muscle weakness and difficulty performing simple tasks such as opening jars, or containers, holding objects), complete paralysis of the arm, muscular atrophy, impaired mobility, and partial dislocation of the shoulder joint.

The exact mechanism of RIBP is not yet completely understood; research indicates that damage to the brachial plexus results from a combination of direct nerve cell damage from ionizing radiation and more progressive damage by the development of scar tissue (radiation fibrosis) in and around the nerves, combined with damage to adjacent vessels that supply these nerves with oxygen and nutrients. Radiation of nerve tissue also causes the nerve cells to shrink, resulting in a decrease in elasticity of nerve fibers, which further aggravates the situation. The extent of damage is associated with the radiation dose and technique, and the concurrent use of chemotherapy.

The progressive damage to vessels and the development of scar tissue continue to evolve significantly in some and gradually in other patients after the initial radiation therapy, which explains why some patients develop RIBP symptoms many years after radiation treatment. Most patients develop symptoms within the first 3 years; however, the average interval between the last dose of radiation and the onset of RIBP symptoms reported in the literature varies widely—it ranges between 6 months and 20 years. The prevalence of RIBP is reported to be between 1.8 and 4.9%; RIBP is more common after radiation in combination with chemotherapy, and the nerve tissue of younger patients seems to be more vulnerable.

3.9.1 The Relationship between RIBP and Lymphedema

Individuals who have had surgery and radiation for breast cancer and do not present with postmastectomy/postlumpectomy lymphedema are considered to be in a latency stage, and are always at risk of developing lymphedema. Any additional stress to the lymphatic system, such as trauma, loss of mobility, or pain, may cause the onset of lymphedema in the upper extremity.

The presence of RIBP, especially in cases with partial or complete loss of mobility, may be a triggering factor for the onset of lymphedema. The return of lymphatic fluid from the upper extremity partially depends on the pumping action the muscles exert to the outside of the lymph vessels. Immobility of these muscles due to pain or partial or complete paralysis has a detrimental effect to the return of lymphatic fluid and causes lymph to stagnate in the extremity. Combined with the adverse effects of gravity, this may cause the onset of lymphedema.

Those individuals who already have lymphedema and develop RIBP may experience an increase in swelling due to pain and partial or complete loss of motor function.

3.9.2 Therapeutic Approach

Although surgical procedures to decompress the brachial plexus and revascularize the nerves and surrounding tissues have been described in the literature, the results are often unsatisfactory.

Unfortunately, RIBP is essentially an incurable condition, and with the absence of satisfactory treatment, emphasis is placed on symptom control and therapeutic exercises specifically addressing the maintenance of movement in the paralyzed extremity for as long as possible. Physical and occupational therapists work as part of a multiprofessional team to address loss of function and flexibility, weakness, pain, and lymphedema. Special adaptive equipment and techniques address basic functions of daily living and suggest ways to modify the home and workplace.

3.9.3 Special Considerations to Address with RIBP in the Presence of Lymphedema

Lymphedema management in patients with RIBP is more challenging, but necessary to help control pain and to decrease the volume of the extremity. Volume reduction lessens the impact of excess weight on the shoulder joint, prevents the build-up of additional fibrotic (scar) tissue, and significantly lowers the risk of infections commonly associated with lymphedema. It is often necessary to adapt compression and exercise protocols to accommodate the special circumstances associated with RIBP.

Compression bandaging: Many patients affected by RIBP experience impaired sensation on the skin and are often unable to provide accurate feedback relating to their individual tolerance to pressure. Therapists applying compression bandages to the affected extremity during the initial sessions of CDT should be very conservative with application pressure and use ample padding to avoid pressure sores; application pressure may be gradually increased in the absence of side effects. Effective compression therapy for lymphedema partially depends on the extent of the interaction between the bandage layers and the musculature working against the resistance of the bandages; this is also known as the working pressure. With partial or complete loss of muscle activity, the working pressure of the bandage is reduced, making the bandage less effective. However, even if compression bandages are applied with less pressure and the day-to-day results of the bandages are not as noticeable, they are still effective in promoting lymphatic return by increasing the pressure in the tissues.

It is also important to consider that some RIBP patients wear arm slings to reduce the degree of subluxation and discomfort of the shoulder joint. In these cases, the elbow should be kept in 90 degrees of flexion during the application of compression bandages.

The possible presence of joint contractures caused by muscular atrophy and immobilization should be addressed with special bandage application techniques.

Compression Garments

The wearing of compression garments is essential to prevent lymphatic fluid from accumulating in the tissues and conserves the results achieved with MLD.

Compression Sleeves and Gauntlets

These are available in several compression classes (see also Chapter 4). The level of compression within the different classes is determined by the value of pressure the garments produce on the skin; these pressure values are measured in units of millimeters of mercury (mm Hg). For a compression garment to work effectively, the pressure needs to gradually decrease from the wrist to the shoulder. This gradient is necessary to avoid tourniquet effects and subsequent obstruction of lymph flow.

In general, compression levels provided by class 2 garments (30–40 mm Hg) will be sufficient to prevent swelling in most patients affected by lymphedema of the upper extremity. However, if lymphedema is combined with RIBP and partial or complete immobility with subsequent loss of normal muscle tone, a lower compression may be required to avoid tourniquet effects. Patients need to be thoroughly educated in the fitting of compression sleeve devices and alternatives for night bandaging.

Exercises

Immobility is detrimental to the lymphatic return. In addition to supporting the return of lymph fluid, the main goal of the exercise protocol is to focus on mobility. Modifications to the usual decongestive exercise program may be necessary to address impaired motor function.

Exercise protocols for RIBP with partial or complete loss of mobility are geared toward the development of strategies that compensate for lost muscle function by using those muscles that still have function. Specific exercises also help maintain and develop any strength and control that remain in the affected musculature. This also helps prevent further shortening of muscle fibers (contracture) and to maintain and regain ROM in the arm. Elevating the arm as often as possible to promote lymphatic return is even more important in patients affected by RIBP. Therapists and doctors

may also suggest adaptive equipment that helps the patient maintain a normal life.

3.10 Imaging of the Lymphatic System

3.10.1 Why Image?

Imaging of the lymphatic system is essential to delineate the underlying anatomic and/or functional disturbances in the lymphatic system. The current classification and staging systems in use today for patients with lymphedema utilize only the outward signs and symptoms of lymphedema without acknowledging that there may be major differences beneath the skin surface. Underlying all cases of lymphedema is a disturbance in the anatomy and/or function of the lymphatic system that produces an imbalance between LL and TC, and the only way to visualize, document, and understand these changes is through imaging. In modern medicine, it would be expected to image an arterial or venous system before treating operatively or nonoperatively the outward sign of arterial or venous disease. Similarly, imaging should be part of the evaluation of lymphatic system disorders. Indeed, we have several reliable, safe, simple, and consistent methods, which are now feasible. Outside of a few cases of clear-cut postmastectomy lymphedema, it should no longer be considered sufficient to evaluate a patient by history and physical examination alone. Even in these "clear-cut" cases, imaging can document the severity and location(s) of the obstruction, which can have an impact on prognosis and treatment planning. In addition, for most patients finally "seeing" for themselves an abnormal functional image of their "invisible" lymphatic system helps explain the underlying physiology of their condition as well as confirms the problem they may have long suspected, but have been told does not exist or is unimportant. In more complicated patients with chylous or nonchylous lymph reflux, unknown causes of swelling, unilateral lymphedema following midline cancer treatment (e.g., prostate, cervical), or possible associated complications in the venous system, imaging is indispensable. Finally, due to the fact that in the United States and Europe the majority of cases of lymphedema occur as a result of cancer treatment, the possibility of cancer must be considered and many of these imaging modalities are useful tools for the oncologist in assessing recurrent disease.

3.10.2 Conceptual Basis of Lymphatic Imaging

Central to almost all types of imaging of the lymphatic system is the use of suitable contrast agents. According to underlying principles governing the movement of fluid, solutes, and particles in the interstitium, contrast agents utilized (or the molecules they tag) need to be of sufficiently large size to ensure their selective absorption into the initial tissue lymphatic vessels rather than into the less permeable venous system. Once the tracers enter the lymphatic system, corresponding imaging modalities can be used to follow the tracer as it moves cephalad up to and through the thoracic duct, providing both anatomic and functional information about the lymphatic system in the patient.

3.10.3 Lymphoscintigraphy

The current gold standard for imaging is LAS. In this technique, a radioactive tracer (technetium) is linked to sulfur colloid and injected in single (commonly) or multiple doses into the skin on the dorsum of the hand or foot in a volume of 0.05 mL (similar to a TB test). Most common protocols image statically for approximately 15 minutes and then perform a "whole-body" scan where the camera moves centrally to follow the flow. This scan is repeated once at about 30 minutes after some nonspecific movement of the hands or feet to stimulate lymph flow and a second time at about 3 hours to examine the clearance of tracer from the system.[160] The total radiation dose is approximately 1/20th of a chest X-ray, and the tracer has a half-life of 6 hours, meaning patients need almost no restrictions (breast feeding a baby is one example). Babies, with sedation to assure immobility, can also be easily imaged.

LAS provides images that demonstrate aplasia or hypoplasia (no or reduced flow); hyperplasia (increased lymphatic channels and nodes); alternative lymphatic channels; site(s) of obstruction and subsequent diffusion of tracer into the tissues as transport to the thoracic duct has been impeded; site(s) of reflux (chylous or nonchylous) into the chest, abdomen, or genitalia; and sites of leakage (e.g., pleural effusion; ▶ Fig. 3.38). See Witte et al[161] for a comprehensive review of multiple LAS examples with corresponding clinical images.

3.10.4 Lymphography

This technique, also known as conventional or direct lymphography, is the original classical method to image the lymphatic system. It utilizes an oily contract medium with iodine, which is directly injected into a cannulated lymphatic vessel exposed in the dorsum of the hand or foot and visualized by X-ray. This technique requires a dye injection to identify the lymph collector and then an incision in the hand or foot to isolate and cannulate the vessel followed by slow infusion of the tracer using a pump. Patients must remain relatively immobile for 60 to 90 minutes. Although there can be some associated problems with the contrast agent causing an inflammatory reaction and a small risk of pulmonary embolism, the technique can also be invaluable for the precise anatomic depiction of the lymphatic vessels and nodes particularly in cases of reflux where a surgeon or interventional radiologist may be required for treatment. Also, lymph node pathology, for instance, can be well delineated.

3.10.5 Ultrasound

The primary use of ultrasound (and venous Doppler) in patients with suspected or known lymphedema is to image the venous system. It is commonly used to assess both the patency and flow of the venous system as well as the competency of the valves for preventing reflux. In addition, ultrasound is useful in assessing the characteristics of the dermis and soft tissues particularly in response to treatment and the presence of fluid pockets or lymphatic lakes in specific conditions. It has also been increasingly used as a screening tool in endemic areas for filariasis to detect asymptomatic worm infestations in the scrotum, which demonstrate a characteristic "dance sign."[162,163]

3.10.6 Magnetic Resonance Imaging

Both contrast-enhanced and noncontrast MRI have been utilized to evaluate patients with lymphedema. The high spatial resolution of MRI provides superior anatomic detail without associated problems of lymphography or the lowered resolution of LAS. The use of heavily T2-weighted, noncontrasted images has been successful for demonstrating pathologic lymphatic vessels. Gadolinium contrast agents have successfully been used outside the United States to clearly depict lymphatic

3

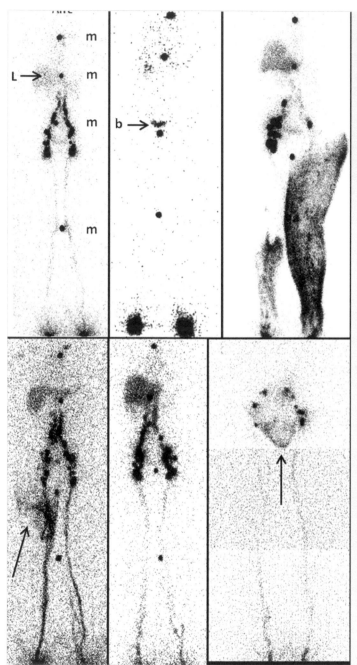

Fig. 3.38 Lymphoscintigraphy **(a)** Normal late (3.5-hour) image of the legs depicting almost complete tracer clearance through the lymphatic vessels following injection into both feet. Symmetric, bilateral inguinal nodes and retroperitoneal nodes are clearly seen. Markers (m) are at the knees, pubis, xiphoid, and sternal notch. Liver (L) can be seen in this later image as the tracer has been successfully transported through the lymphatic system into the blood pool. **(b)** Late image of a patient with Milroy primary lymphedema demonstrating no movement of tracer from the feet due to aplasia or severe hypoplasia of the lymphatic system. There is a slight bladder (B) image seen as the tracer accumulates in the later images. **(c)** Late image of a complicated patient with left leg edema following groin dissection on left for small cell carcinoma, pelvic radiation, and right knee replacement. Image displays severe obstruction on the left with a single groin node and lack of retroperitoneal nodes. The right displays more moderate tracer holdup at the knee. **(d)** Late image of a patient with swelling of the right upper thigh following treatment for sarcoma. The patient developed a seroma which was being treated with a drain (arrow) and both collected tracer as it was transported through the lymphatic system. **(e)** A normal late image of a patient with lipedema depicting tracer clearance from the legs and normal nodal imaging. In later stages of lipedema, secondary changes in the lymphatic system can be seen by lymphoscintigraphy. **(f)** Late image of a patient who developed scrotal swelling with lymphatic fluid leakage clearly depicting tracer filling of the scrotum (*arrow*) following injection in the feet.

vessels and structures in a variety of pathologic lymphatic conditions. The initial studies have included only a small number of patients, and MRI is an expensive modality; in addition, there is some renal toxicity associated with gadolinium, and the volume of the contrast agent injected (milliliters) is much larger than for LAS. Despite these drawbacks, the functional/anatomic images obtained with high spatial resolution may supplant LAS in large medical centers in the future. Recent work with specific MR sequences has demonstrated lymphatic flow within vessels (previously too slow for detection), and this may lead to further advances in the use of MR in the clinic.[21]

3.10.7 Combined Multimodal/ Fusion Imaging Techniques

Although becoming more utilized in the United States, there are imaging systems that combine multiple modalities to produce combination or fusion images. Single-photon emission computed tomography (SPECT) combined with X-ray CT for SPECT-CT brings the advantages of both LAS and higher spatial resolution of CT and may be useful in patients with congenital lymphedema with possible nodal changes, and of particular use for those with clinically more severe disease including chylous and nonchylous reflux where the technique can more precisely demonstrate site(s) of leakage.[164]

3.10.8 Fluorescent Imaging

The recent use of indocyanine green (ICG) fluorescent imaging has been investigated by several groups. Although ICG is not clinically approved by Food and Drug Administration (FDA) in the United States, ongoing research has demonstrated detailed imaging of the superficial peripheral lymphatic vessels. In addition, because the images are captured with highly sophisticated cameras and imaging systems, real-time tracer movement can be monitored, and this feature has allowed analysis of flow rates. While this newer work will need to be replicated in additional centers and the tracer (or a similar tracer) needs FDA approval for this use, the technique may have some future potential. One drawback that has not been overcome yet is the inability of fluorescent imaging to resolve anything deeper than the superficial peripheral lymphatic system and therefore its utility will remain limited for peripheral lymphedema. Surgeons who use ICG intraoperatively to identify lymphatic vessels and nodes are widely using this technique and avoid the problems with depth since the tissue is already open during operation.

3.10.9 Summary and the Future

Imaging should no longer be viewed as purely an investigational or research tool or reserved only for those complicated cases that may confuse the clinician or require surgery. Current imaging modalities are safe and available and allow us to go beyond describing patients as just a collection of outward manifestations. Techniques such as LAS are minimally invasive (one small needle stick),

relatively inexpensive, and provide functional and anatomic information important for diagnosis, prognosis, and treatment of patients with lymphedema. Newer techniques such as MRI (contrasted or noncontrasted) and combination imaging have improved spatial resolution, and the appropriate use of these modalities to evaluate the varied presentations of patients with lymphedema and lymphangiodysplasia syndromes has been delineated.[165]

3.11 Therapeutic Approach to Lymphedema

Therapeutic approaches to lymphedema range from ignorance ("You have to live with it") to numerous surgical procedures. Between these two extremes are several conservative treatments.

CDT is the therapy of choice for the vast majority of patients suffering from primary and secondary lymphedema. In addition to CDT, there are various treatment approaches that may be used to supplement CDT. Some of them will be discussed in the following section; others, such as ultrasound and electrotherapy, will be included in Chapter 4.

3.11.1 Complete Decongestive Therapy

> Because there is currently no cure for lymphedema, the goal of any therapy must be to reduce the swelling and to maintain the reduction, that is, to bring the lymphedema back to a stage of latency.

The only physiological way to achieve this goal is to remove the excess plasma proteins from the tissues via lymph vessels and tissue channels. For a majority of patients, this can be achieved by the skillful application of CDT. CDT shows good long-term results in both primary and secondary lymphedema. The components and techniques of CDT will be described in detail in Chapter 4.

Numerous studies have proven the effectiveness of this therapy, which has been well established in European countries since the 1970s. Although CDT has been practiced in the United States in one form or another since the 1980s, this therapy became accepted only after definitive guidelines and all components of CDT were included in the teaching curricula of schools providing training in lymphedema management in the 1990s.

CDT is applied in two phases. In phase 1, the goal is to mobilize the accumulated protein-rich fluid and to initiate the reduction of fibrosclerotic tissues (if present). The duration of this intensive phase varies and averages 2 to 3 weeks for patients with upper extremity lymphedema and 2 to 4 weeks for patients with lymphedema of the lower extremity. Ideally, the treatment is performed daily, 5 days a week (▶ Table 3.9).

Another important goal in this first phase is to instruct the patient in techniques designed to maintain and improve the achieved success of the treatment (proper skin care, correct application of bandages, wearing of compression garments, etc.).

The first phase of the therapy is immediately followed by phase 2, which is aimed to preserve and improve the success achieved in phase 1. This phase for the most part is continued by the patient. With good patient compliance, the volume reduction can be not only maintained but also improved by progressive reduction of fibrosclerotic tissues in this second phase.

In more severe cases of lymphedema, it may become necessary to repeat phase 1; if lymphedema is associated with other conditions, the individual steps of CDT are modified accordingly.

CDT has been proven to be effective, with excellent long-term results, and it is also noninvasive and safe, that is, without any known side effects to the patient, provided the patient is an appropriate candidate for CDT.

CDT is also cost-effective in that it transfers the care from the medical professional to the patient and/or the patient's family. It significantly reduces the risk factors for developing cellulitis attacks, and improves or reduces lymph cysts, lymphatic fistulas, varicose lymphatics, and fungal infections.

3.11.2 Massage

Massage traditionally has been used to treat edema, but it is not recommended to manage lymphedema. The differences between edema and lymphedema are outlined in Chapter 2, Insufficiency of the Lymphatic System.

The meaning of the word *massage* is "to knead" and is used to describe forms of "classic" or "Swedish" massage, to include such techniques as effleurage, petrissage, tapotement, vibration, and friction.

The word *massage* is frequently misused to describe the techniques of MLD (see Chapter 4).

Table 3.9 Stages of lymphedema and therapeutic approach

Stages	Duration of treatment	CDT-phase I	CDT-phase II
Latency		*Patient Instruction*	
Stage 1	2–3 weeks	• MLD daily	• MLD if necessary
		• Short-stretch bandages	• Compression garments
		• Skin care	• Skin care
		• Decongestive exercises	• Decongestive exercises
Stage 2	3–4 weeks	• MLD daily	• MLD as needed
		• Short-stretch bandages	• Compression garments
		• Skin care	• Bandages at night
		• Decongestive exercises	• Skin care
			• Decongestive exercises
			• Repeat phase I if necessary
Stage 3	4–6 weeks	• MLD daily	• MLD as needed
		• Short-stretch bandages	• Compression garments (if necessary in combination with bandages)
		• Skin care	• Bandages at night
		• Decongestive exercises	• Skin care
			• Decongestive exercises
			• Repeat phase I if necessary
			• Plastic surgery (if indicated)

Abbreviations: CDT, complete decongestive therapy; MLD, manual lymph drainage.

3

MLD includes no kneading elements in its strokes and has nothing in common with traditional massage techniques.

> Traditional massage can have negative effects on lymphedema, including active hyperemia, due to the release of histamine from mast cells in skin areas where those techniques are applied.

Active hyperemia results in an increase of blood capillary pressure and a subsequent increase in capillary filtration. This results in more water accumulating in the interstitial spaces, overloading an already stressed or impaired lymphatic system.

Superficial lymphatics are vulnerable to external pressure. Traditional massage techniques can cause focal damage on anchoring filaments and the endothelial lining of lymph vessels. Massage techniques also increase the LL of water (and often cells) and may further decrease the TC of the lymphatic system by causing additional damage to lymph vessels. The application of traditional massage is therefore contraindicated in extremities (and their ipsilateral trunk quadrants) at risk for lymphedema and in extremities affected by lymphedema.

3.11.3 Thermo Therapy

Ice, heat, thermal ultrasound, hydrotherapy (hot packs), saunas, contrast baths, and paraffin should not be applied on the involved limb and the ipsilateral trunk quadrant as part of lymphedema management. Basic and advanced physiology identifies that active hyperemia occurs with any of the aforementioned modalities. Vasodilation increases blood capillary pressure and in turn will increase the LL of water. Any modality that causes vasodilation to the involved limb, or "limb at risk," and/or ipsilateral trunk quadrant should be avoided.

3.11.4 Elevation

Simple elevation of an extremity affected by lymphedema may help reduce the swelling. This may be the case particularly in stage 1 lymphedema. If the lymphedematous limb decreases by elevation, the effect should be maintained by wearing appropriate compression garments.

3.11.5 Sequential Intermittent Pneumatic Compression

An intermittent pneumatic compression (IPC) device is composed of an inflatable garment consisting of multiple pressure compartments that wraps around the arm or leg and an electrical pneumatic pump, which fills the garment with compressed air. The garment is intermittently inflated and deflated with cycle times and pressures that vary between devices.

First-generation IPCs consisted of an inflatable single compartment pressure chamber that applied a nonsegmented uniform and sustained level of compression to the entire extremity. These nonprogrammable devices did not provide proper pressure distribution or a pressure gradient. To effectively assist the movement of stagnated lymphedematous fluid, a pressure gradient between the lower (higher pressure) and the upper part (lower pressure) of the extremity is imperative—the same principle that is applied by compression bandages and compression garments. Due to the limited amount of control and lack of appropriate pressure gradient, single-chambered devices should not be used in the management of lymphedema.

Multichambered, segmented IPCs are considered to be newer generation compression devices and are equipped with multiple outflow ports on the pneumatic pump leading to distinct segments of the garment that inflate sequentially from the lower part of the extremity to the upper part of the extremity until all segments are inflated. Following this phase, all compartments deflate at the same time (▶ Fig. 3.39).

Two groups of multichambered IPCs can be distinguished—those without or with limited manual control and noncalibrated pressure, and devices equipped with programmable options and calibrated pressure.

Multichambered IPCs without or with Limited Manual Control and Noncalibrated Pressure

In this more traditional group of devices, the pressure present in each chamber is the same, or there is a predetermined gradient in pressure in successive pressure chambers, but no ability to adjust the pressure in each of the chambers independently. The pressure in these pumps is typically determined with a single control on the lowest (most

3

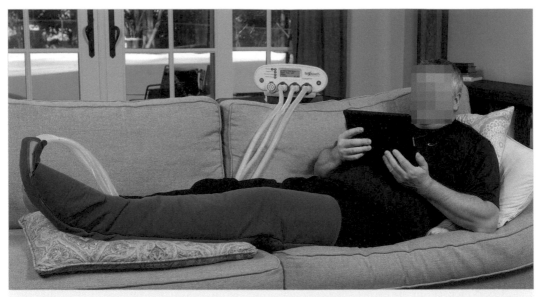

Fig. 3.39 Sequential compression system for the lower extremities. (Reproduced with permission from Tactile Medical.)

distal) pressure segment and applies a sustained pressure in each chamber as the subsequent pressure chambers inflate.

One concern related to the use of these devices is that the applied pressure on the surface of the skin may significantly exceed the pressure value displayed on the device itself. In 2002, Segers et al[166] investigated multichambered pumps to determine if the pressure set on the dial was the actual pressure produced by the chamber on the skin. The authors found that even though the dial was set at 30, 60, 80, and 100 mm Hg, respectively, the pressure applied to the skin in each chamber actually reached 54, 98, 121, and 141 mm Hg.

Considering the anatomic and physiological facts of the lymphatic system, it becomes evident that excessive pressure to the skin may have a harmful, damaging effect on the superficial lymphatic structures.

The pressure garment used with these devices covers only the extremity and has no additional appliances covering the adjacent part of the torso. Subsequently, lymphedematous fluid that is moved from the extremity may accumulate at the top of the limb, resulting in the formation of hardened tissue (fibrotic ring), or may cause the swelling of adjacent parts of the torso (chest, trunk, abdomen) previously not affected by lymphedema. In lower extremity lymphedema, the displaced fluid from the leg may accumulate in the genital area.[167]

Considering the fact that lymphedema of the extremities is often associated with swelling of the adjacent body quadrant and/or external genitalia, these devices are not well suited for the management of lymphedema.

Multichambered IPCs with Programmable Options and Calibrated Pressure

Advanced segmented devices with calibrated gradient pressure are characterized by a manual control on at least three outflow ports of the device that can deliver an individually determined pressure to each compartment of the unit. It is possible to make manual pressure adjustments in the individual compartments and/or adjust the length and frequency of the inflation cycles. These devices are also known as Type III pumps.

The advantage of this system is that the level and location of the compression can be adjusted to meet the patients' specific circumstances in regard to comfort (pressure tolerance, pain) and the need to concentrate on specific areas affected by lymphedema or on areas with excessive fibrotic tissue formation. Nonadjustable and nonprogrammable units do not offer this level of adjustability, which may have negative effects on patient compliance, specifically if sustained pressure is not well tolerated. The programmability of the pressure profile in segmented devices with calibrated gradient pressure reduces the danger of potentially damaging effects on the superficial lymphatic structures.

Pneumatic compression used to treat extremity lymphedema, without treatment of adjacent body quadrants and drainage areas using CDT, bears a significant risk of moving lymphedematous fluid from distal to proximal, where it accumulates. This may cause protein molecules to accumulate in this area, forming a fibrosclerotic ring, which may cause truncal quadrants previously not swollen to fill with fluid, or external genitalia to swell.[167]

More sophisticated models provide additional appliances that allow for treatment of the torso. As mentioned earlier, lymphedema of the extremities is often associated with swelling of adjacent body parts, such as the chest, trunk, or abdomen. These more advanced IPC systems can address these issues and assist in clearing of these areas prior to stimulate the extremity, and thus may be able to prevent the danger of fibrotic cuffs or the onset of additional swelling in other body areas.

An additional concern related to the use of IPCs is that these devices are successful in removing water from the interstitial spaces, but are not effective in removing proteins. The application of pneumatic compression reduces the water content in the lymphedematous limb and the extremity will initially become smaller. However, if the interstitial water content is reduced, but the accumulated protein molecules remain in the tissue, the interstitial fluid colloid osmotic pressure (COP_{IP}) increases. This will result in more water leaving the blood capillaries, exacerbating the swelling. The remaining proteins in the tissue continue to generate new connective tissue.

In 2001, Miranda et al[168] performed a prospective, blind study protocol with sequential intermittent neumatic compression (SIPC). The study evaluated 11 patients who underwent an isotope lymphography before SIPC and 48 hours after a 3-hour session of SIPC. Measuring the lower extremities at six designated points revealed there was a significant reduction of circumference after SIPC below the knee, but not in the thigh. The study concluded that compression increased transport of lymph fluid (e.g., water) without comparable transport of macromolecules (e.g., protein). Alternatively, SIPC reduced lymphedema by decreasing blood capillary filtration rather than by

accelerating lymph return, thereby restoring the balance in lymph kinetics responsible for edema in the first place.

Recommended Pressure Levels and Treatment Times in Programmable and Calibrated Pumps

Unfortunately, consensus in the proper pressure level in IPCs for the treatment of lymphedema is lacking. In general, it can be said that the pressure level should be adjusted to the patient's level of tolerance and response to treatment. Careful instruction of the patient in the use of these devices and surveillance by a practitioner trained on a specialist level in these devices are required. A review of the literature suggests that peak inflation pressure of 25 to 60 mm Hg may be sufficient for most patients.[169,170] There is also no standard consensus on the frequency of IPC treatments. Depending on the individual situation, treatment duration of 30 minutes to 2 hours (1 hour twice a day) is generally recommended. Careful guidance by a practitioner with knowledge in lymphedema treatment is mandatory to determine optimal treatment frequency.

When Are IPCs Contraindicated?

The following contraindications are listed in the Lymphedema Framework's international consensus document "Best Practice Guideline for Lymphedema"[170]:

- Nonpitting chronic lymphedema.
- Known or suspected deep vein thrombosis.
- Pulmonary embolism.
- Thrombophlebitis.
- Acute inflammation of the skin (erysipelas, cellulitis).
- Uncontrolled/severe cardiac failure.
- Pulmonary edema.
- Ischemic vascular disease.
- Active metastatic diseases affecting the edematous region.
- Edema at the root of the extremity or truncal edema.
- Severe peripheral neuropathy.

The use of IPC in the treatment of lymphedema continues to be a topic of discussion, and their use is not accepted as a replacement or component of CDT, the accepted gold standard of lymphedema treatment. However, recent studies suggest that there is a potential place for newer generation IPCs as a beneficial adjunct treatment to effectively control lymphedema, specifically for individuals affected by chronic lymphedema with very limited or no access to medical care, or in those cases when physical limitations of the individual may result in challenges controlling the lymphedema independently in the self-administered maintenance phase directly after CDT treatments. Following discharge from CDT, patients are instructed by the therapist to maintain the results with compression bandages and garments, self-MLD, and decongestive exercise protocols; these conservative therapy modalities are effective for most, but may not be sufficient for some individuals, and an appropriate pneumatic compression device may offer an effective option to control this condition on a more ideal level.

The 2011 Position Statement of the National Lymphedema Network states that IPC is not a "stand-alone" treatment for lymphedema and should not be used without adjunct CDT.

To maintain control of the swelling, it is necessary that compression garments and/or short-stretch compression bandages are worn between treatments with sequential pneumatic compression devices.

More research on the objective clinical benefit and the cost-effectiveness of these systems is needed.

3.11.6 Low-Level Laser Therapy

LLLT devices are infrared lasers, which generate light of a specific wavelength that is able to deeply penetrate the tissue without an increase in tissue temperature. These devices have been introduced to the U.S. market as an additional treatment option for lymphedema, and were cleared by the FDA in 2006.

Several recent studies[171,172] suggest that LLLT may be effective in reducing lymphedema circumference in some patients and may be beneficial in softening the hard tissue in the extremity and help in decreasing pain. While LLLT has shown some promise in relieving some of the symptoms of lymphedema, the exact mechanism by which these effects may be achieved is not clear, and evidence for the effectiveness of LLLT is limited; more studies are required before the usefulness of LLLT as an adjunct modality in the treatment of lymphedema can be confirmed.

3.11.7 Nutritional Aspects in Lymphedema

There is no special diet for lymphedema; patients affected by lymphedema should try their best to achieve and maintain a reasonable weight to reduce the risk factors associated with obesity. Patients should trust their own judgment when it comes to the selection of a proper diet. If there are no other medical conditions present, such as diabetes or heart disease, a healthy and balanced diet should be the goal.

An accepted nutritional approach in the management of lymphedema is to follow a nutrition-balanced and portion-appropriate diet, which, in addition to physical activity and exercises, positively contributes to weight management. Obesity and overweight often worsen the symptoms associated with lymphedema; a recent study[173] indicates that obesity does have an influence on lymph fluid level and extremity volume. A balanced, healthy diet contributes in reducing the risk factors associated with lymphedema.

Many patients are under the impression that lymphedema may be positively affected by limiting protein intake. Although lymphedema is defined as an accumulation of water and protein in the tissues, it is essential to understand that lymphedema cannot be reduced by the limitation of protein ingestion. It is also important not to limit fluid intake in an attempt to reduce the swelling. Good hydration is essential for basic cell function and is especially important before and after lymphedema treatment to assist the body in eliminating waste products.

The Role of Cholesterol in the Management of Lymphedema

Cholesterol is a fatty substance which is produced by the liver and found in food with a high content of saturated fat, such as meat, eggs, and dairy products. Cholesterol has developed a somewhat bad reputation. However, it is the type of fat consumed, rather than the amount of fat, that is linked with disease. Low-density lipoprotein (LDL) consists of saturated and trans fats. LDL, also known as "bad" cholesterol, may stick to the inside wall of arteries and increase the risk of coronary diseases. The "good" fats, monounsaturated and polyunsaturated fats, or high-density lipoprotein (HDL), lower the risk of disease. Eating too many saturated fats can raise the level of "bad" cholesterol and contribute to obesity.

Vitamins and Other Supplements

There are no vitamins, food supplements, or herbs that have been proven to be effective in the reduction of lymphedema. In the United States, dietary supplements are regulated as food, not drugs. Premarket approval by the FDA is not required unless specific disease prevention or treatment claims are made. Because there is no requirement to review dietary supplements for manufacturing consistency, and no specific standards for dosage or purity exist, there may be considerable variation within the products marketed as dietary supplements. However, lymphedema patients are often in need of additional vitamins and supplements, especially if they battle recurrent episodes of infections. To determine which supplements and vitamins are beneficial, individuals with lymphedema should consult with their physicians and/or nutritional specialist.

3.11.8 Pharmaceutical Options in the Treatment of Lymphedema

The use of drugs in the treatment of lymphedema in the western hemisphere is generally limited to antibiotics, which are used to prevent and treat infections commonly associated with lymphedema. As stated in the 2011 Position Paper of the National Lymphedema Network, lymphedema should not be treated exclusively with drugs or dietary supplements. The following is a list of medications, which are mentioned for possible use in the treatment of lymphedema.

Diuretics

Most experts agree that the use of diuretics in the management of uncomplicated lymphedema is ineffective and may lead to worsening of symptoms. Diuretics promote excess fluid in the body to be excreted; although these drugs may be beneficial in the short term, and may be indicated in those cases when lymphedema is associated with systemic conditions (ascites, hydrothorax, protein-losing enteropathy), they may be harmful and contribute to the worsening of lymphedema-related symptoms if used long term.

The reason is that lymphedema is an abnormal accumulation of water and protein molecules in the body's soft tissues, which is caused by a dysfunction of the lymphatic system. Swelling (edema) other than lymphedema may be caused by a variety of conditions, such as CHF, renal diseases, or venous insufficiency. These swellings do not contain a higher level of proteins in the accumulated fluid, and are defined as edemas.

Diuretics used for lymphedema are limited in that they only remove the water content of the swelling, while the protein molecules remain in the soft tissue. The dehydration effect of diuretics causes a higher concentration of the protein mass in the edema fluid, which may cause the tissues to become more fibrotic and increase the potential for secondary inflammation. In addition, the remaining proteins characteristically draw more water to the swollen areas as soon as the diuretic loses its effectiveness and may cause the volume of the lymphedema to increase.

The 2009 Consensus Document of the International Society of Lymphology states: "Diuretic agents are of limited use during the initial treatment phase of complete decongestive therapy (CDT). Long-term administration, however, is discouraged for its marginal benefits in treatment of peripheral lymphedema and potentially may induce fluid and electrolyte imbalance."

Benzopyrones

These drugs include coumarin, hydroxyethylrutin, and flavonoids (diosmin), and have been shown to promote the breakdown of proteins present in lymphedema. Research has shown that their practical usefulness in the treatment of lymphedema is questionable. The United States and Australia abandoned the use of coumarin due to liver toxicity and lack of effectiveness.

The 2009 Consensus Document of the International Society of Lymphology states: "Oral benzopyrones, which have been reported to hydrolyze tissue proteins and facilitate their absorption while stimulating lymphatic collectors, are neither an alternative nor substitute for CPT. The exact role for benzopyrones (which include those termed rutosides and bioflavonoids) as an adjunct in primary and secondary lymphedema treatment including filariasis is still not definitively determined including appropriate formulations and dose regimens. Coumarin, one such benzopyrone, in higher doses has been linked to liver toxicity. Recent research has linked this toxicity with poor CYP2A6 enzymatic activity in these individuals."

3

Diethylcarbamazine Citrate (DEC), Albendazole, and Ivermectin

These medications are used in the treatment of lymphatic filariasis, which is very rare in the United States, but endemic in more than 80 countries in the tropics and subtropics. Filariasis is caused by threadlike, parasitic filarial worms that live almost exclusively in humans. It is estimated that over 120 million individuals are affected by this disease, which is transmitted when a mosquito bites an infected person and then goes on to bite others, thus infecting them with the parasites. The toxicity of the waste products these worms produce results in inflammation and obliteration of the lymphatic system, and often leads to extreme swellings. The goal of these drugs is to eliminate the parasitic worms, so the transmission of the disease by mosquitos consistently can be interrupted.

Antibiotics and Antimycotics

Bacterial (dermatolymphangioadenitis [DLA]) and fungal infections of the skin and nails are common in patients with lymphedema. These complications can be treated effectively with broad-spectrum antibiotics and antimycotic drugs. In cases where cellulitis is a frequent complication, prophylactic antibiotic treatment may be indicated.

3.11.9 Surgical Approaches in the Treatment of Lymphedema

Surgical procedures for the treatment of lymphedema have been practiced for over a century, and advancements in medical technologies and microsurgical techniques have led to increased discussion of the role of surgical treatment as an alternative or additional treatment option for a select group of patients affected by lymphedema. Recent research indicates that the surgical approach to treat lymphedema has beneficial effects for some patients; however, there is a broad consensus that surgical procedures do not eliminate the need of conservative (nonsurgical) therapy, that is CDT pre- as well as postoperatively,[174, 175] and should act as an adjunct to conservative treatment protocols.

CDT is considered the gold standard treatment for lymphedema and, with properly applied treatment techniques and patient compliance, is able to successfully manage lymphedema in the majority of patients.[176] Any surgical approach to treat lymphedema should be reserved for those cases when conservative treatments have clearly been unsuccessful or when the achieved success of conservative measures can no longer be maintained[177] (also refer to Chapter 5, Surgical Treatment of Lymphedema). Other cases where surgery may be a consideration are situations when limb weight contributes to considerable functional impairment and cosmetic deformity, and the occurrence of frequent lymphedema-associated inflammatory attacks.

An important component to determine whether any surgical procedure for lymphedema is indicated is to weigh the potential benefit of the specific surgical procedure against the risks associated with it. Other considerations should include the individual medical needs and goals of the patient, and the medical expertise of the surgical team.[178]

The goal of any surgical approach is to reduce the volume of the area affected by lymphedema to facilitate conservative treatments, improve function, and prevent or remove complications associated with this condition. Literature indicates that after it is determined that the patient will most likely benefit from a surgical procedure, best results are achieved if surgery is performed as part of a comprehensive treatment system, which includes conservative pre- and postoperative lymphedema therapy.[174,175,179]

In general, surgical approaches can be classified as excisional techniques, reconstructive techniques, and tissue transfer procedures.

Excisional techniques remove the tissues affected by lymphedema, and can be further divided into debulking procedures, liposuction, or amputation. Reconstructive techniques include microsurgical attempts to improve or restore lymphatic flow in areas where lymphatic pathways have been damaged or are missing. The goal is to create a bypass for lymphatic fluid beyond or around the area of damaged lymphatic tissue using connections (anastomoses) between two lymph vessels (lymphatic–lymphatic anastomosis), using connections between lymph vessels and veins (lymphatic–venous anastomosis), or using veins as grafts to establish connections to other lymph vessels (lymphatic–venous–lymphatic anastomosis).

Tissue transfer procedures involve the microsurgical transplantation of soft tissues containing lymph nodes and associated lymph vessels with their blood vessels, which are harvested from healthy unaffected donor sites and transferred into the areas with damaged or missing lymphatic tissues (vascularized lymph node transfer).

Debulking and Excisional Operations

Debulking procedures remove the excess skin and subcutaneous tissues down to the muscle fascia of the area affected by lymphedema. The resulting raw surfaces of the excised areas are then covered with skin grafts, which are harvested from the resected area or from other donor sites of the patient.

The most radical technique was first described in 1912 by Sir Richard Charles (Charles procedure). Since then, various less invasive modifications to this procedure have been introduced; however, the results following these procedures are cosmetically very disfiguring and include a long list of complications, such as skin necrosis, chronic wounds, delayed healing, excessive scarring, infections, and excessive hematoma. The major disadvantage of excisional techniques is that, together with the tissue, the subcutaneous lymph vessels are removed or obliterated as well, which seriously interferes with any later attempts to treat the lymphedema with conservative treatments. These procedures do not prevent the reaccumulation of lymph fluid, nor do they improve the function of the compromised lymphatic system.

Fortunately, these invasive procedures are performed with much lower frequency today and are reserved for a small number of very extreme cases of lymphatic elephantiasis, where thickened, pendulous tissues and repeated infections may justify such a radical approach. Other indications may include localized debulking in selected cases of lymphedema to remove excess skin folds with the goal of improving the cosmetic appearance of the decongested limb following successful CDT.

Liposuction

Liposuction is an excisional procedure during which fatty tissue under the skin is removed by a negative atmospheric pressure vacuum tube, which is inserted repeatedly via several incisions made to the areas affected by lymphedema. Not only fatty tissue but also lymph vessels embedded in the fatty tissue are removed during this invasive procedure. Liposuction procedures in the treatment of lymphedema are different from standard cosmetic liposuction, which is not suitable in the treatment of lymphedema. Liposuction for lymphedema should not be attempted by surgeons not trained in this procedure. Other terms to describe this technique include suction-assisted lipectomy (SAL), circumferential suction-assisted lipectomy (CSAL). and suction-assisted protein lipectomy (SAPL).

Liposuction is presently the most common surgical excisional procedure for the treatment of lymphedema. As with other surgical approaches, liposuction should be reserved for those patients where conservative treatments have been shown to be unsuccessful to bringing the lymphedema back to a stage of latency. It should be limited to cases of nonpitting lymphedema, where the excess limb volume is composed of adipose tissue, which is often the case in late-stage lymphedema. Some clinicians, however, report that pitting edema of around 4 to 5 mL in upper extremity lymphedema and 6 to 8 mL in lower extremity lymphedema can be accepted for liposuction if further reduction by means of conservative measures is not possible.[180]

Literature indicates that large amounts of excess volume can be removed successfully in a limited number of patients when performed correctly, and the incidence of cellulitis can be reduced by up to 75%.[181]

The risks of liposuction include bleeding, infection, and abnormal sensation in the skin.

Lymphedema can still recur following liposuction, and patients who underwent this procedure are required to continue lifelong wearing of progressively smaller custom-fitted compression garments. Successful treatment outcome depends largely on close cooperation between the surgeon and a lymphedema therapist with specific experience with this procedure pre- and postoperatively.

Lymphatic Reconstruction

Lymphatic reconstructive procedures attempt to improve the rate of lymphatic return back to the blood circulation. Techniques include autologous transplant of functioning lymph vessels, lymph nodes, or veins from other areas of the body into those areas affected by lymphedema, and the direct connection of lymph vessels and nodes to neighboring veins.

These procedures are mostly used in the earlier stages of lymphedema (before the occurrence of fibrotic and adipose tissues), in which the fluid component is predominantly responsible for the excess volume. Recent advances in microsurgical

3

3

procedures and instruments, as well as improved imaging techniques, have led to continued progress in these procedures, and reductions in limb volume have been reported. However, no long-term studies are currently available on the effectiveness of these techniques, and more research is necessary to properly define indications for microsurgery.

Lymphatic–Lymphatic Anastomosis

This procedure involves the harvesting of healthy, functioning lymph vessels and transferring these vessels to the area affected by lymphedema, where they are sutured directly to the lymph vessels in the lymphedema-affected limb. The goal is to improve or restore lymphatic flow by creating a bridge bypassing the scarred or irradiated area. The healthy lymph vessels used in this procedure are usually taken from the inner thigh region, and there is a theoretical risk of inducing lymphedema at the donor site.

Lymphatic–Venous Anastomosis

This procedure relies on the connection of lymphatic vessels in the lymphedema-affected region to small adjacent subdermal veins (venules), allowing lymph fluid to directly drain into the venous system, thus bypassing areas of obstructed lymph flow. Better results tend to be achieved when numerous lymphatic–venous anastomoses are performed. No donor site is required for this procedure, which makes this procedure the least invasive with the lowest surgical risk.

Vascularized Lymph Node Transfer

In this procedure, autologous soft tissue containing lymph nodes with their arterial and venous blood vessels is harvested from a donor site (groin, chest wall, or neck) and transplanted to the lymphedema-affected area. Here, the blood vessels of the donor tissue are connected to local blood vessels to reestablish blood supply to the transferred nodes. New lymphatic vessels are expected to sprout from the transplanted nodes and remaining lymph vessels are expected to regrow, thus restoring lymphatic drainage and preventing formation of new scar tissue.

It must be stressed that all surgical procedures are invasive, costly, and involve significant risks, and the long-term results are not yet known. Conservative management of lymphedema with CDT is noninvasive, with minimal to no side effects for patients, shows excellent long-term results, and should always be the treatment of choice.

3.12 Chronic Venous and Lymphovenous Insufficiency

3.12.1 Definition of CVI

CVI is an advanced stage of venous disease in which the veins and the muscle pump activity become incompetent, causing blood to pool in the legs and feet. The condition may be caused by repeated damage to the veins due to superficial (severe varicose veins) or deep venous pathology, or a variety of other vein-related conditions, such as the congenital absence of venous valves. CVI is characterized by an increased venous pressure during walking.

> Venous insufficiency directly affects the lymphatic system. Insufficient venous return results in an elevated blood capillary pressure, causing an increase in net filtration. The lymphatic system reacts with its safety factor as an active edema-protective mechanism.

3.12.2 Postthrombotic Syndrome

One of every three patients with deep venous thrombosis (DVT) in the lower extremities or the pelvic area will develop postthrombotic sequelae within 5 years. Most episodes of postthrombotic syndrome (PTS) will occur within 2 years of the thrombosis. Individuals who have had thrombosis more than once (recurrent thrombosis) are at higher risk for PTS.

PTS is one of the most common causes of CVI, and if therapeutic measures are not initiated in the early stages, it is characterized by edema, pigmentation, superficial varicosis, lipodermatosclerosis, ulceration, and pain, especially after ambulation. The long-term effects of PTS are caused by deficient function of the venous valves. DVT typically occurs at the valvular section of the veins, causing irreversible damage and/or obstruction of the deep veins with ambulatory venous hypertension (see 3.12.4 Pathophysiology of CVI later in this chapter).

3.12.3 Venous Dynamics in the Lower Extremities

As with the lymphatic system, the venous system is divided into a superficial (cutaneous) and deep layer, both separated by fascia. The superficial layer communicates with the deep veins, which usually accompany deep arteries, by veins perforating the fascia (perforating veins). A major part of the blood volume, approximately 60%, is contained within the venous system, and for this reason veins are sometimes referred to as capacity vessels (▶ Fig. 3.40).

Venous return to the heart occurs along relatively small pressure gradients. As explained in Chapter 2, Heart and Circulation, the blood pressure value decreases continuously between the

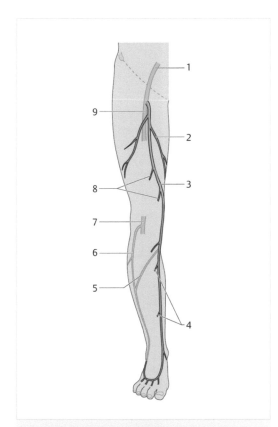

Fig. 3.40 Superficial and deep veins on the lower extremity. 1. External iliac vein; 2. Accessory saphenous vein; 3. Great saphenous vein; 4. Perforating veins; 5. Transverse connection; 6. Small saphenous vein; 7. Popliteal vein; 8. Perforating veins; 9. Femoral vein. (Reproduced with permission from Faller A, Schuenke M. The Human Body. Stuttgart/New York: Thieme; 2004.)

arterial and the venous end of the systemic circulation. In the veins near the heart, the pressure amounts to only 1.5 to 4 mm Hg. The effect of gravity additionally retards venous return.

A sufficient venous return from the lower extremities would not be possible without the help of the muscle and joint pumps (primarily the calf musculature), diaphragmatic breathing, the suction effect of the heart during the diastole, and the pulsation of adjacent arteries enclosed by the same sheath. Together with a functioning valvular system, which prevents retrograde flow, these supporting mechanisms propel the blood within the deep venous system back to the heart. During the relaxation phase of the muscle pump, venous blood from the superficial system reaches the deep veins via the perforating veins.

The normal blood pressure value in venous vessels on the foot amounts to approximately 10 mm Hg in the supine position. When upright and standing motionless (orthostasis), the thin-walled veins dilate, and due to the hydrostatic pressure of the column of blood in the veins below the level of the heart, blood will collect or pool in the feet and legs. The pressure in the foot veins will subsequently increase to approximately 100 mm Hg. During ambulation, pooling is avoided by the muscle and joint pumps, which help propel the venous blood back to the heart. The venous pressure in the same veins on the foot will decrease during ambulation by 70% to roughly 30 mm Hg, provided the valves are sufficient.

3.12.4 Pathophysiology of CVI

The deficient venous valves in CVI fail to prevent retrograde flow of venous blood during muscle pump activity. In the ambulatory phase, the muscle pump forces the venous blood in the deep veins not only toward proximal but also toward distal and via the perforating veins into the superficial venous system (*blow-out syndrome*). This condition is called *ambulatory venous hypertension*, which is thought to cause CVI by the following sequence of events: increased venous pressure transcends the venules to the capillaries, impeding the flow rate. Low-flow states within the blood capillaries cause leukocyte trapping. Trapped leukocytes release proteolytic enzymes and oxygen free radicals, which damage capillary basement membranes. Plasma proteins, such as fibrinogen, leak into the surrounding tissues, forming a fibrin cuff. Interstitial fibrin and resultant edema decrease oxygen delivery to the tissues, resulting in local hypoxia with possible subsequent

3

inflammation and tissue necrosis. High intracapillary pressure causes blood capillary endothelial cells to be stretched away from each other (*stretched-pore phenomenon*). Erythrocytes subsequently leave the blood capillaries, causing the skin to become reddish brown due to hemosiderin deposits.

Effects of CVI on the Lymphatic System

Ambulatory venous hypertension and the subsequent increase in blood capillary pressure result in an increase in net filtration. By activation of its safety factor, the lymphatic system is able to drain the additional amount of water (and protein) for some time. However, without adequate treatment (elevation, compression), the lymphatic system will eventually develop a dynamic insufficiency with subsequent edema, which in most cases will initially recede with elevation and rest.

Over time and without treatment, damage to the lymphatic system, combined with reduction in TC, is unavoidable. The lymphatic system may develop a mechanical insufficiency caused by the constant strain. Due to high intralymphatic pressure and subsequent seepage of proteins into the wall structure, the walls of the lymph angions become fibrotic (mural insufficiency). In addition, the inflammatory process in the deep venous structures may involve adjacent lymph vessels, further reducing the TC.

This condition, described in Chapter 2, Combined Insufficiency (reduced TC in combination with an increase in LLs), has serious consequences and contributes to the signs and symptoms of CVI described in the following section.

3.12.5 Stages of CVI

Without treatment, the symptoms associated with CVI and ambulatory venous hypertension will gradually worsen, and the condition will progress through the following stages (▶ Table 3.10).

Subclinical Stage (Stage 0)

The lymphatic system activates its safety factor as an active edema-protective mechanism. It responds to an increase in LL of water with an increase in lymph formation on the lymph capillary level and with an elevated contraction frequency in lymph collectors and trunks.

> As long as the healthy lymphatic system is able to compensate for the increase in LL of water resulting from venous hypertension, passive vasodilation, and subsequent increase in net filtration, the individual remains free of edema.

Table 3.10 Stages of chronic venous insufficiency and therapeutic approach

Stage	Symptoms	Effects on the superficial lymphatic system				Therapeutic approach
		Lymphatic load of water	Lymphatic load of protein	Status of lymph vessels	Pathology of lymph vessels	
0	None	High	Normal	Normal	LTV increased, lymphatic safety factor	Compression therapy, elevation, exercises
I	Mild (edema)	High	Normal	Normal	Phlebolymphodynamic insufficiency	Compression therapy, elevation, exercises
II	Moderate (pigmentation, varicosis, pain)	High	High	Morphological changes	TC reduced, phlebolymphostatic insufficiency	CDT
III	Severe (hypoxia, necrosis, pain)	High	Very high	Morphological changes	TC reduced, severe phlebolymphostatic insufficiency	CDT and wound care

Abbreviations: CDT, complete decongestive therapy; LTV, lymph time volume; TC, transport capacity.

Stage 1

The lymphatic system is still healthy but fails to drain the elevated lymphatic water load. Edema develops during the course of the day as a result of dynamic insufficiency of the lymphatic system. This stage is also referred to in the literature as *phlebolymphodynamic insufficiency*. Initially, the swelling tends to decrease or completely recede during rest at night. Venous pressure and net filtration return to normal values in the supine position, providing the lymphatic system with a chance to "catch up" with the excess water in the interstitial tissue.

Stage 2

Blood capillaries and lymph collectors with elevated pressure values that remain without treatment for extended periods of time will eventually suffer damage as described in the section Pathophysiology of CVI. The combination of this damage and possible inflammatory processes causes the lymphatic system to develop a mechanical insufficiency, which, with the elevated loads of water and protein, presents as a combined insufficiency. Lymphedema will develop as a result of the venous pathology, and its symptoms are exacerbated by the symptoms associated with CVI (varicosis, pigmentation, pain). Stage 2 of CVI (CVI and lymphedema) is also referred to in the literature as *phlebolymphostatic insufficiency*.

The lymphedema in the early stage appears initially smooth and is pitting. Without treatment, it will progress to a more fibrotic stage (see 3.2.3 previously in this chapter). Regardless of genesis, lymphedema is always a progressive condition.

Stage 3

Typical for this stage are severe changes in the skin associated with the phlebolymphostatic edema. The interstitial fibrin cuff that forms as a result of plasma protein leakage in combination with the increased diffusion distance associated with the swelling decreases oxygen and nutrient delivery to the tissues. This results in local hypoxia and necrosis. Also typical for this stage is *lipodermatosclerosis*. These characteristic skin changes in the lower extremities include capillary proliferation, fat necrosis, and fibrosis of skin and subcutaneous tissues. Pain, especially after ambulation, is present.

Lymphedema resulting from prolonged CVI may show signs and symptoms of elephantiasis. It is important to understand that extremity volume is not considered within the different stages of lymphedema (and phlebolymphedema; see also 3.2.4 previously in this chapter).

> Ulcerations, pigmentation, varicosis, lipodermatosclerosis, and pain may develop in extremities that show minimal swelling.

3.12.6 Complications

The elevated venous pressure in CVI, as well as the delayed clearance of venous blood from the legs, produces a high risk of recurrent thrombophlebitis. Blood clots in the deep veins of the legs are dangerous because they can break free and travel to the lungs. This problem, called pulmonary embolism, can be fatal. It is important that patients and therapists understand the signs and symptoms of pulmonary embolism. Should those signs present, the individual must contact a doctor immediately (see Thrombophlebitis in Deep Veins later in this chapter).

Thrombophlebitis in Superficial Veins

Thrombophlebitis is a blood clot that forms at a certain point in a superficial vein due to irritation or injury to the vein at that point. For example, thrombophlebitis may occur in a vein after an intravenous injection or infusion has been given in that vein. It also may occur as a result of irritation to a varicose vein.

> Symptoms of thrombophlebitis include redness, swelling, and heat in the area of the vein that has been irritated or injured. A vein close to the surface of the skin may appear more noticeable than usual or may feel like a hard piece of rope or cord upon palpation. Pain or discomfort over the involved area as well as fever may be present.

Treatment options for thrombophlebitis may include anti-inflammatory medication (nonsteroidal), antibiotics if an infection of the vein is involved, rest and elevation of the extremity, and the application of moist, warm compresses in the involved area. If lymphedema is associated with thrombophlebitis, the application of warm compresses may supersede the possibility of active hyperemia (vasodilation) and its negative effects on lymphedematous tissue; however, caution should be taken.

Because the blood clot that forms usually stays stuck to the wall of the vein, thrombophlebitis in the superficial veins in most cases is not considered to be a serious condition unless an infection develops. The body will gradually absorb the blood clot as the thrombophlebitis clears up over a period of 1 to 2 weeks. On occasion, however, the blood clot that occurs as a result of thrombophlebitis can contribute to the development of a larger blood clot extending into one of the subfascial veins. This is a more serious condition because the blood clot or a piece of the blood clot in a deep vein may break off and travel to the lungs, causing pulmonary embolism.

Thrombophlebitis in Deep Veins

In DVT, a blood clot forms in a subfascial vein. These clots most often occur as a result of poor or sluggish blood flow through the veins as in CVI, or sitting/standing for long periods of time without moving around, periods of prolonged bed rest, or wearing clothing that interferes with the blood flow. Blood clots may also form as a result of hypercoagulability of the blood (recent surgery, liver diseases, taking oral contraceptives, severe infections, etc.).

Symptoms of thrombophlebitis in deep veins on extremities include
- Redness, swelling, and heat in the area over the path of a deep vein.
- A deep vein feeling like a hard piece of rope or cord.
- Pain or discomfort over the path of a deep vein (usually in the middle of the calf).
- Discoloration or ulceration of the skin over a deep vein.
- Pain in the involved extremity, which increases with coughing, sneezing, or pressing.
- Cramps, which intensify over several days.

Treatment options for thrombophlebitis in deep veins may include restricting activity if there is a

danger of the clot traveling to the lungs, elevating the extremity, taking anticoagulants, and wearing compression garments. Patients should be careful not to rub the affected area as clots may be broken off or dislodged, causing pulmonary embolism.

Many patients with pulmonary embolism have a vague sense that something is wrong but have difficulty describing or defining the problem.

The most common warning signals of pulmonary embolism are
- Unexplained shortness of breath.
- Chest discomfort, usually worse with deep breathing or coughing.
- Anxiety or nervousness.
- Lightheadedness or blacking out.

> Should any sign or symptom of thrombophlebitis in the deep veins or symptoms of pulmonary embolism develop, the patient must see a doctor immediately, and any treatment must be interrupted until the condition is resolved.

Ulcerations

Venous stasis ulcers are the most common form of ulcerations and appear predominantly in the distal third of the lower extremity (usually around the malleoli). Ulcerations generally are persistent and are known to heal slowly (or not at all) if the surrounding environment is edematous. Ulcerations are also a frequent cause for infections in the swollen extremity.

The most important goals in the treatment of venous ulcers is to make sure that the wounds are clean (i.e., free of necrotic tissue, bacteria, yeast, and fungi), that exudate is absorbed while maintaining a moist wound base, and that a normal arterial and venous blood supply is reestablished (decongestion, no constrictive dressings).

3.12.7 Evaluation

The physician's assessment of venous reflux and/or venous occlusion generally consists of noninvasive tests, such as duplex ultrasonography. The evaluation in the lymphedema clinic includes history, inspection, and palpation, as described in 3.6 and 3.7 previously in this chapter.

A major issue in the evaluation of phlebolymphostatic edema is to check skin integrity.

Compromised skin integrity requires additional padding under the compression bandage and meticulous skin care. If ulcerations are present, it is imperative to communicate with the patient's physician or wound specialist to synchronize dressing and wound care issues. It is often more productive if wound care is performed in the lymphedema clinic as part of the treatment protocol.

Therapists should carefully check for any signs and symptoms of superficial or deep thrombophlebitis.

3.12.8 Therapeutic Approach

Prevention

Knowing certain risk factors for venous thrombosis can greatly reduce the likelihood of developing DVT. Maintaining ideal body weight with a healthy nutritional program and exercise regimen, avoiding inactivity or immobility, or wearing support stockings and elevating the legs as often as possible reduce the risk of developing thrombosis. Patients on oral contraceptives who experience symptoms of venous insufficiency should discuss alternatives with the physician due to an elevated risk for DVT.

If signs and symptoms of CVI are present, it is important to prevent it from progressing through its stages by constantly wearing compression stockings prescribed by the physician and by performing meticulous skin care. In the early stages of CVI, it is sufficient to apply compression during the daytime only.

Complete Decongestive Therapy

If CVI remains without adequate treatment (in most cases, compression), the active and passive edema-protective mechanisms (Chapter 2, Safety Factor of the Lymphatic System) of the body will not be able to compensate for the elevated levels of water resulting from ambulatory venous hypertension.

Patients with deficient function of the venous valves in PTS without visible swelling (CVI stage 0) are able to avoid the clinical onset of swelling by the application of daily compression with either bandages or compression garments, provided the compression does not present a contraindication. (Refer to Chapter 4 for contraindications in compression therapy.) The application of cold water on the affected extremity and other noninvasive preventive measures described earlier also assist in preventing the onset of edema (▶ Table 3.10).

If treatment starts in stage 1 of CVI, decongestion of the extremity by elevation precedes the application of compression bandages and/or garments. In some cases, a physician may choose a one-time application of a diuretic to decongest the limb. Because the lymphatic system is healthy (normal TC), although overwhelmed in this stage of the venous pathology, MLD is not indicated.

> The presence of lymphedema in stages 2 and 3 of CVI necessitates the application of the complete spectrum of CDT, including MLD. The goal of the therapy, as in the treatment of uncomplicated lymphedema, is to bring the lymphedema back to a stage of latency. Decongestion of the extremity greatly increases the tendency of venous stasis ulcers to heal.

The treatment protocol of the lymphedema associated with CVI corresponds with the protocol for primary lymphedema.

3.13 Wounds and Skin Lesions

Individuals with chronic lymphedema may present with a variety of skin changes, due to trauma, prolonged tissue hypoxia, fungal infection, immune system dysfunction, or unknown causes (▶ Table 3.11). The skin changes include
- Scarring.
- Dry, scaly skin.
- Skin hyperplasia or plaques.
- Skin fibrosis.
- Hemosiderin staining with accompanying venous insufficiency.
- Papillomas.
- Lymph cysts and varicosities.
- Dystrophic toenails and fingernails.
- Loss of skin appendages (hair, sweat and sebaceous glands).

Another change that may present in individuals with long-standing lymphedema is the development of a vascular tumor (lymphangiosarcoma). These tumors most commonly occur in individuals who have developed chronic lymphedema following mastectomy (Stewart–Treves syndrome). However, tumors have also been reported in individuals with chronic lymphedema of unknown etiology. These tumors are most commonly fatal.

3

Malignant breast cancer is one of the most common malignancies that spread to the skin.[182] Skin metastases most often occur near the breast area, on the trunk, or near the line of surgical incision. Skin metastases commonly present as hardened or rubbery, light pink-red nodules with a surrounding lighter area accompanied by patchy erythema (▶ Fig. 3.41). These nodules may have the appearance of a pimple initially and are usually the size of a grain of rice. They may or may not be painful. These lesions often progress to ulcers and may become frankly infected (▶ Fig. 3.42) and painful. Clinical tips for wound management will be discussed below.

Individuals with lymphedema may also develop lesions or open wounds. These may be related to the dysfunctional lymph vascular system or to other comorbid conditions. They can result from trauma, allergies, or therapeutic procedures such

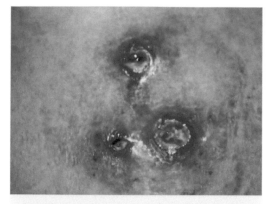

Fig. 3.42 Skin metastases on abdomen presenting with infected ulcerations.

as surgery or radiotherapy. These changes range from simple excoriations to complex wounds with multiple etiologies. Skin wounds in individuals with lymphedema may be classified according to the level of tissue involvement (i.e., depth) and state of the wound (i.e., acute or chronic).

Depending on the location of the dysfunctional lymphatics and coexisting morbidities, individuals may be at greater or lesser risk for particular skin changes or wound types. For example, individuals presenting with lower extremity lymphedema often also present with venous insufficiency in later stages and are at increased risk for wounds related to extremity swelling. Likewise, individuals who have undergone mastectomy with concurrent radiotherapy are at risk for skin breakdown due to radiation burns. Additionally, individuals receiving chemotherapy may also develop infiltration wounds at the intra-arterial catheter site. Wounds that occur in individuals with lymphedema—due to the disease process itself, associated treatments, or related conditions—are listed in ▶ Table 3.11.

3.13.1 Common Skin Changes and Wound Types Associated with Chronic Lymphedema

Vascular Ulcerations

It is estimated that as many as 3.2 million Americans have lower extremity ulcerations due to vascular insufficiency.[183] Vascular ulcerations may result from arterial, venous, or lymphatic dysfunction, or a combination thereof. Vascular ulcerations are most commonly observed in the lower extremity and are associated with long-term

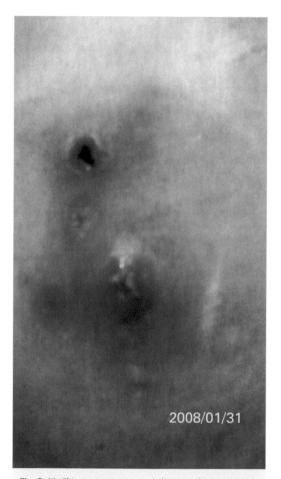

2008/01/31

Fig. 3.41 Skin metastases on abdomen of patient with malignant breast cancer.

Table 3.11 Wound types that may co-occur with lymphedema

Wound type	Wound bed	Characteristics	
		Location	Periwound
Vascular venous	Shallow, irregular	Anterior/medial leg	Hemosiderin staining; scaly, weepy, warm skin
Arterial	Round, deep, necrotic, or pale base	Lateral leg/foot, tips of toes	Tissue pallor; dry, scaly skin; cool to the touch
Mixed	Characteristics of both venous and arterial lesions		Raised, palpable purpura
Inflammatory vasculitis	Small, dark base	Anywhere; common malleolar area	
Pyoderma	Irregular, jagged necrotic base	Mostly leg or trunk	Violaceous wound border, erythema
Fungating	Raised, necrotic; bleeds easily; extremely malodorous	Anywhere; chest	Lip of tissue at wound margin
Chemotherapy (infiltration)	Painful, erythematous, with necroses (eschar and slough)	At site of catheter	Edematous with erythema
Radiation	Exposed dermis; superficial	Skin in treatment field	Erythema; dark black coloration
Minor trauma excoriations	Linear, shallow	Anywhere	Local or advancing erythema
Skin tears	Shallow, linear flap	Arms, hands, legs commonly	Ecchymosis
Failed surgical site	Partial or full thickness, necrotic base	Site of incision	Erythema, edema
Fistulae	Pathological openings between organs/body cavities and the skin	Site of abscess	Opening in wound beds presenting with drainage organs and tissue cavities

vascular compromise. Research indicates that 80 to 90% of these ulcerations have a venous etiology.[184, 185] The prevalence of venous ulceration is approximately 0.16%, or 1% of the general population over 70 years of age,[186,187] and this rate of occurrence increases exponentially with age. The incidence of venous ulceration is also higher in women (62%).

In comparison, skin lesions due to arterial insufficiency account for approximately 5 to 20% of lower extremity ulcers, with as many as 15% of these lesions having both an arterial and venous component. Lesions due solely to lymphedema are poorly discussed in the literature. Other less commonly diagnosed vascular ulcers include those with an underlying genetic or inflammatory etiology.

Venous Ulcerations

Venous ulcerations result from an insufficiency of the venous system, as described previously. They present most often on the anteromedial aspect of the lower leg and ankle, with a high preponderance immediately above the medial malleolus.[183] These ulcerations are typically superficial in nature and are described clinically as being of partial thickness (down to, but not through, the dermis). Venous ulcers have irregular borders and exhibit moderate to heavy exudate. The wound bed often has a ruddy or granular surface that is dull red in appearance. The wound bed is also commonly covered with yellow and/or grayish white slough. Black eschar or necrosis may also be present in the wound. Venous wounds often have strong odors that can be described as foul or putrid. These odors are a result of the high numbers of microorganisms found in necrotic tissue.

Due to the accumulation of blood vascular fluids in the surrounding tissues and the presence of chronic inflammation, the periwound area as well as the entire lower limb typically presents with an

3

increased temperature on palpation. Other periwound characteristics include dry, scaly skin, tissue fibrosis, and loss of skin appendages (hair, glands) with microulcerations or pinpoint openings that allow the passage of accumulated tissue fluids to the skin surface.[183] The skin will often appear to be "weeping." The periwound area both immediately adjacent to and at varied distances from the wound bed is usually discolored (with blue/purple or brown/black staining) due to the deposition of iron (hemosiderin staining). Hemosiderin staining results from the deposition of iron into the interstitial tissue spaces upon lysis of extravasated red blood cells. This finding is not common with lymphedema unless venous compromise has also occurred.

Clinical Tips

The key to successful treatment of wounds that result from the chronic accumulation of interstitial fluids, such as that observed with venous insufficiency or lymphedema, is reduction or clearance of the swollen tissues.[188,189,190] Manual techniques such as MLD, along with the application of short-stretch bandaging for initial reduction of chronic fluid accumulation, followed by maintenance therapy with a compression garment, are necessary for clinical success.[191] However, vascular status should be determined prior to any addition of compression therapy, so that ischemic limbs are not treated inadvertently (see clinical tips on arterial ulceration, below). If an active wound is present, advanced dressing technologies with sufficient fluid-handling characteristics should be used to control exudates and facilitate autolysis of necrotic tissue. Enzymatic preparations may also assist with necrotic tissue reduction and facilitate wound healing. Newer antiseptic technologies that use slow-release iodine or silver preparations will help control the wound bioburden, thus reducing malodor and enhancing wound closure. Charcoal-based dressings may also be applied over a primary dressing to assist with odor control. Exercises that stimulate the calf muscle pump also hasten the reduction of tissue edema and enhance wound healing.[191]

Arterial Ulcerations

Arterial or ischemic ulcerations also commonly present on the lower extremity, but differ significantly in character from venous ulcerations. Arterial ulcerations are typically deep, with even

wound margins.[192] They are located predominantly on the lateral side of the leg or foot, with lesions also occurring over the tips of the toes, between the toes, and over the phalangeal heads. The wound base is usually pale pink in color due to ischemic conditions, unless covered by necrosis. Arterial ulcers are most often dry and covered by a thickened, black eschar. If the eschar is stable, then it is dry and hardened; if the eschar has been penetrated by a significant level of microorganisms, then it may be wet. A wet eschar will often herald the onset of wet gangrene and requires immediate medical attention and debridement.

The periwound skin of individuals with arterial compromise is typically thin, dry, and scaling, with an overt loss of skin appendages such as hair, sweat, and sebaceous glands due to tissue ischemia. The skin is blanched, especially with elevation of the limb, or purpuric when in a dependent position. Depending on the severity and extent of tissue ischemia, muscle and fat atrophy may also be present. Toenails are also usually dystrophic, due to fungal infection. Depending on the level of arterial compromise, the individual may experience pain at rest, with touch, or on exercising.

Clinical Tips

The key to successful treatment of ischemic wounds is revascularization. Revascularization can be achieved through graded exercise programs, medication, surgery, or a combination thereof.[192,193] Before therapy is started, the vascular status of the involved tissues should be established. Without adequate blood flow, arterial wounds simply will not heal. Graded exercise programs have been shown to be successful in facilitating revascularization of an ischemic limb. Some success has also been obtained with the use of cilostazol (Pletal). Walking distances and ankle/brachial indexes improve with cilostazol therapy. However, severely compromised limbs or tissues require surgical interventions such as percutaneous transluminal angioplasty and stenting, as well as bypass procedures. Noninvasive vascular tests can provide extremely useful data on the vascular status of individuals presenting with signs and symptoms of arterial insufficiency. These tests can be performed by most clinicians and do not require extensive equipment or space. Common noninvasive vascular testing involves obtaining peripheral pulses, ankle/brachial index, toe pressures, and transcutaneous oxygen pressures ($tcPo_2$).[193,194] In the lower extremity, the femoral, popliteal, dorsalis pedis, and posterior tibial arteries should be evaluated by examining the pulses. Doppler ultrasound examination can give a more accurate picture, as pulses may be difficult to detect in an ischemic or swollen limb. A variety of scales are available to rate the pulses (e.g., pulse character: 0, no pulse; 1+, very shallow; 2+, decreased; 3+, normal; 4+, bounding).

An ankle/brachial index (ABI) is useful because it provides a picture of systolic blood pressure in the lower limb. The systolic blood pressure is measured at the brachial artery on the same side as the affected lower limb. The systolic pressure from both the dorsalis pedis and the posterior tibial artery should be used separately to calculate the ABI, as they give a clinical picture of different regions of the lower limb and foot. The ABI is calculated using the following equation and is interpreted using the scale shown in ▶ Table 3.12:

$$ABI = \frac{\text{Ankle systolic pressure}}{\text{Brachial systolic pressure}}$$

Systolic ankle pressures of less than 80 mm Hg, along with toe pressures of less than 20 mm Hg and $tcPo_2$ less than 40 mm Hg, are associated with poor healing and require revascularization if possible; otherwise, progression of the condition may require amputation.

Arterial ulcers that present with a stable, dry, adherent eschar on a distal extremity should not be disturbed unless an area of wet necrosis is detected. Ulcers with stable, dry eschars may heal very slowly by re-epithelialization beneath the hardened eschar. A conservative approach to treatment of these intact eschars is warranted, due to their poor prognosis for healing and the risks of

infection and subsequent limb loss. On the other hand, wet necrosis can become rapidly infected in ischemic tissue, due to poor immune surveillance and rapid referral to a vascular surgeon is warranted. In this case, the wet necrosis should be removed as quickly as possible, through surgical debridement. As with venous ulcers, several advanced wound dressings with topical antiseptics are available along with the necessity of systemic therapy. Once the wet necrosis has been effectively reduced, hydration of the wound bed may be necessary to facilitate wound closure. Moisture balance in a wet, necrotic arterial wound requires different interventions from those needed in a dry, clean wound bed. Hydration of desiccated wound-bed tissues is required for cellular migration and subsequent wound closure. Amorphous or sheet hydrogels can provide the moisture required for wound healing processes to occur.

Vascular/Inflammatory Ulcers

While arterial and venous insufficiency ulcerations are the most commonly recognized vascular ulcers, other types do occur. These ulcerations are often painful and heal with difficulty. However, their co-occurrence with lymphedema has not been documented. Their co-occurrence would be expected to be rare. Vascular ulcers that fall into this category include those associated with vasculitis of small or large vessels, sickle-cell anemia, and pyoderma gangrenosum.

Vasculitis

Vasculitis or angiitis of both small and large blood vessels is characterized by the onset of necrotizing inflammation, with subsequent necrosis of blood vessel walls. Evidence of this process is manifested in the development of skin lesions or ulcerations. Small-vessel vasculitis involves the arterioles, capillaries, and venules. Clinical signs of small-vessel vasculitis include urticaria, a palpable purpura (small red lesion or papule that does not blanch with pressure), and the development of nodules, bullae, or ulcers. Small-vessel vasculitis is often associated with hypersensitivity disorders, Henoch–Schönlein purpura, cryoglobulinemia, serum sickness, chronic urticaria, connective-tissue diseases, certain malignancies, and hepatitis type B infection. In comparison, large-vessel vasculitis involves the small and medium-sized muscular arteries. Clinical signs of large-vessel vasculitis include subcutaneous nodules, ulcers, and

Table 3.12 Scale used to interpret the ankle/brachial index (ABI)

ABI value	Level of impairment	Clinical picture
>1.2	Calcification of vessels	Associated with diabetes
0.9–1.0	Normal	
0.8–0.9	Mild disease	No overt symptoms; compress with care in mixed stages
<0.8, >0.5	Moderate disease	Poor healing, claudication pain
<0.5	Severe disease	Revascularization necessary

ecchymosis. Diseases associated with the onset of large-vessel vasculitis include polyarteritis nodosa, Churg–Strauss syndrome, Wegener granulomatosis, and giant cell arteritis.

Clinical Tips

As vasculitic lesions are the result of inflammatory processes, anti-inflammatory or immunosuppressive therapies are required.[195] Sharp debridement should not be used, as it increases the already present inflammation and often leads to a worsening of the ulcerations. Autolytic or enzymatic debridement provides a gentler and more successful intervention. As with other wounds, bacterial numbers need to be controlled and exudate levels need to be balanced for healing to occur. Absorbent dressings that do not produce additional trauma to the wound when removed are therefore recommended. Any product applied to the wound or skin should also be free of common skin sensitizers—as is true for most other wound types, particularly venous ulcerations. Common skin sensitizers include lanolin, balsam of Peru, cetostearyl alcohol, parabens, rosins, latex, and neomycin,[196] and these should be avoided.

Pyoderma Gangrenosum

Another inflammatory condition that involves the skin and vascular system and that can culminate in skin ulcerations is pyoderma gangrenosum (PG). PG is a chronic inflammatory disorder of unknown etiology that often evolves from folliculitis and/or abscess.[195] It may also be associated with a vasculitic condition. PG is associated with the following systemic diseases: inflammatory bowel syndrome, rheumatoid arthritis, systemic lupus erythematosus, acquired immune deficiency syndrome (AIDS), and chronic active hepatitis, among others. Lesions are typically found on the lower extremity, but may occur elsewhere, such as on the thigh and trunk. Initially, pyoderma gangrenosum begins as small, red, sensitive lesions. These lesions may present either as macules, papules, pustules, nodules, or bulla. As the lesion grows in size, the perilesional skin becomes dusky red and indurated. As the inflammatory process that underlies these lesions progresses, purulent, necrotic ulceration(s) develop, with irregular, raised purple/red wound margins and an intense periwound erythema.

Clinical Tips

Pyoderma gangrenosum can be one of the more challenging types of ulcers to treat. The response to therapy can be unpredictable and variable. However, as in vasculitis, anti-inflammatory and immunosuppressive agents are used to control the underlying chronic inflammatory processes.[195] As with the vasculitic lesion, additional trauma should be avoided. Autolytic and enzymatic debridement are preferred, along with nontraumatic cleansing and dressing changes. Exudate and pain control measures are also necessary with pyoderma gangrenosum wounds.

Sickle-Cell Anemia

An additional condition related to the vascular system that also results in the formation of ulcerations is sickle-cell anemia. Ulcerations are painful and tend to produce clinical signs similar to those of both an arterial and venous insufficiency wound.

Fungating Wound/Malignant Ulcerations

Fungating ulcers evolve as a result of a malignant tumor (skin metastasis) invading the skin or a chronic ulcer site. These ulcers can develop either quite rapidly or over a more gradual course. Rapid onset or change in the wound bed is often associated with disease progression, and the individual will often report increased pain.[197,198] When the disease is progressing more rapidly, physical changes are detectable on a daily basis. Another characteristic of fungating wounds is the exuberant development of capillaries in the wound bed. Because of this excessive formation of capillary beds in the wound base and the concomitant deficiency in platelets, the wound is often quite friable. This rapid and excessive formation of blood capillary beds is also associated with focal areas of necrosis. Other characteristics of fungating ulcers include extreme malodor due to tissue necrosis and high levels of bioburden, and a distinct lip of tissue around the wound margin. Fungating wounds may also be associated with fistula development. Fistulas or passages from internal cavities and organs to the skin may occur in areas where malignant tumors give rise to fungating skin lesions. Retrograde drainage from the wound may lead to sepsis, and drainage from internal organs may be carried into the ulcer.

Clinical Tips

As discussed previously, skin metastases present as pink-red nodules much like a pimple. These nodules progress to open ulcers that often develop necrotic bases covered with yellow slough and black eschar (▶ Fig. 3.41, ▶ Fig. 3.42). As the ulcers develop, they often become infected. A hallmark of these fungating lesions is malodor. The quality of life for the individual and family is certainly affected by the strong wound odor. These ulcers are also quite painful. Frequent wound cleansing, removal of necrotic tissue, and control of bacterial content and exudate levels are paramount to decreasing wound odor and assisting with pain control. However, depending on the size of the lesion, this can be a monumental task. Charcoal secondary dressings and topical antimicrobials such as metronidazole or antiseptic dressings that employ ionized silver or slow-release iodine provide some benefit. Hydrofiber dressings are also useful in binding bacteria away from the wound surface. Wound cleansing with gentle irrigation via syringe, pressurized spray, low-frequency ultrasound, or pulsatile lavage on low settings may also be indicated, depending on the risk of further metastasis.

Radiation-Related Skin Changes

Acute skin reactions to radiotherapy may be mild to severe. Because radiotherapy targets rapidly dividing cells, the epidermis is at particular risk for damage due to its intrinsically high rate of cellular proliferation. Skin reactions are related to the dose and dosing schedule, location, total treatment area, radiation type, and individual skin differences.[197,198] The appearance of radiation-induced skin changes is variable; it may present within days or be delayed for months or years after exposure. Skin reactions to radiation can be divided into four categories: erythema, dry desquamation, moist desquamation, and necrosis.

Necrosis, the most severe response of the skin to radiotherapy, results in severe discoloration of the skin, with the development of a nonhealing, necrotic ulcer.[199,200] In contrast, the mildest form of reaction is the development of erythema with concurrent epidermal edema. Successive levels of damage include dry and moist desquamation. With dry desquamation, the epidermis begins to peel, as evidenced by the presence of dry, scaly skin. Skin undergoing this reaction may appear thin and atrophied if epidermal cells are not produced rapidly enough to replace dying and dead cells, or the skin may take on a scaly appearance if new skin cells are accumulating faster than the rate at which dead ones can be shed. The third category of skin reaction that may occur is moist desquamation. Radiotherapy-related damage at this level leads to robust erythema, with subsequent loss of the epidermis and exposure of the dermis. This superficial, partial-thickness lesion is associated with the production of wound exudate and an increased risk for infection due to the often immune-compromised state of the individual. In addition, radiation-induced ulcers may be associated with fistula development, particularly in the area of an abscess. Fistulas require management at a quite different level, depending on the tissue cavities involved.

Clinical Tips

An acute inflammatory reaction may occur in skin over an area that has received radiotherapy. Skin areas that have undergone changes due to radiation and that are subject to trauma or moisture accumulation are at great risk for breakdown. Patients should be informed about the risk for breakdown and encouraged to keep dry any areas that are prone to an excessive build-up of moisture. Padding can be used to absorb moisture and to prevent injury due to frictional forces such as scrubbing by clothing. Maintenance of a dry, clean environment will also aid in preventing fungal infections. Areas that are prone to excessive accumulation of moisture include the axillae and perineal area.

To keep skin that has been exposed to radiotherapy in the healthiest state possible, individuals should be encouraged to use mild, nonfragrant soap for baths and to pat the skin dry, rather than rubbing it, as this may further traumatize the tissues. Use of a basic skin cream that is free of sensitizers or allergens is also recommended to maintain skin hydration. Individuals should also be instructed to drink fluids as this also improves skin hydration.

Open skin areas that are dry can be treated effectively with amorphous or sheet hydrogels, whereas wounds that are producing excessive drainage can be effectively treated with alginates (sheets or ropes, depending on wound shape and depth), foams, or collagen-based wound dressings. Alginate or collagen-based dressings are also useful for establishing hemostasis, as the wounds involved are friable and hence prone to bleeding.

3

Silver alginates may also prove valuable in keeping microorganism levels low as well as hydrofiber dressings impregnated with silver. Atraumatic dressings that use a silicone-based adhesive or a protective gel formation (that forms upon application) are essential to protect the fragile state of irradiated skin. They promote a pain-free approach to dressing removal.

Minor Trauma: Skin Tears/Excoriations

The skin of individuals with lymphedema or edema is at risk for traumatic injury. Minor traumatic injuries such as skin tears, excoriations, and erosions occur with everyday activities. Skin tears or excoriations result from mechanical injury, which can produce either partial-thickness or full-thickness tissue injury in areas where the skin is fragile. Highly edematous tissues are fragile due to the internal pressure associated with highly stretched skin and may burst or "pop" with exposure to minor trauma. Patients often describe "bumping into an object" or being "poked by something." These skin tears are most often shallow in nature, but may present either as a linear injury or as a skin flap that remains partially attached to the surrounding tissues. These skin flaps should be reattached with light compression over a protective bandage such as a foam or film dressing.

Skin excoriations may also be a problem for patients with lymphedema. These typically linear and shallow lesions result commonly from frictional forces, such as scratching due to chronic irritation and/or medication-related side effects. Additionally, the skin of individuals who have received radiation treatment may also be fragile and irritated due to excessive dehydration. The skin of these individuals should be protected from trauma, including constant rubbing produced by clothing such as bras or elastic bands in shirts or pants. A nonsensitizing moisturizing agent should be used to hydrate the skin and maintain the normal pH balance. This will assist in maintaining the skin's normal barriers to dehydration and infection.

Clinical Tips

Fragile skin can be protected using several approaches. Keeping the patient hydrated is a prerequisite for maintaining the skin turgor; dehydrated individuals with dry skin appear to be at greater risk for skin tears. Use of nonsensitizing creams, rather than lotions, produces a longer-lasting moisturizing effect. Arm pads, hydrocolloid, and thin film dressings also confer some level of protection from mechanical injury.

In disoriented individuals, excoriations can also be prevented by having them wear oven mitts, as well as by encouraging fluid intake and the use of moisturizing cream. The frequency with which they take baths may also need to be decreased, as natural skin oils are stripped during bathing. Potential medication issues such as toxicity and side effects should also be investigated.

Failed Surgical Sites

Failed closure of surgical incisions may also be present, due to debulking procedures, removal of tumor masses, implantation of medical devices, or removal of lines and tubes. Wounds that are left to heal by secondary intention may result from infiltration of intravenous lines, dehiscence of sutured incision sites after removal of a tumor, or debulking of skin from an edematous limb. Closed incisional sites commonly fail due to infection or overwhelming mechanical stress resulting from the accumulation of fluids in the operated tissues or excessive weight associated with obesity. Surgical sites can also fail or reopen in association with fistula development due to abscess formation. Fistulas due to deep tissue abscesses allow organs or body cavities to communicate with the skin. As a result, wound exudate may drain to these deep areas, causing sepsis, or bodily fluids such as urine or fecal material may drain to the wound, causing tissue injury and malodor.

Clinical Tips

Dehisced surgical wounds may involve large tissue areas and produce significant amounts of drainage. This copious drainage may result from deep tissue abscesses or fistulae. Because of the factors described above, dehisced surgical wounds often benefit from negative-pressure wound therapy. Negative-pressure wound therapy uses a vacuum to facilitate wound healing by drawing the wound together and reducing exudate levels and bacterial numbers in the wound tissues. Negative-pressure therapy is also particularly useful in allowing early return to functional activities, since wound tissue approximation can be stabilized by the vacuum.

3.13.2 Wound Bed Preparation

Wound bed preparation[201] is a conceptual framework of the basic principles that drive the treatment approach for chronic, open wounds. According to this conceptual framework, there are three basic principles of effective wound bed preparation. These include necrotic tissue removal, bacterial control, and exudate management. Many of these principles have been referred to in the clinical tips sections above.

3.13.3 Wound Necrosis

Removal of necrosis is necessary for wound healing to occur.[202] Necrosis in the wound bed acts as a harbor for microorganisms and impedes cellular migration. There are several methods for removing necrosis from the wound bed, and selection of the appropriate method is based on individual characteristics such as health status, pain tolerance, necrosis type, and vascular status. The four primary methods of debridement are: surgical or sharp, enzymatic, autolytic, and mechanical. A fifth category that is increasingly utilized is biotherapy. Biotherapy involves the use of chemically sterilized maggots. Sterilized maggots have the benefit of delivering the most selective form of debridement available.

Open wounds associated with lymphedema are most often characterized as wet wounds. As such, they typically do not form hardened and dry eschar. They are commonly covered with a slimy, filmy layer characteristic of sloughy wounds. However, wounds that result from damage related to radiation therapy may present as dry or moist wounds and as such may form either a dry, hardened eschar or slough.

The periwound area may also be covered with thickened plaques of epidermal hyperplasia (▶ Fig. 3.43). These plaques may grow to a significant size and form ball-like structures with vascular attachments to the underlying dermis. They often detach on movement and may cause minor bleeding. These plaques reduce with compression and can be easily removed with forceps.

Necrotic tissue in the wound bed can be removed using several different approaches. The debridement approach selected is influenced by the type of necrotic tissue present in the wound bed. The four primary methods of debridement are discussed below.

Surgical or sharp debridement is the most rapid method of removing nonviable tissue. If

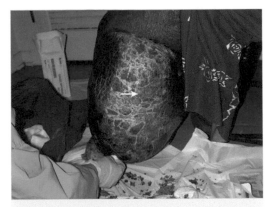

Fig. 3.43 Epidermal hyperplasia (→) associated with grade 4 lymphedema.

large amounts of tissue need to be removed quickly and pain is an issue, then surgical debridement should be used. If the patient is not a candidate for surgery and cannot tolerate the pain associated with sharp debridement, then autolytic, enzymatic, or biotherapy-mediated debridement can be used. Only the collagenase-based enzyme remains on the market. Collagenase debrides wounds with the production of little pain and may be coapplied with antibiotics.

Mechanical debridement via pulsatile lavage, or low frequency ultrasound-assisted debridement for cleansing and removal of both large and small particulate matter, can be used singly or in conjunction with the other debridement procedures. In fact, many of these procedures can be effectively mixed and matched, although reimbursement is typically tied to only one procedure.

3.13.4 Bacterial Control

Bacterial control is another necessary component of advanced wound management.[201] A high wound bioburden may be a factor in nonhealing or chronic wounds and is certainly a major factor in the development of malodorous wounds. Currently, the definition of wound infection is being revised. Wound infection was previously defined as the presence of 10^5 organisms/gram of tissue. This definition is being extended to take account not only of the bacterial dose but also of the virulence of the microorganism and the state of the host or individual's resistance. The relationship among these factors is described by the following equation:

$$\text{Risk of tissue infection} = \frac{\text{Bacterial dose} \times \text{Virulence}}{\text{Host resistance}}$$

The importance of the individual's immune response in fighting tissue infection and the virulence of the offending organism must be fully considered. The above equation indicates that the presence of a small number of highly virulent organisms may produce tissue infection in a normal individual, just as a high number of relatively nonvirulent organisms may produce infection in an immunocompromised individual. Other factors such as tissue hypoxia and impaired circulation also play a role in determining host resistance and as such are important in individuals with conditions such as peripheral vascular disease, diabetes, lymphedema, and venous insufficiency, to name only a few. In individuals with lymphedema, tissues are at particular risk for hypoxia due to the often enormous amounts of fluid present in the interstitial spaces. The accumulation of fluid in the interstitial spaces of the connective tissue (dermis) of the skin progressively increases the diffusion distance for oxygen from dermal capillaries to the avascular outer layer (epidermis) of the skin. The result is the development of tissue hypoxia. This hypoxic state ultimately reduces the ability of the skin to heal or to fight infections. The accumulation of serum proteins also provides a nutritive media for the growth of microorganisms.

When tissue infection is suspected, the clinician has to confirm the diagnosis. The value of culturing wounds versus the use of clinical signs and symptoms in diagnosing wound infection is undergoing serious study. Research indicates that the following signs of local infection are good predictors of localized infection:

• Delayed healing.
• Wound bed color changes.
• Friable granulation tissue.
• Absence or aberrant granulation tissue.
• Strong odor.
• Increased drainage.
• Increased wound tissue pain.

The roles of wound culturing methods, biopsy, and swab are also being debated, and it is currently thought that quantitative swabs as well as tissue biopsy may be useful, especially in determining the best antibiotic to use against spreading tissue infection.

Individuals with lymphedema are at increased risk for cellulitis or acute tissue infection due to tissue hypoxia and a compromised immune system as the result of radiation or chemotherapy. *Staphylococcus aureus*, including methicillin-resistant *S. aureus*, is commonly the offending wound pathogen. Another common wound pathogen, *Streptococcus pyogenes*, often produces a more superficial form of cellulitis (erysipelas) that presents in the papillary or upper layer of the dermis. Individuals with lymphedema can receive prophylactic penicillin treatment due to their propensity to develop erysipelas. High numbers of gram-negative rods have also been detected in wounds in individuals with lymphedema.[203]

Quantitative swab cultures in a patient with grade 3 lymphedema demonstrated large numbers of *Proteus vulgaris*, along with 20 other types of microbes (Conner-Kerr and Sullivan, unpublished data). *P. vulgaris* is a gram-negative rod that is commonly found in the human intestinal tract. It is an opportunistic wound pathogen that is found in large numbers in lower extremity wounds associated with lymphedema. This finding is not surprising, given the difficulty that many individuals experience with personal hygiene due to significant enlargement of the lower extremities and the deep fissures between bulbous skin flaps.

One paper in the literature reports that povidone-iodine (Betadine) solution and ointment were well tolerated and useful in the treatment of infections caused by *S. aureus* and gram-negative rods.[203] There are few published studies regarding the treatment of wounds specifically associated with nonfilarial lymphedema, but best-practice approaches to the care of chronic wounds, especially those related to venous insufficiency,[204,205] can guide the selection of treatment. Several topical antiseptic dressings are available, with some based on a variety of silver technologies and others that use a slow-release formulation of iodine, cadexomer iodine. Cleansing of the skinfolds and the areas between them, along with any open wounds, is also imperative for removing irritants, debris, and microorganisms. These areas should also be dried carefully with a patting motion instead of a rubbing motion, as they are vulnerable to damage.

Some physicians prescribe the drying and antiperspirant agent aluminum hydroxide, prepared in an aqueous solution for heavily exuding areas of the lymphedematous limb. However, there is no literature to support this particular practice and its safety is unknown, especially in relation to the large surface available for absorption, given the micro-openings in lymphedematous skin.

Other therapies that may be useful in controlling bioburden levels include pulsatile lavage with suction, ultrasonic wound therapy systems, ultraviolet C, electrical stimulation, and topical antibiotics such as mupirocin (Bactroban cream).

Moisture Balance

The third critical component of wound bed preparation is moisture balance. Wounds can either be too wet or too dry, so the challenge is to balance the moisture content at the appropriate level for optimizing healing. Wounds such as those that occur due to venous insufficiency and/or lymphatic dysfunction are typically wet in nature and require an absorptive dressing with good fluid-handling characteristics. A variety of dressings are available that can provide absorption, including foams, alginates, super-absorbents, and combination dressings. These dressings have differing abilities to contain and remove excess fluid from the wound bed while preventing maceration of the surrounding tissue. Vertically wicking foam dressings that are semi-permeable with high moisture vapor transmission rates control wound exudates while protecting the periwound from excessive moisture. Large volumes of wound fluid can be effectively controlled by using negative-pressure therapy or baby diapers with super-absorbent materials.

Large volumes of wound fluid are typically observed in individuals who have grade 3[199,200] or gigantic edema, also known as elephantiasis. They may experience large open wounds with copious drainage (▶ Fig. 3.44). The wounds appear to "cry," due to the continuous visible formation of fluid droplets. The fluid production from these wounds is difficult to control, with most bandages becoming saturated within minutes. Several approaches have proved to be helpful in managing this high volume of wound exudate, including the use of baby diapers, adult incontinence pads, and negative-pressure therapy. A contact layer is placed between the open wound and the diaper or incontinence pad material to prevent irritation. The absorptive layer provided by the diaper or incontinence pad is held in place by compression bandaging using short-stretch bandages. Addition of an abdominal binder with its metal stays removed provides additional anchoring and compression for the bandaging.

When negative-pressure therapy (▶ Fig. 3.45) is used to control the copious drainage produced by lymphedema-associated wounds, the clinician

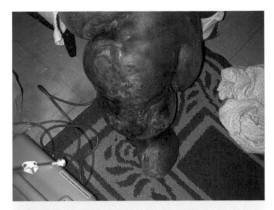

Fig. 3.44 A highly exudative wound associated with grade 4 lymphedema in a patient with chronic lymphedema.

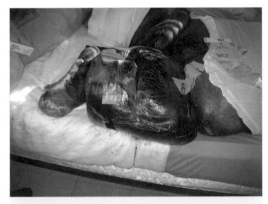

Fig. 3.45 A negative-pressure wound dressing placed over a large, highly exuding lower extremity wound in a patient with grade 4 lymphedema (4,000 mL collected over 2.5 days).

needs to be aware of the substantial amounts of time and materials involved in this method of treatment. Because the skin surrounding the wounds is quite fragile, with micro-openings that allow fluid drainage, it is difficult to secure an attachment site for the transparent film covering of the negative-pressure dressing. Preparations used to protect the skin and enhance attachment of the transparent film dressing also vary in their usefulness, due to the constant fluid leakage through the skin. It may only be possible to achieve a seal for a negative-pressure wound therapy dressing by attaching it to a remote skin site. In the patient shown in ▶ Fig. 3.45, a seal was only achieved using a large plastic bag, which was attached to intact tissues remote from the wounds being treated. With this treatment approach, caution needs to be observed in relation to the patient's safety when moving. A nonslip material (such as Dycem; Dycem Ltd., Warwick, RI) has to be affixed to the bag covering the bottom of the foot so that the patient does not slide during transfers or walking. Additionally, the seal must be maintained at all times so that the suction is not broken. If the suction is broken, the fluid accumulation associated with the wounds will saturate the foam dressing and significantly increase the weight of an already heavy and cumbersome limb.

3.13.5 Chronic Lymphedema Case Study

This 54-year-old woman is ambulatory and community dwelling individual who lives alone but receives daily assistance from a home health aide and family members. She can transfer independently with great exertion (5 minutes of preparation and transfer time) from her bed to standing (prone push-up using bedpost and walk short distances to the bathroom [< 10 feet]). She has chronic lymphedema with bilateral involvement of both lower extremities and lower trunk. She has the following diagnoses: CHF, diabetes mellitus (× 7 years), hypertension, and open superficial wounds bilaterally. Her wounds are partial thickness with max drainage (various modern dressing types tried and saturated within 15 minutes with serosanguinous drainage; very foul/putrid odor, poor quality granulation and minimum amounts of slough). Significant hyperkeratosis can be seen throughout her lower extremities bilaterally.

Patient Problems

- Limited independent ambulation.
- Difficulty with out of bed transfers.
- Difficulty with personal hygiene.
- Unable to prepare food.
- No community ambulation and inability to fit in standard vehicle for transportation to medical care.

Individual has significant foul/putrid smelling odor with copious drainage from extensive superficial wounds to the lower legs bilaterally. Family members and neighbors complain of odor from outside of apartment and talk with patient through the front window of her bedroom. Significant weight of the lower limbs impedes functional ambulation around public housing apartment and makes fitting inside of standard vehicle for transportation in the community difficult. There are safety issues in ambulation due to significant preparatory time for transferring out of bed and copious fluid draining from limbs as well as weight of limbs moved during walking to bathroom across the hall from bedroom. Patient cannot ambulate to kitchen for meal preparation and is dependent on home health aide for assistance with shopping and meal preparation. Patient would have significant difficulty escaping a home fire or protecting herself from home invasion.

Ambulation is further impaired with lack of ankle ROM in dorsiflexion (approximately –5 degrees). Individual uses a hip hiking and circumducting gait pattern to ambulate short distances during swing phase in order for the foot to clear the floor.

Intervention

Superficial wounds were treated with Iodosorb to decreasing bacterial counts (over 20 organisms characterized with *P. vulgaris* identified as the predominant organism) and assist with odor control. Negative pressure wound therapy was initiated to enhance fluid management. Gait training and upper and lower limb strengthening exercises were initiated. Intensive lymphedema management program was implemented with the use of abdominal bind (metal stays removed) to assist in keeping lymphedema wraps in place.

Challenges

The negative pressure wound therapy was difficult to maintain due to micro-openings throughout the skin (▶ Fig. 3.46) in the lower extremity that prevented the thin film dressings from adhering. Solution was to use a plastic trash bag to cover entire lower limb to groin area with Dycem in place to prevent skidding on the floor during ambulation. An associated drop in hematocrit was observed with the removal of more than six (500 mL) containers of fluid per day. Limb volume decreased by 10 cm in first week of treatment.

3.13.6 Lower Extremity Wound Considerations

Patients with lymphedema and CVI are prone to developing skin integrity impairments and wounds. Understanding basic skin integumentary, wound care principles and current evidence-based

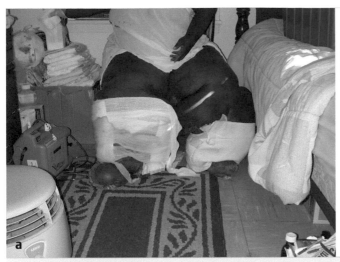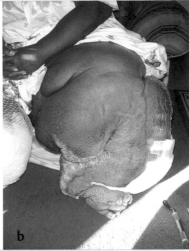

Fig. 3.46 (a) Individual with grade 3 lymphedema. Bilateral buffalo humps are apparent along with deep skin folds and copious drainage from superficial, partial thickness wounds. (b) Dry hyperkeratotic skin with significant hyperplasia and fibrosis (green circle) and abnormal skin folds due to grade 4 lymphedema. Skin located in crevices of skin folds was heavily macerated with significant numbers of microorganisms including fungus and yeast. Silver-based alginate and foam dressings were used to decrease microorganism number and to control moisture. Several papillomas can be seen in the folds located in the medial thigh region. Only the first and portion of the second toes are apparent due to large buffalo hump on dorsum of foot.

practices will allow the lymphedema therapist to communicate and document appropriately with health care professionals. When a wound is not progressing timely, the question should be "Why Not?" Complications can occur and usually could be caused by a vascular insufficiency, infections, nutritional deficits and/or edema to name a few. Wound care may seem simple but in reality there are many components that will challenge the clinician with limited wound care knowledge.

A patient walks into your clinic with the diagnosis of lower extremity edema with orders for CDT. During your assessment you notice a callus on his foot which you already have orders to apply a dressing. There is a difference in circumferential measurements between lower extremities, toes have been amputated and the patient has had this "on and off" wound for 2 years. The patient tells you that he received radiation to the upper anterior thigh and has a history of diabetes. You are convinced that this patient has secondary lymphedema. Are you ready to compress?

The answer may not be as simple as it may seem. This would require prompt communication with a team of professionals as further investigation is warranted before the possibility of compression is considered.

This was an actual patient at our clinic (▶ Fig. 3.47). The results could have been disastrous if the clinician did not assess them properly. Questions that came to mind were how did the wound/callus get there in the first place? Do they have an abnormal gait pattern? Do they use an assistive device? How is their ambulatory balance? Do they have loss of protective sensation? What is their shoe wear? Do they have an appropriate shoe? Do they have foot deformities? What is their ankle/toe/knee/hip ROM? Do they have sufficient muscle strength or is there an imbalance? Asking these questions may lead right to the source.

Patients with diabetes will often have a callus masking a wound. While determining the cause, other important information will include whether there is adequate circulation. Is there a wound infection? If they have clinical signs of infection have we properly cultured them to start antibiotic treatment? Is there bone exposed and do they have osteomyelitis? Is their glucose controlled? What is their blood glucose (HA1C) level? What is the presentation of the wound bed and periwound tissue? Is there swelling? Is the swelling a local inflammatory response, a chronic condition or complicated with a systemic condition (▶ Fig. 3.48)? Does the selected dressing match the

3

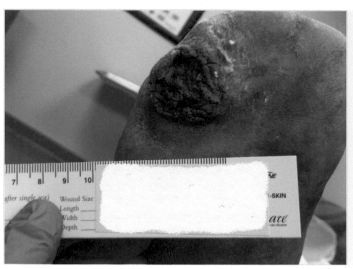

Fig. 3.47 Patient with diabetes complicated by secondary lymphedema with arterial insufficiency. Callus indicates abnormal weight bearing.

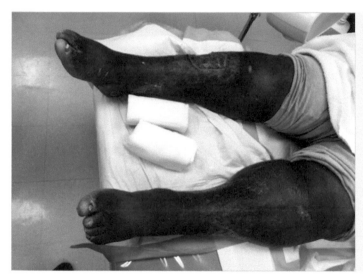

Fig. 3.48 Long-standing chronic venous insufficiency patient with secondary lymphedema complicated with end stage renal disease, arterial insufficiency and on dialysis.

patient & wound characteristics? How can we properly offload? Is there a gait deviation causing the callus? Reaching acceptable results and determining the cause will guide the clinician if compression is a proper intervention.

There are a multitude of factors that influence wound healing. Research indicates that as patient's comorbidities and complexities of wounds continue to increase a team approach is advantageous. A patient-centered model where each team member utilizes their knowledge and skills to the fullest will produce improved outcomes with these challenging patients. Currently health care has been focusing on patient outcomes, which are being tied

to reimbursement. A study by Akesson[206] found a leg ulcer healing rate of 23%, compared with an 82% healing rate after a team approach. Another study found that 72% of patients healed with an average of 12 weeks following a team approach.[207]

A team approach has been discussed but have we truly defined who is on the team and are we underutilizing our team members? For example, physical therapists help patients increase ROM, strength, and assist with ambulation. The reality is that therapists are also trained and able to treat patients with integumentary, musculoskeletal, cardiovascular, lymphatic, and/or neurological problems to name a few. Physical therapists are typically considered the "mobility experts," and able to increase mobility; studies suggest a decrease in function when a patient is wounded. Therapists can also help with wound bed preparation, assist with offloading and treat wounds using various types of compression wraps and/or other devices, able to sharp debride (therapists need to check state practice act and facility policies), utilize modalities such as electrical stimulation, pulse lavage, high & low frequency ultrasound, negative pressure, light therapy, and may attain certifications in CDT, wound care and other specific types of treatment that can have a positive impact with our chronic wound population.

Skin Integrity

The skin, part of the integumentary system, has various important functions as it is considered the largest organ in the human body. Skin consists of the epidermis and the dermal layers and its function is to protect, thermoregulate, and provide sensation. When the integumentary system is damaged, these functions are affected. In our line of work, skin integrity is important because impairments may lead to wounds and/or infections as the protective barrier is damaged.

Impaired skin integrity is defined as an alteration in the epidermis and/or dermis.[208] Understanding this organ, including its anatomic structures, physiological processes while performing a sound assessment of the integumentary system, is critical. When skin integrity is impaired it can lead to chronic wounds which can be difficult to treat.

As the numbers indicate, lower extremity ulcerations of various etiologies continue to increase in our population as we age. Of these, many become chronic in nature creating a significant problem to our health care system. Chronic wounds are defined as those wounds which have failed to proceed through an orderly and timely reparative process to produce anatomic and functional integrity over a period of 3 months.[209]

The Center for Medicare and Medicaid Services (CMS) requested an assessment report from the Agency for Healthcare and Quality Research (AHQR) summarizing the usual care for chronic wound management. On March 8, 2005 this report defined chronic wounds as those wounds that do not heal completely after receiving standard medical treatment for 30 days.[210]

It is estimated that in the US chronic wounds affect 6.5 million Americans with an annual cost of $2.5 billion and rapidly growing due to health care–associated costs, aging of the population and a rise in other conditions such as diabetes.[211]

The population 65 and over will increase from 35 million in 2000 to 55 million in 2020. Those over 85 years old are projected to increase from 4.2 million in 2000 to 7.3 million in 2020.[212] Acute and chronic wounds could be affected with other complications such as arterial disease creating a nonhealing environment. Peripheral arterial disease affects about 8 million Americans and 12 to 20% of Americans age 65 and older.[213]

Wound healing is a complex yet highly orchestrated and sequential cellular process where the injured tissue moves through the phases of healing. The phases of wound healing consist of the inflammatory phase, the proliferative phase and the maturation phase (▶ Fig. 3.49). These phases have important cellular functions in order to

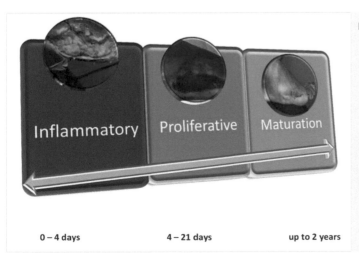

Fig. 3.49 Phases of healing.

Inflammatory   Proliferative   Maturation

0 – 4 days   4 – 21 days   up to 2 years

3

achieve wound closure. In comparison, just like in the stages of human development, we typically learn how to crawl followed by standing and walking. The wounds behave in the same fashion as progression will be dependent on the sequence of events occurring at each phase. Understanding this process and how to properly assess wounds maintaining the focus on the entire patient will be helpful in establishing a successful plan.

These phases overlap and the wounds may regress, remain stagnant, or progress pending on extrinsic and intrinsic factors. The inflammatory phase occurs when there is an injury to the body. Blood vessels dilate and constrict in order to allow essential cells to reach the wounded area followed by clot formation. This phase may last up to approximately 3 to 4 days and the typical signs of inflammation which are redness, warmth, swelling, and pain may be noticed.

The proliferation phase is where new tissue is being formed. Collagen is being laid down and new blood vessels are being developed. The formation of new blood vessels is called angiogenesis. This phase may start 4 days to 3 weeks after injury and granulation tissue growth and/or epithelialization, depending on the severity of the injury, may be noticed.

The maturation phase begins once the wound is closed. Scar tissue, which is only approximately 70% as strong as uninjured skin, is fragile initially and will take some time to mature. Protection of this newly healed area is important for up to 6 weeks after wound closure. Eventually full strength is achieved around 6 months.

A wound is defined as an injury to the body (as from violence, accident, or surgery) that typically involves laceration or breaking of a membrane (as the skin) and usually damage to underlying tissues.[214] Assessment is defined as "information obtained via observation, questioning, physical examination and clinical investigation in order to establish a baseline." This indicates that a wound assessment may not be as simple as it seems; wound assessment contains multiple components that must be considered in order to guide appropriate interventions.

The assessment of the entire patient is imperative in order to determine the cause of the integumentary defect and to have baseline data. This information can help the clinician determine which phase of healing the wound is in, establish if the wound has become chronic in nature, and rule out factors that may impede healing—all of which will lead to establishing an appropriate

diagnosis and available evidence based treatment interventions.

As previously stated in this chapter, if a patient has a wound or an ulcer, communication with the patient's physician and/or wound specialist is imperative. Basic patient and wound assessment will be discussed in order to document and communicate effectively with others. When treating wounds/ulcers, follow your facility policies as well as your state practice acts, rules, and regulations.

Three important aspects need to be considered when taking care of patients with wounds: the patient assessment, the wound assessment, and objective testing (▶ Fig. 3.50). In my opinion, they are all equally important as together they will paint a picture.

Patient Assessment

"The cure of the part should not occur until you take care of the whole." (Unknown)

Patient assessment involves collecting subjective information and objective data during an evaluation. Subjective data collection is defined as information given by the patient (or caretaker) describing the onset, course, and character of the presenting complaint.[215] Objective data can be defined as the information health care professionals collect through observation by touching, seeing, smelling, and hearing.

Combining the patient's subjective and objective data will help in determining the cause,

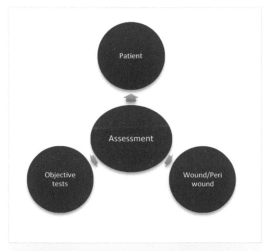

Fig. 3.50 Components of an assessment.

identifying factors that impede healing, and establishing if this is a chronic problem. A proper assessment will drive proper interventions.

A chronic wound is defined as a wound being present longer than 30 days with no progression. Chronic wounds are typically in the prolonged inflammatory phase of healing which will have different characteristics including a higher than normal amount of drainage. It is important to understand how chronic wounds differ from acute wounds (▶ Fig. 3.51).

It has been concluded that chronic wound fluid is cytotoxic, inhibits proliferation of normal cells, and has a decrease number of growth factors. It also promotes a chronic inflammatory response as it contains pro inflammatory cytokines, excessive levels of proteases, and a decrease level of TIMPs (tissue inhibitors of metalloproteinases)▶ Fig. 3.51. These will affect the wound from advancing through the phases of healing.

Chronic Wounds

Chronic wounds are likely to contain biofilm. Garth James et al, identified biofilms in 60% of biopsies of chronic wounds but only 6% in acute wounds.[216] Biofilms are communities of bacteria living inside a protective shield that are suspected to delay healing. Typically, clinicians assess wounds for the classic signs of infection which include erythema, warmth, edema, pain, and purulence. Chronic wounds may have these classic signs of infection but often there will only be subtle secondary signs of delayed healing. When a wound has these secondary signs, it is said to be

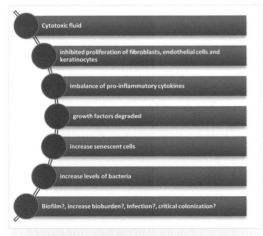

Fig. 3.51 Differentiating chronic wounds.

critically colonized. Critical colonization describes a bacterial invasion delaying wound healing with no host response. The wound will not present with the classic signs of infection but a delay in wound healing is encountered.

Secondary signs of infection include
- Delay of healing.
- Increased exudate.
- Friable tissue.
- Absent or abnormal granulation tissue.
- Increased or abnormal odor.
- Wound deterioration.
- Increased wound pain.

Patient assessment can begin with a patient questionnaire followed by a detailed examination. The questions can be geared toward seeking information on the nature of the problem, onset, any contributing factors, comorbid conditions, medications list, allergies, prior treatments, etc.

Good communication between the patient and health care professionals is important. The literature describes how it improves patient satisfaction, patient adherence to treatment program, and outcomes, but it can also guide the clinician to the correct diagnosis. In the short-term, improved communication leads to more effective diagnosis and treatment of health problems; in the midterm, to greater compliance with treatment programs, better utilization of services, and enhanced feelings of awareness and confidence for both client and provider; in the long term, to greater relief of symptoms, enhanced prevention and reductions in morbidity and mortality.[217] In some cases, overall health care costs are also reduced.[217]

During the patient assessments the health care provider is reviewing the patient's age, weight, vital signs, pain assessment, past and current medical and surgical history, reviewing body systems, looking at physical characteristics, intrinsic and extrinsic factors that may impede healing, etc., as demonstrated in ▶ Fig. 3.52. A determination is being established if the wound is acute or chronic in nature.

Understanding the mechanism of injury or how the wound appeared can help differentiate if the problem began due to pressure, long-standing venous congestion, infection, arterial insufficiency, diabetes, or possibly atypical in nature (▶ Fig. 3.53). This is of utmost importance because treatment interventions will be based on an accurate diagnosis.

Reviewing the body systems is recommended; systems include skeletal, muscular, nervous,

3

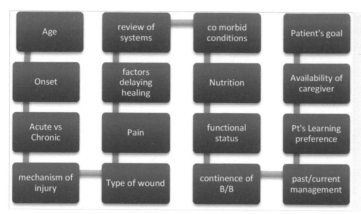

Fig. 3.52 Assessment of the patient.

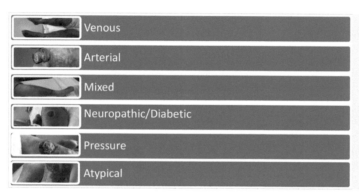

Fig. 3.53 Lower extremity wound etiologies.

respiratory, cardiovascular, lymphatic, endocrine, digestive, urinary, and integumentary systems. Various systems collectively work together in order for organs to function properly. If one system experiences damage, then the human body can become unstable, leading to serious consequences (▶ Fig. 3.54, ▶ Fig. 3.55).

Does the patient have factors that may impede healing such as age, chronic conditions, vascular insufficiency, poor nutrition, history of malignancies, acute versus chronic infections, nicotine use, hypoperfusion, stress, medications, abnormal lab values, excessive/abnormal pressure, dry wound bed environment, infection, and periwound abnormalities (▶ Table 3.13)? When encountering a chronic wound, one must consider these impediments in order to address them and restart the normal repair process (phases of healing).

Contrary to popular belief, time does not heal all wounds but what you do during that time is what matters. If a patient presents with a wound longer than 30 days, it is imperative to ask about any previous treatments received. This will provide

insight as to which products, treatment, and diagnostic tools were used. If products were applied properly, treatment interventions were selected from best practice guidelines and appropriate diagnostic tests were used, one can optimize their use of time by not reinventing the wheel. It should be established if the patient has undergone procedures and/or surgeries, or if they have any allergies, all which can point to contraindications for specific interventions.

Wound care can be affected by the communication that occurs between providers and patients as well as across the continuum of care. Clinical skill and competency also play an important role in wound healing.

Wound care clinicians can pursue various certifications and they are often advantageous. A study determined that nurses certified in wound care, compared to certification in other areas and no certification, demonstrated significantly higher scores on a knowledge test, attended more lectures on the subject and were more up to date with their readings.[218] In

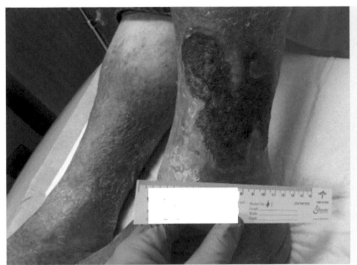

Fig. 3.54 Chronic venous insufficiency patient with ulcerations complicated with rheumatoid arthritis, arterial insufficiency, and liver disease.

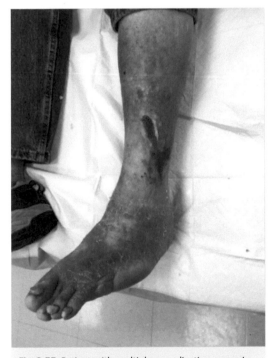

Fig. 3.55 Patient with multiple complications experiencing progress (see ▶ Fig. 3.54 for initial wound appearance). Once edema was appropriately controlled along with wound bed preparation, the patient's wound began to close.

Table 3.13 Factors affecting wound healing

Factors affecting wound healing	
Nutrition	Chemotherapy
Infection	Venous insufficiency
Oxygenation	Stress
Comorbidities	Obesity
Persistent inflammation	Immunocompromised conditions
Clinician's competency	Communication
Swelling	Dressing selection
Inappropriate wound care	Critical colonization
Medications	Activity level
Biofilm	Social environment
Age	Radiation
Patient's adherence to program	Anti-inflammatory steroid medication
Smoking	Pain
Alcohol usage	Malignancy
Trauma	Reduced wound temperature

today's times, with the complexity of wounds, the focus on outcomes, and the delivery of quality care, it behooves clinicians to pursue respective certifications. At the same time, employers are increasingly interested in hiring clinicians with proper training and credentials.

Once we can answer what caused the wound, how long it has been present, which interventions used were successful, which factors impede healing, and the patient's interpretation of their problems, then assessing the wound bed and periwound tissue becomes essential.

As an example, a patient presents to your clinic with diagnosis of lymphedema and classic textbook presentation of a chronic venous hypertension with orders for compression. There is hemosiderin staining (▶ Fig. 3.56), lipodermatosclerosis, a shallow wound bed and it is located in the medial malleolus area. If you skip the subjective assessment you might have missed the fact that the patient's ambulation is limited by pain in her lower extremities, she has resting pain especially when she lies down, and she is a heavy smoker. Her response was that after 10 feet of walking she experiences excruciating pain on her calves. Further testing indicated that this patient had critical limb ischemia, needing revascularization with compression being contraindicated at this point.

Your diagnosis should not be based on the lymphedema presentation without performing a thorough assessment including objective testing. Objective testing may include but not be limited to arterial noninvasive or invasive testing, imaging studies and laboratory testing such as a CMP (comprehensive metabolic panel), a CBC (complete blood count), HA1C (glycated hemoglobin), nutritional markers (albumin, pre albumin), clotting information such as PT (prothrombin time)/INR (international normalized ratio), inflammatory markers such as CRP (C-Reactive Protein) and ESR (Erythrocyte Sedimentation Rate), cultures, etc. (▶ Table 3.14).

Table 3.14 Laboratory testing and their values

Labs	Range	Rationale
WBC	3.8–11 × 10³/mm³	Measure of white blood cells, may detect infection
PT	10–14 s	PT/INR used to monitor anticoagulant effectiveness. Determines bleeding disorders.
INR	0.8–1.1 (if not taking blood thinners)	PT/INR sometimes selected before surgery and other invasive procedures
CRP	0–10 mg/L	C-reactive protein, level increases with inflammation
ESR	Male: up to 15 mm/h Female: up to 20 mm/h	Erythrocyte sedimentation rate, blood test that can reveal inflammatory activity
Albumin	3.5–5.0 g/dL	Used to help with nutrition deficits or as part of a liver panel
Prealbumin	20	Typically used to determine nutritional status
BUN	6–23 mg/dL	Test to determine kidney function
Creatinine	0.6–1.5 mg/dL	Test to determine kidney function
Glucose	65–99 mg/dL	Blood glucose level used to monitor in diabetics
HA1C	4–6%	Glycosylated hemoglobin used to screen & diagnose diabetics

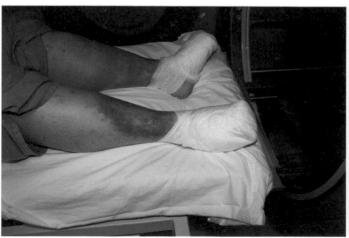

Fig. 3.56 Diabetic patient diagnosed with severe arterial insufficiency and chronic venous insufficiency. Note the hemosiderin staining.

In all essence, good patient assessment skills are usually developed over time with good consistent practice. Those who succeed will be able to communicate well with the patient and provide effective treatment.

Wound Assessment

"If you can't explain it simply, you don't understand it well enough."

Wound assessment is just as important as the patient assessment. The information collected for each assessment will contain valuable information to guide your treatment. The following quotes by Lord Kelvin will describe two similar but varied important components of an assessment. "If you cannot measure it, you cannot improve it." and "When you can measure what you are speaking about, and express it in numbers, you know something about it; when you cannot express it in numbers, your knowledge is of a meager and unsatisfactory kind; it may be the beginning of knowledge, but you have scarcely in your thoughts advanced to the state of science, whatever the matter may be."

A wound following the normal healing trajectory will progress from the inflammatory phase toward the proliferative phase and end with the maturation phase. Each phase has an approximate time frame of occurrence, key turn of events, and they do overlap.

A defect in our integumentary system is repaired by scar tissue. If the defect is superficial, it heals by means of epithelialization. This epithelialization repair process can occur from the wound edges or from intact appendages. If the wound edges are closed, rolled or callused, then healing may be delayed. When the integumentary damage is deeper, the void will need to fill in with granulation formation followed by epithelialization. Once the defect is closed with fragile epithelial tissue, the maturation phase has been reached and it may take up to 2 years for this remodeling process. This newly formed scar tissue strength will be 70 to 80% compared to skin.

A wound in the inflammatory phase will have characteristics of inflammation such as edema, warmth, pain, and redness. This phase occurs as a natural response to injury. After wounding and hemostasis occurs, vasodilation of vessels allows key cells such as white blood cells, enzymes, growth factors and nutrients to enter the site. The main function is for the cells to phagocytize and autolyze devitalized material. Chronic wounds may regress back to the inflammatory phase; characteristic of this regression may be subtle with signs such as friable tissue, abnormal granulation tissue, increased drainage, increased pain, increased odor, or a delay in the healing trajectory.

In the inflammatory phase, as the drainage increases, the selected dressing's absorbing capability and/or frequency of dressing change needs to match. This drainage–dressing mismatch may reveal maceration around the periwound skin and tissue. The wound may necessitate an increase in the frequency of dressing change, select a different dressing, and determine if the wound is critically colonized or if there is an infection needing proper course of treatment.

Wound progress is typically noted by a decrease in surface area and volume but also by improvement in wound characteristics. Several studies suggest a positive wound progression is based on the wound etiology and a 30 to 50% healing rate in 4 weeks.

Being able to collect and measure necessary wound information will help determine the correct course of action. ▶ Table 3.15 demonstrates how wound characteristics can drive the treatment.

An adequate wound assessment will include objective and measurable wound characteristics describing the wound bed, wound edges and periwound skin. Wound characteristics will determine if the wound is critically colonized or infected, if the possibility of an atypical condition exists, and if the wound is progressing, deteriorating or just plain "stuck."

Always keep in mind that a good understanding of basic principles is a must before utilizing advanced products. Concentrating on basic assessment skills is imperative to hone in the actual problem.

Understanding the repair process or the phases of healing with known characteristics of each phase will help determine how to successfully treat the patient's wound. This will partially assist the clinician in selecting treatment interventions. As discussed in this chapter, wound bed preparation is a beneficial component of wound care. If we do not prepare the wound bed properly and start applying expensive dressings, then product failure increases the possibility of leading to poor outcomes. The longer a wound remains open, the higher the opportunity for infection and possible amputation.

Table 3.15 Wound characteristics and rational for treatment

Wound characteristic(s)	Possible rationale
Clinical signs of infection	Appropriate culture to determine organism. Immunocompromised patients may not show typical signs of infection.
Increase wound size/depth	Wound not stable, trauma continues, underlying issue not properly addressed (vascular status, infection, etc.); nonviable tissue removal may increase size
Friable tissue, lack of wound progression	Critical colonization, increase bioburden
Increased drainage/maceration/and-or hypergranulation	Critical colonization, improper dressing category selection—not adequately absorbing exudate, inappropriate frequency of dressing change, infection not addressed
Absence of granulation	Inadequate blood flow, critical colonization/infection, wound in inflammatory phase, trauma
Edema	Decrease nutrient/oxygen supply due to increase diffusion distance, systemic related condition, chronicity/prolonged inflammatory phase, poor calf pump mechanism, lymphedema, improper compression
Odor	Dressing related vs. body part vs. infection
No to minimal change in nonviable tissue	Absence or delay of proper debridement method
Presence of callus	Abnormal weight bearing from improper footwear, offloading not effective, absence of protective sensation, abnormal biomechanics
Presence of redness	Skin irritation, cellulitis, infection, trauma, possible antibiotics not effective against actual organism
Pain	Lack of improper medication during procedure, impaired vascular system, trauma, deep infection
Absence of a pulse, cooler extremity, no hair on toes, thickened nails	Compromised arterial vascular status

A chronic wound in a prolonged inflammatory phase will need assistance progressing to the next phase. Classic signs or delayed signs of healing with the abnormal or absence of granulation tissue may be present; increase in drainage, hypergranulation tissue may be noted as well. The classic signs of infection include pain, swelling, redness, and odor, whereas the secondary signs include delayed progress, friable tissue, decreased, or abnormal granulation tissue.

Gethin reports that main advantages of continuous wound measuring are as follows: it is part of the initial assessment, it aids in re-evaluation, contributes to more accurate communication between professionals, provides objective information for an assessment, it enhances the quality of patient care, it monitors treatment efficacy, it aids in cost justifications for specific treatments, it may help predict healing, and it enhances the overall wound management.[219,220]

The initial wound assessment will provide objective data that serve as reference point to compare subsequent data. The data are used to communicate with other health care workers; it can assist with treatment decisions and select appropriate dressings to match the wound/peri-wound tissue characteristics. Reassessments should occur at regular intervals; at least weekly is recommended. Assessments and reassessments of the wound drive the treatment but will also indicate if the clinician is heading in the right direction. In today's evidence-based environment, there is sufficient available data indicating healing potential based on assessment data at certain endpoints. Studies also suggest outcomes based on etiologies and healing rates.

Basic wound care should emphasize looking for clues to determine what caused the wound (► Table 3.16) in the first place or its etiology. Being able to address the cause of the wound will

Table 3.16 Wound differentiation

	Venous	Arterial	Mixed	Neuropathy/Diabetic	Atypical
Predisposing factor(s)	Hx of DVT, CVI, prior ulcers, valve incompetence, poor calf pump, obesity	Atherosclerosis, diabetes, age, peripheral arterial disease	Venous and arterial ulcer	Diabetes, neuropathy, arterial complications	Vasculitis, inflammatory conditions, infections, malignancy
Location	Medial ankle, near malleolus	Areas where friction/trauma can occur, distal dorsal toes, lateral foot, between toes, over bony prominences		Plantar aspect of foot, heel, metatarsal heads	Wounds with atypical locations described in other categories
Characteristics	Shallow, regular margins, superficial wound, typically no pain, moderate to large drainage, ruddy granular tissue	"Punched out" appearance, deep wound bed, may have gangrene, absent to pale granulation tissue, pain, minimal drainage		Minimal to moderate drainage, possible osteomyelitis	Wounds with atypical characteristics
Patient assessment	Hx of ulcers, LE hemosiderin staining, lipodermatosclerosis, dilated superficial, veins, firm edema, often recurrent, aching/swelling at end of day, pain relieved with elevation	Hx of smoking, intermittent claudication, thin and shiny skin, no hair on toes, thickened nails, decreased temperature, absent/diminished pulses, inadequate foot wear, poor eyesight		Loss of protective sensation, foot deformities, clinical signs of infection (ADA guidelines), dry skin, inadequate foot wear, calluses on foot	Atypical presentation and location. Wound not healing after 3–6 months of appropriate tx should raise flags
Objective testing	Rule out (R/O) DVTs—venous Doppler; R/O arterial insufficiency—ABI/TBI, TCOM/SPP, CTA;R/O soft-tissue infection—punch biopsy/tissue culture; labs including (WBC, hemoglobin/hematocrit, CRP/ESR, PT/INR, kidney function etc.). Measure edema	See venous objective testing plus prolonged capillary refill (>4–5 s), dependent rubor; may also R/O osteomyelitis—probe bone, radiological studies —X-ray/MRI/triple phase bone scan, bone biopsy		See venous and arterial objective testing; HA1C	See objective testing under the venous and arterial section. Biopsy recommended
Possible treatment	If no contraindications: Wound bed preparation, compression, and education. Advanced modalities, possible surgical intervention	Protection, vascular referral depending on vascular testing results. If no contraindications, wound bed preparation and moist wound healing. Advanced modalities		See arterial section plus: glycemic control, offloading, education, if infected—treat. Revascularization if needed. Advanced modalities available.	Treatment varies depending on diagnosis and biopsy results.

help achieve a desirable outcome. It is common knowledge that 70 to 80% of lower extremity wounds are considered to be venous in nature. But we need to do our due diligence and rule out the other 20 to 30% possibilities. If a wound has inadequate arterial circulation, then revascularization will be of importance (▶ Fig. 3.57); if the wound is due to atypical conditions, then it may be controlled by medications, or if it is due to malignancy, then appropriate referral will be needed.

Establishing the cause will also lead to proper wound classification. Diabetic wounds are described by the Wagner scale (▶ Table 3.17) or the University of Texas scale (see Box), pressure ulcers use the National Pressure Ulcer Advisory Panel (NPUAP) pressure ulcer scale (▶ Table 3.18), venous ulcers use the CEAP scale (▶ Table 3.19), skin tears use the Payne-Martin Skin Tear Classification Scale (▶ Table 3.20), and Burns utilize the depth of involvement or degrees (▶ Table 3.21). The NPUAP, in April 2016, renamed pressure ulcers to pressure injuries and redefined their categories (▶ Table 3.22).

Table 3.17 Wagner scale

Grade	Description
0	Preulcerative lesion, healed ulcers, presence of bony deformity
1	Superficial ulcer without subcutaneous tissue involvement
2	Penetration through the subcutaneous tissue—may expose bone, tendon, ligament or joint capsule)
3	Osteitis, abscess, or osteomyelitis
4	Gangrene of the forefoot
5	Gangrene of the entire foot

University of Texas Wound Classification: System of Diabetic Foot Ulcers

Grade I-A: noninfected, nonischemic superficial ulceration.

Grade I-B: infected, nonischemic superficial ulceration.

Grade I-C: ischemic, noninfected superficial ulceration.

Grade I-D: ischemic and infected superficial ulceration.

Grade II-A: noninfected, nonischemic ulcer that penetrates to capsule or bone.

Grade II-B: infected, nonischemic ulcer that penetrates to capsule or bone.

Grade II-C: ischemic, noninfected ulcer that penetrates to capsule or bone.

Grade II-D: infected and ischemic ulcer that penetrates to capsule or bone.

Grade III-A: noninfected, nonischemic ulcer that penetrates to bone or a deep abscess.

Grade III-B: infected, nonischemic ulcer that penetrates to bone or a deep abscess.

Grade III-C: ischemic, noninfected ulcer that penetrates to bone or a deep abscess.

Grade III-A: infected and ischemic ulcer that penetrates to bone or a deep abscess.

Wounds are described based on their characteristics. Noting specific details or characteristics will assist the clinician to communicate with others and select proper interventions. If a

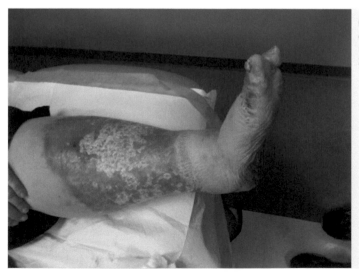

Fig. 3.57 Diabetic patient with Charcot's foot arthropathy, cellulitis, arterial disease, and chronic venous insufficiency.

Table 3.18 Pressure Ulcer Staging (National Pressure Ulcer Advisory Panel's previous staging system)

Stage I	Intact skin with nonblanchable redness over bony prominence
Stage II	Partial thickness loss of dermis—without slough
Stage III	Full-thickness tissue loss
Stage IV	Full-thickness tissue loss with exposed tendon or bone
Unstageable	Full-thickness tissue loss in which wound bed is covered with slough and/or eschar
Suspected deep tissue injury	Purple or maroon localized area of discolored intact skin or blood filled blister

Table 3.20 Payne-Martin Skin Tear Classification

Category IA	Linear type skin tear, epidermis and dermis pulled apart, without tissue loss
Category IB	Epidermal flap completely covers the dermis within 1 mm of the wound margin
Category IIA	Scant tissue loss type < 25% of the epidermal flap loss
Category IIB	> 25% epidermal flap loss
Category III	Epidermal flap absent

Table 3.22 Pressure injury stages (Adapted from National Pressure Ulcer Advisory Panel redefined the staging system on April 2016)

Stage 1	Nonblanchable erythema of intact skin
Stage 2	Partial-thickness skin loss with exposed dermis
Stage 3	Full-thickness skin loss
Stage 4	Full-thickness skin and tissue loss
Unstageable Pressure Injury	Obscured full-thickness skin and tissue loss
Deep Tissue Pressure Injury	Persistent nonblanchable deep red, maroon or purple discoloration

Table 3.19 CEAP

Clinical:	C0: No clinical signs
	C1: Small variocose veins
	C2: Large varicose veins
	C3: Edema
	C4: Skin changes without ulceration
	C5: Skin changes with healed ulceration
	C6: Skin changes with active ulceration
Etiology:	Ec: Congenital
	Ep: Primary
	Es: Secondary (usually due to prior DVT)
Anatomy:	As: Superficial veins
	Ad: Deep veins
	Ap: Perforating veins
Pathophysiology:	Pr: Reflux
	Po: Obstruction

Table 3.21 Burns

First degree		Very painful but not blistered
Second degree	Partial thickness	Extend through the epidermis and may penetrate dermis. Healing by regeneration; full function should be recovered
Third degree	Full thickness	Penetrates the dermis and may involve subcutaneous tissue. Hair follicles, sebaceous glands and sweat glands
Fourth degree		Extends into the subcutaneous tissue. May rapidly lead to infections or sepsis

wound has redness, swelling, and pain, it may indicate clinical signs of infection which will be treated differently from a noninfected wound. Documenting the wound characteristics will also allow the clinician to determine if an intervention is working, if there is adequate progress and insurance companies may request documentation for treatment coverage.

When describing and documenting wound characteristics, consider the following:

Location

- Numbering each wound then naming a wound in relation to an anatomic landmark, such as bony locations, is ideal to maintain consistent reference and documentation. It is also helpful to use a body diagram indicating where wounds are located in addition to their respective number.

Size

- Collecting this information is important as it should be measured accurately, consistently, and with low inter-reliability error. It is recommended to measure in centimeters and each institution should determine their preferred method for measuring length and width. Examples include, linear measurements, measuring the greatest length by greatest width, or the clock method, or a combination of the two, wound tracing, planimetry (measures volume from a photograph or wound tracing), to name a few.
- Clock method (▶ Fig. 3.58)—using numbers on the face of a clock and having reference as the head position at 12 o'clock position and the feet at 6 o'clock position (maintaining the body in anatomic position), your first measurement will be your length taken from 12 to 6 o'clock position and your width will be from 3 to 9 o'clock position capturing the greatest length and perpendicular to this is the greatest width. If the wound margins are irregular in shape, then you can change your reference points as long as length and width are still perpendicular to each other.
- When measuring wounds on the feet, the 12 to 6 o'clock position orientation is heel to toes.
- Surface area will be determined by multiplying the length by the width.

Depth

- Depth is measured by locating the deepest portion in the wound, inserting an appropriate applicator perpendicular to the skin and measuring the distance from the tip of the applicator to where skin should normally exist. Depth is also measured in centimeters.
- If depth is increasing as nonviable tissue is removed, then this would be acceptable and explain the discrepancy.

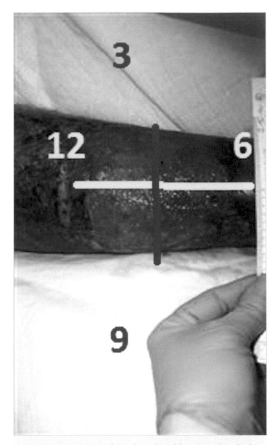

Fig. 3.58 Measuring length and width using the clock method. Length is 12 to 6 o'clock position and width is 3 to 9 o'clock position.

Drainage

- Exudate, another name for drainage, is defined as a fluid with a high content of protein and cellular debris that has escaped from blood vessels and has been deposited in tissues or on tissue surfaces, usually as a result of inflammation.[221]
- As wounds progress, their drainage should decrease to a minimal and manageable amount. An increase of drainage may be indicative of critical colonization, infection, or inappropriate dressing selection.
- Amount:
  - None—skin is intact or eschar covering skin defect.
  - Minimal—tissue is moist or drainage covers less than 25% of dressing.
  - Moderate—drainage covers between 25 and 75% of dressing.

○ Maximal—excessive drainage or drainage covers more than 75% of dressing.
- Type:
  ○ Serous—thin and clear drainage. Drainage consists of protein and fluid in the tissue.
  ○ Serosanguinous—typically pink. Contains small number of blood cells within the serous drainage.
  ○ Bloody—red bloody drainage.
  ○ Purulent—thick drainage most often yellow in color.

Color of Wound Bed

- Describing the color of tissue within the wound bed assists the documenting progress within specific time frames and aids in determining the type of tissue.
- Describing red tissue does not indicate finding healthy granulation tissue in the wound bed.
- The clinician reports the percentage of each color contained within the wound edges in which the sum will equal to 100% (▶ Fig. 3.59).
  ○ Red—could be indicative of healthy or unhealthy tissue
  ○ Yellow—most often slough, nonviable bone, nonviable tendon
  ○ Black—necrotic tissue such as eschar
  ○ Other—Gray, white, dark red

Type of Tissue

- Tendon (▶ Fig. 3.60a)—if exposed, goal is to keep it viable.
- Epithelial tissue—fragile healed tissue that maybe pink in nature.

- Eschar (▶ Fig. 3.60b)—black leathery nonviable tissue.
- Slough (▶ Fig. 3.60c)—yellow stringy adherent or no adherent nonviable tissue.
- Hypergranulation (▶ Fig. 3.60d)—granulation tissue with excess moisture (see picture).
- Granulation (▶ Fig. 3.60e)—beefy red viable tissue.
- Fibrin—fibrinous tissue.
- Adipose tissue—exposed tissue may be nonviable.
- Bone—if bone is exposed rule out osteomyelitis and must keep it viable.

Tunnels or Sinus Tracts

- Tunnels can be described as any pathways under the skin that may run in various directions. They may connect other wounds under the skin. It is important to locate these as proper irrigation and packing is warranted.
  ○ Proper irrigation should be utilized when cleaning tunnels. The cleansing method should provide enough pressure to remove debris yet not cause trauma to the wound bed. The optimal pressure to cleanse is between 4 and 15 psi. A 35 mL syringe with 19-gauge angiocath creates an 8-psi irrigation pressure stream, which may be used to remove adherent material in the wound bed.[222]
  ○ Common causes include but are not limited to foreign materials, trauma, infection and surgical interventions.
  ○ Tunnels are measured in centimeters.
  ○ Describe location of tunnel by using the face of the clock for reference (clock method).
  ○ Use a proper applicator and measure.

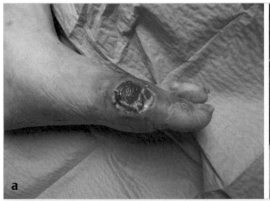
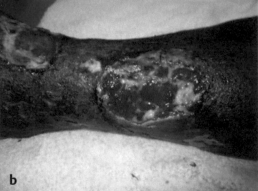

Fig. 3.59 Determining wound bed color. **(a)** Tissue: red, 70%; yellow, 20%; black, 10%. Diabetic ulcer complicated with arterial insufficiency and osteomyelitis. **(b)** Tissue: red, 60%; yellow, 20%; grey, 20%. Venous insufficiency wound with severe pain. Biopsy revealed severe vasculitis.

3

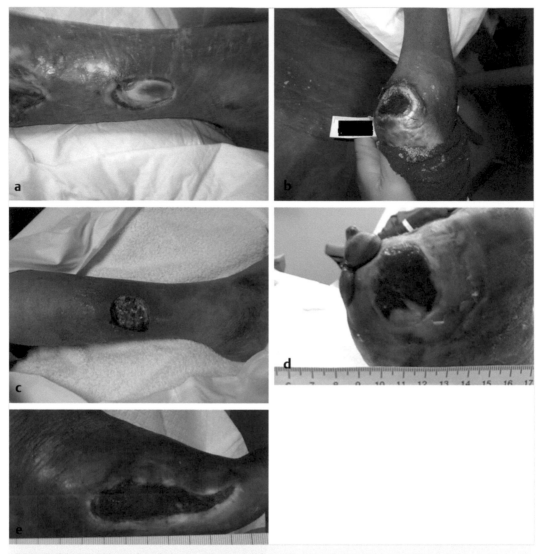

Fig. 3.60 (a) Nonviable tendon. (b) Eschar. (c) Slough. (d) Hypergranulation tissue. (e) Granulation.

Undermining

- Undermining can be described as a pocket extending from the wound bed under skin/tissue. Typically, these are found in pressure ulcers caused by friction and shear.
  - Describe location based on the clock method providing a starting and ending location of pocket. For example, + undermining from 1 to 4 o'clock measuring 4 cm.
- Measure deepest part of pocket in centimeters.

Wound Edges

- It is imperative to assess the wound edges. A superficial wound heals by epithelialization as the epithelial cells migrate from the wound edges to close defect. If wound edges are closed, then the chances of it becoming a chronic wound increase. The following list describes various possibilities of wound edges encountered:
  - Well defined
  - Open

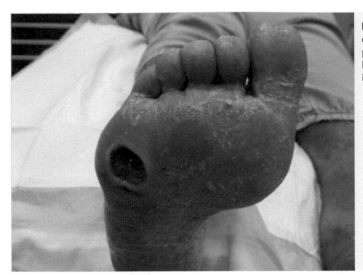

Fig. 3.61 Diabetic patient with a chronic ulcer complicated with neuropathy, closed wound edges, exposed bone, and infection. No clinical signs of infection but biopsy was positive.

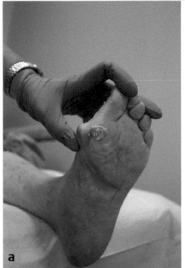

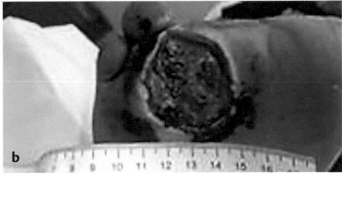

Fig. 3.62 A diabetic patient with neuropathy. **(a)** Callus covering defect. **(b)** Necrotic tissue under callus (silver nitrate used in wound bed).

- ○ Closed (▶ Fig. 3.61)
- ○ Rolled
- ○ Callused (▶ Fig. 3.62)

Periwound assessment includes

Redness

- Redness can indicate inflammation, infection, skin irritation, etc. Being able to compare serial measurements will determine if current treatment is appropriate (▶ Fig. 3.63).

- Measure redness extending from edge of the wound, measure in centimeters. Describe location using the clock method.

Induration

- Defined as the hardening of a tissue, particularly the skin, caused by edema, inflammation, or infiltration by a neoplasm.[223]
  - ○ Measure hardened tissue starting at the edge of the wound to the where the skin becomes normal.

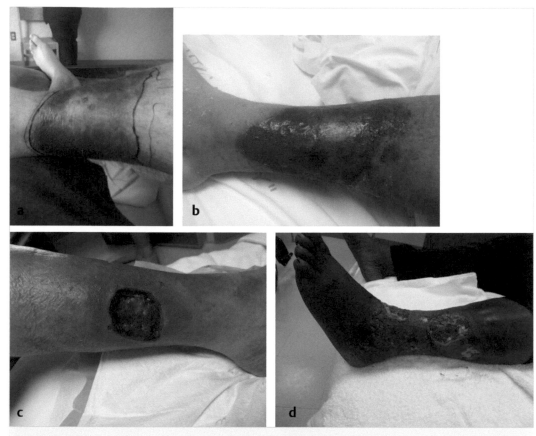

Fig. 3.63 Redness: **(a)** periwound from a spider bite; **(b)** spider bite redness decreasing; **(c)** from an infection; **(d)** from inflammatory process—redness on a dark pigmented individual is noted by darker periwound skin tone.

○ Measure in centimeters and describe the location of induration using the clock method.

Odor

- When assessing odor, it is recommended to cleanse the wound and then assess. Sometimes the location, body odor, incontinence or the dressing reacting with wound exudate will provide you with unpleasant or unfamiliar odors.
  ○ Strong or Foul—may indicate infection.
  ○ Sweet—typically indicative of Pseudomonas. Sometimes accompanied by a blue-greenish drainage residue found on the dressing.

Temperature

- Skin temperature can be measured by palpation or with an infrared thermometer. Infrared thermometer will be able to pick up slight skin differences compared to palpation. Differences in

mirror-image readings using the Fahrenheit scale are easier to detect a 3 °F to 4 °F temperature difference related to deep and surrounding infection, deep inflammation, or unequal vascular supply.[224]
- Good indicator for evaluating circulatory response, repeated trauma and inflammation.
- When assessing the temperature, it is a great idea to compare the involved with uninvolved extremity.

Pain

- Pain is an unpleasant feeling that is conveyed to the brain by sensory neurons. Wound pain is common, highly subjective[225,226,227,228] and can be particularly distressing for both patients and clinicians. It has multiple causes and, unfortunately, is often managed inadequately.[229,230,231] Pain that a patient experiences is influenced by many factors and there are studies indicating that pain is often underestimated or mismanaged by health professionals.[232,233]

- Pain may be indicative of an infection. Pain may also be experienced during dressing changes and with certain procedures such as debridement.
- There are a few pain scales available such as
  ○ Wong-Baker FACES Pain Rating Scale – used for ages 3 and older (▶ Fig. 3.64).
  ○ Numerical Rating Scale – 0, being no pain through 10 being worst possible pain.
  ○ Visual Analogue Scale – patient's subjective feeling of pain.

Maceration

- Excess moisture over intact skin results in the softening and destruction of skin. The skin will have a white appearance initially and with prolonged exposure it will continue to deteriorate (▶ Fig. 3.65).
- Measured in centimeters.
- Measure same way as induration. Use the clock method to determine location and measure the distance from the edge of the wound to where maceration ends.
- An increase in moisture may be due to infection, inappropriate dressing selection, infrequent dressing change

Sensation

- Testing sensation is important in order to determine if patients have protective sensation.
- Nerves are responsible for sensory, autonomic and motor functions. Sensory usually tested with the monofilament and when impaired trauma may occur. When autonomic is impaired, dry skin is noted and skin care is a must. And when motor is affected, muscle imbalances exist as well as weight bearing structural changes.
- Loss of protective sensation will warrant a prompt referral to an appropriate specialist and evaluation for proper footwear
- Protective Sensation can be tested using the Semmes Weinstein 5.07 (10g) Monofilament level (▶ Fig. 3.66).

Instructions for test on foot for loss of protective sensation:

- Explain the procedure.
- Test monofilament on upper extremity for patient understanding.
  ○ Touch the monofilament to the skin on the foot for 1 to 2 seconds, until the monofilament bends (do not use over wounds, callus or scars). Multiple locations on both feet tested (dorsum of mid foot, heel, 1st/3rd/5th toes - plantar area of toes then metatarsal heads, and plantar mid foot). Document whether or not the patient feels the monofilament.

Fig. 3.64 Wong-Baker FACES Pain Rating Scale (© 1983 Wong-Baker FACES Foundation. www.WongBakerFACES.org. Used with permission. Originally published in Whaley & Wong's Nursing Care of Infants and Children. © Elsevier Inc.)

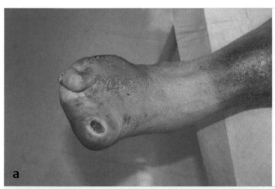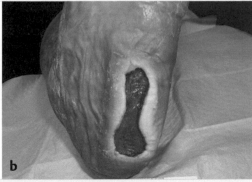

Fig. 3.65 Maceration periwound. **(a)** Hypergranulation noted, **(b)** no granulation noted.

3

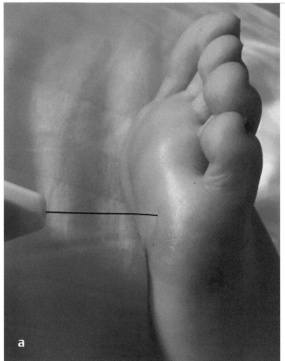 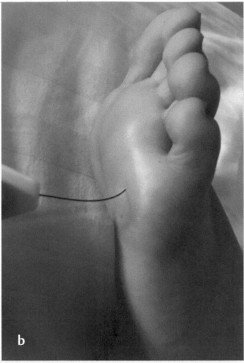

Fig. 3.66 Semmes Weinstein monofilament testing.

Edema

- Edema is usually caused by fluid leaking from the capillaries into the nearby tissue.
- It can be caused by venous congestion, trauma, faulty calf pump mechanism, lymphedema and systemic diseases, such as kidney damage, heart failure, liver disease and others.

Edema affects wound healing due to a decreased amount of oxygen and nutrients being transported to the tissue.

- Edema can be described as pitting or nonpitting. Pitting edema can be described by the indentation; see ▶ Table 3.23.
- Typically measured circumferentially at predetermined points. Measures in centimeters and on initial assessment recommend to measure other extremity if available for comparison. Other forms of measurements are available such as water displacement, volumetric measurements, etc.
- Patient must be cleared by the physician and adequate vascular testing needed before providing compression.

Table 3.23 Description of pitting edema. Adapted from the *Guelph General Hospital Congestive Heart Failure Pathway*

Pitting Edema	Description
1+	2 mm or less
	Slight pitting, no visible distortion, disappears rapidly
2+	2–4 mm
	Somewhat deeper pit, no readably detectable distortion, disappears in 10–15 s
3+	4–6 mm
	Pit is noticeably deep, lasts > 1 min, dependent extremity looks fuller and swollen
4+	6–8 mm
	Pit is very deep, last as long as 2–5 min, dependent extremity is grossly distorted

- CVI patients benefit from ruling out a DVT in the involved extremity.

Range of Motion (ROM)

- ROM can be defined as the available movement of a joint. Typically measured in degrees by an instrument called a goniometer.
- When evaluating musculoskeletal injuries and wounds, physical therapist typically concentrates on available ROM. When ROM is limited it will have an effect at a functional level as you will see in the examples listed below. Research indicates that musculoskeletal impairments are related to function[234] and disability.[235]
- Limitations in lower extremity ROM will affect the patient's gait and decrease the calf-pump mechanism which may delay wound healing if not addressed (▶ Fig. 3.67).
- When ankle dorsiflexion is limited (▶ Fig. 3.68), the calf pump mechanism is not effective which will increase venous hypertension. With prolonged hypertension the patient may experience valvular failure leading to CVI and if not treated lymphedema.
- Patients with diabetes will experience Achilles tendon stiffness (▶ Fig. 3.69) leading to a decrease ROM at the ankle. During the gait cycle,

a decrease ankle ROM will lead to abnormal biomechanics creating an excessive force on the distal plantar foot.

Documenting wound characteristics (▶ Table 3.24) and describing them will provide the clinician a starting point, guide interventions, and—equally important—it will help with reimbursement. Health care is transitioning from a volume based system to a system that will be focused on quality and outcomes. The impressive results that we come across on a regular basis can be captured with our documentation. In other words, tell the story of each patient to others via your documentation.

Vascular Testing

A patient walks into your clinic with lower extremity edema with orders for CDT and application of hydrogel ointment. During your assessment a small wound is noticed on his foot, there is a difference in circumferential measurements between lower extremities, a positive Stemmer's sign, and the patient has had the wound for 2 years. The

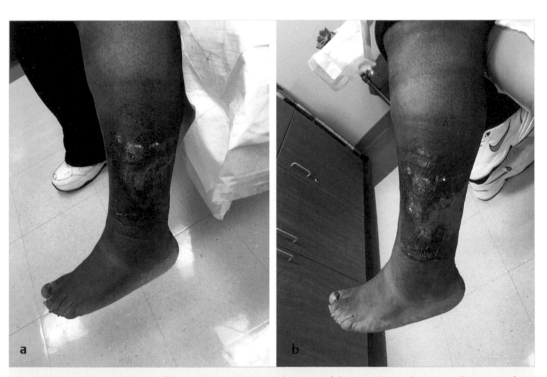

Fig. 3.67 **(a)** Chronic venous insufficiency ulcer with maximal amount of drainage. Patient has an antalgic gait with a poor muscle function calf pump. During ambulation patient is not able to achieve dorsiflexion. **(b)** Ulcer healed after appropriate level of compression applied.

3

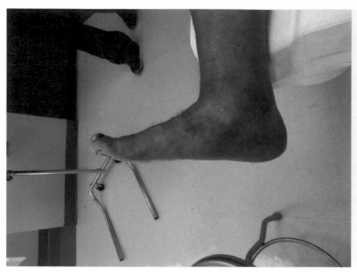

Fig. 3.68 Diabetic patient with limited ankle dorsiflexion altering his gait biomechanics and increasing plantar peak forces.

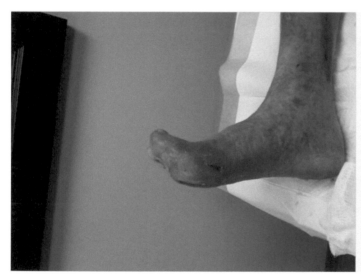

Fig. 3.69 Diabetic patient with stiff Achilles tendon and decreased range of motion (ROM). Unable to straighten toes to normal.

patient tells you that he received radiation to the upper anterior thigh and has a history of diabetes. You are convinced that this patient has secondary lymphedema. Are you ready to compress?

The answer would be *no*. Red flags are popping everywhere. A lower extremity vascular assessment must be performed. He had diabetes prior to his new onset of lymphedema. Patients may have conditions where the arterial system is compromised. His vascular testing indicated that he had critical limb ischemia and urgent vascular referral was needed.

Vascular testing is typically ordered with lower extremity wounds to confirm your clinical diagnosis as well as to establish adequate arterial blood flow in order to proceed with treatment interventions. Remember that 70–80% of lower extremity wounds are noted to be venous related making the other 20–30% wounds to possibly have an arterial component (▶ Fig. 3.70) or be atypical in nature. As mentioned before, wounds will not heal without adequate blood flow. Treatments such as compression, debridement of stable wounds, total contact cast and advanced biological products, to name a few are contraindicated if there is not adequate arterial flow.

During the assessment, the clinician begins with palpating arterial pulses such as the popliteal,

Table 3.24 Wound assessment/characteristics

Wound assessment	
Location:	Use bony landmark as reference.
Wound type:	Arterial, venous, neuropathy, pressure, atypical, etc.
Size: length and width	Measure in centimeters. Various methods exist.
Depth:	Measure depth perpendicular to skin and in centimeters.
Drainage: amount Type	None/min/mod/max Serous, bloody, serosanguinous, purulent
Color of wound bed:	Red, pink, yellow, black, grey, white. Describe in %
Odor:	None/mild/sweet/foul
Type of tissue:	Granulation, hypergranulation, eschar, slough, fibrin, etc.
Undermining:	Location described by clock method and measured in cm
Tracts:	Location described by clock method and measured in cm
Periwound:	
Induration	Location described by clock method and measured in cm
Redness	Location described by clock method and measured in cm
Warmth	Compare LEs temp w/palpation or infrared thermometer
Maceration	Document if present
Sensation	Light touch, Semmes Weinstein monofilament, vibration
Edema	Circumferential measurements, volumetric, others
Pain	Subjective, address prior to dressing changes/procedures
Wound edges	Open, closed, rolled, calloused
ROM	Any limitations affecting function or calf pump mechanism

dorsalis pedis, and posterior tibial vessels (▶ Fig. 3.71, ▶ Fig. 3.72). The dorsalis pedis pulse is reported to be absent on 8.1% of healthy individuals and the posterior tibialis pulse is absent on 2% of the population. The absence of both pedal pulses, when assessed by an experienced clinician, strongly suggest the presence of pedal vascular disease.[228] As you are palpating for pulses it is a good practice to determine if there is a difference in temperature between lower extremities. A cooler to touch distal extremity may be indicative of poor circulation.

In the wound care clinic, patients with lower extremity wounds will undergo noninvasive arterial testing to establish adequate blood flow. Further testing and prompt referrals will be obtained if abnormal values are encountered. During the patient assessment, examination of pulses has been established by palpation and/or use of a Doppler ultrasound. But you must not stop here. Some clinicians are satisfied with the palpation of lower extremity pulses. A study by Lundin M et al showed a high proportion of misdiagnosis of peripheral arterial disease using distal extremity pulse palpation as a single diagnostic method. The degree of underdiagnosis was unacceptably high at more than 30%.[236] Collins et al concluded that pulse palpation is not sensitive for the detection of peripheral arterial disease (PAD) compared to an ankle-brachial index test (ABI). More than two thirds of the patients with PAD had a detectable pulse.[237] Studies suggest that 60% of patients with a palpable pulse had adequate circulation, effectively making the other 40% of patients having an inadequate lower extremity arterial circulation.

Selecting proper vascular tests for our patients is now being tied to reimbursement. Available advanced products and treatments are not being reimbursed on the outpatient arena if vascular assessment data is not available. In all essence, if vascular assessments are not being ordered as the "right thing" to do for our patients, clinician's outcome/quality scores, as well as their reimbursement will suffer.

Assessment of the circulatory system (large and small vessels) is a priority anytime patients have a lower extremity wound. Noninvasive tests are available to determine the macro vascular circulation. These tests include ABI, toe indices, toe pressures, pulse volume recording, ultrasounds, and segmental leg pressures. Noninvasive microvascular tests include transcutaneous oximetry (TCOM) and Skin Perfusion tests (SPP). Further investigation is warranted and proceeding with a screening tool such as the ABI. An ABI will provide baseline information for reference as well as intervention guidelines; refer to ▶ Table 3.12 for levels of impairments and clinical picture.

3

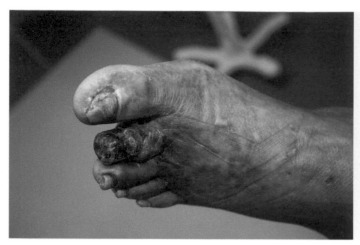

Fig. 3.70 Arterial wound complicated with arterial insufficiency and dialysis.

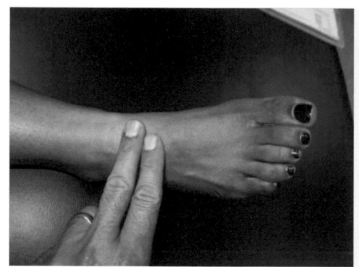

Fig. 3.71 Palpation of dorsalis pedis arterial pulse.

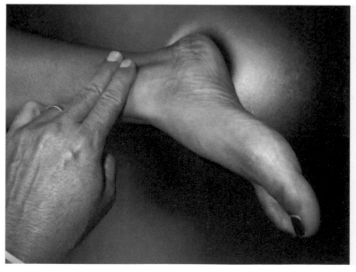

Fig. 3.72 Palpation of the posterior tibialis arterial pulse. This patient does not have a wound or skin impairments. If patient has a wound, Personal Protective Equipment (PPE) is required.

It is important to mention that the ABI is only a screening tool and further testing is needed if abnormal ABI values are encountered. In the literature we recognize severe arterial disease if the value is below 0.5 but it is also considered to have a noncompressible vessel if the ABI is higher than 1.2, therefore unable to attain a satisfactory systolic pressure.

Arterial vessels, when calcified, yield a higher than normal ABI value, warranting further testing and prompt referral. It must also be noted that these patients may need a referral with a cardiologist especially if an ABI is higher than 1.4 because they may have calcification in other locations such as in the carotid vessels.

A toe brachial index (TBI) is also attained with an ABI. TBIs are used when ABIs are noncompressible since digital arteries are rarely calcified.

If a patient has a great toe, a TBI can be established; see ▶ Table 3.25 for TBI values. A TBI is performed just like an ABI but using the great toe and selecting the digital arteries.

To calculate a TBI, divide the highest toe pressure by the highest brachial pressure.

TBI = Toe systolic pressure/brachial systolic pressure

A toe systolic pressure greater than 30 mm Hg may be an indicator that there is healing potential in a foot with ulcers.

Transcutaneous Oximetry (TcPO2)

Transcutaneous oximetry (TcPO2), or TCOM measures excess oxygen diffusion in the periwound skin. It measures the oxygen molecules within the periwound tissue. This is not an oxygen perfusion test as a pulse oximeter. This test is used for assessing wound healing potential, screening for vascular disease, assessing after revascularization, predicting amputation level and predicting benefits of hyperbaric oxygen therapy (HBOT).

Normal limb TcPO2 values are 50- 60 mm Hg (▶ Fig. 3.73), though values greater than 55 mm Hg

Table 3.25 TBI interpretations

TBI Interpretation[15]	
0.64 ± 0.20	Limbs normal
0.52 ± 0.20	Claudication in limbs
0.23 ± 0.19	Limbs with ulcers or ischemic rest pain

Table 3.26 Transcutaneous oxygen measure values

TcPO2 Value	Interpretation
> 50 mm Hg	Normal
40 mm Hg	Unimpaired wound healing
< 30 mm Hg	Impaired wound healing
20 mm Hg	Predicted rest pain, ischemic ulceration, gangrene.
< 20 mm Hg	Amputation likely

at any site regardless of age are considered normal.[238] Wound healing is considered unimpaired at pressures less than 40 mm Hg.[239] Pressures of 20 mm Hg are seen in legs with rest pain, ischemic ulcers, and/or gangrene, while pressures below 20 mm Hg usually require amputation (▶ Table 3.26).[240]

Provocative testing during the TCOM is performed in order to determine possible reasons for low baseline values. Low baseline values may be due to edema, inflammation and micro vascular involvement. When testing patients baseline results are obtained when the patient is supine. They must lie still for 15 minutes while the machine performs calibration tests and warms the electrodes to 45 degrees C. Patients with pulmonary disease, heart failure and PVD can also have low values. Once you obtain the baseline values in supine you proceed with leg elevation for 15 minutes. If the reading drops greater than 10 mm Hg, or 20% more than baseline, then it may indicate macro vascular disease. Followed by testing with a non-rebreather mask with oxygen, which is used to determine if vascular issues exist or if it is related to edema or infection. An increase in TcPO2 to 100 mm Hg or 100% from baseline during the oxygen challenge indicates low baseline values may be due to edema or inflammation and not peripheral arterial disease.

TcPO2 testing may require approximately 45 to 60 minutes. Avoidance of placing electrodes over bony prominences, vessels, calloused areas, and plantar foot is important. The disadvantage is not being able to apply over most digits due to electrode size because a tight seal is needed. Patients that are on continuous oxygen will experience limitations for this test.

TCPO2 has a wound healing predictive accuracy of 83%.[241] It can also predict response to revascularization. TCOM values that increase at least 30 mm

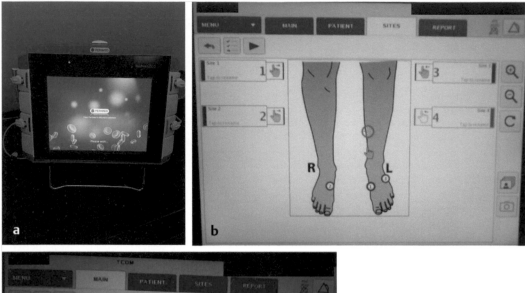

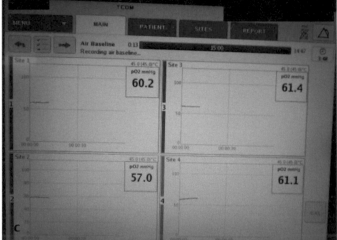

Fig. 3.73 **(a)** TCOM machine. **(b)** Electrode location and placement. **(c)** Actual test.

Hg after either endovascular or surgical revascularization are associated with a successful revascularization procedure and with a high likelihood of healing an open wound.[116] It was also found that an optimal waiting period of at least three days but optimally one week before TcPO2 measurements after surgical interventions.[242] Ballard and colleagues found that a trans metatarsal TcPO2 level of 30 mm Hg or greater successfully predicted healing with conservative care in 31/36 (86%) of diabetic patients.[243] Katsamouris and colleagues found that a level of 40 mm Hg at the anterior skin surface was predictive of successful healing after partial foot and lower leg amputations.[244]

It is always good practice to utilize data from various noninvasive testing. Another valuable test utilized is the skin perfusion pressure test (SPP). Along with TCOM, SPP is measured in the same units—mm Hg, but measures different objectives.

This test measures the pressure when blood volume returns after controlled release of occlusion combining a laser Doppler and a blood pressure cuff. SPP is a noninvasive test which assesses microcirculation and is not affected by calcification, edema, or callused areas. It measures capillary perfusion.

SPP measurement is an objective, noninvasive method that can be used to diagnose critical limb ischemia with approximately 80% accuracy.[245] It has been established in earlier studies that healing may occur with SPP levels of > 30 mm Hg but other recent studies have determined that healing was likely if values were > 40 mm Hg. The probability of wound healing with SPP values > 30 mm Hg were 69.8% compared to 40 mm Hg–86.3% respectively.[246] Another group also found a threshold of 40 mm Hg as predictive of healing ulceration or gangrene.[247]

A study compared TCOM versus SPP and determined skin perfusion pressure was more sensitive in its ability to predict wound healing relative to TcPO2 (90% versus 66%). SPP is a measure of the capillary pressure, while TCOM measures the oxygen molecules in the peri-wound tissue. Both tests are useful in predicting wound healing.

In conclusion, arterial testing should be a priority with lower extremity wounds. The clinician can look for signs and symptoms that indicate periph-eral arterial problems such as resting pain, inter-mittent claudication, wound presentation, lack of hair over toes and/or foot, thickened nails, cool skin temperature and absence of pedal pulses, to name a few. It is only when you utilize a noninva-sive test that you can be certain if patients have peripheral arterial problems given that some patients may be asymptomatic. Patients with rest-ing pain are said to be experiencing 90% occlusion in the respective artery. If the noninvasive testing has abnormal values, it is highly recommended to proceed with more in depth tests such as CT's and MRI's. The noninvasive tests discussed above will not be able to determine where exactly the prob-lems exist. Noninvasive testing will provide a pic-ture of the macro and micro vascular system without an exact location of the problem.

Diabetic Standard of Care

In the United States it has been estimated that 29.1 million or 9.3% of the population has diabetes (21 million diagnosed and 8.1 million undiagnosed) with a total care cost of 245 billion dollars ($176 billion directly (medical expenditure) and $69 bil-lion indirectly (loss of work, disability).[248]

Standard of care for diabetic wounds as sug-gested by the wound healing society include diag-nosis, offloading, infection control, wound bed preparation, appropriate dressing selection, glyce-mic control, proper wound documentation, and prevention strategies (▶ Fig. 3.74).[249] During the recommended diagnosis, you are ruling out an arterial component, infection and loss of protec-tive sensation. Loss of protective sensation on a diabetic patient typically leads to ulcers which may become infected needing hospitalization and

depending on the severity combined with arterial hypo-perfusion will lead to amputations. Approxi-mately 15% of diabetic foot ulcers (DFU) result in lower-extremity amputation.[249,250] More than 85% of lower-extremity amputations in patients with diabetes occur in people who have had an antece-dent foot ulcer.[213,251] 5-year mortality rates after lower-extremity amputation range from 50% to 76%.[252,253] Contralateral limb amputation was at a rate of 50% that contralateral limb will be ampu-tated within specified time.

Offloading is important for patients with dia-betic wounds. Typically, patients will have wounds on the plantar aspect of the foot. As the diabetes process progresses it will affect the nerves in the foot; it will damage the nerve functions which are sensation, autonomic and motor components. Experiencing the loss of protective sensation, the ability to keep the skin lubricated and structural changes is normal for these patients. These changes, if not addressed, can delay the healing process.

Infection is diagnosed based on your clinical assessment findings. The bedside wound evalua-tion is the most important diagnostic tool in deter-mining infection. A culture is performed to determine which organism is present in order to provide the proper antibiotics. Diabetics will not demonstrate the typical signs of infections such as warmth, erythema, edema, and pain as they have an immune compromised system. The American Diabetes Association recommends that if the pres-ence of purulent drainage or two or more signs of inflammation then the wound is noted to be infected.[254] In a diabetic, infection can be classified as limb threatening or non–limb threatening. Non–limb threatening will include characteristics such as cellulitis less than 2 cm periwound as well as the absence of osteomyelitis, peripheral arterial disease and gangrene. A limb threatening infection will have extensive cellulitis beyond 2 cm from periwound, a deep abscess, osteomyelitis and gan-grene. Keep in mind that more than half of the time, the surface bacteria will differ from the deeper bacteria. Deeper bacteria in a diabetic pa-tient is usually limb threatening if not addressed promptly.

Once the clinician determines the wound to be infected via bedside clinical evaluation, a proper culture is recommended. The gold standard cultur-ing method is a biopsy followed by a tissue culture. Swab cultures are usually discouraged as the wound bed may be contaminated with various bacteria which could misrepresent the actual

3

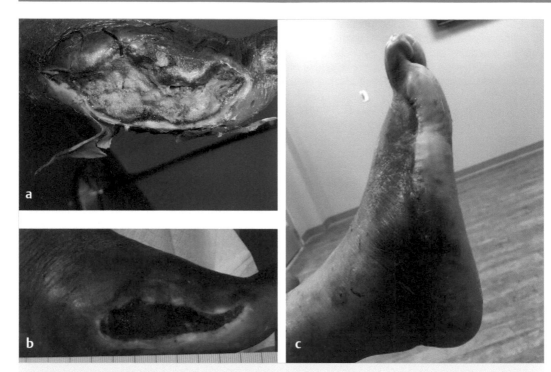

Fig. 3.74 Diabetic wound progressing through the phases of healing. This patient was to have her foot amputated. Pictures depict the three phases of healing: (a) inflammatory, (b) proliferative, and (c) maturation phase. This patient had complications due to poor arterial blood flow, uncontrolled glycemic level, extensive necrotic tissue, and improper dressing selection, to name a few. Treatment consisted of wound bed preparation (debridement, exudate management, and bacterial control), revascularization, glycemic control, offloading, and advanced modalities.

pathogen causing the infection. It has been estimated, on diabetic patients, that the surface bacteria are different from the deeper bacteria. Some other studies demonstrated that the wound bed has to be cleansed and prepared prior to the culture.

Offloading is imperative when diabetic patients have a wound on the plantar aspect of the foot (▶ Fig. 3.75, ▶ Fig. 3.76). In this author's experience, as the foot structures change, Achilles tendon stiffness and ongoing trauma is encountered, offloading becomes essential for a neuropathic/diabetic patient. There are various offloading choices for patients but the gold standard is considered to be the total contact cast.

Glycemic control is important because it has a tremendous impact on wound care. When elevated blood glucose levels are experienced, the arteries become stiffer and create narrowing of the blood vessels. This narrowing of blood vessels leads to decreased arterial circulation which negatively impacts wound healing. Poor glycemic control can lead to nerve injuries where sensation is

lost and can cause the immune cells to function ineffectively increasing risk of infection. Patient education is important and patient must be an active participant taking an active role with managing their diabetes.

Wound Infections

The history of surgical site infections has shed multiple theories on its occurrence. It was once the standard of care to allow pus to form as a natural component of healing. Hippocrates believed that pus was not a natural component in the healing process and suppuration should be avoided. In 130 AD, a respected surgeon, Claudius Galen's assertion, a deviation from Hippocrates, of promoting the formation of pus being essential in wound healing proved to be incorrect thousand years later.

Galen's views of promoting "laudable pus" were challenged in the 1200s by Theodoric Borgognoni as he was looking for ideal conditions for wound healing. Borgognoni's four essential conditions included control of bleeding, removal of contaminated or necrotic material, and avoidance of dead space and careful application of the wound dressing. His views were not accepted and the practice of continuing to encourage the wound to suppurate continued until the 16th century by Ambroise Pare.

In today's times successful chronic wound management not only incorporates Borgognoni's essential conditions for avoiding surgical site infections but also aims at finding the cause, treating infection, understanding colonization versus critical colonization and establishing adequate blood flow.

Wounds have the potential to develop bacterial proliferation which can affect the healing process. When these wounds are identified, prompt action is required given that there are many variables that will potentially delay healing.

Normally, we have bacteria throughout our body. These bacteria can infiltrate defects in our skin such as fissures and wounds. The longer the wound is open the higher the chance of bacteria colonizing.[255] In fact, the type of bacteria present and whether the bacteria have infected the wound depends on the type, depth, location, level of perfusion and the efficacy of the host response.[255]

A wound that is colonized will have bacteria present but their number is not growing enough to affect the host; there will not be any visual signs of this. As this colonized bacterium continues to grow, but does not show signs of infection, it is said that critical colonization is present. Critical colonization is a stage where wound healing is delayed without the overt signs and symptoms of infection.[254] When the bacteria multiply beyond 10^5 organism per gram of tissue, then it will affect the host and clinical signs of infection will be noticeable.

Vincent Falanga in the 1990s also defined the new term "critical colonization." Vincent Falanga in 1994[256] identified the concept of critical colonization with fresh insights into chronic wound healing and nonhealing wounds.

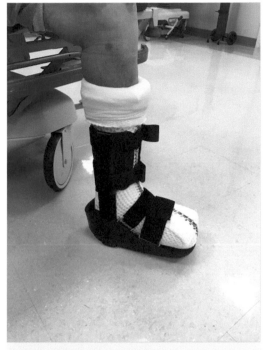

Fig. 3.75 Diabetic patient wearing a total contact cast (TCC) to offload plantar wound.

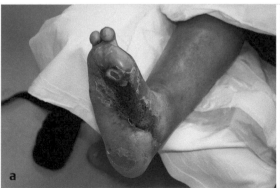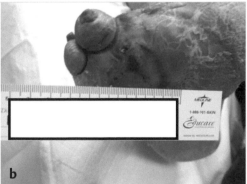

Fig. 3.76 (a) Diabetic patient with a chronic ulcer, neuropathy, prior amputations. Note the dark skin on the foot—this is a previous skin graft and not necrotic tissue. (b) Diabetic/neuropathic ulcers treated with wound bed preparation principles and offloaded with total contact cast (TCC). For initial wound prior to offloading see ▶ Fig. 3.62.

3

- Wound contamination: the presence of bacteria within a wound without any host reaction[257]
- Wound colonization: the presence of bacteria within the wound which do multiply or initiate a host reaction[257]
- Critical colonization: multiplication of bacteria causing a delay in wound healing, usually associated with an exacerbation of pain not previously reported but still with no overt host reaction[256,258]
- Wound infection: the deposition and multiplication of bacteria in tissue with an associated host reaction[257]

Various factors that will affect a wound's defense mechanism include the diffusion distance, local perfusion, necrotic tissue, immune system, and length of time that wound has been open. Microbial proliferation is increased at PO2 levels < 20 mm HG.[259] Treatment goals should be to optimize perfusion levels as well as adequately remove necrotic tissue which harbors bacteria and treat the wound that is infected or critically colonized.

Cutting and Harding described signs of infection in a granulating wound: delayed healing, friable tissue, offensive odor, secretion of pus, increase in lesion size pain or discomfort and prolonged exudate production (▶ Fig. 3.77).[260]

Classical Signs of Infection

- Erythema
- Pain
- Warmth
- Swelling

Signs and Symptoms of Sepsis

- Body temperature above 101F or below 96.8 F
- Heart rate higher than 90 beats a minute
- Respiratory rate higher than 20 breaths a minute
- Abrupt change in mental status
- Significantly decreased urine output
- Septic shock

Edema

Edema plays a role in wound healing as it is found in the inflammatory phase of healing. This is a normal process where the body is protecting itself and sending the necessary cells to the injured area. Edema is defined as an accumulation of an excessive amount of watery fluids in cells or interstitial tissues.[261] Edema or a prolonged inflammatory phase will have detrimental effect to healing.

Excessive edema will cause pain, stiffness, and increase risk of infection (▶ Fig. 3.78) decreasing circulation. An article describes severe edema as creating an environment for nonhealing as the area is deprived of local blood supply.

As noted in earlier chapters, the body maintains a fluid balance whether the location is within the blood vessel system or in the tissues. The normal occurrence is for water to leave the circulatory system at the capillary level where necessary oxygen and nutrients are being delivered to the tissues followed by the body reabsorbing the water back into the circulatory system. The lymphatic system, which is involved at the capillary level as well, also assists in transporting fluid back to the circulatory system including the larger molecules that are not able to be picked up by the blood vessels. Edema can be caused by either too much water leaving the blood vessels or the lymphatic system not being able to remove protein and fluid from the tissue.

Common conditions that will damage or slow down this fluid balance are as follows:

- Heart failure

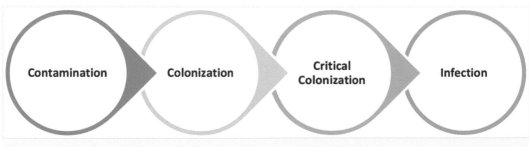

Fig. 3.77 Contamination to infection continuum model.

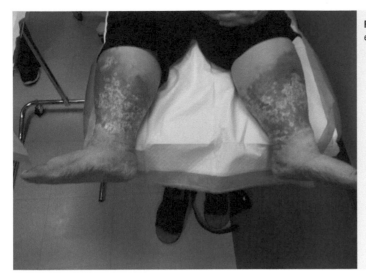

Fig. 3.78 Bilateral lower extremity edema with cellulits.

- Kidney disease
- Liver disease
- Malnutrition
- Blood clots
- Infection
- Inflammation
- Lymphedema
- CVI
- Decrease calf pump mechanism/immobility
- Heat
- Medications
- Tumors
- Diet related—too much salt in diet
- Hormonal related
- Trauma

Patients that have wounds as well as edema need prompt assessment to rule out systemic problems, DVTs, infections and establishing adequate blood flow in order to implement proper interventions (▶ Fig. 3.79). Knowing when to appropriately compress and selecting an appropriate method of compression is important. Compression will increase the tissue pressure therefore promoting reabsorption of excess fluid, decreasing the diffusion distance allowing oxygen and nutrients to reach cells timely, and decrease pressure on blood vessels improving local blood supply.

Dressings

Wound care clinicians must have a good understanding of how to establish and maintain an optimal wound bed environment. An optimal environment consists of a wound bed with an adequate vascular supply, proper temperature, proper pH level and a moist environment to promote cellular activity. Although not all wounds benefit from a moist wound bed environment, such as dry stable ischemic toes, wounds heal 50% faster when a moist wound bed in present. Wounds heal in a complex and well-orchestrated fashion therefore establishing the right environment will allow key cellular function to occur timely.

In order to establish this ideal wound bed environment, the clinician must be able to match the dressing to specific wound characteristics as well as other important components. These include appropriately assessing the patient and the wound, ordering appropriate diagnostic tests, understanding each phase of healing with differentiating characteristics, following established clinical guidelines based on etiology, effective wound bed preparation, understanding reimbursement and coding, knowing when to use available advanced modalities, using research to determine if adequate progress is occurring, coordinating treatment and communicating effectively with other disciplines, and finally being able to select an appropriate wound dressings to match your patient and wound bed needs.

Dressings can promote a moist wound environment and are used to help with wound bed preparation. The aim for utilizing dressings is to maintain a moist wound environment at the proper temperature while maintaining the periwound tissue dry, being cost effective with dressing selection, and protect from bacteria.

3

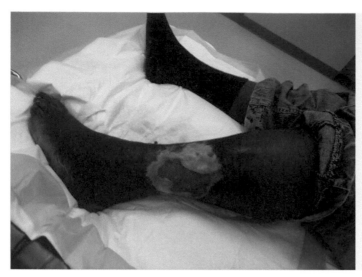

Fig. 3.79 Bilateral lower extremity edema. Patient with CVI from history of DVTs.

Dressing selection should be based on each patient's individual needs. A dressing will compliment and speed up your treatment but it should not be your only source of intervention. Wound bed preparation is of utmost importance along with targeting the cause. For example, in general, a chronic venous ulcer that may have nonviable tissue with lower extremity edema treatment focus may include establishing adequate vascular supply to rule out an arterial component, ruling out infection and DVTs in order to remove nonviable tissue, apply an appropriate dressing with an adequate compression dressing/modality.

Clinicians must keep in mind that wound healing is an active well thought out process. The dressing will complement the actual active treatment and goals for each specific wound. In other words, the dressing should not be the only considered form of treatment. Dr. Armstrong's article said it best, "It's not what you put on a wound that heals it, but what you take off." I want to emphasize the importance of this statement as selected dressing should not be the only form of treatment to our patients. To put it in perspective and expand this message, wounds have the ability to improve when the following is "taken off" promptly: abnormal mechanical forces such as pressure and shear, necrotic nonviable tissue, a hypoxic state, edema, protein rich edema, soft-tissue/bone infection, chronic wound fluid, etc., in which dressings may support above purposes but should not be the only source of treatment.

Normal intact skin pH ranges from 4.8 to 6.0 while interstitial fluid had a neutral ph. Chronic wounds are said to have an alkaline or neutral pH level. The role of wound bed pH has proven to be of fundamental importance during the healing of chronic wounds, and prolonged chemical acidification of the wound bed has been shown to increase the healing rate in chronic venous leg ulcers.[262]

Dressings assist with maintaining the proper pH level as noted in a study where the wounds shifted from an alkaline to an acidic level and maintained this level for up to 72 hours when the dressing was removed.[263] The ability of dressings to absorb fluids and maintain an ideal wound environment will promote wound healing.

So how do you decipher through the thousands of available dressings and their functions? How do I know which one to use and when? When consulting with health care entities the first step I strongly recommend is to concentrate on the basics. In other words, do they know the fundamentals ensuring that concentration is not on advance treatment but on the basics? Do they know how to assess the wound and periwound skin as well as documenting it properly? This is important because the dressing and needed functions are based on wound characteristics. In my opinion failure is achieved when we select a "magical" dressing without considering the wound characteristics.

I had the pleasure of reviewing charts at a new agency to assist them with their dressing formulary. I was noting that antimicrobial dressings were being used but the documentation did not indicate that the wound had neither an infection nor a critically colonized state. On one chart the cause of the wound was noted as a venous ulcer caused by a prior injury to lower extremity with no active calf pump mechanism while adequate vascular supply was established. Because of the edema, increased diffusion distance, oxygen and nutrients were not effectively reaching the wound but compression was not being applied creating a delay in healing. This is an example of mismatching the dressing to the wound and not treating the cause which escalates the treatment cost without achieving expected results.

To understand how to match dressings to wound characteristics, let's review moist wound healing and its advantages, an ideal dressing and dressing categories

Dr. George Winter is credited with the concept of moist wound healing. In 1962, he demonstrated that wounds left to dry formed scabs while others covered with a polymer film epithelialized twice as quickly.[264] Wounds covered with the film healed in about 12–15 days while wounds covered with a scab healed in about 25 – 30 days.[208] In other words, creating the proper moist wound environment will allow cells to migrate faster whereas wounds that scabbed over took longer time to epithelialize as they traveled downward searching for moist viable tissue. This began a large wound care product industry promoting moist wound healing.

At the same time, it was found that the usage of wet to dry dressings were diminishing and considered not an appropriate dressing selection for most applications. Gauze dressings dry out the wound surface, delay wound healing, may involve more wound pain, interfere with the wound healing process as cells need moisture to survive, therefore not providing the most optimal moist wound bed environment.

Moist wound environment speeds up healing when compared to dry wounds, promotes cell growth and proliferation, increases the synthesis of collagen and the proliferation of fibroblasts. Additional benefits include prevention of tissue dehydration and cell death, accelerated angiogenesis, increased breakdown of dead tissue and fibrin, and reduction of pain.[260] Dressings will also provide a bacterial barrier, decreasing infection rates, decrease scar formation, and proper selection will lead to a significant decrease in cost.

Cellular function is optimized when the wound maintains proper temperature. A low tissue temperature of the wound bed has been shown to slow healing, mainly by causing a decrease in oxygen release.[265] Wound bed temperature in chronic leg ulcers ranges between 24 and 26 °C when the ulcer is left uncovered. It has been studied that upon dressing removal and application, the wound will take hours to regain its proper temperature. A drop in a few degrees can negatively affect the wound healing process. So if dressings, such as wet to dry, are not able to maintain normal temperature, healing will be delayed.

When thinking of moist wound healing, considering the proper amount of moisture is important. The best example of the proper amount of moisture can be illustrated by the picture on ▶ Fig. 3.80. The beach sand located above the sea water remains moist instead of fully saturated or in a dry state.

There are some signs that will alert you if your dressing is not maintaining an adequate amount of

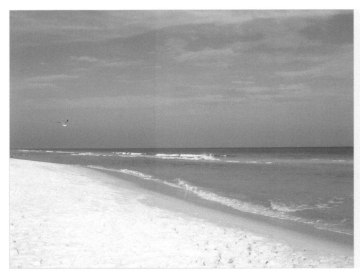

Fig. 3.80 Example of the proper amount of moisture illustrated by the beach sand located above the sea water, which remains moist instead of fully saturated or in a dry state.

moisture. Inappropriate dressing selection is noted when the wound bed is dry upon dressing removal. Either the dressing is absorbing too much drainage (absorbency) or a high degree of moisture is escaping through the dressing. The ability for dressings to control moisture is known in the dressing industry as the moisture vapor transport rate (MVTR). MVTR is defined as a measure of the passage of gaseous H2O through a barrier. Dressings will have varying amount of MVTR.

Frequent patient monitoring and dressing changes is required based on the level of exudate and type of wound. It must be mentioned that if you have a poorly vascularized area with eschar with no clinical signs of infection, otherwise labeled as stable, and it's dry, then vascular referral is warranted timely while protecting it from trauma, keeping it dry, and free from infection.

If your dressing is draining excessively it may be caused by an occult infection, a wound that is critically colonized, edema or sometimes an inappropriate dressing selection or frequency of dressing changes. Typically, inappropriate dressings may exhibit the inability to absorb wound exudate and have the proper MVTR due to having a wound with an increase bioburden state or proper dressing frequency not followed. Typical signs of increase drainage include maceration of the periwound skin, hypergranulation tissue, clinical signs of infection and secondary signs of delayed healing. On the opposite end, if you have an infected wound or one with excessive drainage, you do not want to apply an occlusive dressing or a dressing with a low MVTR especially for prolonged duration.

A dressing will be ideal when its function is utilized to maintain an ideal moist wound environment. A new clinician will have difficulty deciphering through the thousands of available products to select the appropriate one. The dressing choice is also dependent on availability as well as being on the facility product formulary.

An ideal dressing can be described as one that will promote a moist wound environment, provides mechanical protection and thermal insulation, allows gaseous exchange, easy to use, cost-effective, allows removal without pain or trauma, conformable, acts as a barrier to bacteria, nontoxic, and have a variable wear time.

Dressing selection is based on the desired frequency after an assessment/reassessment of the wound has been completed. One must understand the current phases of healing as well as periwound characteristics, frequency of dressing changes to maintain optimal environment, product availability, desired purpose for dressing, and the patient-centered goal of closure or maintenance/palliative and patient compliance.

As the wound progresses or regresses through the phases of healing, your dressing should change based on your reassessment. In this author's opinion, there has not been a single dressing that has been able to manage and optimize the wound characteristics throughout each phase of healing.

For example, a wound in the inflammatory phase most likely will have excessive exudate where an absorbent dressing may be needed with frequent dressing changes, or it may be in a high bioburden state where a topical antimicrobial dressing may aid other forms of treatment. A wound in the proliferative phase may need less frequent dressing changes while a wound in the maturation phase will need protection.

Clinicians that expect the dressing to be the sole form of treatment and forgo wound bed preparation steps may not reach positive outcomes.

Before selecting the "right" dressing, the clinician needs to determine what is the purpose or goal and match the wound characteristics to the desired dressing in order to have the optimal wound environment. Factors such as wound etiology, present healing phase, response to prior used dressings, and adequate blood flow as well as infection will also determine appropriate dressing selection. Variables such as dressing frequency changes also need to be determine based on the product insert recommendations, reassessments, evidence-based research, and your clinical experience.

Dressings can be divided into product categories. Each category typically has a main function with indications and contraindications. The clinician should concentrate on what expected function is expected from the dressing based on your patient and wound assessment.

Characteristics of an ideal dressing:
- Maintains a moist wound environment:
  - Absorbs when there is excessive drainage.
  - Hydrates in the presence of desiccation.
  - Allows the exchange of gases and vapors as desired.
- Matches specific ulcer etiology needs.
- Protects the surrounding skin.
- Comfortable.
- Provides thermal protection.
- Protects the wound from infiltrating bacteria.
- Does not create trauma upon removal.
- Eliminates dead space.

- Conforms to anatomic area.
- Controls odor.
- Minimizes pain.
- Assists other forms of debridement when necrotic tissue is present.
- Cost effective.

The product category list and their usage are as follows (▶ Table 3.27).

Gauze

Characteristics: Gauze dressings are made in both woven and nonwoven materials. There are multiple variations that can be used on infected wounds, as a postsurgical pressure dressings, draining wounds, wounds with tunnels/tracts, for protection or used as a secondary dressing. Even though they are inexpensive they may not be the best choice to maintain a moist wound bed environment.

  Indication:
- May be used as a primary or secondary dressing.
- Often used as a means of mechanical debridement but not utilized appropriately.
- Used for protection.
- Dry application for heavily draining wounds.
- Sometimes impregnated with antimicrobial agents or hydrogel.

Contraindication:
- Often not able to maintain a moist wound environment.
- Not effective as a bacterial barrier.

Composite

Characteristics: Dressing which combines two or more product types. Typically, you will find a combination of gauze and a moisture retentive dressing.

Table 3.27 Dressing categories

Gauze	Antimicrobials
Composite	Honey
Transparent film	Antiseptics
Foam	Collagen
Hydrocolloid	Fillers
Hydrogel	Negative Pressure
Calcium Alginate	Compression
Hydrofiber	Cellular tissue products

  Indication:
- Used as a primary or secondary dressing.
- Use varies pending on combination of products—see package inserts for details.

Contraindication:
- Sizes vary needing ample storage space.

Transparent Film

- Characteristics—protective clear film layer allowing visualization of the wound, able to slow moisture transport rate but it does not absorb, and is not permeable to water and bacteria.
- Indication(s):
  ○ Maintains moisture.
  ○ Partial thickness wounds with minimal drainage.
  ○ May be used in areas of shear to prevent friction.
  ○ May be used for promoting autolytic debridement.
  ○ Used on minor injuries (i.e., lacerations).
- Contraindication:
  ○ Fragile skin.
  ○ Wounds with moderate to maximal drainages.

Foam

Characteristics: semi permeable dressings that protect and insulate while promoting a moist wound environment. Foams may come in an adhesive, nonadhesive, and silicone adhesive form while others may be shaped for specific anatomic sites such as heels and sacral areas.

  Indication:
- Partial or full thickness.
- Moderate to maximal draining wounds.
- Minimal drainage used with thinner foams.

Contraindication:
- Dry wounds.
- Third degree burns.

Hydrocolloid

Characteristics: Promotes moist wound environment and autolytic debridement. An occlusive dressing preventing infiltration of bacteria.

  Indication:
- Low to moderate draining wounds.
- Various shapes for various anatomic areas.

Contraindication:
- Infected wounds.

- Dry eschar especially if there is arterial insufficiency.

Hydrogel

Characteristics: Hydrogel dressings are made mostly of water or glycerin used to hydrate and maintain a moist wound environment. Available in a gel or a sheet.
  Indication:
- For dry wounds.
- Granulating wounds.
- Necrotic wounds.
- Promotes autolytic debridement.

Contraindications/disadvantages:
- Wounds with moderate to high exudate.
- Requires secondary dressing.
- Infected wounds where dressing will not be changed frequently.

Alginate

Characteristics: a woven or nonwoven natural material derived from seaweed utilized for absorbing moderate to heavy amount of drainage turning into a gel. Available in a rope or sheet form.
- Indication:
  ○ Highly absorbent.
  ○ Promotes hemostasis action on minimal bleeding wounds.
  ○ Could be used on infected wounds.
  ○ Rope form useful for tunneling wounds.
- Contraindication:
  ○ Wounds with minimal drainage.
  ○ Over tendons and bone as it may desiccate them.
  ○ Requires a secondary dressing.
  ○ Heavy bleeding.
  ○ Dry eschar.
  ○ Third degree wounds.
  ○ Do not apply saline to make alginate gel on minimal draining wounds.

Hydrofiber

Characteristics: Similar to alginates, synthetic fibers used for absorption of moderate to heavy draining wounds.
- Indications:
  ○ Highly absorbent.
  ○ Rope form useful for tunneling wounds.
- Contraindication:
  ○ Dry wounds.

○ Third degree wounds.
○ Requires a secondary dressing.
○ Heavy bleeding.
○ Used over tendons and bone.
○ Minimal draining wounds.

Antimicrobial

Characteristics: Topical dressings used to reduce bioburden at the wound surface. When wounds are infected, antibiotics should be first line of treatment.
- Silver:
  ○ Nanocrystals.
  ○ Ionized.
- Cadoxer iodine.
- Polyhexamethylene biguanide (PHMB).

Indication:
- Reduce bioburden in infected wounds.
- Reduce bioburden in wounds that are critically colonized.
- Used in conjunction with debridement to reduce biofilm.

Contraindication:
- Allergies to product.

Honey

Characteristics: Medical grade honey used for various types of wounds. These dressings are used for creating a moist wound environment, debriding action, and odor control. The literature also describes its antibacterial properties but refer to product manufacturer's recommendation for this. Honey is available in ointments, gels, as well as in other delivery systems such as alginates, hydrocolloids, and contact layers.
  Indications:
- Can be used as a primary or secondary dressing.
- Various types of wounds—see product insert.

Contraindications:
- Wounds with minimal drainage.
- Dry necrotic wounds.
- Patients with allergies to honey or dressing materials.

Antiseptic

Characteristics: The use of antiseptic has been controversial. It has been accepted to use on intact skin while studies indicate that they are cytotoxic on nonintact skin. A wound in a chronic state may not have healthy cells. Examples include Povidone Iodine, chlorhexidine, etc.

Indication/contraindication: refer to product insert/manufacturer's guidelines.

Collagen

Characteristics: Dressing derived from porcine or bovine collagen material typically used when a wound has stalled. Available in powder, sheets, gel, and some products are made with an antimicrobial component.

Indication:
• Used for wounds that have failed to progress.

Contraindication:
• Third degree burns.
• Wounds with heavy exudate.
• Wounds covered with slough or eschar.
• Allergies to collagen.

Wound Fillers

Characteristics: Fillers function to maintain a moist wound environment and manage exudate.

Contraindication:
• Requires a secondary dressing.

Negative Pressure Wound Therapy Device (NPWT)

Characteristics: NPWT (▶ Fig. 3.81) is used in preparing the wound bed for closure, enhancing healing, decreasing edema, removal of exudate, granulation formation, and enhancing angiogenesis

and tissue perfusion. Foam and gauze dressings are available. Need to be careful and follow product insert recommendations when there is exposed bone or tendon, when there is a clotting disorder and wounds with a fistula.

Indication: acute surgical and traumatic wounds, subacute and dehisced wounds, pressure ulcers, chronic wounds, meshed grafts, adjunct to skin grafts/flap procedures.

Contraindication: fistulas to organs, wounds with untreated osteomyelitis, wounds with necrotic tissue, do not use silver products if patient is allergic to silver, wounds exposing blood vessels or organs, wounds with open joint capsules, skin malignancy

Compression

Characteristics: Compression is used to promote a decrease in swelling. It enhances the calf muscle pump function. Long stretch bandages contain elastic fibers allowing to stretch to approximately 160% its original length (Ace wraps) versus short stretch bandages which stretch approximately 40%. Precaution needs to be taken with spinal cord injury patients, CHF, and neuropathy.

Indication:
• CVI.
• Edema.
• Lymphedema.

Contraindication:
• Contraindicated on patients with arterial insufficiency (see product insert for details).
• Long stretch bandage contraindicated on patients with arterial insufficiency.

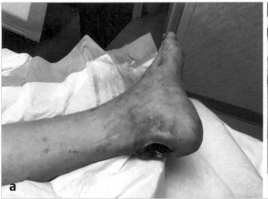 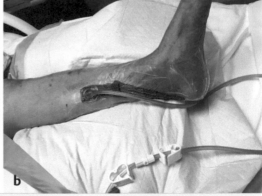

Fig. 3.81 Nonhealing chronic diabetic ulcer caused by trauma two months earlier. (a) Status post surgical debridement of soft tissue and partial calcanectomy (osteomyelitis). (b) Application of NPWT using a bridging technique to avoid pressure injury while supine.

- Infection.
- Blood clot.
- Uncontrolled CHF.
- Weeping dermatitis.
- Typically, when patients have small ankles (see product insert for details).

Cellular Tissue Products

Characteristics: Bioengineered tissue derived from human tissue, nonhuman tissue, synthetic materials or a composite. May be cellular or acellular.
  Indication:
- See manufacturer's recommendation as it may be pending on diagnosis and coverage.
- Some cellular tissue products are only covered for certain diagnosis (i.e., diabetes and/or venous problems).
- Ulcers have been present for 1 to 3 months prior (pending on insurance).
- Ulcers have failed to respond to conservative measures for 1 month.

Contraindication:
- See manufacturer's recommendation.
- Typically, must have adequate arterial blood flow (some need at least an ABI of 0.65 or greater).
- Ulcer must be free from infection.

Case Study

The following case study will demonstrate the importance in determining the cause and using evidence.

An 80-year-old woman presents to the clinic with a nonhealing heel ulcer (▶ Fig. 3.82, ▶ Table 3.28). This patient is wheelchair bound and resides at a local nursing home. According to the patient, the left heel ulcer began in mid-December due to her restless leg syndrome. There was a history of diabetes, CABG, pacemaker, valve replacement, neuropathy, and edema affecting the left lower extremity.

The patient's goal was to not have an amputation.
  Objective testing:
- Labs:
  - Prealbumin, 7.
  - H&H, low.
- Vascular:
  - ABI: left, 1.12; right, 1.49.
  - Doppler: indicates monophasic waveforms bilateral feet.
  - TBI: left 0.23, right, 0.84.

  - TCOM: < 31 mm Hg.
  - CTA: heavy calcification bilateral lower extremities. Left lower leg with heavy calcification.
- Culture:
  - Clinical signs of infection and tissue culture indicating organism.
  - No osteomyelitis on imaging but + bone biopsy.

Other: Due to patient's current health, diagnostics, and prior history, physicians determined that revascularization is not an option.
  Problem list:
1. Unstable heel unstageable pressure ulcer complicated with diabetes and arterial insufficiency.
2. Vascular insufficiency.
3. Clinical signs of infection.
4. Poor nutritional status (based on prealbumin and food intake).
5. Positive osteomyelitis.
6. Decrease functional mobility.

▶ Fig. 3.82 and ▶ Fig. 3.83 document the patients' progress.

Wound Progression

An important wound care principle is being able to collect objective data and analyze it to determine wound progression. Often, wound progress may be described subjectively and inaccurately. A thorough wound assessment documents objective wound characteristics in order to have actual comparative data to make decisions on current treatment. This information will determine if the wound is progressing or not. This data will also assist in predicting a possible outcome.

The wound assessment must be consistently performed, valid, accurate, reliable, and reproducible. An assessment will occur on the first visit, after surgical/sharp debridement, with wound deterioration and/or prior to discharge from the facility. It is recommended that clinicians follow their institution's policies and procedures regarding initial and subsequent assessments. A reassessment should also be performed on a regular basis because this will provide data to determine wound progression.

Wound measurements will yield wound bed surface area in cm^2 by multiplying the length and width. Volume is determined in cm^3 by multiplying length, width, and depth. There are various studies that predict healing rates at certain endpoints based on wound etiology and surface area.

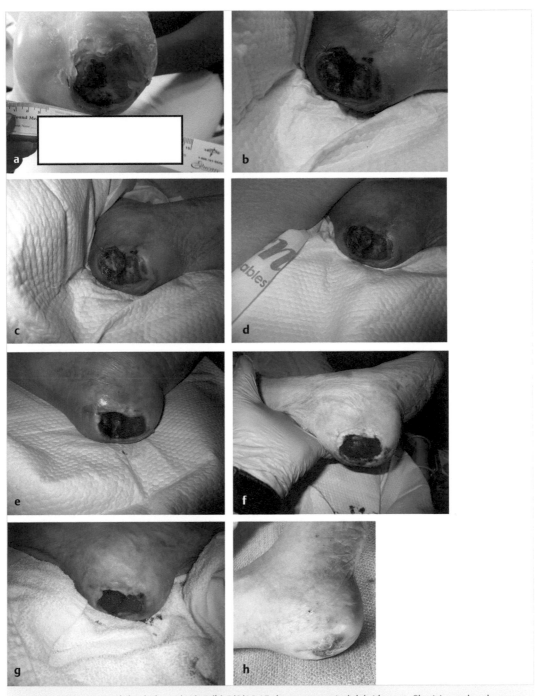

Fig. 3.82 (a) Patient with heel ulcer 1/15/16 (b) 2/8/16:15 days post surgical debridement. Physician ordered a gauze dressing 2/1/16. (c) 2/8/16 post sharp debridement. Physician ordered for bedside sharp debridement, contact low frequency ultrasound and remove suture. (d) 2/8/16 post contact low frequency ultrasound debridement. (e) 2/15/16 physician ordered to continue gauze dressing. Size 5 cm × 3.1 cm × 1.4 cm. (f) 2/24/16. Physician ordered negative pressure and collagen dressing to "jump" start wound on 2/22/16. Edema is also resolved. Picture taken only after 2 days of advanced products. Advanced modalities assisted this poor healing wound. (g) 3/7/16 size 4.5 cm × 2.8 cm × 0.7 cm. (h) 5/1/16 Closure achieved on a complex wound with initial poor healing.

Table 3.28 Case study wound characteristics/assessment

WOUND ASSESSMENT:	
Location:	Left Heel
Etiology:	Pressue Injury complicated with Diabetes
Classification:	Unstageable Pressure Injury
Size:	6.9 cm x 6 cm
Depth:	0.8 cm
Drainage:	Moderate serosanguineous
Tissue Color:	60% Black, 30% Pink, 10% Yellow
Tissue:	+ Eschar, Slough, no granulation
Tract(s):	?
Undermining:	?
Redness:	+
Induration:	None
Palpation:	Minimal Warmth
Pain:	None
Odor:	+
Maceration:	None
Edema:	+. Girth incr 6 cm at ankle and calf
Sensation:	No protective sensation

Cardinal M et al, found patients with venous leg ulcers (VLU) to have a higher healing rate when serial debridement was performed (46 vs. 30%).[128] Margolis study based wound outcomes on size and duration of the venous ulcer stating long-standing ulcers (> 12 months) and larger ulcers (> 10 cm²) only have a 29% chance of healing at 24 weeks versus 78% chance for smaller ulcers (< 10 cm²) and of more recent duration (< 12 months).[266] Barwell reported 20% of venous ulcers remain unhealed after more than 50 weeks of appropriate compression. Mostow concluded that wounds treated with an extracellular matrix and debridement healed 63% at 12 weeks compared to 40% receiving only standard of care. Other studies indicate that VLU require an average of 24 weeks to heal; approximately 15% never heal; and recurrence is found once or multiple times in 15 to 71% of cases.[267,268]

Healed ulcerations possibly can have a 5-year recurrence rate as high as 40%.[269]

A study proposes that 30% or greater closure in 4 weeks is a good predictor of healing in venous leg ulcers and diabetic foot ulcers.[270,271]

Sheehan et al suggested that the diabetic foot ulcer area change at 4 weeks is a robust predictor of healing at 12 weeks. The results showed that a > 53% reduction in ulcer area at four weeks indicated healing at 12 weeks.[270] There are algorithms available, based on the Sheehan study, stating that at four weeks of standard diabetic wound care that if percentage of area reduction is less than 53% then its recommended to reassess vascular status, check for infection, consider advance modalities. In this study the group that had this reduction in area, healing rate was 58 versus 9% for those not reaching this percentage in area reduction.

This assessment of wound progression within a 3- to 4-week period is important. A wound may deteriorate for many reasons such as if patient develops an infection, if the antibiotic given is not targeting the correct organism, if patient is not controlling their nutrition, etc., making frequent assessments valuable. Prompt response to these changes and appropriate referrals can make a difference to the overall outcome.

In conclusion, accurate wound measurement is essential because it will determine how the wound may or may not be progressing, which interventions are beneficial. It will assist with proper communication between health care workers, guide the use of advance modalities and the ability to predict healing potential based on current evidence base practices.

Compression

We fully understand how tissues are affected when the diffusion distance increases because it delays the delivery of needed oxygen and nutrients as well as decreasing the ability for the wound to progress. Being able to determine edematous and lymphedema related edema through a good thorough assessment is paramount in order to drive the interventions. As evidence base practice indicates, compression should be the treatment of choice for these patients, yet it is not utilized appropriately and consistently throughout clinics. Each patient will present with unique characteristics and this is where we must not only evaluate their wound but their functional mobility, assistance, financial constraints, educational

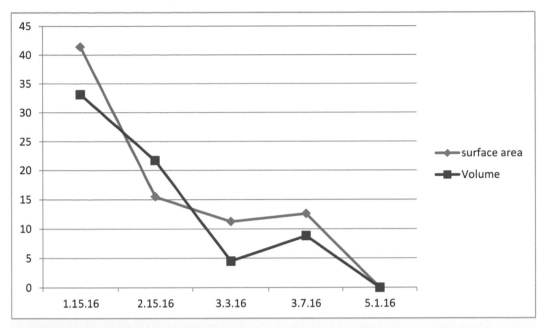

Fig. 3.83 Case study surface area and volume graph.

barriers, etc. Currently there are at least 9 different methods of compression for our patients.

Methods of compression include
- Inelastic (Unna boots).
- Short stretch bandage (short stretch bandages—layers).
- Multicomponent short stretch (light compression, e.g., two-layer wraps).
- Multicomponent long stretch (e.g., four-layer wraps).
- Long stretch wrap elastic (ace wraps).
- Compression stocking elastic (various products with degrees of compression).
- Ulcer stockings (double stockings. One holds dressing, other wear during day).
- Velcro devices (compression garments).
- Pumps (multiple products to choose from).

A Cochrane review determined that patients with VLU heal with compression than without, and that a multi component compression device achieves improved healing outcomes.[272]

Adequate compression is an important component for treating ulcers on CVI and lymphedema patients. Assessment of the lower arterial system is crucial before compression begins. The ankle-brachial index (ABI) test, a screening tool, may not be reliable particularly on patients with diabetes. Vascular consultation is warranted when an abnormal ABI is noted. Noninvasive vascular testing is advisable before compression, post revascularization, and when wound/ulcer characteristics deteriorate or fail to progress. An ABI greater than 0.5 but less than 0.8 precludes high levels of sustained compression.[273] Sustained compression is contraindicated in the presence of severe peripheral vascular disease, an ABI ≤ 0.6, because this sustained tissue pressure could further compromise tissue perfusion and potentially cause ischemic tissue death.[74] Patients with venous insufficiency and ABI ≤ 0.5 needing compression should be managed with IPC.[273] Arterial calcification may exist and falsely elevate the results of an ABI. Depending on protocol, it may start at an ABI ≥ 1.2, which precludes compression and further testing is required. Doppler waveforms, TBI, toe pressures, transcutaneous oxygen, and skin perfusion pressure test will provide a better picture when ABI is abnormal. These tests are useful in determining arterial status but do not show exactly where the blockage is located. Once these tests show arterial insufficiency, further diagnostic tests are warranted and referral indicated.

A wound in an edematous lower extremity with no contraindications will benefit from adequate sustained compression. When combining the appropriate compression, following manufacturer's recommendation, with MLD techniques wound healing is optimized on patients diagnosed with CVI and lymphedema.

3.13.7 A Rationale for MLD in Wound Healing

MLD is helpful in wound healing. This is because skin wounds inherently involve a disruption of normal lymphatic function and because of the unique ability of MLD to enhance otherwise impaired lymphatic drainage. Literature supports that insufficiency of lymph drainage and interstitial fluid stagnation contributes to sluggish wound healing and recurrence of ulcers.

It has been demonstrated that lymph vessel anatomy is adversely affected by development of skin ulceration. The valves and smooth muscle activity of lymphangions are disrupted during ulcer development. CVI causes obliteration of part of the superficial skin lymphatic capillary network, and causes dilatation and increased permeability of remaining lymphatics, resulting in dermal back flow of lymph fluid. The skin around an ulcer demonstrates collapse of lymph capillaries and closed interendothelial junctions of the capillaries. PTS demonstrates similar findings. This impedes the process of lymph formation in the skin surrounding the wound. Microscopic examination of wound and surrounding tissue samples shows a decrease in or absence of lymph capillaries and larger lymph vessels. Dilated lymph vessels are found in the periwound tissue as much as 20 cm from the ulcer base, in both normal-looking skin as well as intact lipodermatosclerotic skin. Damage to lymph vessels includes edema in the vessel walls and damage to the smooth muscle cells of the internal media. Therefore lymphatic microangiopathy and insufficient lymph drainage contribute to delayed ulcer healing and likely lead to later recurrence of the ulcer with minimal insult[274]. Either very localized lymphedema exists around an ulcer or the lymphedema may be more generalized in the limb, but in either case lymphedema is present and a primary factor impeding wound healing.

Even if lymph transport were to remain normal, the wound itself contributes to potential lymphatic insufficiency. The accumulation of waste products generated by the process of wound healing causes an increased LL and potential outflow obstruction, slowing the removal of wastes from the wound site, which is a further likely inhibitory factor in wound healing. Locally, the increase in interstitial fluid compromises the blood microvascular system, decreasing delivery of oxygen and nutrients. Conversely, the removal of lymphedema results in a significant increase in transcutaneous oxygen tension and increased density of blood capillaries in the skin. The fluids that remain in chronic wounds, due to stagnated lymph drainage, suppress proliferation of the healing constituents of the inflammatory cascade (i.e., keratinocytes, fibroblasts and vascular endothelial cells).[275] This suppression of the inflammatory cascade contributes to the delayed-healing status of chronic wounds.

One author[275] states that lymphedema is the underlying pathology that contributes to the formation of a venous ulcer and also that lymphedema is evident in nonvenous wounds (wounds due to ischemia, diabetes, and trauma) as well. Therefore, controlling periwound lymphedema will result in enhanced wound healing. Another author states that indurated edema and dermatosclerosis of skin are at least in part the result of lymphatic involvement that may be aggravated by recurrent infections.[276] Localized secondary lymphedema from CVI is characterized by microangiopathy of both blood *and* lymph capillaries.

Wounds therefore have lymphedema. The treatment of lymphedema requires the dispersal of accumulated interstitial proteins. MLD results in improved filling of initial lymphatics (lymph capillaries and pre-collectors capable of lymph formation), and increases the rate of lymphangion contraction while facilitating compensatory pathways for the decongestion of accumulated interstitial fluid. MLD also increases macrophage activity that helps degrade interstitial proteins. This aids in the dispersal of interstitial proteins.[277] If we consider the significant reduction in lymph TC due to the extensive damage to lymph vessel structure and function caused directly by skin ulcerations, and that wounds inherently increase LL, it follows that MLD would be a beneficial intervention in wound healing.

3.14 Lipedema

Lipedema, meaning fluid in fat, is an easy bruising painful, weight loss resistant symmetric subcutaneous adipose tissue (SAT) disorder found primarily in women that can be confused with obesity. While conservative and other medical therapies are available, liposuction remains the definitive treatment at this time. Lipedema SAT feels different than nonlipedema SAT having small sometimes firm frozen pea-sized nodules that can be palpated just under the skin but also deeper in the tissue. Estrogen, leaky vessels, inflammation and fibrosis are thought to be important in the growth of lipedema SAT. Lymphedema is often confused with lipedema but the hands and feet are not swollen with fluid in lipedema as in lymphedema. Women with lipedema can go on to develop lymphedema called lipo-lymphedema making conservative treatment of lipedema important including healthy eating, exercise, CDT and intermittent sequential pneumatic compression pumps. Medications and supplements that improve lymphatic pumping (lymphagogues) and mucolytics are nonstandard treatments of lipedema and are discussed in this chapter. Interestingly, lipedema SAT is primarily in the gynoid distribution, thought to be healthy SAT, and diabetes in this population is low. This chapter provides a comparison of lipedema to obesity, venous disease, Dercum's disease, Madelung's disease, familial multiple lipomatosis and fibromyalgia. This chapter also addresses liposuction of lipedema SAT including medical necessity and insurance coverage.

3.14.1 Definition of Lipedema

Lipedema, meaning fluid in fat, is a symmetric painful fat disorder found primarily in women affecting subcutaneous adipose tissue (SAT) in the gynoid distribution (hips, buttocks, legs, and arms). Lipedema SAT holds onto fluid preventing it from passing down the body dependently to the hands and feet so that lipedema SAT tends to stop abruptly at the wrist and ankle. This is very different from lymphedema in which free lymph fluid causes swelling on the hands or feet so that the Stemmer's sign is positive; Stemmer's sign is negative in > 90% of women with lipedema. Lipedema is, however, a risk factor for lymphedema which makes treatment with CDT for lipedema SAT important. The fluid in lipedema SAT is located in the interstitium (between and around adipocytes and other cells) and contains nutrients to induce adipocytes (fat cells) to grow. The SAT can grow to such great extents that it restricts mobility and damages blood and lymphatic vessels resulting in significant disability.

The hallmark of lipedema is the presence of SAT that cannot be lost by extreme dieting or over-exercise as first described by Drs. Allen and Hines in 1940.[278] Case reports describing women with a typical lipedema distribution of increased SAT on the thighs and lower legs with the appearance of a stove-pipe lower limb were published prior to this date but were labeled as having Dercum's disease, also a painful fat disorder with additional signs and symptoms of a systemic metabolic or inflammatory disorder.[279] Lipedema occurs primarily in women and usually begins around the time of puberty with a rapid growth in SAT in the gynoid distribution. However, some women share pictures of stove pipe-shaped legs as toddlers, and in agreement, lipedema has been noted in the pediatric population[280]; others notice lipedema SAT after childbirth or at menopause. When lipedema SAT is noticed later in life, it may be an initial appearance or an exacerbation of the underlying disease that was already present but not recognized.

The prevalence of lipedema in the female population has been cited as high as one out of every 2.6 women affected (39%)[281] to as low as one out of every 72,000[281]; the most common number cited in the literature is one out of every nine women or 11%,[282,283] none of these studies provide accurate prevalence data. Amongst providers who see many of these patients, lipedema is considered common.

3.14.2 Pathophysiology of Lipedema

Histology

Published descriptions of lipedema histopathology have been reviewed[284] and include hypertrophy and hyperplasia of adipocytes, dilation of capillaries and venules, fibrosis of arterioles and venules, increased numbers of capillaries and venules, perivascular cells which appear to be lymphocytes similar to those seen in massive localized lymphedema,[285] clusters of macrophages, and oily cysts. Histopathology of the lipedema SAT by stage would be helpful in clarifying this disease.

Etiology of Lipedema

At this time, the underlying cause of lipedema is not known. Speculation as to the underlying etiology has focused on

1. Leaky vasculature (blood vessels and lymphatics) under the control of estrogen. Lymphatic vessel aneurysms and dilated lymphatics in lipedema SAT are documented supporting the role of vessel leak in lipedema pathophysiology.[286,287,288]

3

2. Estrogen-induced abnormal expansion (number and size) of adipocytes, moving the cells away from their local blood supply inducing hypoxia.[289] Activation of tyrosine kinase receptors such as fibroblast growth factor, epidermal growth factor or platelet derived growth factor that are important in cell growth do not seem to be involved.[290]
3. Innervation abnormalities coexisting with inflammation of sensory nerves.[291]
4. Metabolic alterations in electrolytes such as sodium; macromolecules are not cleared as quickly from obese compared to lean fat which may affect electrolyte concentration in the interstitium.[292]

Hypothetical Development of Lipedema SAT

Lipedema SAT is more friable and therefore subject to damage[293]; it does not have the structure to hold fluid in all its compartments resulting in leakage. The greater the leak, the more extensive the hypoxia (low oxygen) in the tissues as cells are restricted by excess fluid from their oxygen source, capillaries. Hypoxia induces growth of new blood vessels under the guidance of vascular endothelial growth factor (VEGF) also known as vascular permeability factor, so that any new vessels made are leaky; VEGF levels are elevated in women with lipedema compared to women with cellulite.[294] Bruises are common in lipedema and signify fragility of vessels in the lipedema SAT. MLD is known to reduce capillary fragility in lipedema[202] confirming that fluid in the tissue contributes to destabilization of vessels. The body responds to leaky vessels by recruiting immune cells to the tissue for repair. These immune cells include lymphocytes around blood vessels and macrophages that circle dead adipocytes and consume the fat inside.[283,295] When contents of blood capillaries including proteins, cells and nutrients spill in excess into the interstitium, then combine with cell waste materials and other interstitial components, the result is a protein-rich, edematous and fibrotic interstitium that retards flow through the tissues. Receptors (protein-molecules that receive chemical-signals from outside the cell) become subject to the inflammatory process and are cleaved by activated matrix metalloproteinases (MMP) that line vessel walls near adipocytes.[296,297] Adipocytes that lose their connection to the environment due to destruction of the receptors, take up more fat than they should, becoming enlarged or hypertrophic,[295] then lose function and die; macrophages become activated and ingest the leftover fat in the dead adipocytes. The macrophages recruit fibroblasts to fill in the damaged tissue with scar tissue resulting in fibrosis. Fibrosis around lobules of adipocytes becomes palpable as nodules under the skin. Inflamed lymphatics and veins develop fibrosis of the vascular walls so they too become palpable under the skin and have reduced function.[298] The inflamed fibrotic SAT can clump further and stick to skin, bone, muscle, tendons, and ligaments further inhibiting flow into and out of the tissue and inducing pain signals in nerves.

Lipedema SAT Nodules and Elasticity

Lipedema SAT tissue nodules range in size from a grain of sand to a frozen pea; these nodules feel rounded, and elastic or hard, unless the overlying skin and fascia becomes edematous or fibrotic masking the presence of the nodules. Areas on the body where the nodules can easily be palpated include the area around the cubit nodes (inside of the elbow) and the medial knee. At least 80% of women with lipedema have small nodules on their arms in addition to nodules in the gynoid distribution.[299,300] The lower abdomen under the umbilicus is a common area for lipedema nodules. Careful palpation of the tissue with the tips of the fingertips in a rolling manner can help find the nodules; just looking at the body without touching the tissue can result in missing pockets of lipedema SAT. Nodules are prevalent in more tissue areas in Stage 3 > Stage 2 > Stage 1.[299] The lipedema SAT can also feel and look more gel-like especially on the upper inner thigh when there is a loss of elasticity in the skin; loss of skin elasticity can occur in other areas as well, especially the upper arm (▶ Fig. 3.84).

Lipedema Pain

Pain is notable in most women with lipedema but not 100%. A history of significant growing pains affecting the legs, premenstrual and menstrual pain, and pain to the touch are common complaints from women with lipedema. Pain in the tissue can be excruciating, occurring after the slightest pressure such as a cat walking on the affected legs or a light touch. In the absence of stated pain, pain can be elicited by rotating a finger over a small nodule in the fat. The cause of the

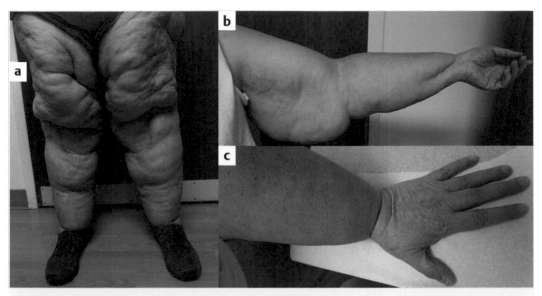

Fig. 3.84 Stage 3 Type III and V lipedema. Extensive excess heavy tissue on the upper arm which with loss of elasticity and thinning of the skin. There is a cuff at the ankle and at the wrist and the hand is obviously completely unaffected.

pain is not clear at this time but compression of nerves by enlarged fibrotic vessels and SAT, and nerves sitting in a caustic interstitial fluid are two plausible hypotheses. Average pain levels in women with lipedema can be very high, 7 out of 10 on a visual analogue scale (VAS; zero = no pain and 10 = the worst pain ever).[299] Pain scores significantly reduced from an average of 7.2 ± 2.2 by VAS, to 2.1 ± 2.1 ($p < 0.001$) after liposuction.[301]

3.14.3 Imaging

Lymphangioscintigraphy (LAS)

The diagnosis of lipedema is made clinically but imaging modalities are useful for visualizing the structure of the lymphatics and to assess for obstruction or lymphedema. Whole body LAS is the first-line imaging modality for visualization of the lymphatic vasculature and for assessment of lymphatic flow in lipedema. Transport of lymph through lymphatics can be normal in lipedema[161] but the lymphatics tend to be tortuous especially below the knee and lymphedema can be present (▶ Fig. 3.85). Others have found a marked slowness and asymmetry of the lymphatic system as compared with normal subjects.[287,302] Clinical phenotyping of lipedema and correlation with LAS is important to understand when and why the lymphatic system slows in lipedema.

Dual Energy X-ray Absorptiometry Scans

Dual energy X-ray absorptiometry (DEXA) scans for whole body composition demonstrate significantly higher amount of fat adjusted for BMI in the legs and in the gynoid region in women with lipedema group compared to women without lipedema.[303] Interestingly, this increase in gynoid fat in lipedema is independent of obesity; no matter the size, gynoid SAT is evident. An optimal cutoff for leg fat mass adjusted for BMI was proposed as 0.46 with a good sensitivity (0.87), helpful for ruling out lipedema, but a low specificity (0.68) raising the number of women who would be misdiagnosed with lipedema.

Magnetic Resonance Imaging (MRI)

In advanced lipedema Stage 3, MRI shows massive circumferential enlargement of SAT lobules and fibrous septa without subcutaneous edema.[304] Dilated lymphatic vessels were found in the lower leg of 40% and upper leg in 20% of women with lipedema by MR lymphography yet lymphatic flow was normal.[288]

Indirect Lymphography

Demonstration of initial lymphatics has been performed in lipedema using indirect lymphography.

3

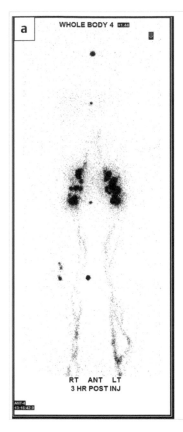 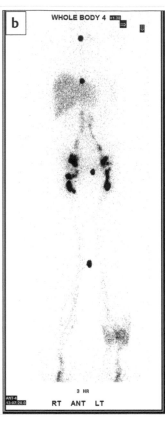

Fig. 3.85 Lymphangioscintigraphy in two women with lipedema. In both cases, following the bilateral intradermal toe webspace injections of approximately 1 mCi of filtered Technetium 99 m sulfur colloid, immediate dynamic images demonstrate prompt superior migration of radiotracer up the legs. Multiple lymphatic channels are seen in both lower extremities with relatively tortuous course particularly below the knee. The delayed images show continued normal migration of radiotracer superiorly visualization of the abdominal nodes. Radiotracer uptake in the liver is also identified at 3 hours. (a) A 50–year-old woman with local dilatation of lymphatic vessels seen in the right lateral leg at the level of knee of uncertain clinical significance. (b) A 69-year-old woman with lipolymphedema. Edema is seen in the distal left lower extremity.

Radio contrast media is injected intradermally and visualized under a fluoroscopic monitor. In a healthy lower extremity, imaging of the injection site appears rounded and normal linear lymphatics fill from this area. In lipedema, the contrast medium depots are flame-shaped instead of circular and tonguelike projections taper and end in normal appearing lymph collectors.[305] These data suggest that the tissue in lipedema is more pliable or hyperextensible which may correlate with hypermobility in lipedema.[299]

3.14.4 Stages and Types of Lipedema

Stages of Lipedema

Stages describe changes seen within lipedema SAT and skin (▶ Table 3.29), but absolute progression between Stages is not required. In **Stage 1**, the subcutaneous adipose tissue (SAT) expands on the lower body in the gynoid distribution but can also occur on the arms; the skin appears remarkably smooth without a cellulite appearance (▶ Fig. 3.86**a**); nodules can be palpated within the SAT. So much

SAT can grow under the skin that it can balloon out over the ankle forming a "cuff" (Table 3.29). A cuff can also develop on the wrist. Many women with SAT cuffs complain about the inability to wear boots and some shoes. Compression can also cause pain in the cuff area and foam pads or inserts are required to prevent damage to the skin and tissue. The SAT can be very painful in Stage 1, and easy bruising can be prominent; lymphedema can also develop but the occurrence is less than with Stage 2 or Stage 3 lipedema.

In **Stage 2**, the fibrous septae between fat lobules contract pulling the skin down in a mattress pattern (▶ Fig. 3.86**b,c**). In addition to easy bruising and pain, the SAT nodules can become stuck together, likely secondary to inflammation-induced fibrosis, forming a mass of SAT akin to a lipoma. These masses can occur anywhere in the SAT but often on the ankle anterior to the lateral malleolus, on the medial knee, thighs and hips. Lymphedema occurs more often in Stage 2 lipedema than Stage 1.[306]

In **Stage 3** lipedema, the tissue becomes flush with macrophages, especially around adipocytes in crown like structures, and fibrosis develops

Table 3.29 Stages and types of lipedema

Stage	Skin	Hypodermis			Risk of lymphedema[34]
		Expanded	Nodular	Folded	
1	Smooth	X	X		+
2	Indented—"mattress"	X	X		+ +
3	Folded	X	X	X	+ + +
4	Variable—based on stage	X	X	Variable	Lymphedema present
Type	**Lipedema tissue location**				
I	Hip and buttock region; ankle cuff not present				
II	Hips down to the knees; ankle cuff not present				
III	Hips and buttocks down to the ankles; cuff usually present; "harem pant" appearance				
IV	Arms are affected; usually along with legs				
V	Knees to ankle				

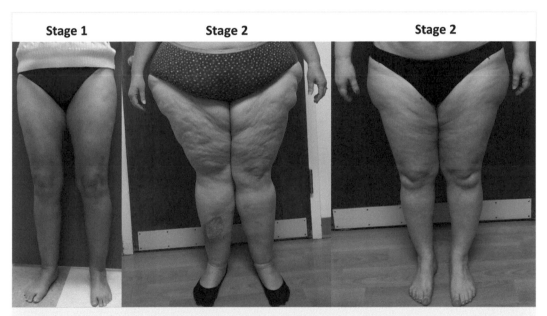

Stage 1 **Stage 2** **Stage 2**

Fig. 3.86 Comparison of Stage I and Stage II lipedema. (a) Expanded hypodermis and smooth skin in Stage I. (b) Valgus stance in a woman with Stage 2 Type III lipedema and Ehlers Danlos Hypermobility Type; cuff at the ankle. A scar is present on the right lower leg from an injury. (c) Stage 2 Type II lipedema without an ankle cuff. Notice the fullness of the subcutaneous adipose tissue on the anterior shin under the knee most visible on the right leg.

around cells and in the lobular septae surrounding fat lobules.[295] It is not known whether macrophages are prevalent in all stages, and all areas of lipedema SAT. Edema is also found around fat cells and lymphedema can occur in Stage 3. The dermis can lift from the hypodermis forming "bubbles" in the skin especially notable on the thigh

(▶ Fig. 3.84**a**). What is most striking about Stage 3 lipedema SAT tissue is that it creates folds or stretches into lobules that cause deformations in the lymphatic vessels and other structures, which may impede the flow of lymph fluid in the tissue. Walking can become difficult in Stage 3 due to the weight of the legs, pain in the knees, and interference by large amounts of SAT, including the lobules. The medial thigh and knee lipedema SAT commonly push the lower legs apart causing a knock-knee stance (genu valgum). The lower ankle is a common place for fibrosis to develop in the skin and underlying tissue due to excess fluid that leaks in this dependent area in a pre-lymphedema condition, and from venous involvement (phlebolipedema). Fibrosis also develops deep in the SAT tissue commonly on the upper buttocks and hips and along the groin causing tenderness to palpation and pain in this area with sitting for prolonged periods or when compression is applied. The large clumps of fat contort the shape of the tissue and on lymphangioscintigraphy, the lymphatic vessels are described as tortuous. Early on in the disease the lymphatics increase their function but over time wear out forming microaneurysms which eventually leak.[284,286,287,288] Women can rapidly progress to Stage 3 lipedema seemingly bypassing earlier stages. There are three conditions that appear to promote the development of Stage 3 lipedema including (1) polycystic ovarian syndrome (PCOS) in which women have high testosterone levels and android but also gynoid obesity[307]; (2) lymphedema; and (3) the connective tissue disorder, Ehlers Danlos Syndrome Hypermobility Type (EDS-HT); indeed, in one study, approximately half of women with lipedema had hypermobile joints consistent with EDS-HT.[306]

Types of Lipedema

There are five types of lipedema (Table 3.29). The type of lipedema refers to the location of the lipedema SAT tissue on the body. Joints are used to demarcate lipedema SAT on the leg but it is not absolute. For example, women with Type II where lipedema SAT extends from the waist to the knees can also have mounds of nodular lipedema SAT on the anterior lower legs just under the knees even though the lower leg and ankle are not involved. Women with Type V lipedema can also have nodular lipedema SAT on the thighs despite the huge amount of fat on the lower leg compared to the thighs. Types of lipedema SAT also do not take into account the location of fat in other areas. For example, many women with lipedema have nodular lipedema SAT below and above the umbilicus, sparing the lateral abdomen. The suprapubic area can also become nodular and tender with lipedema SAT and intercourse can become painful due to involvement of the genitalia.

3.14.5 Genetics

The gene or genes underlying lipedema are not known but inheritance has been described in up to 60% of families.[308,309,310] Inheritance of lipedema is considered autosomal dominant with incomplete penetrance.[281] This means that a mother or father can pass lipedema down to a child, and that each child has a 50% chance of inheriting the gene or genes for lipedema, but that the expression of lipedema may vary amongst the women; in addition, men who pass on lipedema do not seem to have lipedema SAT. Men reported with lipedema in the literature tend to have low testosterone or liver disease, both of which are associated with a relative increase in estrogen levels and therefore a higher estrogen to testosterone ratio. These data suggest that higher testosterone levels or a low estrogen to testosterone ratio may be protective against lipedema, at least in men, but not women with PCOS.

Approximately 50% of women with lipedema have hypermobile joints by the Beighton score[299] suggesting that genes important in joint hypermobility may also be important in lipedema. A putative gene for Ehlers Danlos hypermobility type is *TNXB* producing tenascin X[311,312,313]; mutations in this gene have not been assessed in women with lipedema.

As lipedema is primarily a disorder of gynoid SAT, genes expressed exclusively in this area should be of interest. Developmental genes exclusive to gynoid SAT include *Shox2*, *HOXA10* and *HOTAIR*.[314,315] Deletion of *Shox2* protects mice against high-fat-diet-induced obesity, and adipocytes in these mice demonstrate increased expression of the β3 adrenergic receptor and increased rates of lipolysis; over-expression of *Shox2* results in decreased β3 adrenergic receptor expression and rates of lipolysis which would be more likely in lipedema.[316] *HOXA10* gene expression is regulated by progesterone and estrogen,[317] regulates the production of bone marrow stem cells[318] and is down-regulated in adipocytes by insulin.[319] Epigenetics appears to be important in the depot-specific expression of *HOTAIR*[314] and it might be a gluteal-specific adipogenic regulator that contributes to the expansion of this SAT depot.[320] More data is needed to better understand if these genes also are important in lipedema. Additional gene candidates for lipedema have been reviewed.[291]

3.14.6 Comorbid Conditions in Lipedema

In addition to Ehlers Danlos syndrome, 38% of women with lipedema were reported to have arthritis or dyslipidemia and 48% of the women had undergone abdominal or pelvic surgery.[299] Musculoskeletal complications include gait disturbance, change in posture and arthritis especially of the knees. Soft-tissue abnormalities include obesity, which may be in part due to a slower metabolic rate,[321] decreased skin elasticity, lipomas, thinning of the skin, cellulite, unusual fatty deposits and cysts that form due to increased shearing forces around skin adnexa (hair, sebaceous glands). Vascular complications include lymphedema, bruising, edema especially in warm weather or after standing for long periods, and varicose veins noted in 35%.[321] Shortness of breath, cellulitis especially with underlying lymphatic dysfunction, and psychological distress and anxiety are also notable in women with lipedema.

3.14.7 Differentiating Conditions of Obesity and Other Edematous Disorders from Lipedema

Obesity

Lipedema is often confused with lifestyle-induced obesity.[284] However women with lipedema tend to restrict caloric intake developing anorexia and other eating disorders; they may also over-exercise,[322] the opposite of lifestyle-induced obesity, and none of these attempts induce loss of the lipedema SAT; women with lipedema have lifestyle-resistant SAT. A woman with lipedema and obesity can reduce obesity SAT under restrictive lifestyle changes, leaving a disproportion of lipedema SAT on the lower part of the body and much less fat on the trunk. Under restrictive lifestyle changes, women with obesity and lipedema notice *some* loss of fat in the areas of lipedema SAT, suggesting that lipedema SAT and obese SAT are intermixed, or that some aspect of lipedema fat does respond to restricted lifestyle changes, but not enough to reduce the large amounts of lipedema SAT. Inability to lose SAT from the gynoid area after lifestyle changes with evident loss of SAT on the trunk, easy bruising, and painful and nodular SAT can all be used to distinguish between lipedema and lifestyle-induced obesity (▶ Table 3.30). A family history of female relatives with excess gynoid SAT

and stovepipe legs, often-time with cuffs, are also helpful in identifying lipedema.

Lymphedema

Lipedema can be confused with other edematous conditions, and edematous conditions can coexist with lipedema, including lymphedema. While lymphedema tends not to have significant pain unless untreated, lipedema can be painful even in Stage 1. Stemmer's sign is positive in lymphedema and not in lipedema until lipo-lymphedema develops. Both limbs are affected in lipedema while unilateral affected limbs are more common in lymphedema though hereditary lymphedema cases can be bilateral (▶ Table 3.31).

Venous Disease

Venous insufficiency and venous dilation increase edema in tissues localized to the lower leg and foot. Red blood cells leak out of veins and deposit hemosiderin in tissues causing the skin to become brown in color while the skin color in lipedema is normal on the leg and foot. Lipedema can be differentiated from venous insufficiency due to the lack of browning in the skin and lack of a positive Stemmer's sign on the feet (▶ Table 3.30). It is thought that approximately 25% of women with lipedema have venous insufficiency, or lipophlebedema therefore an assessment of venous insufficiency by a venous duplex ultrasound is warranted in lipedema to rule out simultaneous venous disease.

Table 3.30 Differentiating lipedema from obesity

	Lipedema	Obesity
Onset puberty	√	Any decade
Painful fat	√	
Easy bruising	√	
Fat unaffected by lifestyle	√	
Responds to diet		√
Disproportion legs > trunk	√	
Nodular fat	√	+/-
Malleolar fat	√	+/-
Involvement of feet	+/-	√

3.14.8 Comparison of Lipedema to Other SAT Disorders and Fibromyalgia

Lipedema can be mistaken for other SAT disorders such as Dercum's disease, familial multiple lipomatosis, Madelung's disease, lipodystrophy and fibromyalgia. Specific signs and symptoms help in differentiating these disorders (▶ Table 3.32).

Dercum's Disease

Women with lipedema have been diagnosed simultaneously with Dercum's disease (DD). There are three types of DD:
- Diffuse Type—small nodules palpated in SAT diffusely over the body;
- Nodular Type—larger nodules big enough to be called lipomas, including angiolipomas, are present on the arms, lower abdomen, flank and

Table 3.31 Differentiating lipedema from lymphedema and venous disease

Sign or symptom	Lipedema	Lymphedema	Venous disease
Sex	Female	Male or female	Male or female
Laterality	Bilateral	Unilateral	Bilateral
Foot edema	No	Yes	Yes
Pain Fat	Yes	No	In area of edema
Tissue fibrosis	Diffuse but subclinical until lymphedema	Present if longstanding untreated	Liposclerosis possible
Skin coloration	Normal	Normal; may darken	Brownish
Stemmer's sign - foot	Negative	Positive	Positive

Table 3.32 Comparison of lipedema to other fat or pain disorders

Characteristic	Lipedema	DD	MSL	FML	Fibromyalgia
Abnormal SAT location	Legs, arms, low abdomen	Global	Upper body	Arms, thighs, abdomen	Global
Diet-resistant SAT	Yes	Yes	Yes	Yes	Unknown
Lipomas	Yes	Common	Common	Common	No
Time SAT change	Puberty; 3rd decade	Child - adult	Adult; child rare	Child - adult	Any age
Painful SAT	Yes	Yes	Not usually	Not usually	Yes
Sex	Female	Female	Male	Male=Female	2:1 F:M[161]
Lymphatic dysfunction	Yes	Yes	Yes	Yes	Benefit from MLD
Prevalence	Common	Rare	Rare	Rare	Common
Associated conditions	Lymphedema	Autoimmune; diabetes	Neuropathy	Moles; neuropathy	Similar to DD
Inheritance Pattern	Autosomal dominant; incomplete penetrance	Autosomal dominant; sex-specific influence	Autosomal dominant or recessive	Autosomal dominant	Polygenic[165]
Gene	None	None	Rare tRNALys	None	No standard[94]
Biomarkers	None	None	None	None	No standard

thighs can disfigure. This type of DD was formerly called Type III;

- Mixed Type—both small and larger nodules are present.

Pain is generally more intense in people with DD, and they have more co-morbid conditions including diabetes, autoimmune disease, IBS, shortness of breath, and exercise intolerance[6] to name a few.

Diffuse Dercum's Disease

Women who have Diffuse DD have SAT in the same gynoid distribution as lipedema, but they have more fat and larger nodules and masses in the abdominal and trunk area especially over the lower ribs in the lateral and anterior aspects of the body. Similar to lipedema, there is a large firm pad or fold of SAT on the back under where the lower aspect of a brassiere presses into the tissue. The pressure on the tissue by the brassiere likely inhibits lymphatic flow through the area resulting in hypoxia, inflammation and fibrosis. Women with lipedema plus diffuse DD usually have a BMI in the overweight to obese range.[299,323] The SAT in Diffuse DD can also appear by MRI similar to massive localized lymphedema.[324]

Nodular and Mixed Dercum's Disease

Women and men with Nodular DD have larger SAT masses or lipomas as a dominant feature on the body. The lipomas can be disfiguring and are found in similar areas as lipomas in the nonpainful disorder familial multiple lipomatosis (FML), i.e., the abdomen, flanks, low back, arms and thighs.[325] People with nodular DD can gain weight that they find hard to lose masking the location of the lipomas; the SAT gained by women with Nodular DD can look similar to lipedema and then it is considered Mixed DD. The lipomas are visible by MRI and ultrasound which can be helpful in the diagnosis when excess lipedema SAT masks accurate palpation of lipomas.[326]

Madelung's Disease (Launois–Bensaude Syndrome)

Madelung's disease is excess SAT that occurs around the face and neck (horsecollar lipomata) primarily in men after alcohol use, or as symmetric masses of SAT on the back, supraclavicular area, abdomen and flank in men and women.[284,327] Women with Madelung's disease can have a large

excess of upper arm SAT similar to lipedema Type IV.[284] The Madelung SAT is not usually painful but can be so enlarged that it causes pain in the skin and prevents movement of the arms similar to lipedema. What is notable in women with Madelung SAT is that they have normal legs.

Fibromyalgia

The pain associated with lipedema can lead to a misdiagnosis of fibromyalgia instead of lipedema. Women with Dercum's disease are more likely to be diagnosed with fibromyalgia than women with lipedema. In fact it has been suggested that people with Nodular DD are on the spectrum with fibromyalgia.[328] Discrete and measurable "geloid masses" in fibromyalgia are described as rubbery and pliable or hard in an extremely taut area of dense tissue without associated edema.[329] The masses can be small, or larger than 2.5 cm in diameter. It is likely that these masses are in muscle and fascia therefore are not equal to the nodules palpated in lipedema and DD. Dysregulation of blood flow in cutaneous arteriole–venule shunts (AVS) in glabrous skin in fibromyalgia patients has been noted to occur as a consequence of an excessive sympathetic and sensory innervation, with the potential to compromise regulation of blood flow in other areas of the body.[330] Fibromyagia may therefore be a vascular disorder similar to lipedema and DD, and these highly innervated AVS should be examined for in lipedema and Dercum's disease.

3.14.9 Standard Treatment of Lipedema

The goals of treatment of lipedema can be met with a multipronged approach (▶ Table 3.33). The Dutch guidelines for the diagnosis and treatment of lipedema recommend stimulating vascular or lymphatic pumping by caloric balance, a meticulous exercise program aimed at strength training and conditioning, and weight loss if needed. MLD is not recommended by these guidelines as a treatment for lipedema unless combined with lymphedema[331,332,333]; in agreement, in one study out of Germany, half of women with lipedema did not respond to MLD.[323]

The percent of women with lipedema in the US that respond by reducing tissue volume and pain with CDT is not known. The main difference in CDT for lipedema compared to lymphedema is that the entire body should be treated, meaning head,

Table 3.33 Multipronged approach to accomplish treatment goals for lipedema

Goals	Effectors							
	CDT and/or ISPCP	Anti-inflammatory medication or supplement	Metformin	Low processed carbohydrate food	Move-ment	Lympha-gogues	Venoton-ics	Liposuc-tion
Decrease capillary fragility/leak	•	•		•	•			
Improve venous dysfunction[82]	•	•		•	•	•	•	
Decrease SAT edema	•	•		•	•	•		•
Decrease insulin resistance	•	•	•	•	•	•		
Decrease lipedema SAT								•
Halt growth of new lipedema SAT	•	•		•	•	•	•	•
Improve mobility	•	•		•	•	•		•
Reduce pain	•	•		•	•	•	•	•

neck, all four limbs, pelvis, trunk, back and abdomen. This might be different for therapists who are used to treating legs or arms only for lymphedema. Women with lipedema may have painful sexual intercourse due to affected tissue or swelling requiring pelvic physical therapy including intra-vaginal MLD.

Compression Garments

If a patient with lipedema responds to CDT, she is a candidate for compression garments which help support skin that has lost its elasticity, reduce fluid accumulation in lipedema SAT, and prevent return of fluid after MLD or other therapies. In the absence of lymphedema, the compression garment strength for lipedema SAT can be as light as 8–15 mm Hg and as high as 20–30 mm Hg. Even if high compression is warranted, a woman with very painful lipedema may not be able to tolerate the higher compression levels and therefore lower compression levels should be suggested; it is better to have some compression rather than none at all. The abdomen should always be treated along with the legs to prevent fluid accumulating in the abdominal tissue when just thigh high compression stockings are prescribed. High waist leggings are the preferred lower compression garment with ankle length or open or closed toes per patient preference and location of SAT. The cuff at the ankle can be difficult to compress requiring foam or other inserts to prevent damage to the tissue from the compression garments. Changes in the skin including loss of elasticity and edema may alter the ability for initial lymphatics in the skin to take up the excess fluid in lipedema, therefore patterned compression garments that help engorge and stimulate the initial lymphatic endings may be very effective in treating the edema component of lipedema. Women with nodular lipedema SAT on the hands should be offered gauntlets if the hands swell. Arm compression is also needed in lipedema and the one-piece dual arm compression garments are ideal to treat the axillary area which becomes engorged and tender in lipedema. Trunk compression is also warranted to provide extra support to the abdomen and the lower back, areas which become involved in lipedema to a greater extent in Stage 2 and 3.

Sequential Pneumatic Compression Pumps

A number of studies have shown the benefit of intermittent sequential pneumatic compression pumps (ISPCP) in the treatment of lymphedema. There are also a number of studies on the use of ISPCP in the treatment of lipedema. ISPCP therapy does not adversely affect lipedema[202]; when secondary lymphedema is present, ISPCP improves wounds in women with lipedema.[275] Important for lipedema where leaky capillaries are proposed as underlying pathology for lipedema,[283,310] ISPCP decreases capillary[334] making vessels healthier, meeting a goal in lipedema treatment (▶ Table 3.33). ISPCP is also recommended in conjunction with liposuction surgery for lipedema.[323] A clinical trial is needed to determine which women with lipedema clearly benefit from ISPCP; this study could also supply information on fluid retention in the SAT. If a woman with lipedema responds well to MLD as part of CDT, or she tries an ISPCP and has a reduction in tissue volume, she should be offered ISPCP therapy to continue treatment at home when insurance will no longer cover CDT or when distance or commitments prevent regular professional visits. The ISPCP should be an E0652 device with a segmented, multiported pump that allows for individual pressure calibration at each port. This allows the patient to alter pressure in areas of severe pain or for different shaped tissue. Pump garments should wrap around and treat the abdomen and pelvis when the legs are pumped, and the chest when the arms are pumped. If basic compression pumps, usually reserved for prevention of deep venous thromboses or for treatment of cardiovascular edema (E0650; E0651) are the only alternative, pressure should be kept low so as to not damage the valves of the lymphatic vessels, and compression garments to protect the abdomen, pelvis, chest and/or head should be worn during pumping. Without these compression garments, fluid is pushed up the leg into the abdominal and pelvic area where it accumulates due to lymphatic dysfunction. As this fluid sits in the tissue with all its nutrients and protein, fat grows.[335] With an E0652 pump, the abdomen is treated along with the leg and the chest is treated along with the arm preventing dangerous pooling of lymph fluid.

Lifestyle

Exercise

Even though lipedema SAT will not reduce, exercise and eating healthy foods are the standard of care for lipedema. Exercise improves lymphatic and venous pumping by the action of muscle contraction and strengthens and increases muscle groups that feed on blood fats and take up blood sugar.[336] Weight loss is not required to improve lymphatic pumping; for example, aerobic exercise training of high-fat diet-induced obese mice results in improved lymphatic function, *independent of weight loss*[337]; these changes correlated with decreased perilymphatic inflammatory cell accumulation and normalization of lymphatic endothelial cell gene expression. Types of exercise important in lipedema care include walking in compression garments, Nordic walking, swimming or any kind of water movement where the water acts as compression around the entire body thereby stimulating lymph flow, whole body vibration, mini-trampoline with handles for safety, spinning or biking, Pilates, yoga, dancing, etc. The goal is to maintain daily movement without generating lactic acid and reactive oxygen species causing a burning feeling and damage to the tissue. If a burning feeling does occur with exercise, exercise should be halted or slowed and then resumed once the burning feeling has dissipated. A new form of therapy that may be beneficial in lipedema is the use of an underwater stationary bike.[338] Another unique form of exercise is the Cyclic Variations in Adaptive Conditioning (CVAC®) Process which improved pain and mental function while reducing weight and body fluid in people with Dercum's disease.[339] The CVAC Process form of exercise is ideal for a woman with lipedema who has trouble ambulating as she simply sits comfortably in the CVAC Pod while air cycles around her, likened to a touch free sequential pneumatic pump but for the entire body. The CVAC Process has been shown to improve metabolism in sedentary men.[340]

Healthy Eating Plan

There are no diet studies evaluating changes in SAT tissue in women with lipedema. Instead, the goal of food choices should be to lower inflammation or the generation of inflammation, while providing optimal nutrition (▶ Table 3.33). Women with lipedema eating rainbow colored fruits and vegetables and lean meats, primarily fish, while lowering processed food and simple carbohydrates

3

such as those from white flour and sugar,[341] feel well, have less pain, and more energy. Some women also find benefit from an Atkins (high fat and protein) type diet. In either case, processed simple carbohydrates are kept to a minimum. Meat should be a condiment in the meal (small portion) and eating meats such as grain-fed beef or grain-fed chicken should be avoided due to the prevalence of inflammatory omega-6 fatty acids from the grain in the meat. Grass fed beef and chicken are available which are good alternatives if meat is eaten. Grains should also be a condiment at meals where brown or wild rice improves insulin sensitivity compared to white rice,[342] and old grains such as quinoa, and teff should be considered. Vegetable smoothies containing spinach, kale, ginger, lemon, green apple and berries are a great way to get good nutrition quickly. Many women with lipedema seem to do well with reducing gluten and dairy in their diet, substituting goat and sheep cheese, high protein yogurt and kefir which all seem to be tolerated better than dairy. Resources on nutrition for lipedema are available.[341]

3.14.10 Nonstandard Treatment of Lipedema

Lipedema fat is resistant to diet and exercise. There is nothing that reliably reduces lipedema SAT except excision by liposuction (discussed below). Supplements, medications, and other therapeutic modalities have been used in clinical practice and have been discovered by patients on their own to reduce limb heaviness, pain, and fibrosis and improve mobility and mentation. Clinical studies on nonstandard treatment modalities are needed to better understand how to improve lipedema.

Lymphagogues

A lymphagogue is an agent that increases the function of lymphatic vessels. There are multiple medications and supplements available that are documented to improve lymphatic flow (▶ Table 3.34). Most of the known lymphagogues that are available as medications increase lymphatic function through alteration of the sympathetic nervous system. Amphetamines such as dextroamphetamine, increase the release of norepinephrine and other transmitters from nerves innervating lymphatic vessels[343]; phentermine is a sympathomimetic amine with pharmacologic activity similar to amphetamine and has been used successfully to treat the obesity component

of SAT in women with lipedema. Unfortunately, the amphetamine-type medications tend not to be available in Europe. Plant derivatives also can affect the sympathetic nervous system. The ruscogenins in the Butcher's broom plant (*Ruscus aculeatus*) bind to α1 and α2 adrenergic receptors and augment the release of norepinephrine from sympathetic nerves[344] increasing oncotic pressure in the lymphatic system and venous tone without affecting arteries.[345] Citrus peel-derived diosmin (synthetically converted from hesperidin), inhibits catechol-O-methyltransferase decreasing the metabolism of norepinephrine enhancing sympathetic activity.[346] A hydrolysis product of rutin, quercetin,[347] acts synergistically with epinephrine on beta-adrenergic receptors stimulating lipolysis in adipocytes.[348]

Anecdotally, lymphagogues have been used in the clinical setting and each has shown benefit in some women with lipedema; not all women benefit from each of the lymphagogues; clinical trials are needed to confirm the effectiveness of lymphagogues in lipedema and to figure out why some women respond well and others do not.

Anti-Inflammatories for the Vascular System

Lymphatic vessels originate from embryonic veins (lymphangiogenesis) except for some dermal lymphatics,[351] therefore both lymphatics and veins tend to benefit from similar therapies. Many natural compounds have anti-inflammatory properties that can be important in maintaining the integrity of veins and lymphatics in women with lipedema. These include L-arginine, an amino acid known to restore aberrant nitrous oxide signaling by reducing phosphodiesterase 3 and therefore lymphatic vessel leakage,[352] Pycnogenol, or French maritime pine bark extract that improves venous insufficiency and venous tone,[353] and beta aescin from horse chestnut seed extract and other seeds that strengthen venous tone[354] and increase venous pressure thus promoting venous and lymphatic return.[355] Anecdotally the anti-inflammatory products work well in women with lipedema reducing pain and tissue fluid, but all need formal testing in women with lipedema.

Selenium

Selenium is a mineral that when taken internally inhibits matrix metalloproteinase (MMP)-2,[356] an enzyme important in lymphatic vessel remodeling

Table 3.34 Lymphagogues

Medication Plant Derivative	Lymphatic Effect	Other Uses	Side Effects
Medications			
Dextroamphetamine, amphetamine, amphetamine salts	Indirect through release of norepinephrine and inhibition of reuptake from nerves[112]	Attention deficit, hyperactivity disorder	Hypertension, palpitations, tachycardia, CNS overstimulation, gastrointestinal disturbances, urticaria, impotence
Ketoprofen	Improves experimental lymphatic insufficiency in rats[182]	Pain[183]	Nausea and vomiting[185]
Phentermine	Increases sympathetic activity[185]; effect on lymphatics is unknown but likely similar to ampheatmine	Weight loss[186]	Hypertension, palpitations, tachycardia, CNS overstimulation, gastrointestinal disturbances, urticaria, impotence[187]
Plant derivatives			
Butcher's broom root (*Ruscus aculeatus*)	Reduced secondary lymphedema[188];improved lymphatic flow and intensity[189]; reduced vascular permeability[190]; antielastase[191]	Venous insufficiency[192]; premenstrual syndrome[168]; hemorrhoids[167]; orthostatic hypotension[166]	Nausea[171] and vomiting[349]; edema, abdominal pain[171]
Diosmin	Increased lymphatic vessel contractility[172,193,350]	Vein health[194]; hemorrhoids[195]; protects gastric mucosa[196]	Two cases: increased creatine phosphokinase; increased lactate dehydrogenase[197]
Quercetin-3-O-rutinoside (rutin)	Increases lymph flow[198] and heavy legs[201]	Venous health[194,203]; diabetes[204]; cramps[201]	Abdominal pain, diarrhea, flatulence, nausea, epistaxis[201]

and vessel damage[357]; selenium improved limb volume in combination with Butcher's broom in a woman with lipedema.[358] Selenium is recommended for the excess fluid component of lymphedema and lipedema because it decreased lymphedema in two placebo controlled trials for postmastectomy and head and neck cancer,[359,360] and increased the efficacy of physical therapy while reducing the incidence of erysipelas infections in patients with chronic lymphedema.[359] Additional anti-inflammatory mechanisms of selenium include lowering oxygen radical[361] and reducing glycoprotein adhesion molecules (P-selectin, intercellular *adhesion* molecule-1, vascular cell adhesion molecule-1, endothelial leukocyte adhesion molecule-1) in a dose-dependent manner.[362] Average amounts of selenium taken in clinical trials of lymphedema range from 500–600 micrograms daily. The US National Research Council has defined the individual maximum safe

dietary intake for selenium as 600 mcg daily and the no adverse effect level as 800 mcg daily.[358,363] Selenium may be obtained from Brazil nuts containing 200 micrograms selenium per nut. High selenium levels have been associated with diabetes in a large database[364] therefore checking blood levels of selenium under the care of a health care provider during supplementation is important.

Metformin

The hypoglycemic medication, metformin, is reserved for the treatment of insulin resistance or diabetes. Metformin is a useful medication in women with lipedema who have or are developing metabolic syndrome as it improves inflammation,[365] reduces weight, improves gut bacteria,[366] which is known to impact obesity, and improves longevity.[367] As diabetes and therefore metabolic syndrome is common in Dercum's disease (incidence of 16%),[279] women with Dercum's disease and women with lipedema who are developing signs and symptoms of the metabolic dysfunction associated with Dercum's disease should be considered for metformin treatment (▶ Table 3.33).

Whole Body Vibration

Whole body vibration (WBV) by a powerful motor transmitted to the entire body of a person standing on a platform excites stretch receptors and tendon reflexes in joints. Whole body vibration improves peripheral circulation[368,369] and increases lymphatic flow raising the threshold level for edema formation in the legs.[370] Anecdotally, women with lipedema who use WBV even just minutes a day experience improvement in the feeling of heaviness of the legs and have experienced weight loss of nonlipedema SAT. Studies are needed to better understand how WBV can help women with lipedema.

3.14.11 Surgical Treatment of Lipedema

Liposuction of lipedema SAT with an aim to spare any damage to lymphatic and blood vessels, has been performed in Europe, especially in Germany, since the 1990s.[301,371,372,373] In power liposuction, the SAT is tumesced with a combination of saline, a local anesthetic such as lidocaine or prilocaine, a small amount of buffer[374] and with or without steroid[375] firming up the turgor of the tissue to the consistency of a watermelon to allow the blunt microcannulae to slide in the tissue avoiding the creation of shearing forces and vessel damage. Tiny, rapid vibrations of the microcannulae break up fat which is then suctioned out of the tissue. Water jet assisted liposuction (WAL) uses jets of saline and local anesthesia to release the fat for suction into a blunt cannulae that is held and moved like a violin or cello bow across strings, a gentle procedure that can leave cells and vessels intact.[372] The WAL equipment can also be used to tumesce the tissue. Laser assisted liposuction is usually reserved for more fibrotic areas of the tissue such as the posterior thighs or lower leg.

Surgical Approaches

Removal of the lipedema SAT by liposuction can be performed (1) circumferentially on the thigh, lower leg, upper and lower arms; or (2) by removal of the lipedema SAT in sections including medial thigh and knee in one operation, then outer thigh and hips in a second operation and the circumferential lower leg in the second or a third operation (▶ Fig. 3.87); the average number of surgeries for a women with Stage II lipedema was 2.6 in one practice[323]; in another clinic in Germany, women with stage II lipedema needed two to three surgeries but in some, more than five sessions were necessary due to the amount of SAT.[376] Arms and touch-up can be performed in a final operation.[323] Both the circumferential and the strip methods aim to remove as much of the lipedema SAT in the safest manner. Patients are usually awake during the liposuction procedure working with the surgeon to move on the table into positions, including standing, that allow the best outcome for the part of the body undergoing liposuction; some physicians choose to have anesthesiologists or anesthetists provide twilight sedation, for example, intravenous diazepam[301] or low dose propofol.[377] Conscious sedation with sublingual valium, intravenous fentanyl or midazolam, or nitrous oxide are alternatives[378] however some patients and physicians prefer general anesthesia especially if the patient is very sensitive or has high anxiety about the procedure. If liposuction is performed under general anesthesia, the observation period after surgery must be extended. The benefit of the patient being completely awake during the surgery or with twilight sedation includes a rapid recovery.[377] It should be noted that propofol (Diprivan) significantly decreases the amplitude of spontaneous activity of lymphatic vessels.[379] In terms of general anesthesia, the contractility of mesenteric lymphatics was suppressed in a dose-dependent manner by halothane.[380] Pentobarbitone and halothane together inhibited bovine lymphatic contractility.[381] Lymph flow was suppressed by general anesthesia most in peripheral regions (skin, tendon, muscular areas) while lymph draining soft tissues in central regions (kidney, liver) was less affected.[382] Prior to undergoing liposuction by a qualified surgeon, a patient should have a thorough knowledge of the surgeon's technique, whether the surgeon uses general anesthesia along with the type of analgesia, the number of surgeries performed by the surgeon and outcomes and complications.

Qualitative Measures of Liposuction

Two surgeons in Germany in different clinics have assessed signs and symptoms after power

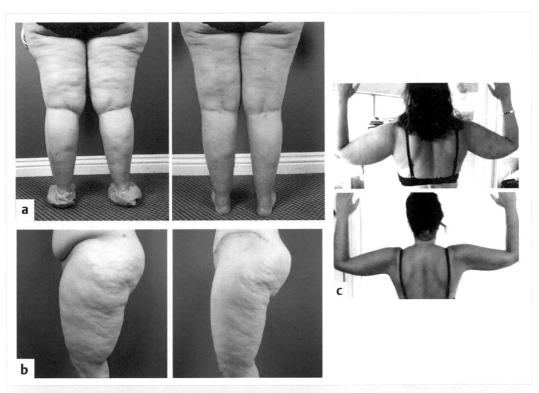

Fig. 3.87 Pre- and postliposuction pictures. **(a)** Stage II lipedema of the lower extremities. Before (left) and after (right) combination liposculpture with water-assisted (Body-Jet), laser-asissted (SmartLipo), and power-assisted (MicroAire PAL) devices. Disproportion and contour improved after 3 months; pain and swelling resolved after 6 months. **(b)** Stage II lipedema of the lower extremities. Before (left) and after (right) combination liposculpture with water-assisted (Body-Jet), laser-asissted (SmartLipo), and power-assisted (MicroAire PAL) devices. Disproportion and contour improved after 3 months on circumferential thighs. Note improvement in size and cellulite. The torso (back and stomach) were also treated with liposculpture followed by skin removal (tummy tuck) without any complications. **(c)** Stage II Lipedema of the upper extremities. Before (top) and after (bottom) combination liposculpture with water-assisted (Body-Jet), ultrasound-asissted (VASER), and power-assisted (PowerX) devices. Disproportion and contour improved after 1 month. Notice the significant skin retraction and decrease in size. Photos and procedure text courtesy of Jason Emer, MD, FAAD, FAACS, The Roxbury Institute, Beverly Hills, CA.

liposuction in significant numbers of women with lipedema. Twenty-five women treated in the clinic of Dr. Stefan Rapprich had significant improvements in pain, tension in the legs, excessive warmth, muscle cramps, leg heaviness, legs that feel tired, swelling, itching and general involvement of the skin, difficulty walking, quality of life and appearance of the legs six months postsurgery.[301] A larger study of 85 women from the same clinic again demonstrated significant improvements six months after surgery for all complaints with the greatest improvement in quality of life[323] similar to the previous study.[301] Dr. Wilfred Schmeller's clinic followed twenty-one women for an average of 3 years and 8 months after the first power liposuction and 2 years and 11 months after

the second surgery showing improvement in the parameters of body disproportion, swelling, edema and quality of life, except for bruising which improved in all but two of the women.[371] A retrospective study on women with Stage I or II lipedema (only 2% had Stage III) from the same clinic, four, and eight years after liposuction, for parameters including pain, sensitivity to pressure, edema, bruising, restriction of movement, cosmetic impairment, reduction of overall quality of life and overall impairment, demonstrated an almost identical maintenance of significantly improved scores at both time points.[383] Women who have Stage II and III lipedema tend to do better in qualitative assessments after liposuction because they have a greater extent and number of complaints than women with Stage I therefore more room to improve.[376] The most interesting data from the qualitative studies of signs and symptoms after liposuction was the reduced need for combined decongestive therapy four years after liposuction that decreased even further eight years after surgery[376]; similar to data from Dr. Rapprich.[301,323] Interestingly, in the latter study by Dr. Schmeller, after liposuction, trouser size decreased by one size in 38% of the patients, 25% had a decrease of two sizes and 11% a three size decrease; but 23% of the patients did not notice any change and 2% experienced an increase of one size.[376] It will be important to determine which women do not benefit from liposuction. Outside of Germany, in terms of long-term studies, improvement in pain and mobility along with the aesthetic component of lipedema has been reported four years after liposuction for a single case.[384] The number of surgeons performing liposuction for lipedema in the United States dramatically increased in 2015–2016. Documenting patient baseline characteristics and outcomes by these surgeons will be important to understand the benefits of liposuction for lipedema in the US population compared to Europe.

Medical Necessity for Liposuction Surgery in Lipedema

The majority of women with lipedema have medically necessary reasons for undergoing liposuction of lipedema SAT. Common indications for liposuction surgery for lipedema include

- Loss of mobility as assessed by a functional questionnaire[385] especially when documented over time, or loss of mobility requiring use of an assistive device such as a cane, walker, wheelchair or scooter.
- Reduced quality of life especially when lymphedema is present[101]
- Joint damage or altered gait: These include degenerative disc disease of the spine, significant arthritis of the spine due to lordosis, and/or knee damage with or without the need for total knee replacement from the valgus stance due to lipedema SAT on the medial leg.
- Chronic pain requiring medication, imaging, clinic visits, and/or resulting in missed opportunities inside and outside the home or at work, or a significantly reduced quality of life.
- Failure to improve signs and symptoms associated with lipedema despite conservative therapy.

Preparing for Surgery

CDT including MLD, compression garments, a healthy eating plan, and movement are requirements before liposuction for surgery. The surgeon will order lab tests which include a complete blood count (CBC) with platelet level, electrolyte assessment and kidney function (basic metabolic panel), liver panel to ensure the liver is not inflamed and that it is properly functioning, as well as coagulation labs to include activated prothrombin time (aPTT), prothrombin time (PT), thrombin time (TT), fibrinogen. People with normal coagulation labs and easy bruising can have hereditary and acquired platelet defects, hereditary disorders of vascular and perivascular tissues including Ehlers Danlos Syndrome and disorders of blood clotting. Any woman with lipedema and a personal or family history of bleeding or clotting should work with a health care provider to determine additional testing needed well before liposuction surgery.[386]

Insurance Coverage for Liposuction

Any surgery, including liposuction, requires a case be established to prove medical necessity to the insurance company. Insurance approvals for nonliposuction emergent surgeries are commonplace and nonliposuction elective surgeries have strong evidence-based data in the literature. Surgical resection of lipedema SAT is elective, has minimal supporting evidence-based data in the published literature, and is therefore confused with the aesthetic need to improve body shape without a specific medical need. As more case reports, case series and benefits are reported on liposuction for lipedema in the literature, emergent liposuction cases are likely to occur, and insurance is more likely to cover liposuction procedures. Surgeons agree that quality of life is strongly and consistently improved by liposuction.[301,323,383,387]

The patient can immensely improve the chance of insurance coverage of liposuction for lipedema by collecting evidence in a concise and clear manner (notebook with tabs, pdf file with index, historical and current pictures, etc.).

Suggested materials to collect:
- **Patient's self-description** of their life with lipedema including obstacles.
- **Documentation of conservative therapy** including MLD, us of compression garments, use of ISPCP, activity such as swimming, WBV, healthy food eating patterns, supplements, and medications taken specifically for lipedema.

- **Consultation reports**: Documentation of issues due to lipedema:
  - Orthopaedic surgeon: Spine, knee and other bone and joint problems; include imaging.
  - Podiatry: Abnormal gait and bone and joint damage of the feet; need for orthotics, specialized shoes or surgery.
  - Lymphedema therapy trained physical or occupational therapist report: Measurements of limb volume and response to therapy aimed at reducing fluid in the limbs (includes MLD).
  - Physical therapy or physical medicine and rehab: Functional assessment of gait, strength, mobility, fatigue.
  - Lymphedema/lipedema physician specialist: Physical exam and recommendations; letter of medical necessity.
  - Surgeon consulted for liposuction (dermatology, plastic, vascular, general, other): Exam and agreement by the surgeon for need for therapy, location of lipedema amenable to liposuction, along with an estimate on the number of operations, the amount of SAT likely to be removed, and the specific areas targeted for removal.

Complications of Liposuction for Lipedema

Complications after liposuction for lipedema are rare, especially when women are mobilized immediately after surgery. There is a single report of acute pulmonary edema and pneumonia in a woman who had 2600 mL of lipedema SAT suctioned from her bilateral thighs.[388] A patient with lipedema who had a previous DVT developed a DVT one week after liposuction.[301] In 112 women who underwent 349 liposuctions, 1.4% of patients developed postoperative infections despite prophylactic antibiotics, and one patient had a significant amount of blood loss.[376] The need for choosing a liposuction surgeon with medical experience and technical expertise is demonstrated by reported complications after liposuction procedures (not necessarily for lipedema specifically) including necrotizing fasciitis, toxic shock syndrome, hemorrhage, perforation of inner organs and pulmonary embolism.[389] The Dutch lipedema guidelines agree that liposuction and/or reductive surgery "should take place in specialized centers, where these procedures should be performed by a multidisciplinary team in accordance with standard protocols and with the backing of good clinimetrics."[331] Protocols to improve outcomes of liposuction for lipedema should include conservative therapy before and after liposuction.[301]

Anecdotal reports of women with lipedema developing breast enlargement after surgery have been shared among lipedema liposuction surgeons. Breast enlargement after liposuction of the abdominal wall has been reported in up to 40% of patients.[390] Other studies do not report breast enlargement after liposuction with or without abdominoplasty.[391] Volumetrics including measurement of breast volume before and after liposuction for lipedema should be considered to determine if women with lipedema have a different propensity for fat redistribution after liposuction than women without lipedema.

Does Lipedema SAT Return After Liposuction

Liposuction cannot remove all of the lipedema SAT; some remains and if it behaves like lipedema SAT, it will continue to grow over time. According to Dr. Rapprich, of 50 women with lipedema five years after power liposuction, 30% of women had no return of lipedema SAT, 46% had a slight return, 16% had a moderate return, and 8% had almost complete return of lipedema SAT (Dr. med Stefan Rapprich in prep). Standardized methods of measuring lipedema SAT are needed to determine what kind of SAT is being removed by liposuction and what kind of SAT is returning in the years following.

Psychological Support After Liposuction

There are anecdotal reports of women with lipedema developing depression after liposuction; women with lipedema have to adapt to the dramatic changes in shape that occur over a very short period of time after liposuction. Women who have been starving themselves to try and lose lipedema SAT may also struggle with anorexia after liposuction and it is these women that tend to have a return of lipedema SAT.[392] Support of family and friends is needed before and after liposuction because a woman with lipedema undergoes a major transition and transformation in her life. Underlying psychological issues in women with lipedema should not be taken lightly; one in eight women with lipedema in Germany who presented to a surgeon for liposuction had attempted suicide.[393] Women with significant depression should seek professional help because people with higher scores in optimism and coping have better outcomes after surgery.[394] Women with lipedema should view their lipoaspirate after liposuction because patients who were allowed to view their diseased specimens also had better outcomes after surgery.[395]

Benefits of Liposuction Before Other Surgeries

Total Knee Replacement

Most surgeons agree that liposuction should be performed prior to total knee replacement in women with lipedema who have a significant amount of SAT around the knee. Many orthopaedic surgeons have refused to replace knees because of the fear of infection and difficulty in accessing the knee joint when it is surrounded by a large amount of painful lipedema SAT, and because of the weight load on a newly replaced knee. The goals of reduction of lipedema SAT go beyond the desire to improve body shape. Liposuction removes abnormal exquisitely sensitive tissue, improves flow through tissue from blood capillary to interstitium to lymphatic to vein, and improves mobility preventing the need for single or double knee replacements. Conservative treatment along with liposuction of lipedema SAT located above, overhanging, and/or surrounding the knee that occludes lymph and blood flow to the knee, should be performed prior to knee surgery to decrease the risk of infection, reduce healing time, and improve outcomes. Surgery can also improve the misalignment caused by the excess lipedema SAT.[396]

Bariatric Surgery

Bariatric surgery is not a treatment for lipedema—it does not reduce lipedema SAT. However, bariatric surgery can treat the morbid obesity that accompanies lipedema in some women. Most liposuction surgeons prefer to remove lipedema SAT prior to bariatric surgery for a number of reasons. These include the fact that liposuction can decongest the SAT resulting in weight loss that had been hindered by poor flow through the tissue, mobility can improve after liposuction which will impact weight loss, and loose skin after bariatric surgery may make liposuction more difficult. Women with lipedema who have undergone weight loss prior to liposuction may achieve good results along with skin tightening despite lower yields of fat removed per volume of lipoaspirate solution.[397]

Inpatient Treatment of Lipedema with Lipo-Lymphedema

Women with lipedema who develop lymphedema and obesity are at risk for progression of their disease above and beyond usual care. When a woman with lipo-lymphedema loses her ability to perform activities of daily living, her weight is rising rapidly and is no longer controlled by MLD, compression, diet and exercise, she has a wound that is not resolving due to the presence of lymphedema, she has recurrent infections due to her lymphedema, or she develops fluid overload, she is a candidate for inpatient care for lymphedema. Inpatient care centers for lipedema and lymphedema are available in Europe and the United States. Cost of inpatient care is very high in the US and some inpatient facilities may not have the equipment or rooms to accommodate a larger patient. Women with lipedema and lymphedema who are admitted to an inpatient facility tend to undergo extensive intravenous diuresis to reduce fluid in the tissues, improve mobility, reduce risk of infection and improve outcomes after CDT. Kidney function must be carefully monitored to prevent damage, and electrolytes need to be monitored closely. Many women with lipedema use mucolytics such as N-acetyl cysteine (NAC) or guaifenesin to improve diuresis of lipedema SAT (Herbst KL, unpublished). A woman with lipo-lymphedema who was admitted as an inpatient for recurrent sepsis, developed progressive shortness of breath, fluid overload and declining kidney function on intravenous diuresis. She was offered hospice care. Her hospitalist was contacted and he started both NAC and guaifenesin; the patient had a remarkable diuresis and was eventually discharged to inpatient intensive lymphedema care and then home. Mucolytics should be considered for inpatient and outpatient therapy when available; some women with lipedema do not respond to either mucolytic.

New programs are needed to help women with lipedema and lymphedema that are hospitalized to improve care including sensitivity training for all health care staff on how to maintain patient dignity and respect when delivering care.

Conclusion

Awareness of lipedema is on the rise which means that more health care providers will be treating women with lipedema. Research on lipedema is under way which should open up treatment options as the pathophysiology is clarified. Until medical alternatives are available to reduce the lipedema SAT, liposuction will remain the dominant treatment option.

3.14.12 Complete Decongestive Therapy for Lipolymphedema

General

If lipolymphedema is associated with obesity, nutritional guidance must be provided to reduce the weight and avoid further weight gain. Patients should be physically active and exercise regularly. Some younger patients report improvements following rigorous exercise routines; for most patients, however, the reduction in fatty tissues from the hip down is disappointing. Any hormonal imbalance should be corrected through medical management.

CDT shows good long-term results in removing the fluid components in lipolymphedema. However, the patient needs to understand that, although the lymphedematous component responds well and relatively fast to CDT, the lipedema itself responds more slowly, and sometimes not at all.

The MLD treatment protocol should include the entire body; treatment of the extremities in lipolymphedema corresponds with that for primary lymphedema, that is, regional lymph nodes are included in the treatment. The pain and hypersensitivity often associated with lipolymphedema may mandate lighter pressures in MLD and compression techniques during the initial treatment sessions. In some cases, it may be necessary not to apply a compression bandage in the first few treatments. Patients often require more padding under the compression bandages, particularly in the anterior tibial area, and generally do not tolerate denser materials, such as Komprex or chip bags (see Chapter 5: Required Materials). The pain typically diminishes after several treatments.

After the decongestion of the lymphedematous component during the intensive phase of CDT, the patient should be fitted with a compression garment, which in the majority of cases needs to be custom made. The preferred garment is a pantyhose type of a higher compression class.

According to several authors, some reduction of the excessive fatty tissue in lipedema is possible if the compression garments are worn constantly and if short-stretch compression bandages are applied at night.

3.15 Pediatric Lymphedema

Pediatric lymphedema may be uncomplicated in its presentation, akin to adult primary lymphedema, or prove very medically complex. One must assume, in any new onset pediatric swelling, that either a defect in the normal development of lymphatic tissue or an undiagnosed malignant disease are the most likely causal factors to investigate. Immediate clarification as to the presence or absence of cancer must be attained so that appropriate therapy can commence for either benign primary or malignant secondary lymphedema (▶ Fig. 3.88).

3.16 Classification: Primary and Secondary Lymphedema

3.16.1 Milroy's Disease

Benign primary lymphedema occurring at birth or within the first year of life is classified as Type 1 Nonne-Milroy syndrome, or Milroy's disease. This "congenital hereditary" form of lymphedema (meaning that it is present at or near birth, sometimes inherited) is generally described as involving the lymphatic hypoplasia of vessels and regional nodes of the lower extremities, and sometimes the arms, hands, and face.

In some, Milroy's disease may further involve malformations of the intestinal lymphatics (omentum), leading to congestion of digested fat molecules (long chain triglycerides) which rely upon lymphatic vessels for absorption. If clinically apparent, this intestinal involvement results in the malabsorption of proteins, fats, and other nutrients into the blood stream. Symptoms may include bloating of the abdomen (ascites), oily stool, low blood albumin levels (hypo-proteinemia), high protein in the stool (protein losing enteropathy) and, in advanced cases, a malnourished appearance. Some Milroy's patients may require infusions of protein or special dietary guidelines involving less complex fatty acids (medium chain triglycerides), which are often successful in alleviating the congested intestinal lymphatic system (▶ Fig. 3.89).

Meige's Disease

Another form of primary lymphedema occurring in children includes Type 2 Primary Lymphedema, or Meige's syndrome (Meige's disease). This

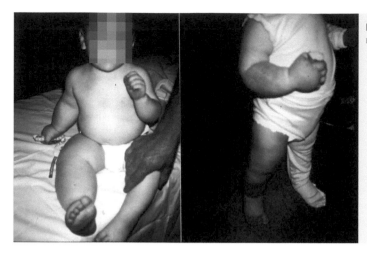

Fig. 3.88 Milroy's disease child, age 15 months.

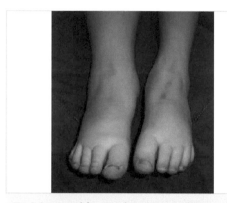

Fig. 3.89 Dorsal foot involvement, asymmetry.

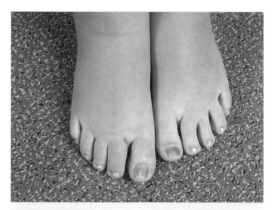

Fig. 3.90 Meige's disease. Stemmer's sign positive.

noncongenital, familial form (not present at birth, sometimes inherited) is associated with the hormonal changes of puberty and occurs primarily in females. As in Milroy's disease, this form is also a hypoplasia of lymphatic tissue that generally presents as lower-extremity lymphedema; in rare cases, however, it also involves the upper quadrant or face. Both diseases are chronic and progressive if ignored, and Meige's disease does not involve intestinal lymphatic malformations.

Both Type 1 and Type 2 primary lymphedema can be grouped as lymphedema praecox, which is an umbrella classification used to describe any primary lymphedema occurring before the age of 35. Of the two, Milroy's disease accounts for only 6–7% of all lymphedema praecox cases, making type 2, Meige's disease, a far more common clinical presentation (▶ Fig. 3.90).

Distichiasis Syndrome

This variant of peripubertal primary lymphedema is not a subset of Meige's or Milroy's diseases. A double row of "accessory" eyelashes (distichiasis) appears along the posterior border of the eyelid margins and, unlike the formerly described primary lymphedemas, involves hyperplasia of superficial vessels. Lymphedema may not be expressed in all cases, particularly those in which distichiasis appears as solely a problem of the eye that is treated in infancy. However, with this knowledge, the physician may investigate for concomitant limb swelling that appears later in the teenage years. Hyperplasia creates "lakes" of lymph fluid on imaging studies, as well as larger diameter and/or more numerous collectors in the involved areas.

Pediatric Primary Lymphedema: Pure, Benign Forms

- Milroy's disease
  - A congenital, hereditary lymphedema, present at birth or shortly thereafter, usually involving one lower extremity, which occurs more frequently in males. The arms, face, and genitals are sometimes involved. This form involves hypoplasia, mainly of the lymph capillaries. Chylous ascites causing hypoproteinemia may occur.
- Meige's disease
  - A noncongenital, hereditary (familial) lymphedema presenting near puberty. Meige's is more common in girls involving one or both legs, typically but not exclusively sparing the arms and face. This form involves hypoplasia of lymphatic tissues.
- Distichiasis syndrome
  - A variant of peripubertal primary lymphedema affecting females, which involves a double row of "accessory" eyelashes and the hyperplasia of superficial vessels.

Secondary Lymphedema in Children

It should be noted that lymphedema in children can be acquired by the same traumatic external circumstances as those which lead to adult onset cases. These include

- Surgeries near to or directly targeted at lymph nodes or vessels.
- Malignant tumor obstructions (active cancer).
- Cancer therapies involving lymphadenectomy and radiation therapy.
- Significant trauma to any body region (or cumulative trauma).
- Limb tourniquet.
- Infection (acute or chronic).

Akin to adult-onset secondary lymphedema, it is incumbent upon the diagnostician to assess the gravity of any particular lymphatic trauma to correctly classify lymphedema as either primary or secondary. For example, pregnancy at any age is not the cause of lymphedema but rather the triggering event within an already insufficient lymphatic system. As such pregnancy-related lymphedema is considered primary not secondary lymphedema.

3.16.2 Differentiation

Diseases associated with pediatric lymphedema include Klippel–Trenaunay–Weber Syndrome (KTWS), otherwise termed angio-osteohypertrophy syndrome, Noonan's syndrome, Turner's syndrome (3 chromosomal disorders), amniotic band syndrome, and nearly 40 others. Of these syndromes, KTWS is frequently encountered in a busy lymphedema clinic attracting all types of referrals related to limb enlargement. Depending upon its severity and precise variant, KTWS may be a serious medical disorder involving overgrowth of veins, arteries, bones, and lymphatic tissues. Practicing lymphedema therapists and diagnosticians must identify this condition correctly, adjusting treatment to accommodate the associated complications of this disease. It is recommended that pediatric patients with KTWS and associated lymphedema seek expert physician supervision, preferably from a vascular surgeon or hematologist with additional training in lymphology (▶ Fig. 3.91) (see below, "3.16.6.").

Diagnostic Considerations: Imaging

After ruling out malignant disease, a correct diagnosis is generally ascertained by physical examination and relies in large part upon skilled observation, palpation, and historical analysis. One safe and minimally invasive imaging procedure currently used to diagnose primary lymphedema is called lymphangioscintigraphy (LAS). This procedure involves subcutaneous (within the dermis)

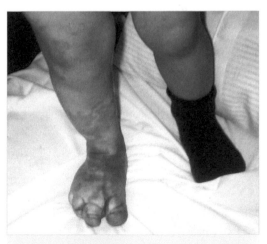

Fig. 3.91 Klippel–Trenaunay–Weber syndrome (KTWS).

injections of radioisotope-labeled proteins, which are photographed at set intervals to show rates of uptake and regional transport within the superficial lymphatic system. If primary lymphedema is accurately diagnosed clinically, LAS is unnecessary, given it will not change the course of treatment. Clearly, LAS is of great academic value and, more importantly, may contribute to supporting the accuracy of the clinical diagnosis (▶ Fig. 3.92). Many times, as in the case of pediatric lymphedema, a clear image verifies insufficient lymphatic drainage, putting to rest parental concerns that lymphedema is not an accurate or complete diagnosis.

Other testing procedures such as venography and lymphography, which involve injections of dye, are painful, potentially damaging to vessels, and associated with severe allergic reactions (anaphylaxis) in some. In more complicated cases involving combination forms of lymphedema, MRI, Computer Tomography (CT scan) and venous Doppler/duplex studies may be required to assist in designing a successful treatment plan. In uncomplicated cases, they are not necessary, and only incur additional expense.

The consequence of primary lymphedema is always mechanical insufficiency (low output failure) and, as with other body systems, this tendency for subnormal TC further degrades with aging, due to such factors as hormones or minor injury, which can trigger a late onset of lymphedema in some individuals (lymphedema tardum).

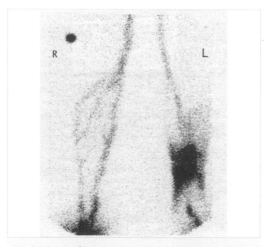

Fig. 3.92 Lymphscintogram. Bilateral lower extremities from feet to midthigh.

3.16.3 Imaging Studies Reveal Primary Lymphedema

In the case of Milroy's and Meige's disease inguinal lymph node volume and structure (aplasia, hypoplasia) are abnormal on the affected side, with a decrease of 16%–38%. Similar observations apply to the asymptomatic leg, but with less severity. Morphological alterations in structure are more distinct in the regions of greater severity.

- Node malformation includes fibrosclerosis, fibrosis, fatty degeneration, and hyalinization, with other morphological changes.
- Characteristics are more pronounced in the inguinal lymph nodes than in the iliac nodes, although both are observed.

Milroy's disease may involve lymphostatic enteropathy, which leads to hypoproteinemia and generalized edema with ascites and worsening limb involvement. This malformation of the intestinal lymphatics has also been observed in Meige's disease (less common) and other disorders where lymphedema accompanies a genetic syndrome. Since hypoproteinemia may have no association with defective lymphatic tissues, the edema caused should be accurately characterized and assessed for its impact on other body systems including the at-risk lymphedema patients' insufficient regions.

3.16.4 Severity and Extent

Even when lymphedema is the only physical finding (benign, pure lymphedema) extent and severity can vary widely. In some instances a mild, distal unilateral foot involvement is the only presentation. And unlike typical secondary lymphedema due to regional lymphadenectomy, which if unchecked, progresses to involve the entire limb, primary lymphedema may remain localized within distinct margins (i.e. foot only, foot and calf only) into adulthood. This finding verifies local developmental abnormalities within an intact systemic lymphatic anatomy. Imaging studies of this example may reveal abnormal lymph formation (lymph capillaries) or transport (lymph collectors) defined to this region, with normal uptake and transport in all other body regions. It should be noted that a trait such as this might be inherited. Father and son, or grandmother, mother, daughter may all possess precisely the same clinical presentation.

Conversely a high variability exists in pediatric presentations borne out by time, growth and development. In some cases the unilateral dorsal foot involvement progresses to the calf and thigh. Or an uninvolved leg begins to show involvement upon standing erect and achieving walking milestones. As such in the absence of gravity the lymphatic deficiency was not yet challenged to reveal the underlying mechanical insufficiency.

When a child graduates from breast milk or formula to more complex adult foods containing long chain fats, a bloated abdomen may appear for the first time. In such cases genital lymphedema may precipitate due to reflux of retroperitoneal and deep lymphatic congestion originating at the intestinal trunk or thoracic duct. Reflux from the deep system into superficial regional nodes and collectors render less productive drainage leading to limb worsening. Alternately reflux may act as a triggering event for an uninvolved, yet predisposed limb.

Some children express lymphedema on one side of the body (left face, neck, chest, arm, leg) limited by the body's midline axis, which corresponds to the mid-sagittal superficial watershed.

These findings verify dysplasia consistent with the architecture of the superficial lymphatic anatomy, which observes developmental and functional boundaries to lymph absorption and transport. In others a checkerboard pattern may be seen whereby right head and neck, left upper quadrant, and right lower quadrant are involved, again segregated by the watersheds (boundaries).

As the above examples reveal, primary lymphedema is distinct in comparison to a known trauma to a previously healthy lymphatic system (secondary lymphedema). Understanding the extent and location of acquired traumas allows the clinician to predict the regions requiring treatment and monitoring with some certainty. However primary lymphedema, which is due to developmental abnormalities, cannot be easily assessed for risk of involvement or potential severity early in life. For this reason clinicians should be cautious when assessing the ongoing clinical picture and summarizing the complete medical outlook for parents.

3.16.5 Pathologies Contributing to Edema Formation: Adults and Children

All of the following medical concerns cause generalized edema so may accompany or even mask an underlying lymphedema. In cases of primary lymphedema it is prudent to rule out additional causes of edema due to organic disease processes.

If blood albumin levels are subnormal, colloid osmotic pressure of the plasma (COPp) decreases, resulting in increased ultrafiltration as Blood Capillary Pressure (BCP) exceeds COPp with mounting force. In the case of pediatric retroperitoneal (intra-abdominal) ascites, protein deficiency must be identified at the source and medically managed. Once stabilized, the underlying regional lymphatic impairments of primary lymphedema in the limbs or face can be treated with greater success. All primary and secondary lymphedema patients are similarly managed where this diagnosis coexists.

Protein-Losing Enteropathy: Bowel Disease

A malabsorption syndrome caused by dilated (hyperplastic/lymphangiectasia) lymph vessels of the bowel, resulting in hypoproteinemia (hypoalbuminemia), and eventual abdominal ascites with systemic edema. Protein-losing enteropathy causes a "combined insufficiency," since it coexists with underlying regional lymphatic hypoplasia—mechanical insufficiency of the legs, arms, and face.

Treatment Considerations

Once protein-losing enteropathy is diagnosed, Milroy's patients must be placed on a high-protein diet supplemented with MCT (medium chain triglycerides) oil. Long chain triglycerides congest the intestinal lymphatics, reducing absorption of nutrients such as protein, fats, and fat-soluble vitamins. Hypocalcaemia (low blood calcium) is also seen due to poor absorption of vitamin D and calcium, and secondary to low protein-binding of calcium. Protein and/or blood plasma infusions are sometimes indicated. The drug Octreotide may also be prescribed. Lymphocytopenia is also a sign of intestinal lymphatic dysplasia.

Proteinuria and Renal Failure

Although not characteristic of primary lymphedema syndromes abnormal protein levels and generalized edema should prompt renal testing for thoroughness. Loss of proteins with the urine—usually albumin—may result in hypoproteinemia and systemic swelling, including abdominal ascites. A dynamic insufficiency prevails if there were no preexisting suspicions of lymphedema; therefore, with successful medical management, edema should resolve.

Treatment Considerations

Proteinuria indicates renal dysfunction and nephrotic syndrome, and requires medical management. If the underlying cause is related to hypertensive renal lymphatic drainage, chyluria, or chyle in the urine, may be present.

Liver Failure

Although not characteristic of primary lymphedema syndromes, abnormal protein levels should prompt hepatic testing for thoroughness. With liver disease, protein synthesis is impaired, leading to hypoproteinemia, abdominal ascites, and generalized edema in some (▶ Fig. 3.93).

Treatment Considerations

Liver disease may indicate poor protein synthesis, but also involves venous congestion, as found in

cirrhosis. Blood filtration is slowed by fibrosis, causing venous hypertension that leads to increased (BCP) and increased ultrafiltration. A dynamic insufficiency can be treated with compression, but medical management is the only solution to address underlying liver disease. Along with generalized edema, these patients have a pronounced ascites and bilateral lower quadrant venous edema due to gravity and dependency.

Pleural Effusion (Pulmonary Failure)

A rare associated condition of primary lymphedema in which low oncotic pressure (COPp) causes serous fluid to leak in the area between the viscera and parietal pleura. It should be noted that primary lymphangiectasia (vessel malformation) may involve the thoracic duct leading to chylous effusion (chylothorax).

Treatment Considerations

Pulmonary distress may worsen during treatment for limb lymphedema. Consult a knowledgeable physician before commencing CDT. Medical management is the only appropriate therapy for

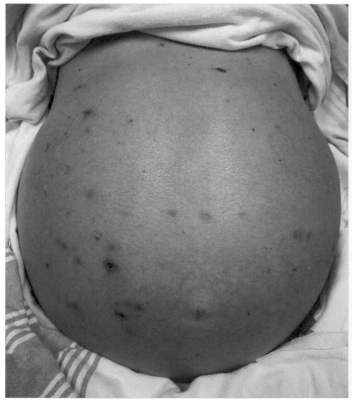

Fig. 3.93 Abdominal ascites caused by cirrhosis.

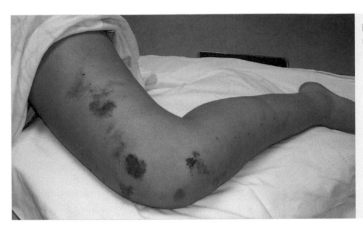

Fig. 3.94 Hemangiomas and vascular malformations (KTWS).

pleural effusion and its underlying cause. However, to the extent that decongestive therapy can influence a positive recovery and stabilization long-term, therapy for the deep lymphatic system (breathing, abdominal MLD) may be indicated.

3.16.6 Vascular Anomalies Involving Lymphedema in Children

Swelling of the subcutaneous space as seen with extremity lymphedema is not always the cause of asymmetrical limb girth discrepancies. In some cases, bony and/or soft-tissue hypertrophy will substantiate additional volume in the absence of notable edema. Since lymphatic dysplasia is closely related to vascular dysplasia syndromes, both conditions can coexist, which necessitates the therapist's familiarization with precautions, contraindications, and modifications to therapy that may apply. Since lymphedema clinics treat conditions of "limb enlargement," they attract patients desperate for reduction therapy. As such, clinicians will encounter rare associated diseases such as Klippel–Trenaunay–Weber Syndrome or KTWS.

Klippel–Trenaunay–Weber Syndrome

(Also Named Angio-Osteohypertrophy Syndrome)

KTWS is a rarely occurring impairment of embryonic development associated with numerous anomalies. Klippel–Trenaunay–Weber syndrome is a condition characterized by a triad of findings:

- A port-wine stain or "birthmark" caused by capillary malformations in the skin.
- Vascular anomalies, such as congenital varicose veins.

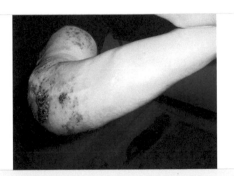

Fig. 3.95 Multifocal superficial vascular lesions of the upper extremity.

Hemangiomas of the skin and hypertrophy of the bones and other soft tissues in one or several extremities (▶ Fig. 3.94).

Other characteristics of KTWS:

- Occurs twice as frequently in females as in males.
- May also include visceral and neurogenic vascular malformations.
- Possible involvement of congenital lymphatic dysplasia—aplasia, hypoplasia and hyperplasia—of vessels and nodes.

May also involve lymphangioma and/or lymphangiomatosis: the congenital benign cystic malformation of lymphatic tissue.

- Can also involve arterio-venous fistulae—the abnormal interconnection of separate vascular networks (▶ Fig. 3.95, ▶ Fig. 3.96).

Clinical Considerations

Since vascular anomalies are highly varied and potentially complex, patients must be medically

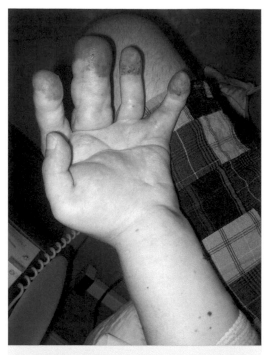

Fig. 3.96 Osteohypertrophy (gigantism of the digits).

cleared for complications to CDT. In many cases an apparent girth discrepancy cannot be accounted for by lymphedema, venous edema, or a combination form of edema alone. Soft-tissue and bone hypertrophy can contribute significant volume, and will not change with MLD and compression therapy. Once cleared for therapy, the treatment plan and goals must be modified according to a realistic expectation for volume reduction.

The following list of findings applies to the KTWS patient and represents a highly complex diagnosis, with multiple considerations for administration of CDT. Physical examination may reveal one or all of them.

- *Hemangioma.* A benign and usually self-involuting tumor composed of the endothelial cells that line blood vessels. They are characterized by increased numbers of normal or abnormally formed blood vessels. Hemangiomas usually appear during the first weeks of life, generally resolve by age 10, and are not uncommon, affecting 13% of newborns.
  - ○ Some lesions are simply cosmetic defects, inconsequential to therapy and appearing as superficial stains on the skin. These superficial hemangiomas are common and do not substantiate a precaution to therapy, except that their presence indicates a potential for

associated deep hypertrophic anomalies. Hemangiomas are not always apparent superficially as discolorations but can also be palpated below the skin; while others may involve organ structures, and require imaging studies to determine extent, type and severity.

- *Arterio-Venous Malformation (AVM).* An abnormal connection (fistula) between veins and arteries, usually of congenital origin. AVMs are lesions of the vasculature such that blood flows directly from the arterial limb to the venous system without passing through a capillary network.
  - ○ Precaution: Compression may disturb rather than enhance arterial perfusion and venous return, since regional hemodynamics are abnormal. Consult vascular medicine whenever there are known AVMs, to discern the efficacy of compression therapy.
- *Ulceration.* AVM may occur superficially, leading to skin ulceration caused by the disruption of oxygenated blood to the skin, in what is called the steal syndrome. Secondly, skin at the site of hemangioma may be thin and dry, and therefore prone to injury from mechanical stresses of compression. Bleeding and ulceration are common with these forms of vascular anomalies.
  - ○ Precaution: Infection and disturbed healing can occur from the stresses of compression bandaging or MLD. Special care must be taken to avoid these complications. If a lymphatic malformation coexists, immune response may be delayed.
- *Bone and Soft-Tissue Hypertrophy.* "Gigantism," of entire limbs or, more commonly, the digits, may accompany KTWS and is caused by increased blood supply to the epiphyseal plates. Soft tissues that experience abnormal and disproportionate growth may indicate the presence of lymphangioma, lymph varicosities, hyperplasia of veins and arteries, fatty depositions, and more. Treatment must be modified accordingly.
  - ○ Precaution: Baseline volume is impossible to calculate by comparison to the contralateral limb. However, edema is always responsive to therapy so should be treated. Attempting to achieve normalcy as compared to the uninvolved limb is futile and proves a lack of understanding of the underlying disease.
- *Thrombus.* Hyperplasia of arteries and veins with extreme anatomic variations disturb normal hemodynamics, allowing for increased clot formations. KTWS and other vascular anomalies must be carefully assessed for the presence or risk of thrombi to avoid present emergency,

assess the optimal start of therapy, and predict the likely response to the modalities of CDT.

- Precaution: MLD or compression may dislodge Deep Vein Thrombosis at the risk of pulmonary embolism. Acute DVT is a strict contraindication, with therapy resuming following physician approval. KTWS patients are always considered high-risk, so are approached with caution.

- *Lymphangioma.* These benign lymphatic tumors are not uncommon in KTWS and other vascular anomalies. Lymphagiomas consist of hyperplastic lymphatic vessels and are spongy upon palpation, with either diffuse or distinct margins. Some are suitable for surgical excision in the hands of a knowledgeable specialist. Lymphagiomas can be massive, and account for large volume discrepancies between limbs. They respond spontaneously to compression and without compression these spongy vessel networks rapidly fill with lymph and again assume full size.

Precaution: A thorough medical work-up may indicate lymphangiomatosis of the viscera or bones, which can be a serious complication. One example, Gorham syndrome, or "disappearing bone disease," is caused by lymphatic hyperplasia of the bones.

Therapeutic combinations

Considering the above complications comingled with primary lymphatic and or vascular syndromes, CDT may be an absolute contraindication for a high-risk patient in general or in a localized body region. In other instances medical supervision may allow for careful low intensity conservative therapy to commence taking into consideration particular precautions, such as open wound sites, skin fragility, ischemic tissues, risk of infection, thrombus or areas of sensory disturbance caused by debulking surgeries.

Potential complimentary medical management may include

- Surgery:
  - To debulk benign masses such as a lymphangiomas or excess soft-tissue "bulk."
  - To address bone growth at the epiphyseal plates, to shorten bones or to remove vestigial digits.
  - To remove or repair vascular malformations.
  - In concert with but not related to the enlarged limb (heart defects, craniofascial, other).

- Using paracentesis to alleviate excessive fluid accumulations in the body cavities
- Sclerotherapy:
  - To address arteriovenous malformations.
  - To assist closure of superficial wound sites, fistulas.
  - To assist closure of wound site related to lymphatic cysts, chylous reflux, lymph fistulas, or varicosities.
  - To alter the drainage pathway of the deep trunks or ducts related to pulmonary effusion or retroperitoneal ascites.
- Anticoagulant therapy:
  - For patients at high risk of pulmonary embolism or with a history of DVT.
- Albumin infusions:
  - For those with low plasma protein levels which lead to generalized edema, retroperitoneal and pulmonary effusions, and lymphedema exacerbations.
- Dietary alteration:
  - Medically supervised nutritional supplementation such as medium chain triglyceride (MCT oils) substitutes to decrease the burden on absorption of digested fats in the intestinal lymphatics.

3.16.7 Summary

Vascular anomalies are not as rare as formerly thought and accompany pediatric lymphedema with frequency since the formation of blood and lymph vascular tissues occur simultaneously in utero.

When identified, a comprehensive diagnosis will investigate to rule out possible grave comorbidities, or to identify complications or precautions as they pertain to therapeutic intervention with CDT. Soft-tissue hypertrophy as seen in KTWS (with or without lymphedema) constitutes abnormal and added limb volume that may distract from edema amenable to treatment. Adaptation of CDT and in particular compression must be carefully considered, since the vasculature may be radically altered. Never proceed to administer CDT without a vascular specialist's approval of the proposed plan of care.

Clinical strategies appropriate for pediatric patients (pure lymphedema or combined) can be found in Chapter 5, "Adaptations of Complete Decongestive Therapy for Pediatric Patients".

3.17 Pediatric Syndromes

3.17.1 Amniotic Band Syndrome

The congenital disorder amniotic band syndrome is caused by intrauterine constriction rings or bands that cause tissue depressions or strangulation marks on the digits, extremities, and sometimes the thorax, neck, and abdomen. These constriction rings are caused by strands of amniotic tissues adherent to the embryo or fetus and often cause the onset of swelling.

3.17.2 Turner's Syndrome and Noonan's Syndrome

The genetic disorder Turner's syndrome involves girls and is characterized by the absence of an X chromosome. Turner's syndrome is associated with multiple malformations, such as deformed fingernails, anomalies of the ears and palate, skeletal deformities, dwarfism, and dysplasia of the ovaries and kidneys. Lymphedema may present in the extremities, head, trunk, and other areas.

Noonan's syndrome resembles Turner's syndrome; however, Noonan's syndrome involves males and females, and no chromosomal abnormality is present.

3.17.3 Klippel–Trénaunay Syndrome and Parkes Weber Syndrome

Klippel–Trénaunay syndrome (KTS) and Parkes Weber syndrome (PWS) are two distinct conditions that involve diffuse vascular malformations with limb overgrowth.[398] KTS is a slow-flow malformation including a triad of cutaneous capillary malformations (port wine stain), venous malformations, and overgrowth of bone and soft tissue.[398,399] Complicating factors may include lymphatic abnormalities, coagulopathy, cellulitis, venous thrombosis, pulmonary embolism, hand and feet anomalies, or involvement of the abdominal and pelvic organs. Occasionally a patient may present with atrophy of an affected area instead of enlargement.

Parkes Weber syndrome is a fast-flow anomaly that can resemble KTS but has the additional characteristic of arteriovenous malformation associated with true tissue hypertrophy. It can be associated with high output cardiac failure which does not occur in KTS patients. The comparison between KTS and PWS is outlined in ▶ Table 3.35.[398]

Recent studies have indicated KTS is associated with a somatic mutation of the PIK2CA gene.[400]

Table 3.35 Klippel–Trénaunay syndrome and Parkes Weber syndrome comparison (From Cohen MM Jr. Klippel–Trénaunay syndrome. Am J Med Genet A. 2000;93(3):171–175. Reprinted with permission.)

	Klippel–Trénaunay syndrome	Parkes Weber syndrome
Types of vascular malformations	Slow flow: capillary, lymphatic, venous	Fast flow: capillary; arterial; venous
Color of cutaneous malformations	Bluish to purplish	Pink and diffuse
Arterio-venous fistulas	Insignificant	Significant
Lateral venous anomaly	Very common	Not found
Lymphatic malformations	Common	Rare
Lymphatic vesicles	Present	Not found
Venous flares	Present	Not found
Limb affected		
• Upper	5%	23%
• Lower	95%	77%
Limb enlargement	Usually disproportionate, involving soft-tissue and bone; macrodactyly, particularly of toes, is common	Arm or leg length discrepancy
Prognosis	Usually good; pulmonary embolism encountered in ~10% of children; risk is increased postoperatively	More problematic, particularly in those who develop heart failure resulting in cardiac enlargement and cutaneous ischemia, requiring limb amputation

Other conditions with similar symptoms of overgrowth have also been identified with the PIK3CA gene and are referred to as PIK3CA Related Overgrowth Syndromes (PROS).[401] These conditions are CLOVES syndrome, M-CM (Macrocephaly-capillary malformation), and FAVA (Fibro adipose vascular anomaly). These overgrowth conditions are referred to as PIK3CA Related Overgrowth Syndromes (PROS). PWS has been identified to have a mutation in the RASA1 gene.[402]

Each individual has unique characteristics with varying degrees of symptoms ranging from mild port wine stains to life-threatening pelvic or rectal bleeding.[403] KTS characteristics may not be apparent at birth and become more evident as a person develops. It may be difficult to diagnose KTS due to the complexity and lack of awareness of the syndrome and therefore some patients are not diagnosed until later in life. KTS has a negative impact on quality of life affecting function, social, and psychological aspects of the disease.[404]

Lower extremity involvement tends to be the most common area affected, followed by upper extremity, pelvic and abdominal, thorax, and rarely head and neck involvement. The lower extremity KTS venous malformations are frequently related to persistent embryonic veins.[405] The lateral marginal vein (vein of Servelle) and the sciatic vein are two common embryonic veins that are expected to disappear during normal development but often persist in KTS patients.[405,406,407] The lateral margin vein presents along the lateral part of the foot and leg. Significant venous malformations of the leg can lead to syncope and lightheadedness when standing for which compression may be helpful in reducing the symptoms.

Pain is a common complaint especially in the lower extremity. Pain has been identified to be caused by multiple factors including CVI, cellulitis, superficial thrombophlebitis, deep vein thrombosis, calcification of vascular malformations, growing pains, intraosseous vascular malformation, arthritis, and neuropathic pain.[408] Therapeutic modalities may be helpful in pain reduction.

Epiphysiodesis is a surgical procedure used to treat limb length discrepancy. It involves slowing down the growth of the longer extremity by damaging the growth plate. This procedure may be indicated for a leg discrepancy of more than 2 cm and is usually performed of age between the ages of 10 and 14 years. Shoe lifts can be used with limb length discrepancies less than 2 cm.

Lymphatic involvement is common in KTS patients but is often overlooked because of the difficulty in proper diagnosis.[409,410] CDT is indicated in individuals with lymphedema. Compression, MLD, elevation, exercise, and a compression pump may be beneficial in improving lymphatic and venous drainage. Awareness of the increased risk of venous thrombosis and pulmonary embolism needs to be considered throughout treatment.

Patients with KTS are prone to infections, skin issues, and blood clots because of the circulatory involvement. The skin temperature is often elevated in an affected area. Skin breakdown, draining wounds, blood filled blebs, and weeping ulcerations are common and therefore wound and skin care education is important. Anticoagulants may be recommended by a doctor to reduce risk of clotting. A compression garment can help protect the skin in addition to facilitating venous and lymphatic flow to reduce risk of blood clots. In some patients, compression may irritate the skin due to the fragility of the skin. In a small number of KTS patients, the deep venous system may be absent or hypoplastic and therefore the application of compression may increase venous stasis and cause pain. Careful evaluation of the appropriate treatment and compression garment needs to be assessed to obtain the best results.

3.17.4 Treatments

Laser therapy has been used to address lymphatic blebs and port wine stains. Varicose veins have been treated with endovascular and surgical intervention.[399,407,411] Surgical procedures may also be indicated to remove excessive tissue and address limb overgrowth. Recent studies have reported sirolimus has been helpful in treating some cases of KTS.[412] A multidisciplinary approach is highly recommended to provide a full comprehensive evaluation for KTS and other conditions that involve a vascular malformation. A conservative approach such as compression, lymphedema treatment, and proper wound care is typically advised.

3.18 Traumatic Edema

As discussed previously in this chapter, physical trauma may cause a reduction of the TC of the lymphatic system to a level below the normal LL. If the lymphatic system was healthy before the traumatic event, severe trauma with excessive scarring is usually necessary to cause posttraumatic secondary lymphedema. In a lymphatic system with an already reduced TC (and FR), as is the case in congenital malformations, the balance between LLs and TC is often very fragile. Even minor trauma can cause the onset of posttraumatic primary lymphedema in these cases.

> Swelling after traumatic events should be distinguished from general edema or posttraumatic lymphedema.

3.18.1 Definition

Traumatic events (surgery, blunt trauma, burns) result in inflammatory reactions accompanied by high-protein edema. The majority of these soft-tissue swellings are temporary, and the tissue returns to normal over time, but it is also possible that the inflammatory process causes permanent damage to the lymphatic system with long-lasting results.

The purpose of the following sections is to discuss inflammatory processes and their possible damaging effects on the tissues and the lymphatic system.

3.18.2 Pathophysiology

Inflammation is a nonspecific, localized immune response elicited by physical trauma with destruction of tissues. This process serves to destroy injured cells and to repair the damaged tissues.

Inflammation is characterized in the acute form by the classical signs of rubor (redness), calor (heat), dolor (pain), tumor (swelling), and functio laesa (functional disorder) with rapid onset (▶ Fig. 3.97). In its chronic form, these signs are usually less intense and have a prolonged duration. Increased leukocytes, pain, and low-grade fever may also present in chronic inflammation.

The initial step in the inflammatory process is a local vasodilation, which increases the blood flow, followed by an increase in the permeability of the blood capillaries toward plasma protein. These reactions cause redness, heat, and swelling, as well as pain secondary to pressure on nerve endings. Often clotting of the interstitial fluid occurs due to large amounts of fibrinogen and other proteins leaving the blood capillaries. White blood cells (neutrophil granulocytes) and monocytes leave the blood capillaries into the injured tissues. The neutrophils and tissue cells release mediators (histamine, kinin, serotonin), which continue the inflammatory response. Within a few hours, macrophages devour the damaged tissue cells. Tissue repair starts after the damage is controlled.

Whereas these inflammatory processes are important for tissue healing, they may also cause secondary damage to the tissues. Macrophages may further injure the still living tissue cells and surrounding structures. The lymphatic system may become involved in the inflammatory process or may be otherwise damaged due to a proliferation of macrophages in a localized area.

There are three possible results from the inflammatory process: complete healing, chronic inflammation, or additional tissue damage.

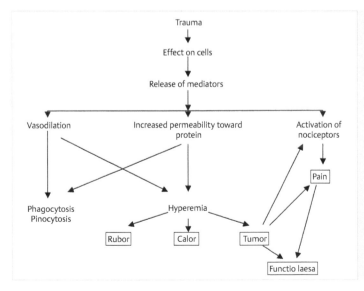

Fig. 3.97 Pathophysiology of trauma.

3.18.3 Effects of Inflammation on the Lymphatic System

The increased amount of LL of water (as well as protein and cells) triggers an increase in lymph time volume of the lymph collectors in the affected area (lymphatic safety factor). Either the lymphatic system is able to drain the excess fluid without the visible onset of edema, or it develops a dynamic insufficiency. Because of the increased amount of proteins leaving the blood capillaries in inflammation, the swelling resulting from the dynamic insufficiency is protein-rich.

> Involvement of the lymphatic system in the inflammatory process (lymphangitis) and spasms of the smooth musculature in the lymph collectors caused by pain (lymphangiospasm) are factors that may contribute to permanent damage to the lymphatic system.

The vicious pain cycle includes lymphangiospasm, increased swelling, and further pain (in combination with immobility), which can greatly exacerbate the symptoms.

The TC may also be permanently reduced by the development of valvular and mural insufficiency due to the constant strain, especially in chronic inflammations.

The consequence of the TC of the lymphatic system falling below the normal LL (mechanical insufficiency) as a result of inflammation is a combined insufficiency (increased LLs, decreased TC) of the lymphatic system (see Chapter 2, Combined Insufficiency).

3.18.4 Therapeutic Approach

The goals of treatment in traumatic edema are to eliminate edema and to support wound healing.

Traumatic edema results in increased tissue pressure and an extended diffusion distance between the blood capillaries and tissue cells, with the following negative effects:

- Lack of oxygen and nutrients in the traumatized area.
- Impeded drainage of wound components from the traumatized area, causing delay in the healing process.

- Irritation of pain receptors.
- Delayed scar healing and/or increased scar formation.

MLD in combination with other modalities improves lymph vessel activity proximal to the trauma and in the traumatized area itself, thus reducing the swelling. The subsequent decrease in diffusion distance improves local oxygenation and nutrition, thereby accelerating the drainage and elimination of wound components. Decongestion reduces tissue pressure and subsequently the pain associated with the inflammation.

Complete Decongestive Therapy in Blunt Trauma

CDT applied early following blunt trauma improves absorption of edema fluid and accelerates wound healing. These are important aspects especially in athletic care, where quick resolution and return to performance are of importance.

Severe injuries, such as fractures or compartment syndrome, must be ruled out before MLD can be initiated. The individual must consult a doctor if severe pain or dizziness is present.

Cryotherapy (Ice) and Compression

Ice packs can be made by placing ice cubes or crushed ice in a self-closing plastic bag or by using a commercial frozen gel pack. Ice should be applied as soon as possible following the traumatic event. Long-term cooling decreases local metabolism, disengages nociceptors to reduce pain, and promotes vasoconstriction. Cryotherapy also reduces the muscle spindle activity responsible for mediating local muscle tone. Peripheral nerve injury and local frostbite secondary to prolonged cryotherapy have been reported, emphasizing the need for monitoring during the use of cryotherapy. To avoid frostbite, ice packs should not be placed directly on the skin, they should be placed over a wet washcloth or towel. To decrease filtration and to promote reabsorption, ice should be applied in combination with compression bandages for a minimum of 15 minutes over a period of 3–4 hours (refer to Chapter 4, Contraindications for Compression Therapy). An additional effect of compression bandages is stabilization and immobilization of the traumatized area.

Manual Lymphatic Drainage

MLD is applied with the ice/compression bandage in place and the individual placed in a comfortable position, promoting venous and lymphatic return during the treatment. MLD is applied to the regional lymph nodes and the lymph vessels proximal to the trauma. In the case of an injury below the knee, the treatment includes the inguinal lymph nodes and basic MLD techniques on the anteromedial thigh and knee. Following MLD (duration of the treatment is ~15–20 minutes), the ice/compression bandages are renewed. MLD may be repeated 2–3 hours after the initial treatment, if necessary. If edema is still present, the treatment should be followed by a padded compression bandage (no ice).

Postsurgery Application of Complete Decongestive Therapy

In addition to the effects of MLD outlined above, scar management plays an important role in the early treatment of postsurgical conditions.

In 1989, Hutzschenreuther and Bruemmer[413] showed in an experimental study that MLD applied in the area of fresh scars promotes lympho-lymphatic regeneration of interrupted lymph vessels in scar tissue.[169] The connective tissue fibers seem to be more organized, and the consistency of the scar tissue treated with MLD seems to be softer than in untreated scars.

Manual Lymphatic Drainage

To avoid any disturbance of the wound healing process, it is important to apply MLD techniques in the first 5–7 days postoperatively only proximal to the scar tissue. For example, after knee surgery, the inguinal lymph nodes are stimulated, and basic techniques on the anterior, medial, and lateral thigh are performed. It is important to observe a safe distance from the scar tissue to avoid any tension on the edges of the scar. After 5–7 sessions, the general scar area may be carefully incorporated into the treatment area. It is important not to disturb the approximation of the wound edges; therefore, only mild pressure should be applied. Gentle stationary circles using the distal phalanges of the fingers or thumb can be applied directly around the scar tissue after the sutures are removed (usually after 1–2 weeks). Stationary circles are directed away from the wound edges,

but again, to avoid disturbance of wound healing, only very light pressure should be applied. Pretreatment of the regional lymph nodes and the thigh precedes scar treatment.

General Considerations

As always in postsurgical care, signs and symptoms of DVT and pulmonary embolism should be observed. During the treatment the extremity is placed in a comfortable position, promoting venous and lymphatic return. Mild compression using padded short-stretch bandages or compression stockings may be applied with the physician's permission. Sterile gloves should be worn while working in the area of the scar.

3.19 Inflammatory Rheumatism

3.19.1 Definition

> Inflammatory rheumatism or rheumatoid arthritis is a chronic, systemic, inflammatory disease that mostly affects the synovial membranes of multiple joints.

Because of its systemic nature, there are many extra-articular symptoms of rheumatism, or rheumatoid arthritis (RA), such as fever, loss of energy, loss of appetite, and anemia. RA can attack any synovial joint in the body. The small joints of the hand (excluding the distal inter-phalangeal joints), wrist, and foot are the most commonly affected joints. Joints that are actively involved with the disease are usually symmetrically tender and swollen and demonstrate reduced motion. To better understand the effects of RA on a joint, a brief anatomic review of a synovial joint follows.

3.19.2 Anatomy of a Synovial Joint

A synovial joint has the following components: The *joint capsule,* which isolates the joint cavity from the surrounding tissue, is composed of an outer fibrous layer and an inner synovial layer. The outer layer is poorly vascularized but contains a large number of joint receptors; the opposite is true for the synovial layer (▶ Fig. 3.98**a**). In

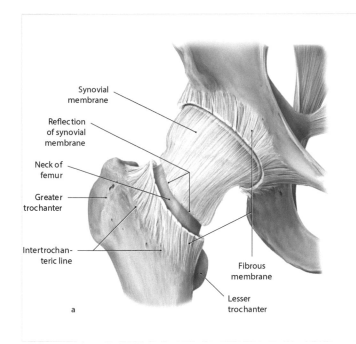

Fig. 3.98 **(a)** The ligaments of the right hip joint, anterior view. Removed: Fibrous membrane (at level of femoral neck). Exposed: Synovial membrane. (Reproduced with permission from Thieme Atlas of Anatomy, General Anatomy and Musculoskeletal System. © Thieme 2005. Illustration by Karl Wesker.)

3

Synovial membrane

Reflection of synovial membrane

Neck of femur

Greater trochanter

Intertrochan-teric line

Fibrous membrane

Lesser trochanter

a

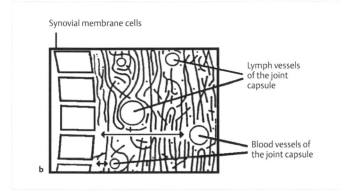

Synovial membrane cells

Lymph vessels of the joint capsule

Blood vessels of the joint capsule

b

(b) Cross section through the joint capsule (the arrows indicate the diffusion distance between the blood capillaries and the synovial membrane cells).

addition to a large number of blood vessels, the synovial layer contains lymph vessels (▶ Fig. 3.98**b**). The joint capsule forms the *joint cavity* containing synovial fluid. Synovial fluid is the medium by which nutrients are carried to, and waste products are removed from, the avascular hyaline (articular) cartilage. Synovial fluid is secreted by the synovial layer and not only is responsible for carrying oxygen and nutrients but also serves as a lubricant for the joint. The *hyaline cartilage* covers and protects the ends of long bones participating in the joint and minimizes friction and wear between the opposing joint surfaces during movement. It also dissipates the forces on the joint over a wider area, thus decreasing stress on the joint surfaces.

3.19.3 Pathophysiology

Despite many years of intensive investigation, the etiology of rheumatoid arthritis remains unknown. Metabolic and nutritional factors, the endocrine system, and geographic, psychological, and occupational data have been studied extensively without conclusive findings. It appears that an unknown antigen initiates the autoimmune response; that is, the body's immune system attacks healthy joint tissue and initiates a process of inflammation and joint damage, resulting in RA.

Early in the course of RA several changes in joint structures occur. Inflammation of the synovial layer, with the typical signs of heat, redness, swelling, pain, and loss of function, is present (inflammatory phase). Additionally, changes in the ends of the bones forming the joint (osteoporosis) may occur early in the disease process. As the disease progresses, the synovial layer may grow considerably larger, eventually forming tissue called *pannus*. Pannus can be considered the most destructive element affecting joints in the patient with rheumatoid arthritis. It attacks and destroys articular cartilage (destructive phase). Pannus can also destroy the soft subchondral bone, after the protective articular cartilage is gone. The destruction of bone eventually leads to laxity in tendons and ligaments. Under the strain of daily activities and other forces, these alterations in bone and joint structure result in the deformities frequently seen in patients with rheumatoid arthritis.

3.19.4 Effects on the Lymphatic System

In addition to the effects of inflammatory processes on the lymphatic system as described previously in this chapter (see Pathology and Pathophysiology of Lipedema), including the vicious cycle of pain generated by these effects, additional problems contribute to the swelling associated with RA.

Lymphangiographic imaging has shown that clotted fibrin obliterates channels in the tissues through which the protein-rich tissue fluid reaches the initial lymph vessels, thus inhibiting lymph formation. The lymphatic system in rheumatoid arthritis is involved in both the inflammatory and the chronic phases of the disease; therefore, lymphedema can be associated with RA.

3.19.5 Therapeutic Approach

The significance of a systemic disease like RA is that it is pervasive, leaving almost no part of the patient's life untouched. Attempting to maintain one's lifestyle while dealing with the effects of a chronic disease can be difficult. The financial burdens placed on patients with RA magnify the emotional and physical stress. Yet, with appropriate, accurate guidance from health care practitioners, many patients with RA can live the lifestyle of their choice for many years.

To cover all aspects of physical therapy (mobilization, thermotherapy, etc.) in RA would extend beyond the scope of this text. The following covers the role of CDT as an adjunct to other modalities used in the treatment and management of rheumatoid arthritis.

Complete Decongestive Therapy in the Treatment of Rheumatoid Arthritis

The goal of MLD is to reduce the intra- and extra-articular swelling, thereby interrupting the vicious pain cycle previously described. With the reduction of pain, the patient is able to move the affected joints more freely, thus improving nutrition and oxygenation of the articular cartilage.

If possible, MLD should be applied daily in the subacute phase of RA and should be avoided in the inflammatory phase. Basic MLD stroke sequences are used to treat the regional lymph nodes and the extremity, including the affected joints. For example, if RA is present on the hand and wrist, the therapist should utilize the axillary lymph nodes, collectors of the upper arm, elbow, and forearm, as well as wrist, hand, and finger techniques. As always, during the treatment the extremity should be placed in a comfortable position for the patient, promoting venous and lymphatic return.

Mild compression bandages may be applied in this stage with the physician's approval and should be worn only for short time periods (several hours, if possible). Bandages must not cause pain or considerably restrict movement. If the RA is located on the fingers/wrist, padded bandages are applied on the hand and arm; fingers are bandaged unpadded.

Complete Decongestive Therapy in the Treatment of Lymphedema Associated with Rheumatoid Arthritis

The goals of the therapy—to reduce the swelling and to maintain the reduction—correspond with those outlined in uncomplicated primary or secondary lymphedema (refer to Chapter 4).

In the case of a combination of lymphedema and RA in the subacute stage, the treatment protocol in the intensive phase of CDT is modified in such a way as to accommodate the considerations and guidelines outlined above (the bandages must never cause pain or discomfort and should only be worn for short time periods). Compression garments of a lighter compression class are recommended for lymphedema patients with a combination of RA. If possible, treatments should be provided daily for maximum benefit.

If lymphedema is associated with chronic RA, special padding is necessary under the compression bandages to accommodate areas of deformity, muscle atrophy, or possible tendon ruptures.

In most cases of RA, the patient has remissions and exacerbations of the symptoms; therefore, it is important to observe any signs or symptoms of increased disease activity or worsening of symptoms (flare-ups or flares).

3.20 Reflex Sympathetic Dystrophy

3.20.1 Definition

Reflex sympathetic dystrophy (RSD), also known as complex regional pain syndrome, is most often initiated by trauma to a nerve, neural plexus, bone, or soft tissue. It is one of the most frequent complications after surgery to extremities. RSD includes other medical diagnoses, such as causalgia, Sudeck's dystrophy, shoulder-hand syndrome, and posttraumatic osteoporosis.

The five components of RSD are pain, edema, autonomic dysfunction, movement disorder, and trophic changes. If not treated, RSD can cause stiffness and loss of use of the affected part of the extremity.

3.20.2 Pathology and Stages

RSD arises from a disturbance in the sympathetic nervous system affecting all tissue levels—skin, subcutaneous tissue, fascia, muscle, synovial layer, and bone. The disease shows simultaneous involvement of nervous tissue, skin, muscle, blood vessels, and bones. The only common denominator in all patients is pain, which is often described as burning in nature. It should be noted that RSD is a condition that affects not only adults but children as well.

The condition evolves in stages that progress insidiously over time. Some patients remain in one stage or another for many months or even years. They may never progress, or they may progress quickly through the stages.

Stage I (acute or inflammatory) may last up to 3 months. During this stage, the symptoms include severe pain closely localized to the site of injury and more severe than would normally be expected from the injury, localized pitting edema, increased warmth in the affected body part/limb, and excessive sweating. There may be faster than normal nail and hair growth and joint pain, as well as muscle spasms during movement of the affected area.

Stage II (dystrophic or degenerative) can last 3–12 months (usually 3-6 months). The edema spreads and becomes firmer, skin wrinkles disappear, and the skin temperature becomes cooler. The fingernails become brittle and cracked. The pain is more severe and more widespread. Hand or foot dryness becomes prominent, and atrophy in skin, subcutis, and muscle tissue develops. Stiffness develops, and there may be diffuse osteoporosis.

In stage III (atrophic), the pain spreads proximally, involving the entire limb. Although it may diminish in intensity, pain remains the prominent feature in this stage. The skin of the affected area is now pale, dry, tightly stretched, and shiny. Atrophy of muscle tissue and contractures in flexor tendons may also be present. Subluxations in interphalangeal joints are occasionally produced. Edema is absent, and deossification of bone tissue has now become marked and diffuse. Flare-ups may occur spontaneously.

3.20.3 Lymphatic Involvement

The LL of water (and protein) exceeds the TC of the lymphatic system, resulting in dynamic insufficiency (stages I and II). Accumulation of protein-rich fluid affects the subcutaneous tissues but may also be present in muscle tissue, tendons, and joint cavities.

3.20.4 Therapeutic Approach

After the diagnosis of RSD is established, several therapeutic approaches that have been proven helpful are available. RSD is treated by neural blockage (surgically or chemically), drug therapy, thermotherapy, and electrotherapy. Physical therapy shows good results, particularly in children.

Goals of treatment include controlling and minimizing the pain. Studies have shown that breaking through the pain cycle early precipitates a better outcome, preventing progression of the disease, restoring function of the limb affected by RSD, and improving the patient's quality of life.

Complete Decongestive Therapy in RSD

MLD is applied in stages I and II of RSD. The goal of the therapy is to reduce the pain and to increase lymphatic drainage, thereby reducing or eliminating the swelling associated with the early stages of

RSD. The resulting decrease in diffusion distance improves the trophic situation.

The extremity is placed in a comfortable and elevated position to promote venous and lymphatic return. The treatment must never cause or increase pain. Treatments should be given daily (if possible) and include basic MLD stroke sequences on the regional lymph nodes and the extremity to the proximal joint. If RSD is present on the hand, strokes on the axillary lymph nodes, upper arm, and elbow should be utilized. The forearm may be included in later treatments and only if comfortable for the patient. The application of compression bandages is contra-indicated in the treatment of RSD.

3.20.5 Cyclic Idiopathic Edema

Cyclic idiopathic edema is a syndrome characterized by soft (pitting) symmetric edema and weight gain. The cause of this condition is unclear. It occurs in menstruating females (not present before the menarche or after the menopause) and in the absence of cardiac, renal, or hepatic disease. The swelling involves the entire body and appears in cycles (premenstrual syndrome), or the edema is constantly present and varies in volume. In premenstrual syndrome, the swelling starts with the ovulation and recedes spontaneously after the beginning of the menstruation.

With orthostatic-ambulatory cyclic idiopathic edema, the swelling is dependent on gravity. The face and hands are swollen in the morning, and lower extremities and trunk, including the often painful mammary gland, become involved during the day.

Many women experience excessive weight gain during the day in the edema phase, with heat and orthostasis aggravating the symptoms. Altered vascular permeability may also be part of the disorder.

Cyclic idiopathic edema is often associated with other conditions, such as lipedema, CVI, and lymphedema. The symmetric involvement of the swelling in cyclic idiopathic edema makes it difficult to distinguish this from other conditions in which CDT may be contraindicated (cardiac edema).

3.20.6 Complete Decongestive Therapy

In the edema phase, MLD should be applied daily, if possible. The treatment involves the neck, face, thorax (including axillary lymph nodes), and legs (including inguinal lymph nodes), using basic stroke sequences. Following the MLD treatment, compression bandages are applied on the lower extremities and the abdomen.

Patients should be fitted with a compression garment (pantyhose style), which should be worn continuously. In premenstrual syndrome, the compression garment is worn between the ovulation and the beginning of the menstruation. Compression garments increase the tissue pressure, which results in reduced net filtration. Compression garments reduce, or may even prevent, the onset of swelling in the edema phase of this condition. If lymphedema is associated with cyclic idiopathic edema, the treatment protocol for lymphedema has priority.

References

[1] Norman SA, Localio AR, Potashnik SL, et al. Lymphedema in breast cancer survivors: incidence, degree, time course, treatment, and symptoms. J Clin Oncol. 2009; 27(3):390–397

[2] Ostby PL, Armer JM. Complexities of adherence and post-cancer lymphedema management. J Pers Med. 2015; 5 (4):370–388

[3] Rockson SG, Rivera KK. Estimating the population burden of lymphedema. Ann N Y Acad Sci. 2008; 1131:147–154

[4] Smeltzer DM, Stickler GB, Schirger A. Primary lymphedema in children and adolescents: a follow-up study and review. Pediatrics. 1985; 76(2):206–218

[5] Stamatakos M, Stefanaki C, Kontzoglou K. Lymphedema and breast cancer: a review of the literature. Breast Cancer. 2011; 18(3):174–180

[6] Cormier JN, Askew RL, Mungovan KS, Xing Y, Ross MI, Armer JM. Lymphedema beyond breast cancer: a systematic review and meta-analysis of cancer-related secondary lymphedema. Cancer. 2010; 116(22):5138–5149

[7] Whiting P, Rutjes AW, Reitsma JB, Bossuyt PM, Kleijnen J. The development of QUADAS: a tool for the quality assessment of studies of diagnostic accuracy included in systematic reviews. BMC Med Res Methodol. 2003; 3:25

[8] Milroy QW. An undescribed variety of hereditary oedema. NY Med J. 1892; 56:505–508

[9] Witte MH, Dellinger MT, Bernas MJ, Jones KA, Witte CL. Molecular lymphology and genetics of lymphedema-angiodysplasia syndromes. In: Földi M, Földi E, eds. Földi's Textbook of Lymphology. 2nd ed. Munich: Elsevier; 2006:497–524

[10] Brouillard P, Boon L, Vikkula M. Genetics of lymphatic anomalies. J Clin Invest. 2014; 124(3):898–904

[11] Johns Hopkins University, Baltimore, MD. Online Mendelian Inheritance in Man. OMIM(™). Available at: http:www.ncbi.nlm.nih.gov/omim. Accessed June 14, 2012

[12] Northup KA, Witte MH, Witte CL. Syndromic classification of hereditary lymphedema. Lymphology. 2003; 36(4):162–189

[13] Evans AL, Brice G, Sotirova V, et al. Mapping of primary congenital lymphedema to the 5q35.3 region. Am J Hum Genet. 1999; 64(2):547–555

[14] Ferrell RE, Baty CJ, Kimak MA, et al. GJC2 missense mutations cause human lymphedema. Am J Hum Genet. 2010; 86 (6):943–948

[15] Fang J, Dagenais SL, Erickson RP, et al. Mutations in FOXC2 (MFH-1), a forkhead family transcription factor, are responsible for the hereditary lymphedema-distichiasis syndrome. Am J Hum Genet. 2000; 67(6):1382–1388

[16] Alders M, Hogan BM, Gjini E, et al. Mutations in CCBE1 cause generalized lymph vessel dysplasia in humans. Nat Genet. 2009; 41(12):1272–1274

[17] Irrthum A, Devriendt K, Chitayat D, et al. Mutations in the transcription factor gene SOX18 underlie recessive and dominant forms of hypotrichosis-lymphedema-telangiectasia. Am J Hum Genet. 2003; 72(6):1470–1478

[18] Au AC, Hernandez PA, Lieber E, et al. Protein tyrosine phosphatase PTPN14 is a regulator of lymphatic function and choanal development in humans. Am J Hum Genet. 2010; 87(3):436–444

[19] Ostergaard P, Simpson MA, Brice G, et al. Rapid identification of mutations in GJC2 in primary lymphoedema using whole exome sequencing combined with linkage analysis with delineation of the phenotype. J Med Genet. 2011; 48 (4):251–255

[20] Ostergaard P, Simpson MA, Mendola A, et al. Mutations in KIF11 cause autosomal-dominant microcephaly variably associated with congenital lymphedema and chorioretinopathy. Am J Hum Genet. 2012; 90(2):356–362

[21] Rane S, Donahue PM, Towse T, et al. Clinical feasibility of noninvasive visualization of lymphatic flow with principles of spin labeling MR imaging: implications for lymphedema assessment. Radiology. 2013; 269(3):893–902

[22] Brice G, Ostergaard P, Jeffery S, Gordon K, Mortimer PS, Mansour S. A novel mutation in GJA1 causing oculodentodigital syndrome and primary lymphoedema in a three generation family. Clin Genet. 2013; 84(4):378–381

[23] McClelland J, Burgess B, Crock P, Goel H. Sotos syndrome: an unusual presentation with intrauterine growth restriction, generalized lymphedema, and intention tremor. Am J Med Genet A. 2016; 170A(4):1064–1069

[24] Joyce S, Gordon K, Brice G, et al. The lymphatic phenotype in Noonan and Cardiofaciocutaneous syndrome. Eur J Hum Genet. 2016; 24(5):690–696

[25] Gordon K, Schulte D, Brice G, et al. Mutation in vascular endothelial growth factor-C, a ligand for vascular endothelial growth factor receptor-3, is associated with autosomal dominant milroy-like primary lymphedema. Circ Res. 2013; 112(6):956–960

[26] Michelini S, Vettori A, Maltese PE, et al. Mutation screening in a large cohort of Italian patients affected by primary lymphedema using a next generation sequencing (NGS) approach. Lymphology. 2016:In press

[27] Heppner PP, Armer JM, Mallinckrodt B. Problem-solving style and adaptation in breast cancer survivors: a prospective analysis. J Cancer Surviv. 2009; 3(2):128–136

[28] Mak SS, Mo KF, Suen JJS, Chan SL, Ma WL, Yeo W. Lymphedema and quality of life in Chinese women after treatment for breast cancer. Eur J Oncol Nurs. 2009; 13(2):110–115

[29] Tsuchiya M. Patient education, upper-limb symptom perception, and quality of life among Japanese breast cancer survivors. Qual Life Res. 2014; 23(8):2327–2332

[30] Wanchai A, Stewart BR, Armer JM. Experiences and management of breast cancer-related lymphoedema: a comparison between South Africa and the United States of America: LE experiences and management: SA and USA. Int Nurs Rev. 2012; 59(1):117–124

[31] Deng J, Fu MR, Armer JM, et al. Factors associated with reported infection and lymphedema symptoms among individuals with extremity lymphedema. Rehabil Nurs. 2015; 40 (5):310–319

[32] Fu MR, Ridner SH, Hu SH, Stewart BR, Cormier JN, Armer JM. Psychosocial impact of lymphedema: a systematic review of literature from 2004 to 2011. Psychooncology. 2013; 22 (7):1466–1484

[33] Cancer Facts and Figures 2016. Available at: http://www.cancer.org/acs/groups/content/@research/documents/document/acspc-047079.pdf. Accessed March 14, 2016

[34] Fu MR, Rosedale M. Breast cancer survivors' experiences of lymphedema-related symptoms. J Pain Symptom Manage. 2009; 38(6):849–859

[35] Velanovich V, Szymanski W. Quality of life of breast cancer patients with lymphedema. Am J Surg. 1999; 177(3):184–187, discussion 188

[36] Huggenberger K, Wagner S, Lehmann S, Aeschlimann A, Amann-Vesti B, Angst F. Health and quality of life in patients with primary and secondary lymphedema of the lower extremity. Vasa. 2015; 44(2):129–137

[37] Okajima S, Hirota A, Kimura E, et al. Health-related quality of life and associated factors in patients with primary lymphedema. Jpn J Nurs Sci. 2013; 10(2):202–211

[38] McWayne J, Heiney SP. Psychologic and social sequelae of secondary lymphedema: a review. Cancer. 2005; 104 (3):457–466

[39] Ridner SH, Dietrich MS, Kidd N. Breast cancer treatment-related lymphedema self-care: education, practices, symptoms, and quality of life. Support Care Cancer. 2011; 19 (5):631–637

[40] Paskett ED, Dean JA, Oliveri JM, Harrop JP. Cancer-related lymphedema risk factors, diagnosis, treatment, and impact: a review. J Clin Oncol. 2012; 30(30):3726–3733

[41] Augustin M, Bross F, Földi E, Vanscheidt W, Zschocke I. Development, validation and clinical use of the FLQA-I, a disease-specific quality of life questionnaire for patients with lymphedema. Vasa. 2005; 34(1):31–35

[42] Hulett JM, Armer JM, Stewart BR, Wanchai A. Perspectives of the breast cancer survivorship continuum: diagnosis through 30 months post-treatment. J Pers Med. 2015; 5 (2):174–190

[43] Sherman KA, Miller SM, Roussi P, Taylor A. Factors predicting adherence to risk management behaviors of women at increased risk for developing lymphedema. Support Care Cancer. 2015; 23(1):61–69

[44] Leventhal H, Meyer D, Nerenz D. The common sense representation of illness danger. In: Rachman S, ed. Contributions to Medical Psychology. Vol 2. New York, NY: Pergamon Press; 1980:7–30

[45] Keeley V, Crooks S, Locke J, Veigas D, Riches K, Hilliam R. A quality of life measure for limb lymphoedema (LYMQOL). J Lymphoedema. 2010; 5(1):26–37

[46] Klernäs P, Johnsson A, Horstmann V, Kristjanson LJ, Johansson K. Lymphedema Quality of Life Inventory (LyQLI)-Development and investigation of validity and reliability. Qual Life Res. 2015; 24(3):427–439

[47] Ostby PL, Armer JM, Dale PS, Van Loo MJ, Wilbanks CL, Stewart BR. Surveillance recommendations in reducing risk of and optimally managing breast cancer-related lymphedema. J Pers Med. 2014; 4(3):424–447

[48] Armer JM, Shook RP, Schneider MK, Brooks CW, Peterson J, Stewart BR. Enhancing supportive-educative nursing systems to reduce risk of post-breast cancer lymphedema. Self Care Depend Care Nurs. 2009; 17(1):6–15

3

[49] Armer JM, Hulett JM, Bernas M, Ostby P, Stewart BR, Cormier JN. Best practice guidelines in assessment, risk reduction, management, and surveillance for post-breast cancer lymphedema. Curr Breast Cancer Rep. 2013; 5(2):134–144

[50] Armer JM. The problem of post-breast cancer lymphedema: impact and measurement issues. Cancer Invest. 2005; 23 (1):76–83

[51] Fu MR. Women at work with breast cancer-related lymphoedema. J Lymphoedema. 2008; 3(1):20–25

[52] Radina ME, Armer JM. Post-breast cancer lymphedema and the family: a qualitative investigation of families coping with chronic illness. J Fam Nurs. 2001; 7(3):281–299

[53] Radina ME. Breast cancer-related lymphedema: implications for family leisure participation. Fam Relat. 2009; 58(4):445–459

[54] Armer JM, Radina ME, Porock D, Culbertson SD. Predicting breast cancer-related lymphedema using self-reported symptoms. Nurs Res. 2003; 52(6):370–379

[55] Cormier JN, Xing Y, Zanaletti I, Askew RL, Stewart BR, Armer JM. Minimal limb volume change has a significant impact on breast cancer survivors. Lymphology. 2009; 42 (4):161–175

[56] Ridner SH. Quality of life and a symptom cluster associated with breast cancer treatment-related lymphedema. Support Care Cancer. 2005; 13(11):904–911

[57] Armer J, Fu MR, Wainstock JM, Zagar E, Jacobs LK. Lymphedema following breast cancer treatment, including sentinel lymph node biopsy. Lymphology. 2004; 37(2):73–91

[58] Fu MR, Axelrod D, Cleland CM, et al. Symptom report in detecting breast cancer-related lymphedema. Breast Cancer (Dove Med Press). 2015; 7:345–352

[59] Bernas M, Askew R, Armer J, Cormier J. Lymphedema: how do we diagnose and reduce the risk of this dreaded complication of breast cancer treatment? Curr Breast Cancer Rep. 2010; 2(1):53–58

[60] Howlader N, Noone AM, Krapcho M, et al. Surveillance, Epidemiology, and End Results Program (SEER) Cancer Statistics Review, 1975–2012. Bethesda, MD: National Cancer Institute; 2015

[61] Nazarko L. Understanding lymphoedema in older people. Nursing and Residential Care. 2006; 8(6):254–258

[62] Armer JM, Stewart BR, Wanchai A, Lasinski BB, Smith K, Cormier JN. Rehabilitation concepts among aging survivors living with and at risk for lymphedema: a framework for assessment, enhancing strengths, and minimizing vulnerability. Top Geriatr Rehabil. 2012; 28(4):260–268

[63] Konecne SM, Perdomo M. Lymphedema in the elderly: a special needs population. Top Geriatr Rehabil. 2004; 20 (2):98–113

[64] Wilson IB, Cleary PD. Linking clinical variables with health-related quality of life. A conceptual model of patient outcomes. JAMA. 1995; 273(1):59–65

[65] Ware JE, Jr, Sherbourne CD. The MOS 36-item short-form health survey (SF-36). I. Conceptual framework and item selection. Med Care. 1992; 30(6):473–483

[66] Basta MN, Fox JP, Kanchwala SK, et al. Complicated breast cancer-related lymphedema: evaluating health care resource utilization and associated costs of management. Am J Surg. 2016; 211(1):133–141

[67] Shih YCT, Xu Y, Cormier JN, et al. Incidence, treatment costs, and complications of lymphedema after breast cancer among women of working age: a 2-year follow-up study. J Clin Oncol. 2009; 27(12):2007–2014

[68] Radina ME, Armer JM. Surviving breast cancer and living with lymphedema: resiliency among women in the context of their families. J Fam Nurs. 2004; 10(4):485–505

[69] Radina ME, Armer JM, Stewart BR. Making self-care a priority for women at risk of breast cancer-related lymphedema. J Fam Nurs. 2014; 20(2):226–249

[70] Shigaki CL, Madsen R, Wanchai A, Stewart BR, Armer JM. Upper extremity lymphedema: presence and effect on functioning five years after breast cancer treatment. Rehabil Psychol. 2013; 58(4):342–349

[71] Stanton AW, Modi S, Mellor RH, Levick JR, Mortimer PS. Recent advances in breast cancer-related lymphedema of the arm: lymphatic pump failure and predisposing factors. Lymphat Res Biol. 2009; 7(1):29–45

[72] Stanton AW, Modi S, Bennett Britton TM, et al. Lymphatic drainage in the muscle and subcutis of the arm after breast cancer treatment. Breast Cancer Res Treat. 2009; 117 (3):549–557

[73] Stout NL, Pfalzer LA, Levy E, et al. Segmental limb volume change as a predictor of the onset of lymphedema in women with early breast cancer. PM R. 2011; 3(12):1098–1105

[74] Stout Gergich NL, Pfalzer LA, McGarvey C, Springer B, Gerber LH, Soballe P. Preoperative assessment enables the early diagnosis and successful treatment of lymphedema. Cancer. 2008; 112(12):2809–2819

[75] Stout NL, Binkley JM, Schmitz KH, et al. A prospective surveillance model for rehabilitation for women with breast cancer. Cancer. 2012; 118(8) Suppl:2191–2200

[76] Soran A, Finegold DN, Brufsky A. Lymphedema prevention and early intervention: a worthy goal. Oncology (Williston Park). 2012; 26(3):249–249, 254, 256

[77] Shah C, Arthur DW, Wazer D, Khan A, Ridner S, Vicini F. The impact of early detection and intervention of breast cancer-related lymphedema: a systematic review. Cancer Med. 2016; 5(6):1154–1162

[78] Breastcanzcer.org. Available at: http://www.breastcancer.org/treatment/lymphedema/evaluation/diagnosis. Accessed April 18, 2016

[79] AHRQ. Available at: http://www.cms.gov/medicare-coverage-database/details/technology-assessments-details.aspx?TAId=66&bc=BAAgAAAAAAAA&. Accessed April 18, 2016

[80] Yost KJ, Cheville AL, Weaver AL, Al Hilli M, Dowdy SC. Development and validation of a self-report lower-extremity lymphedema screening questionnaire in women. Phys Ther. 2013; 93(5):694–703

[81] Armer JM, Stewart BR, Shook RP. 30-month post-breast cancer treatment lymphoedema. J Lymphoedema. 2009; 4 (1):14–18

[82] NLN. Position Statement of the National Lymphedema Network: Screening and measurement for early detection of breast cancer related lymphedema. Available at: http://www.lymphnet.org/pdfDocs/nlnBCLE.pdf. Accessed April 18, 2016

[83] Northern Ireland Cancer Network. Crest Guidelines Lymphoedema 2008. Available at: http://www.gain-ni.org/Publications/Guidelines/CrestGuidelines.pdf. Accessed April 19, 2016

[84] Mayrovitz HN, Macdonald J, Davey S, Olson K, Washington E. Measurement decisions for clinical assessment of limb volume changes in patients with bilateral and unilateral limb edema. Phys Ther. 2007; 87(10):1362–1368

[85] Stanton A, Modi S, Mellor R, Levick R, Mortimer P. Diagnosing breast cancer related lymphedema in the arm. J Lymphoedema. 2006; 1(1):12–15

[86] Killaars RC, Penha TR, Heuts EM, van der Hulst RR, Piatkowski AA. Biomechanical properties of the skin in patients with breast cancer-related lymphedema compared to healthy individuals. Lymphat Res Biol. 2015; 13(3):215–221

3

[87] Hacard F, Machet L, Caille A, et al. Measurement of skin thickness and skin elasticity to evaluate the effectiveness of intensive decongestive treatment in patients with lymphoedema: a prospective study. Skin Res Technol. 2014; 20 (3):274–281

[88] Shah C, Arthur DW, Wazer D, Khan A, Ridner S, Vicini F. The impact of early detection and intervention of breast cancer-related lymphedema: a systematic review. Cancer Med. 2016; 5(6):1154–1162

[89] ImpediMed. http://www.impedimed.com/products/l-dexu400/. Accessed April 18, 2016

[90] Williams A. Breast and trunk odema after treatment for breast cancer. J Lymphoedema. 2006; 1(1)

[91] Degnim AC, Miller J, Hoskin TL, et al. A prospective study of breast lymphedema: frequency, symptoms, and quality of life. Breast Cancer Res Treat. 2012; 134(3):915–922

[92] Deng J, Ridner SH, Dietrich MS, et al. Prevalence of secondary lymphedema in patients with head and neck cancer. J Pain Symptom Manage. 2012; 43(2):244–252

[93] WHO. Lymphatic filariasis. Available at: http://www.who. int/topics/filariasis/en/. Accessed April 18, 2016

[94] Tam EK, Shen L, Munneke JR, et al. Clinician awareness and knowledge of breast cancer-related lymphedema in a large, integrated health care delivery setting. Breast Cancer Res Treat. 2012; 131(3):1029–1038

[95] Ferguson CM, Swaroop MN, Horick N, et al. Impact of ipsilateral blood draws, injections, blood pressure measurements, and air travel on the risk of lymphedema for patients treated for breast cancer. J Clin Oncol. 2016; 34(7):691–698

[96] Miller CL, Specht MC, Skolny MN, et al. Sentinel lymph node biopsy at the time of mastectomy does not increase the risk of lymphedema: implications for prophylactic surgery. Breast Cancer Res Treat. 2012; 135(3):781–789

[97] Jeffs E, Purushotham A. The prevalence of lymphoedema in women who attended an information and exercise class to reduce the risk of breast cancer-related upper limb lymphoedema. Springerplus. 2016; 5:21

[98] Bar Ad V, Cheville A, Solin LJ, Dutta P, Both S, Harris EE. Time course of mild arm lymphedema after breast conservation treatment for early-stage breast cancer. Int J Radiat Oncol Biol Phys. 2010; 76(1):85–90

[99] Morgan P, Moffatt C. Lymphoedema Framework. Template for Management: Developing a Lymphedema Service. London: MEP Ltd; 2007

[100] National Lymphedema Network. Patient Questionnaire. Available at: http://www.lymphnet.org/questionnaire.htm. Accessed June 15, 2012

[101] Weiss J, Daniel T. Validation of the Lymphedema Life Impact Scale (LLIS): a condition-specific measurement tool for persons with lymphedema. Lymphology. 2015; 48(3):128–138

[102] Devoogdt N, Van Kampen M, Geraerts I, Coremans T, Christiaens MR. Lymphoedema Functioning, Disability and Health questionnaire (Lymph-ICF): reliability and validity. Phys Ther. 2011; 91(6):944–957

[103] Viehoff PB, van Genderen FR, Wittink H. Upper limb lymphedema 27 (ULL27): Dutch translation and validation of an illness-specific health-related quality of life questionnaire for patients with upper limb lymphedema. Lymphology. 2008; 41(3):131–138

[104] Földi E, Földi M. Földi's Textbook of Lymphology. 3rd ed. Munich: Mosby/Elsevier; 2012

[105] Stout NL, Pfalzer LA, Springer B, et al. Breast cancer-related lymphedema: comparing direct costs of a prospective surveillance model and a traditional model of care. Phys Ther. 2012; 92(1):152–163

[106] Fu MR, Chen CM, Haber J, Guth AA, Axelrod D. The effect of providing information about lymphedema on the cognitive and symptom outcomes of breast cancer survivors. Ann Surg Oncol. 2010; 17(7):1847–1853

[107] Shaitelman SF, Cromwell KD, Rasmussen JC, et al. Recent progress in the treatment and prevention of cancer-related lymphedema. CA Cancer J Clin. 2015; 65(1):55–81

[108] Petlund CF. Volumetry of limbs. In: Olszewski WL, ed. Lymph Stasis: Pathophysiology, Diagnosis and Treatment. Boca Raton, FL: CRC Press; 1991:443–452

[109] Armer JM, Stewart BR. A comparison of four diagnostic criteria for lymphedema in a post-breast cancer population. Lymphat Res Biol. 2005; 3(4):208–217

[110] National Accreditation Program for Breast Centers. Breast Center Standards Manual 2011. Available at: http://www. accreditedbreastcenters.org/standards/2011standardsmanual.pdf. Accessed June 15, 2012

[111] Armer JM, Stewart BR. Post-breast cancer lymphedema: incidence increases from 12 to 30 to 60 months. Lymphology. 2010; 43(3):118–127

[112] Meek AG. Breast radiotherapy and lymphedema. Cancer. 1998; 83(12) Suppl American:2788–2797

[113] Petrek JA, Heelan MC. Incidence of breast carcinoma-related lymphedema. Cancer. 1998; 83(12) Suppl American:2776–2781

[114] Chance-Hetzler J, Armer J, Van Loo M, et al. Prospective lymphedema surveillance in a clinic setting. J Pers Med. 2015; 5 (3):311–325

[115] Ridner SH, Fu MR, Wanchai A, Stewart BR, Armer JM, Cormier JN. Self-management of lymphedema: a systematic review of the literature from 2004 to 2011. Nurs Res. 2012; 61(4):291–299

[116] Passik SD, McDonald MV. Psychosocial aspects of upper extremity lymphedema in women treated for breast carcinoma. Cancer. 1998; 83(12) Suppl American:2817–2820

[117] Olson JA, Jr, McCall LM, Beitsch P, et al. American College of Surgeons Oncology Group Trials Z0010 and Z0011. Impact of immediate versus delayed axillary node dissection on surgical outcomes in breast cancer patients with positive sentinel nodes: results from American College of Surgeons Oncology Group Trials Z0010 and Z0011. J Clin Oncol. 2008; 26(21):3530–3535

[118] Giuliano AE, Hunt KK, Ballman KV, et al. Axillary dissection vs no axillary dissection in women with invasive breast cancer and sentinel node metastasis: a randomized clinical trial. JAMA. 2011; 305(6):569–575

[119] Petrek JA, Pressman PI, Smith RA. Lymphedema: current issues in research and management. CA Cancer J Clin. 2000; 50(5):292–307, quiz 308–311

[120] Gebruers N, Verbelen H, De Vrieze T, Coeck D, Tjalma W. Incidence and time path of lymphedema in sentinel node negative breast cancer patients: a systematic review. Arch Phys Med Rehabil. 2015; 96(6):1131–1139

[121] Cheville AL, McGarvey CL, Petrek JA, Russo SA, Taylor ME, Thiadens SRJ. Lymphedema management. Semin Radiat Oncol. 2003; 13(3):290–301

[122] Wilke LG, McCall LM, Posther KE, et al. Surgical complications associated with sentinel lymph node biopsy: results from a prospective international cooperative group trial. Ann Surg Oncol. 2006; 13(4):491–500

[123] Clark B, Sitzia J, Harlow W. Incidence and risk of arm oedema following treatment for breast cancer: a three-year follow-up study. QJM. 2005; 98(5):343–348

[124] Runowicz CD, Leach CR, Henry NL, et al. American Cancer Society/American Society of Clinical Oncology Breast Cancer

Survivorship Care Guideline. CA Cancer J Clin. 2016; 66 (1):43–73

[125] National Cancer Institute. Lymphedema PDQ. 2015. Available at: http://www.cancer.gov/cancertopics/pdq/supportivecare/lymphedema/healthprofessional

[126] Brown JC, Cheville AL, Tchou JC, Harris SR, Schmitz KH. Prescription and adherence to lymphedema self-care modalities among women with breast cancer-related lymphedema. Support Care Cancer. 2014; 22(1):135–143

[127] Alcorso J, Sherman KA, Koelmeyer L, Mackie H, Boyages J. Psychosocial factors associated with adherence for self-management behaviors in women with breast cancer-related lymphedema. Support Care Cancer. 2016; 24(1):139–146

[128] Manne S, Ostroff J, Sherman M, et al. Buffering effects of family and friend support on associations between partner unsupportive behaviors and coping among women with breast cancer. J Soc Pers Relat. 2003; 20(6):771–792

[129] Armer JM, Brooks CW, Stewart BR. Limitations of self-care in reducing the risk of lymphedema: supportive-educative systems. Nurs Sci Q. 2011; 24(1):57–63

[130] Mallinckrodt B, Armer JM, Heppner PP. A threshold model of social support, adjustment, and distress after breast cancer treatment. J Couns Psychol. 2012; 59(1):150–160

[131] Armer JM, Heppner PP, Mallinckrodt B. Post breast cancer treatment lymphedema: the hidden epidemic. Scope Phlebol Lymphol. 2002; 9(1):334–341

[132] Armer JM, Henggeler MH, Brooks CW, Zagar EA, Homan S, Stewart BR. The health deviation of post-breast cancer lymphedema: symptom assessment and impact on self-care agency. Self Care Depend Care Nurs. 2008; 16(1):14–21

[133] Gerber LH. A review of measures of lymphedema. Cancer. 1998; 83(12) Suppl American:2803–2804

[134] Swedborg I. Voluminometric estimation of the degree of lymphedema and its therapy by pneumatic compression. Scand J Rehabil Med. 1977; 9(3):131–135

[135] Callaway CW, Chumlea WC, Bouchard C, et al. Circumferences. In: Lohman TG, Roche AF, Martorell R, eds. Anthropometric Standardization Reference Manual. Champaign, IL: Human Kinetics Books; 1988:39–51

[136] Tierney S, Aslam M, Rennie K, Grace P. Infrared optoelectronic volumetry, the ideal way to measure limb volume. Eur J Vasc Endovasc Surg. 1996; 12(4):412–417

[137] Impedimed.com. Medical applications for lymphedema 2016. Available at: https://healthcare.impedimed.com/knowledge-center/medical-applications/lymphedem. Accessed May 26, 2016

[138] Ridner SH, Bonner CM, Doersam JK, Rhoten BA, Schultze B, Dietrich MS. Bioelectrical impedance self-measurement protocol development and daily variation between healthy volunteers and breast cancer survivors with lymphedema. Lymphat Res Biol. 2014; 12(1):2–9

[139] Fu MR, Cleland CM, Guth AA, et al. L-dex ratio in detecting breast cancer-related lymphedema: reliability, sensitivity, and specificity. Lymphology. 2013; 46(2):85–96

[140] Tobin MB, Lacey HJ, Meyer L, Mortimer PS. The psychological morbidity of breast cancer-related arm swelling. Psychological morbidity of lymphoedema. Cancer. 1993; 72 (11):3248–3252

[141] Ridner SH, Rhoten BA, Radina ME, Adair M, Bush-Foster S, Sinclair V. Breast cancer survivors' perspectives of critical lymphedema self-care support needs. Support Care Cancer. 2016; 24(6):2743–2750

[142] Andersen BL, Kiecolt-Glaser JK, Glaser R. A biobehavioral model of cancer stress and disease course. Am Psychol. 1994; 49(5):389–404

[143] Holahan CH, Moos RH, Schaefer JA. Coping, stress resistance, and growth: conceptualizing adaptive functioning. In: Zeidner M, Endler NS, eds. Handbook of Coping: Theory, Research, Applications. New York, NY: Wiley; 1996

[144] Lazarus RS, Folkman P. Stress, Appraisal, and Coping. New York, NY: Springer; 1984

[145] Zeidner M, Endler NS. Handbook of Coping: Theory, Research, Applications. New York, NY: Wiley; 1996

[146] Rose KE, Taylor HM, Twycross RG. Long-term compliance with treatment in obstructive arm lymphoedema in cancer. Palliat Med. 1991; 5(1):52–55

[147] Zeissler RH, Rose GB, Nelson PA. Postmastectomy lymphedema: late results of treatment in 385 patients. Arch Phys Med Rehabil. 1972; 53(4):159–166

[148] Ancukiewicz M, Russell TA, Otoole J, et al. Standardized method for quantification of developing lymphedema in patients treated for breast cancer. Int J Radiat Oncol Biol Phys. 2011; 79(5):1436–1443

[149] Hyngstrom JR, Chiang YJ, Cromwell KD, et al. Prospective assessment of lymphedema incidence and lymphedema-associated symptoms following lymph node surgery for melanoma. Melanoma Res. 2013; 23(4):290–297

[150] Swartz RJ, Baum GP, Askew RL, Palmer JL, Ross MI, Cormier JN. Reducing patient burden to the FACT-Melanoma quality-of-life questionnaire. Melanoma Res. 2012; 22(2):158–163

[151] Harvey NL, Srinivasan RS, Dillard ME, et al. Lymphatic vascular defects promoted by Prox1 haploinsufficiency cause adult-onset obesity. Nat Genet. 2005; 37(10):1072–1081

[152] Demark-Wahnefried W, Peterson BL, Winer EP, et al. Changes in weight, body composition, and factors influencing energy balance among premenopausal breast cancer patients receiving adjuvant chemotherapy. J Clin Oncol. 2001; 19(9):2381–2389

[153] Rock CL, Demark-Wahnefried W. Nutrition and survival after the diagnosis of breast cancer: a review of the evidence. J Clin Oncol. 2002; 20(15):3302–3316

[154] Oremus M, Walker K, Dayes I, Raina P. Diagnosis and treatment of secondary lymphedema: technology assessment report 2010. Available at: https://www.cms.gov/Medicare/Coverage/DeterminationProcess/downloads//id66aTA.pdf. Accessed April 6, 2012

[155] MEDCAC. Lymphedema policy review. 2009. Available at: https://www.cms.gov/Regulations-and-Guidance/Guidance/FACA/Downloads/id51a.pdf. Accessed May 27, 2016

[156] Lasinski BB, McKillip Thrift K, Squire D, et al. A systematic review of the evidence for complete decongestive therapy in the treatment of lymphedema from 2004 to 2011. PM R. 2012; 4(8):580–601

[157] Lasinski BB. Complete decongestive therapy for treatment of lymphedema. Semin Oncol Nurs. 2013; 29(1):20–27

[158] Green JM, Paladugu S, Shuyu X, Stewart BR, Shyu C-R, Armer JM. Using temporal mining to examine the development of lymphedema in breast cancer survivors. Nurs Res. 2013; 62 (2):122–129

[159] Shyu C-R. Smart Infoware: Providing University Research Stakeholders Soft Power to Connect the Dots in Information Haystacks. Information Systems as Infrastructure for University Research Now and in the Future; 2012:55

[160] McNeill GC, Witte MH, Witte CL, et al. Whole-body lymphangioscintigraphy: preferred method for initial assessment of the peripheral lymphatic system. Radiology. 1989; 172(2):495–502

[161] Witte CL, Witte MH, Unger EC, et al. Advances in imaging of lymph flow disorders. Radiographics. 2000; 20(6):1697–1719

[162] Amaral F, Dreyer G, Figueredo-Silva J, et al. Live adult worms detected by ultrasonography in human Bancroftian filariasis. Am J Trop Med Hyg. 1994; 50(6):753–757

[163] Shetty GS, Solanki RS, Prabhu SM, Jawa A. Filarial dance-sonographic sign of filarial infection. Pediatr Radiol. 2012; 42(4):486–487

[164] Weiss M, Schwarz F, Wallmichrath J, et al. Chylothorax and chylous ascites. Clinical utility of planar scintigraphy and tomographic imaging with SPECT/CT. Nucl Med (Stuttg). 2015; 54(5):231–240

[165] Bourgeois P. Combined role of lymphoscintigraphy, X-ray computed tomography, magnetic resonance imaging, and positron emission tomography in the management of lymphedematous disease. In: Lee B-B, Bergan J, Rockson SG, eds. Lymphedema: A Concise Compendium of Theory and Practice. London: Springer; 2011:167–182

[166] Segers P, Belgrado JP, Leduc A, Leduc O, Verdonck P. Excessive pressure in multichambered cuffs used for sequential compression therapy. Phys Ther. 2002; 82(10):1000–1008

[167] Boris M, Weindorf S, Lasinski BB. The risk of genital edema after external pump compression for lower limb lymphedema. Lymphology. 1998; 31(1):15–20

[168] Miranda F, Jr, Perez MC, Castiglioni ML, et al. Effect of sequential intermittent pneumatic compression on both leg lymphedema volume and on lymph transport as semi-quantitatively evaluated by lymphoscintigraphy. Lymphology. 2001; 34(3):135–141

[169] Feldman JL, Stout NL, Wanchai A, Stewart BR, Cormier JN, Armer JM. Intermittent pneumatic compression therapy: a systematic review. Lymphology. 2012; 45(1):13–25

[170] International Best Practice Guideline for Lymphedema. Available at: http://www.woundsinternational.com/media/issues/210/files/content_175.pdf

[171] Carati CJ, Anderson SN, Gannon BJ, Piller NB. Treatment of postmastectomy lymphedema with low-level laser therapy: a double blind, placebo-controlled trial. [erratum appears in Cancer 2003;98:2742]. Cancer. 2003; 98(6):1114–1122

[172] Lawenda BD, Mondry TE, Johnstone PA. Lymphedema: a primer on the identification and management of a chronic condition in oncologic treatment. CA Cancer J Clin. 2009; 59 (1):8–24

[173] Fu MR, Axelrod D, Guth AA, et al. Patterns of obesity and lymph fluid level during the first year of breast cancer treatment: a prospective study. J Pers Med. 2015; 5(3):326–340

[174] Cormier JN, Rourke L, Crosby M, Chang D, Armer J. The surgical treatment of lymphedema: a systematic review of the contemporary literature (2004–2010). Ann Surg Oncol. 2012; 19(2):642–651

[175] International Lymphedema Framework Position Document. Best Practice for the Management of Lymphoedema. 2nd ed. Surgical Intervention. Available at: http://www.lympho.org/mod_turbolead/upload/file/Resources/Surgery%20-%20final.pdf. Accessed January 28, 2016

[176] Cormier JN, Cromwell KD, Armer JM. Surgical treatment of lymphedema: a review of the literature and a discussion of the risks and benefits of surgical treatment. LymphLink;24 (2):1–3

[177] International Society of Lymphology. The diagnosis and treatment of peripheral lymphedema: 2013 Consensus Document of the International Society of Lymphology. Lymphology. 2013; 46(1):1–11

[178] Position Statement of the National Lymphedema Network on the Diagnosis and Treatment of Lymphedema. http://www.lymphnet.org/pdfDocs/nlntreatment.pdf. Updated February 2011

[179] Granzow JW. The current state of surgery for lymphedema. LymphLink;28(4):3–6

[180] Brorson H. Circumferential suction-assisted lipectomy is the only surgical procedure that can normalize a large chronic non-pitting lymphedema. LymphLink;28(4):7–9

[181] Granzow JW, Soderberg JM, Kaji AH, Dauphine C. Review of current surgical treatments for lymphedema. Ann Surg Oncol. 2014; 21(4):1195–1201

[182] Helm TN, Lee TC. Metastatic carcinoma of the skin. Available at: http://www.emedicine.medscape.com/article/1101058-overview. Accessed October 19, 2012

[183] Corbett LQ, Burns PE. Venous ulcers. In: Milne CT, Corbett LQ, Dubuc DL, eds. Wound, Ostomy, and Continence Nursing Secrets. Philadelphia, PA: Hanley & Belfus; 2003:163

[184] Young JR. Differential diagnosis of leg ulcers. Cardiovasc Clin. 1983; 13(2):171–193

[185] Callam MJ, Harper DR, Dale JJ, Ruckley CV. Arterial disease in chronic leg ulceration: an underestimated hazard? Lothian and Forth Valley leg ulcer study. Br Med J (Clin Res Ed). 1987; 294(6577):929–931

[186] Nelzén O, Bergqvist D, Lindhagen A. Venous and non-venous leg ulcers: clinical history and appearance in a population study. Br J Surg. 1994; 81(2):182–187

[187] Andersson E, Hansson C, Swanbeck G. Leg and foot ulcers. An epidemiological survey. Acta Derm Venereol. 1984; 64 (3):227–232

[188] Reichardt LE. Venous ulceration: compression as the mainstay of therapy. J Wound Ostomy Continence Nurs. 1999; 26 (1):39–47

[189] Capeheart JK. Chronic venous insufficiency: a focus on prevention of venous ulceration. J Wound Ostomy Continence Nurs. 1996; 23(4):227–234

[190] Kunimoto B, Cooling M, Gulliver W, Houghton P, Orsted H, Sibbald RG. Best practices for the prevention and treatment of venous leg ulcers. Ostomy Wound Manage. 2001; 47 (2):34–46, 48–50

[191] Orsted HL, Radke L, Gorst R. The impact of musculoskeletal changes on the dynamics of the calf muscle pump. Ostomy Wound Manage. 2001; 47(10):18–24

[192] Bozeman PK. Arterial ulcers. In: Milne CT, Corbett LQ, Dubuc DL, eds. Wound, Ostomy, and Continence Nursing Secrets. Philadelphia, PA: Hanley & Belfus; 2003:168–172

[193] Patterson GK. Vascular evaluation. In: Sussman C, Bates-Jensen BM, eds. Wound Care: A Collaborative Practice Manual for Physical Therapists and Nurses. 2nd ed. Gaithersburg, MD: Aspen; 2001:177–193

[194] Myers BA. Wound Management: Principles and Practice. Upper Saddle River, NJ: Prentice Hall; 2004:201–228

[195] Slachta PA, Burns PE. Inflammatory Ulcerations. In: Milne CT, Corbett LQ, Dubuc DL, eds. Wound, Ostomy, and Continence Nursing Secrets. Philadelphia, PA: Hanley & Belfus; 2003:193–197

[196] Sibbald RG, Cameron J. Dermatological aspects of wound care. In: Krasner DL, Rodeheaver GT, Sibbald RG, eds. Chronic Wound Care: A Clinical Source Book for Healthcare Professionals. 3rd ed. Wayne, PA: HMP Communications; 2001:273–285

[197] Barton P, Parslow N. Malignant wounds: holistic assessment and management. In: Krasner DL, Rodeheaver GT, Sibbald RG, eds. Chronic Wound Care: A Clinical Source Book for Healthcare Professionals. 3rd ed. Wayne, PA: HMP Communications; 2001:699–710

[198] Naylor W, Laverty D, Mallett J, Eds. The Royal Marsden Hospital Handbook of Wound Management in Cancer Care. Malden, MA: Blackwell Science; 2001:73–122

3

[199] McPherson T, Fay MP, Singh S, Penzer R, Hay R. Health workers' agreement in clinical description of filarial lymphedema. Am J Trop Med Hyg. 2006; 74(3):500–504

[200] Ananthakrishnan S, Das LK. Entry lesions in bancroftian filarial lymphoedema patients–a clinical observation. Acta Trop. 2004; 90(2):215–218

[201] Sibbald RG, Williamson D, Orsted HL, et al. Preparing the wound bed–debridement, bacterial balance, and moisture balance. Ostomy Wound Manage. 2000; 46(11):14–22, 24–28, 30–35, quiz 36–37

[202] Szolnoky G, Borsos B, Bársony K, Balogh M, Kemény L. Complete decongestive physiotherapy with and without pneumatic compression for treatment of lipedema: a pilot study. Lymphology. 2008; 41(1):40–44

[203] Daróczy J. Antiseptic efficacy of local disinfecting povidone-iodine (Betadine) therapy in chronic wounds of lymphedematous patients. Dermatology. 2002; 204 Suppl 1:75–78

[204] Kunimoto BT. Management and prevention of venous leg ulcers: a literature-guided approach. Ostomy Wound Manage. 2001; 47(6):36–42, 44–49

[205] Hansson C, Cadexomer Iodine Study Group. The effects of cadexomer iodine paste in the treatment of venous leg ulcers compared with hydrocolloid dressing and paraffin gauze dressing. Int J Dermatol. 1998; 37(5):390–396

[206] Akesson H, Bjellerup M. Leg ulcers: report on a multidisciplinary approach. Acta Derm Venereol. 1995; 75(2):133–135

[207] Buttler T. Interdisciplinary chronic-wound care services involving podiatry – a strengthened model of care? Wound Pract Res. 2011; 19(4):229–233

[208] Impaired Skin Integrity. Miller-Keane Encyclopedia and Dicitonary of Medicine, Nursing, and Allied Health. 7th ed. 2003. Available at: http://medical-dictionary.thefreedictionary.com/impaired + skin + integrity. Accessed April 24 2016

[209] Mustoe TA, O'Shaughnessy K, Kloeters O. Chronic wound pathogenesis and current treatment strategies: a unifying hypothesis. Plast Reconstr Surg. 2006; 117(7) Suppl:35S–41S

[210] Technology Assessment. March 3, 2005 AHQR

[211] Sen CK, Gordillo GM, Roy S, et al. Human skin wounds: a major and snowballing threat to public health and the economy. Wound Repair Regen. 2009; 17(6):763–771

[212] Administration on Aging. Services DoHaH. A profile of older Americans 2007; 1–19. Available at: http://www.wvseniorservcises.gov/Portals/0/pdf/Profiles of older Americans pdf

[213] American Heart Association. Peripheral Arterial Disease Statistics – 2008 Update. American Heart Association; 2008

[214] "Wound." Merriam-Webster.com. Merriam-Webster.

[215] "subjective data collection." Mosby's Medical Dictionary, 8th edition. 2009. Elsevier 25 Feb. 2016 http://medicaldictionary.thefreedictionary.com/subjective + data + collection

[216] Garth James et al. Wound Repair Regen 2008

[217] De Negri B, et al. Improving interpersonal communications between health care providers and clients. Available at: http://pdf.usaid.gov/pdf_docs/PNACE294.pdf

[218] Zulkowski K, Ayello EA, Wexler S. Certification and education: do they affect pressure ulcer knowledge in nursing? Adv Skin Wound Care. 2007; 20(1):34–38

[219] Gethin G. Evidence base for wound measurement. World Ir Nurs. 2005; 13(8):S6–S8

[220] Gethin G, Cowman S. Comparison of acetate tracing and digital planimetry to obtain area measurement of superficial leg ulcers. Poster presented at Wounds UK Conference; November 14–16, 2005; Harrogate

[221] Exudate. (n.d.) Miller-Keane Encyclopedia and Dictionary of Medicine, Nursing, and Allied Health, Seventh Edition. (2003). Retrieved April 9 2016 from http://medical-dictionary.thefreedictionary.com/exudate

[222] Institute for Clinical Systems Improvement (ICSI). Pressure Ulcer Prevention and Treatment Protocol. Health Care Protocol. Bloomington, MN: Institute for Clinical Systems Improvement (ICSI); 2012

[223] Miller-Keane Encyclopedia and Dictionary of Medicine, Nursing, and Allied Health, 7th ed. 2003. Available at: http://medical-dictionary.thefreedictionary.com/induration. Accessed April 10, 2016

[224] Sibbald RG, Mufti A, Armstrong DG. Infrared skin thermometry: an underutilized cost-effective tool for routine wound care practice and patient high-risk diabetic foot self-monitoring. Adv Skin Wound Care. 2015; 28(1):37–44, quiz 45–46

[225] Charles H. The impact of leg ulcers on patients' quality of life. Prof Nurse. 1995; 10(9):571–572, 574

[226] Ebbeskog B, Ekman S-L. Elderly people's experiences. The meaning of living with venous ulcer. EWMA J. 2001; 1(1):21–23

[227] Rich A, McLachlan L. How living with a leg ulcer affects people's daily life: a nurse-led study. J Wound Care. 2003; 12(2):51–54

[228] Mudge E. Tell me if it hurts: the patients perspective of wound pain. Wounds UK. 2007; 3(1):6–7

[229] Mudge E, Orsted H. Wound infection and pain management made easy. Wounds International 2010;1(3): Available at: http://www.woundsinternational.com

[230] Brennan F, Carr DB, Cousins M. Pain management: a fundamental human right. Anesth Analg. 2007; 105(1):205–221

[231] Scholten W, Nygren-Krug H, Zucker HA. The World Health Organization paves the way for action to free people from the shackles of pain. Anesth Analg. 2007; 105(1):1–4

[232] Herr K, Coyne PJ, McCaffery M, Manworren R, Merkel S. Pain assessment in the patient unable to self-report: position statement with clinical practice recommendations. Pain Manag Nurs. 2011; 12(4):230–250

[233] Hirsh AT, Jensen MP, Robinson ME. Evaluation of nurses' self-insight into their pain assessment and treatment decisions. J Pain. 2010; 11(5):454–461

[234] Bergström G, Aniansson A, Bjelle A, Grimby G, Lundgren-Lindquist B, Svanborg A. Functional consequences of joint impairment at age 79. Scand J Rehabil Med. 1985; 17(4):183–190

[235] Jette AM, Branch LG, Berlin J. Musculoskeletal impairments and physical disablement among the aged. J Gerontol. 1990; 45(6):M203–M208

[236] Lundin M, Wiksten JP, Peräkylä T, et al. Distal pulse palpation: is it reliable? World J Surg. 1999; 23(3):252–255

[237] Collins TC, Suarez-Almazor M, Peterson NJ. An absent pulse is not sensitive for the early detection of peripheral arterial disease. Fam Med. 2006; 38(1):38–42

[238] Cina C, Katsamouris A, Megerman J, et al. Utility of transcutaneous oxygen tension measurements in peripheral arterial occlusive disease. J Vasc Surg. 1984; 1(2):362–371

[239] White RA, Nolan L, Harley D, et al. Noninvasive evaluation of peripheral vascular disease using transcutaneous oxygen tension. Am J Surg. 1982; 144(1):68–75

[240] Oh PI, Provan JL, Ameli FM. The predictability of the success of arterial reconstruction by means of transcutaneous oxygen tension measurements. J Vasc Surg. 1987; 5(2):356–362

[241] Padberg FT, Back TL, Thompson PN, Hobson RW, II. Transcutaneous oxygen (TcPO2) estimates probability of healing in the ischemic extremity. J Surg Res. 1996; 60(2):365–369

[242] Arroyo CI, Tritto VG, Buchbinder D, et al. Optimal waiting period for foot salvage surgery following limb revascularization. J Foot Ankle Surg. 2002; 41(4):228–232

[243] Ballard JL, Eke CC, Bunt TJ, Killeen JD. A prospective evaluation of transcutaneous oxygen measurements in the management of diabetic foot problems. J Vasc Surg. 1995; 22 (4):485–490, discussion 490–492

[244] Katsamouris A, Brewster DC, Megerman J, Cina C, Darling RC, Abbott WM. Transcutaneous oxygen tension in selection of amputation level. Am J Surg. 1984; 147(4):510–517

[245] Castronuovo JJ, Jr, Adera HM, Smiell JM, Price RM. Skin perfusion pressure measurement is valuable in the diagnosis of critical limb ischemia. J Vasc Surg. 1997; 26(4):629–637

[246] Utsunomiya M, Nakamura M, Nagashima Y, Sugi K. Predictive value of skin perfusion pressure after endovascular therapy for wound healing in critical limb ischemia. J Endovasc Ther. 2014; 21(5):662–670

[247] Yamada T, Ohta T, Ishibashi H, et al. Clinical reliability and utility of skin perfusion pressure measurement in ischemic limbs–comparison with other noninvasive diagnostic methods. J Vasc Surg. 2008; 47(2):318–323

[248] Centers for Disease Control and Prevention. National Diabetes Statistics Report: Estimates of Diabetes and Its Burden in the United States, 2014. Atlanta, GA: U.S. Department of Health and Human Services; 2014

[249] Sanders LJ. Diabetes mellitus. Prevention of amputation. J Am Podiatr Med Assoc. 1994; 84(7):322–328

[250] Ramsey SD, Newton K, Blough D, et al. Incidence, outcomes, and cost of foot ulcers in patients with diabetes. Diabetes Care. 1999; 22(3):382–387

[251] Pecoraro RE, Reiber GE, Burgess EM. Pathways to diabetic limb amputation. Basis for prevention. Diabetes Care. 1990; 13(5):513–521

[252] Ghanassia E, Villon L, Thuan Dit Dieudonné JF, Boegner C, Avignon A, Sultan A. Long-term outcome and disability of diabetic patients hospitalized for diabetic foot ulcers: a 6.5-year follow-up study. Diabetes Care. 2008; 31(7):1288–1292

[253] Resnick HE, Carter EA, Lindsay R, et al. Relation of lower-extremity amputation to all-cause and cardiovascular disease mortality in American Indians: the Strong Heart Study. Diabetes Care. 2004; 27(6):1286–1293

[254] American Diabetes Association. Concensus Conference on Diabetic Foot Management. 1999

[255] American Diabetes Association (ADA). Standards of medical care in diabetes-2011. Diabetes Care. 2011; 33:S11–S61

[256] Falanga V, Grinnell F, Gilchrest B, Maddox YT, Moshell A. Workshop on the pathogenesis of chronic wounds. J Invest Dermatol. 1994; 102(1):125–127

[257] Ayton M. Wound care: wounds that won't heal. Nurs Times. 1985; 81(46):16–19

[258] Kingsley A. A proactive approach to wound infection. Nurs Stand. 2001; 15(30):50–54, 56, 58

[259] Edwards R, Harding KG. Bacteria and wound healing. Curr Opin Infect Dis. 2004; 17(2):91–96

[260] Cutting KF, Harding KG. Criteria for identifying wound infection. J Wound Care. 1994; 3:198–201

[261] Mosby's Medical Dictionary. 8th edition. S.v. "Hydropsy." Retrieved March 3, 2016 from http://medical-dictionary. thefreedictionary.com/Hydropsy

[262] Wilson IAI, Henry M, Quill RD, Byrne PJ. The pH of varicose ulcer surfaces and its relationship to healing. Vasa. 1979; 8 (4):339–342

[263] Romanelli M, Schipani E, Piaggesi A, Barachini P. Evaluation of surface pH on venous leg ulcers under Allevyn dressings. In: Suggett A, Cherry G, Mani R, Eaglstein W, eds.

International Congress and Symposium Series. No. 227. London: Royal Society of Medicine Press, 1998:57–61

[264] Winter GD. Formation of the scab and the rate of epithelization of superficial wounds in the skin of the young domestic pig. Nature. 1962; 193:293–294

[265] Ring EFJ. Skin temperature measurement. Bioeng Skin. 1986; 2:15–30

[266] Margolis DJ, Allen-Taylor L, Hoffstad O, Berlin JA. The accuracy of venous leg ulcer prognostic models in a wound care system. Wound Repair Regen. 2004; 12(2):163–168

[267] Kurz N, Kahn SR, Abenhaim L, et al, eds. VEINES Task Force Report, The management of chronic venous disorders of the leg (CVDL): an evidence based report of an international task force. McGill University. Sir Mortimer B. Davis-Jewish General Hospital. Summary reports in: Angiology. 1997;48 (1):59–66; and Int Angiol. 1999;18(2):83–102

[268] Heit JA. Venous thromboembolism epidemiology: implications for prevention and management. Semin Thromb Hemost. 2002; 28 Suppl 2:3–13

[269] Margolis DJ, Berlin JA, Strom BL. Risk factors associated with the failure of a venous leg ulcer to heal. Arch Dermatol. 1999; 135(4):920–926

[270] Sheehan P, Jones P, Caselli A, Giurini JM, Veves A. Percent change in wound area of diabetic foot ulcers over a 4-week period is a robust predictor of complete healing in a 12-week prospective trial. Diabetes Care. 2003; 26(6):1879–1882

[271] Kantor J, Margolis DJ. A multicentre study of percentage change in venous leg ulcer area as a prognostic index of healing at 24 weeks. Br J Dermatol. 2000; 142(5):960–964

[272] O'Meara S, Cullum NA, Nelson EA. Compression for venous leg ulcers. Cochrane Database Syst Rev. 2009(1):CD000265

[273] Kelechi TJ, Bonham PA. Measuring venous insufficiency objectively in the clinical setting. J Vasc Nurs. 2008; 26 (3):67–73

[274] Eliska O, Eliskova M. Morphology of lymphatics in human venous crural ulcers with lipodermatosclerosis. Lymphology. 2001; 34(3):111–123

[275] Macdonald JM, Sims N, Mayrovitz HN. Lymphedema, lipedema, and the open wound: the role of compression therapy. Surg Clin North Am. 2003; 83(3):639–658

[276] Bollinger A, Fagrell B. Clinical Capillaroscopy. Toronto: Hogrefe & Huber; 1990:104

[277] Weissleder H, Schuchhardt C, eds. Lymphedema Diagnosis and Therapy. 3rd ed. Koln: Viavital Verlag GmbH; 2001:337–342

[278] Allen EV, Hines EAJ. Lipedema of the legs: a syndrome characterised by fat legs and orthostatic edema. Ann Intern Med. 1951; 34(5):1243–1250

[279] Herbst KL, Asare-Bediako S. Adiposis dolorosa is more than painful fat. Endocrinologist. 2007; 17(6):326–344

[280] Schook CC, Mulliken JB, Fishman SJ, Alomari AI, Grant FD, Greene AK. Differential diagnosis of lower extremity enlargement in pediatric patients referred with a diagnosis of lymphedema. Plast Reconstr Surg. 2011; 127(4):1571–1581

[281] Child AH, Gordon KD, Sharpe P, et al. Lipedema: an inherited condition. Am J Med Genet A. 2010; 152A(4):970–976

[282] Beninson J, Edelglass JW. Lipedema–the non-lymphatic masquerader. Angiology. 1984; 35(8):506–510

[283] Foldi E, Foldi M. Lipedema. In: Foldi M, Foldi E, eds. Foldi's Textbook of Lymphology. Munich: Elsevier GmbH; 2006:417–427

[284] Herbst KL. Rare adipose disorders (RADs) masquerading as obesity. Acta Pharmacol Sin. 2012; 33(2):155–172

[285] Bogusz AM, Hussey SM, Kapur P, Peng Y, Gokaslan ST. Massive localized lymphedema with unusual presentations: report of 2 cases and review of the literature. Int J Surg Pathol. 2011; 19(2):212–216

[286] Amann-Vesti BR, Franzeck UK, Bollinger A. Microlymphatic aneurysms in patients with lipedema. Lymphology. 2001; 34(4):170–175

[287] Bilancini S, Lucchi M, Tucci S, Eleuteri P. Functional lymphatic alterations in patients suffering from lipedema. Angiology. 1995; 46(4):333–339

[288] Lohrmann C, Foeldi E, Langer M. MR imaging of the lymphatic system in patients with lipedema and lipo-lymphedema. Microvasc Res. 2009; 77(3):335–339

[289] Fife CE, Maus EA, Carter MJ. Lipedema: a frequently misdiagnosed and misunderstood fatty deposition syndrome. Adv Skin Wound Care. 2010; 23(2):81–92, quiz 93–94

[290] Schneble N, Wetzker R, Wollina U. Lipedema – lack of evidence for the involvement of tyrosine kinases. J Biol Regul Homeost Agents. 2016; 30(1):161–163

[291] Szél E, Kemény L, Groma G, Szolnoky G. Pathophysiological dilemmas of lipedema. Med Hypotheses. 2014; 83(5):599–606

[292] Arngrim N, Simonsen L, Holst JJ, Bülow J. Reduced adipose tissue lymphatic drainage of macromolecules in obese subjects: a possible link between obesity and local tissue inflammation? Int J Obes. 2013; 37(5):748–750

[293] Stallworth JM, Hennigar GR, Jonsson HT, Jr, Rodriguez O. The chronically swollen painful extremity. A detailed study for possible etiological factors. JAMA. 1974; 228(13):1656–1659

[294] Siems W, Grune T, Voss P, Brenke R. Anti-fibrosclerotic effects of shock wave therapy in lipedema and cellulite. Biofactors. 2005; 24(1–4):275–282

[295] Suga H, Araki J, Aoi N, Kato H, Higashino T, Yoshimura K. Adipose tissue remodeling in lipedema: adipocyte death and concurrent regeneration. J Cutan Pathol. 2009; 36(12):1293–1298

[296] DeLano FA, Schmid-Schönbein GW. Proteinase activity and receptor cleavage: mechanism for insulin resistance in the spontaneously hypertensive rat. Hypertension. 2008; 52(2):415–423

[297] Mazor R, Schmid-Schönbein GW. Proteolytic receptor cleavage in the pathogenesis of blood rheology and co-morbidities in metabolic syndrome. Early forms of autodigestion. Biorheology. 2015; 52(5–6):337–352

[298] Wollina U, Heinig B, Schönlebe J, Nowak A. Debulking surgery for elephantiasis nostras with large ectatic podoplanin-negative lymphatic vessels in patients with lipo-lymphedema. Eplasty. 2014; 14:e11

[299] Herbst K, Mirkovskaya L, Bharhagava A, Chava Y, Te CH. Lipedema fat and signs and symptoms of illness, increase with advancing stage. Arch Med. 2015; 7(4):1–8

[300] Cornely M. Lipoedema of arms and legs. Part 2: Conservative and surgical therapy of the lipoedema, Lipohyperplasia dolorosa. Phlebologie. 2011; 40:146–151

[301] Rapprich S, Dingler A, Podda M. Liposuction is an effective treatment for lipedema-results of a study with 25 patients. J Dtsch Dermatol Ges. 2011; 9(1):33–40

[302] Tiedjen KV, Knorz S. Different methods of diagnostic imaging in lymphedema, lipedema and venous disorders: indirect lymphography, xeroradiography, CT and isotope lymphography. In: Cluzan RV, Pecking AP, Lokiec FM, eds. Progress in Lymphology: XIII International Congress of Lymphology. Amsterdam: Elsevier Science Publishers B.V.; 1992

[303] Dietzel R, Reisshauer A, Jahr S, Calafiore D, Armbrecht G. Body composition in lipoedema of the legs using dual-energy X-ray absorptiometry: a case-control study. Br J Dermatol. 2015; 173(2):594–596

[304] Fonder MA, Loveless JW, Lazarus GS. Lipedema, a frequently unrecognized problem. J Am Acad Dermatol. 2007; 57(2) Suppl:S1–S3

[305] Partsch H, Stöberl C, Urbanek A, Wenzel-Hora BI. Clinical use of indirect lymphography in different forms of leg edema. Lymphology. 1988; 21(3):152–160

[306] Herbst KL, Coviello AD, Chang A, Boyle DL. Lipomatosis-associated inflammation and excess collagen may contribute to lower relative resting energy expenditure in women with adiposis dolorosa. Int J Obes. 2009; 33(9):1031–1038

[307] Kozakowski J, Zgliczyński W. Body composition, glucose metabolism markers and serum androgens - association in women with polycystic ovary syndrome. Endokrynol Pol. 2013; 64(2):94–100

[308] Schmeller W, Meier-Vollrath I. Lipödem-aktuelles zu einem weitgehend unbekannter Krankheitsbild. Akt Dermatol. 2007; 33:1–10

[309] Greer KE. Lipedema of the legs. Cutis. 1974; 14:98

[310] Földi E, Földi M. Das Lipödem. In: Földi M, Földi E, Kubik S, eds. Lehrbuch der Lymphologie für Mediziner, Masseure und Physiotherapeuten. Munich: Elsevier, Urban & Fischer; 2005:443–453

[311] Sakiyama T, Kubo A, Sasaki T, et al. Recurrent gastrointestinal perforation in a patient with Ehlers-Danlos syndrome due to tenascin-X deficiency. J Dermatol. 2015; 42(5):511–514

[312] Mackenroth L, Fischer-Zirnsak B, Egerer J, et al. An overlapping phenotype of Osteogenesis imperfecta and Ehlers-Danlos syndrome due to a heterozygous mutation in COL1A1 and biallelic missense variants in TNXB identified by whole exome sequencing. Am J Med Genet A. 2016; 170A(4):1080–1085

[313] Morissette R, Chen W, Perritt AF, et al. Broadening the spectrum of Ehlers Danlos syndrome in patients with congenital adrenal hyperplasia. J Clin Endocrinol Metab. 2015; 100(8): E1143–E1152

[314] Pinnick KE, Nicholson G, Manolopoulos KN, et al. MolPAGE Consortium. Distinct developmental profile of lower-body adipose tissue defines resistance against obesity-associated metabolic complications. Diabetes. 2014; 63(11):3785–3797

[315] Shungin D, Winkler TW, Croteau-Chonka DC, et al. ADIPO-Gen Consortium, CARDIOGRAMplusC4D Consortium, CKDGen Consortium, GEFOS Consortium, GENIE Consortium, GLGC, ICBP, International Endogene Consortium, LifeLines Cohort Study, MAGIC Investigators, MuTHER Consortium, PAGE Consortium, ReproGen Consortium. New genetic loci link adipose and insulin biology to body fat distribution. Nature. 2015; 518(7538):187–196

[316] Lee KY, Yamamoto Y, Boucher J, et al. Shox2 is a molecular determinant of depot-specific adipocyte function. Proc Natl Acad Sci U S A. 2013; 110(28):11409–11414

[317] Taylor HS, Arici A, Olive D, Igarashi P. HOXA10 is expressed in response to sex steroids at the time of implantation in the human endometrium. J Clin Invest. 1998; 101(7):1379–1384

[318] Magnusson M, Brun AC, Miyake N, et al. HOXA10 is a critical regulator for hematopoietic stem cells and erythroid/megakaryocyte development. Blood. 2007; 109(9):3687–3696

[319] Singh S, Rajput YS, Barui AK, Sharma R, Datta TK. Fat accumulation in differentiated brown adipocytes is linked with expression of Hox genes. Gene Expr Patterns. 2016; 20(2):99–105

[320] Karpe F, Pinnick KE. Biology of upper-body and lower-body adipose tissue–link to whole-body phenotypes. Nat Rev Endocrinol. 2015; 11(2):90–100

3

[321] Wold LE, Hines EA, Jr, Allen EV. Lipedema of the legs; a syndrome characterized by fat legs and edema. Ann Intern Med. 1951; 34(5):1243–1250

[322] Shin BW, Sim YJ, Jeong HJ, Kim GC. Lipedema, a rare disease. Ann Rehabil Med. 2011; 35(6):922–927

[323] Rapprich S, Baum S, Kaak I, Kottmann T, Podda M. Treatment of lipoedema using liposuction. Results of our own surveys. Phlebologie. 2015; 44:121–133

[324] Petscavage-Thomas JM, Walker EA, Bernard SA, Bennett J. Imaging findings of adiposis dolorosa vs. massive localized lymphedema. Skeletal Radiol. 2015; 44(6):839–847

[325] D'Ettorre M, Gniuli D, Guidone C, Bracaglia R, Tambasco D, Mingrone G. Insulin sensitivity in Familial Multiple Lipomatosis. Eur Rev Med Pharmacol Sci. 2013; 17(16):2254–2256

[326] Tins BJ, Matthews C, Haddaway M, et al. Adiposis dolorosa (Dercum's disease): MRI and ultrasound appearances. Clin Radiol. 2013; 68(10):1047–1053

[327] Nisi G, Sisti A. Images in Clinical Medicine. Madelung's Disease. N Engl J Med. 2016; 374(6):572–572

[328] Stormorken H, Brosstad F, Sommerschid H. The fibromyalgia syndrome: a member of the painful lipo[mato]sis family? In: Pederson JA, ed. New Research on Fibromyalgia. New York, NY: Nova Science Publishers, Inc.; 2006

[329] Starlanyl DJ, Roentsch G, Taylor-Olson C. The effect of transdermal T3 (3,3′,5-triiodothyronine) on geloid masses found in patients with both fibromyalgia and myofascial pain: double-blinded, N of 1 clinical study. Myalgies International: Supplement Scientifique 2001–2002;2(2):8–18

[330] Albrecht PJ, Hou Q, Argoff CE, Storey JR, Wymer JP, Rice FL. Excessive peptidergic sensory innervation of cutaneous arteriole-venule shunts (AVS) in the palmar glabrous skin of fibromyalgia patients: implications for widespread deep tissue pain and fatigue. Pain Med. 2013; 14(6):895–915

[331] Halk AB, Damstra RJ. First Dutch guidelines on lipedema using the international classification of functioning, disability and health. Phlebology. 2016; 12:0268355516639421

[332] Langendoen SI, Habbema L, Nijsten TE, Neumann HA. Lipoedema: from clinical presentation to therapy. A review of the literature. Br J Dermatol. 2009; 161(5):980–986

[333] Reich-Schupke S, Altmeyer P, Stücker M. Thick legs - not always lipedema. J Dtsch Dermatol Ges. 2013; 11(3):225–233

[334] Szolnoky G, Nagy N, Kovács RK, et al. Complex decongestive physiotherapy decreases capillary fragility in lipedema. Lymphology. 2008; 41(4):161–166

[335] Schneider M, Conway EM, Carmeliet P. Lymph makes you fat. Nat Genet. 2005; 37(10):1023–1024

[336] Witte CL, Witte MH. Contrasting patterns of lymphatic and blood circulatory disorders. Lymphology. 1987; 20(4):171–178

[337] Hespe GE, Kataru RP, Savetsky IL, et al. Exercise training improves obesity-related lymphatic dysfunction. J Physiol. 2016; 594(15):4267–4282

[338] Giacomini F, Ditroilo M, Lucertini F, De Vito G, Gatta G, Benelli P. The cardiovascular response to underwater pedaling at different intensities: a comparison of 4 different water stationary bikes. J Sports Med Phys Fitness. 2009; 49(4):432–439

[339] Herbst KL, Rutledge T. Pilot study: rapidly cycling hypobaric pressure improves pain after 5 days in adiposis dolorosa. J Pain Res. 2010; 3:147–153

[340] Marquez JL, Rubinstein S, Fattor JA, Shah O, Hoffman AR, Friedlander AL. Cyclic hypobaric hypoxia improves markers of glucose metabolism in middle-aged men. High Alt Med Biol. 2013; 14(3):263–272

[341] Erlich C, Iker E, Herbst KL, et al. Lymphedema and Lipedema Nutrition Guide. Foods, Vitamins, Minerals, and Supplements. San Francisco, CA: Lymph Notes; 2015

[342] Mohan V, Spiegelman D, Sudha V, et al. Effect of brown rice, white rice, and brown rice with legumes on blood glucose and insulin responses in overweight Asian Indians: a randomized controlled trial. Diabetes Technol Ther. 2014; 16(5):317–325

[343] Westfall TC, Westfall DP. Adrenergic agonists and antagonists. In: Brunton LL, Lazo JS, Parker KL, eds. Goodman and Gilman's The Pharmacological Basis of Therapeutics. 11th ed. New York, NY: McGraw-Hill Medical Publishing Division; 2006:237–295

[344] Marcelon G, Vanhoutte PM. Mechanism of action of Ruscus extract. Int Angiol. 1984; 3 Suppl 1:74–76

[345] Bouskela M. Microcirculatory responses to Ruscus extract in the hamster cheek pouch. In: Vanhoute PM, ed. Return Circulation and Norepinephrine: An Update. Paris: John Libby Eurotext; 1991:207–218

[346] Boudet C, Peyrin L. Comparative effect of tropolone and diosmin on venous COMT and sympathetic activity in rat. Arch Int Pharmacodyn Ther. 1986; 283(2):312–320

[347] Wang J, Zhao L-L, Sun G-X, et al. A comparison of acidic and enzymatic hydrolysis of rutin. Afr J Biotechnol. 2011; 10(8):1460–1466

[348] Kuppusamy UR, Das NP. Potentiation of beta-adrenoceptor agonist-mediated lipolysis by quercetin and fisetin in isolated rat adipocytes. Biochem Pharmacol. 1994; 47(3):521–529

[349] Kaviani A, Fateh M, Yousefi Nooraie R, Alinagi-zadeh MR, Ataie-Fashtami L. Low-level laser therapy in management of postmastectomy lymphedema. Lasers Med Sci. 2006; 21(2):90–94

[350] Brorson H. Liposuction gives complete reduction of chronic large arm lymphedema after breast cancer. Acta Oncol. 2000; 39(3):407–420

[351] Martinez-Corral I, Ulvmar MH, Stanczuk L, et al. Nonvenous origin of dermal lymphatic vasculature. Circ Res. 2015; 116(10):1649–1654

[352] Scallan JP, Hill MA, Davis MJ. Lymphatic vascular integrity is disrupted in type 2 diabetes due to impaired nitric oxide signalling. Cardiovasc Res. 2015; 107(1):89–97

[353] Gulati OP. Pycnogenol® in chronic venous insufficiency and related venous disorders. Phytother Res. 2014; 28(3):348–362

[354] Berti F, Omini C, Longiave D. The mode of action of aescin and the release of prostaglandins. Prostaglandins. 1977; 14(2):241–249

[355] Yu Z, Su P. Effect of beta-aescin extract from Chinese buckeye seed on chronic venous insufficiency. Pharmazie. 2013; 68(6):428–430

[356] Conley SM, Bruhn RL, Morgan PV, Stamer WD. Selenium's effects on MMP-2 and TIMP-1 secretion by human trabecular meshwork cells. Invest Ophthalmol Vis Sci. 2004; 45(2):473–479

[357] Rutkowski JM, Boardman KC, Swartz MA. Characterization of lymphangiogenesis in a model of adult skin regeneration. Am J Physiol Heart Circ Physiol. 2006; 291(3):H1402–H1410

[358] Nourollahi S, Mondry TE, Herbst KL. Bucher's Broom and Selenium Improve Lipedema: A Retrospective Case Study. Altern Integr Med. 2013; 2(4):1–7

[359] Micke O, Bruns F, Schäfer U, et al. Selenium in the treatment of acute and chronic lymphedema. Trace Elem Electrolytes. 2000; 17:206–209

[360] Kasseroller RG, Schrauzer GN. Treatment of secondary lymphedema of the arm with physical decongestive therapy and sodium selenite: a review. Am J Ther. 2000; 7(4):273–279

[361] Lewin MH, Arthur JR, Riemersma RA, et al. Selenium supplementation acting through the induction of thioredoxin reductase and glutathione peroxidase protects the human endothelial cell line EAhy926 from damage by lipid hydroperoxides. Biochim Biophys Acta. 2002; 1593(1):85–92

[362] Horváthová M, Jahnová E, Gazdík F. Effect of selenium supplementation in asthmatic subjects on the expression of endothelial cell adhesion molecules in culture. Biol Trace Elem Res. 1999; 69(1):15–26

[363] Selenium in Nutrition: Revised. Washington, DC: National Research Council;1983

[364] Laclaustra M, Navas-Acien A, Stranges S, Ordovas JM, Guallar E. Serum selenium concentrations and diabetes in U.S. adults: National Health and Nutrition Examination Survey (NHANES) 2003–2004. Environ Health Perspect. 2009; 117 (9):1409–1413

[365] Woo SL, Xu H, Li H, et al. Metformin ameliorates hepatic steatosis and inflammation without altering adipose phenotype in diet-induced obesity. PLoS One. 2014; 9(3):e91111

[366] Shin NR, Lee JC, Lee HY, et al. An increase in the Akkermansia spp. population induced by metformin treatment improves glucose homeostasis in diet-induced obese mice. Gut. 2014; 63(5):727–735

[367] Bannister CA, Holden SE, Jenkins-Jones S, et al. Can people with type 2 diabetes live longer than those without? A comparison of mortality in people initiated with metformin or sulphonylurea monotherapy and matched, non-diabetic controls. Diabetes Obes Metab. 2014; 16(11):1165–1173

[368] Lohman EB, III, Petrofsky JS, Maloney-Hinds C, Betts-Schwab H, Thorpe D. The effect of whole body vibration on lower extremity skin blood flow in normal subjects. Med Sci Monit. 2007; 13(2):CR71–CR76

[369] Kerschan-Schindl K, Grampp S, Henk C, et al. Whole-body vibration exercise leads to alterations in muscle blood volume. Clin Physiol. 2001; 21(3):377–382

[370] Stewart JA, Cochrane DJ, Morton RH. Differential effects of whole body vibration durations on knee extensor strength. J Sci Med Sport. 2009; 12(1):50–53

[371] Schmeller W, Meier-Vollrath I. Tumescent liposuction: a new and successful therapy for lipedema. J Cutan Med Surg. 2006; 10(1):7–10

[372] Stutz JJ, Krahl D. Water jet-assisted liposuction for patients with lipoedema: histologic and immunohistologic analysis of the aspirates of 30 lipoedema patients. Aesthetic Plast Surg. 2009; 33(2):153–162

[373] Wollina U, Goldman A, Heinig B. Microcannular tumescent liposuction in advanced lipedema and Dercum's disease. G Ital Derm Venereol. 2010; 145(2):151–159

[374] Gadelha AdR, de Miranda Leão TL. Rule of four: a simple and safe formula for tumescent anesthesia in dermatologic surgical procedures. Surg Cosmet Dermatol. 2009; 1(2):99–102

[375] Sattler G, Rapprich S, Hagedorn M. Tumeszenz-Lokalanästhesie – Untersuchung zur Pharmakokinetik von Prilocain. Z Hautkr. 1997; 7:522–525

[376] Schmeller W, Hueppe M, Meier-Vollrath I. Tumescent liposuction in lipoedema yields good long-term results. Br J Dermatol. 2012; 166(1):161–168

[377] Pollock H, Forman S, Pollock T, Raccasi M. Conscious sedation/local anesthesia in the office-based surgical and procedural facility. Clin Plast Surg. 2013; 40(3):383–388

[378] Amron D. Liposuction Panel. Living with Lipedema and Dealing with Dercum's Disease. St. Louis, MO: Fat Disorders Research Society; 2016

[379] Hattori J, Yamakage M, Seki S, Okazaki K, Namiki A. Inhibitory effects of the anesthetics propofol and sevoflurane on spontaneous lymphatic vessel activity in rats. Anesthesiology. 2004; 101(3):687–694

[380] Takeshita T, Morio M, Kawahara M, Fujii K. Halothane-induced changes in contractions of mesenteric lymphatics of the rat. Lymphology. 1988; 21(2):128–130

[381] McHale NG, Thornbury KD. The effect of anesthetics on lymphatic contractility. Microvasc Res. 1989; 37(1):70–76

[382] Quin JW, Shannon AD. The effect of anaesthesia and surgery on lymph flow, protein and leucocyte concentration in lymph of the sheep. Lymphology. 1975; 8(4):126–135

[383] Baumgartner A, Hueppe M, Schmeller W. Long-term benefit of liposuction in patients with lipoedema: a follow-up study after an average of 4 and 8 years. Br J Dermatol. 2016; 174 (5):1061–1067

[384] Peled AW, Slavin SA, Brorson H. Long-term outcome after surgical treatment of lipedema. Ann Plast Surg. 2012; 68 (3):303–307

[385] Binkley JM, Stratford PW, Lott SA, Riddle DL, North American Orthopaedic Rehabilitation Research Network. The Lower Extremity Functional Scale (LEFS): scale development, measurement properties, and clinical application. Phys Ther. 1999; 79(4):371–383

[386] Neutze D, Roque J. Clinical evaluation of bleeding and bruising in primary care. Am Fam Physician. 2016; 93(4):279–286

[387] Rapprich S, Loehnert M, Hagedorn M. Therapy of lipoedema syndrome by liposuction under tumescent local anaesthesia. Ann Dermatol Venereol. 2002; 129:711

[388] Wollina U, Graf A, Hanisch V. Acute pulmonary edema following liposuction due to heart failure and atypical pneumonia. Wien Med Wochenschr. 2015; 165(9–10):189–194

[389] Sattler G, Eichner S. Complications of liposuction [in German]. Hautarzt. 2013; 64(3):171–179

[390] van der Lei B, Halbesma GJ, van Nieuwenhoven CA, van Wingerden JJ. Spontaneous breast enlargement following liposuction of the abdominal wall: does a link exist? Plast Reconstr Surg. 2007; 119(5):1584–1589

[391] Swanson E. No increase in female breast size or fat redistribution to the upper body after liposuction: a prospective controlled photometric study. Aesthet Surg J. 2014; 34(6):896–906

[392] Stutz JJ. Liposuction Panel. Living with Lipedema and Dealing with Dercum's Disease. St. Louis, MO: Fat Disorders Research Society; 2016

[393] Stutz JJ. All about lipedema. human med AG. 2015

[394] Busse JW, Bhandari M, Guyatt GH, et al. SPRINT Investigators & the Medically Unexplained Syndromes Study Group. Development and validation of an instrument to predict functional recovery in tibial fracture patients: the Somatic Pre-Occupation and Coping (SPOC) questionnaire. J Orthop Trauma. 2012; 26(6):370–378

[395] Tait MJ, Levy J, Nowell M, et al. Improved outcome after lumbar microdiscectomy in patients shown their excised disc fragments: a prospective, double blind, randomised, controlled trial. J Neurol Neurosurg Psychiatry. 2009; 80 (9):1044–1046

[396] Stutz JJ. Liposuction of lipedema to prevent later joint complications [in German]. Vasomed. 2011; 23:1–6

[397] Boeni R. Weight loss and its relation to fat aspiration yields in liposuction: a survey in 48 patients. Dermatology. 2012; 224(4):320–322

[398] Cohen MM, Jr. Klippel-Trenaunay syndrome. Am J Med Genet. 2000; 93(3):171–175

[399] Gloviczki P, Driscoll DJ. Klippel-Trenaunay syndrome: current management. Phlebology. 2007; 22(6):291–298

[400] Luks VL, Kamitaki N, Vivero MP, et al. Lymphatic and other vascular malformative/overgrowth disorders are caused by somatic mutations in PIK3CA. J Pediatr. 2015; 166(4):1048–54.e1, 5

[401] Vahidnezhad H, Youssefian L, Uitto J. Klippel-Trenaunay syndrome belongs to the PIK3CA-related overgrowth spectrum (PROS). Exp Dermatol. 2016; 25(1):17–19

[402] Eerola I, Boon LM, Mulliken JB, et al. Capillary malformation-arteriovenous malformation, a new clinical and genetic disorder caused by RASA1 mutations. Am J Hum Genet. 2003; 73(6):1240–1249

[403] Jacob AG, Driscoll DJ, Shaughnessy WJ, Stanson AW, Clay RP, Gloviczki P. Klippel-Trénaunay syndrome: spectrum and management. Mayo Clin Proc. 1998; 73(1):28–36

[404] Oduber CE, Khemlani K, Sillevis Smitt JH, Hennekam RC, van der Horst CM. Baseline quality of life in patients with klippel-trenaunay syndrome. J Plast Reconstr Aesthet Surg. 2010; 63(4):603–609

[405] Mattassi R, Vaghi M. Management of the marginal vein: current issues. Phlebology. 2007; 22(6):283–286

[406] Cherry KJ, Gloviczki P, Stanson AW. Persistent sciatic vein: diagnosis and treatment of a rare condition. J Vasc Surg. 1996; 23(3):490–497

[407] Servelle M. Klippel and Trénaunay's syndrome. 768 operated cases. Ann Surg. 1985; 201(3):365–373

[408] Lee A, Driscoll D, Gloviczki P, Clay R, Shaughnessy W, Stans A. Evaluation and management of pain in patients with Klippel-Trenaunay syndrome: a review. Pediatrics. 2005; 115 (3):744–749

[409] Schook CC, Mulliken JB, Fishman SJ, Alomari AI, Grant FD, Greene AK. Differential diagnosis of lower extremity enlargement in pediatric patients referred with a diagnosis of lymphedema. Plast Reconstr Surg. 2011; 127(4):1571–1581

[410] Liu NF, Lu Q, Yan ZX. Lymphatic malformation is a common component of Klippel-Trenaunay syndrome. J Vasc Surg. 2010; 52(6):1557–1563

[411] Malgor RD, Gloviczki P, Fahrni J, et al. Surgical treatment of varicose veins and venous malformations in Klippel-Trenaunay syndrome. Phlebology. 2016; 31(3):209–215

[412] Adams DM, Trenor CC, III, Hammill AM, et al. Efficacy and safety of sirolimus in the treatment of complicated vascular anomalies. Pediatrics. 2016; 137(2):e20153257

[413] Hutzschenreuther P, Bruemmer H, Silberschneider K. Die Vagotone Wirkung der Manuellen Lymphdrainage nach Dr. Vodder. LymphForsch. 2003; 7(1):7–14

Recommended Reading

Lymphedema

Brennan MJ. Lymphedema following the surgical treatment of breast cancer: a review of pathophysiology and treatment. J Pain Symptom Manage. 1992; 7(2):110–116

Cheville AL, Tchou J. Barriers to rehabilitation following surgery for primary breast cancer. J Surg Oncol. 2007; 95(5):409–418

Erickson VS, Pearson ML, Ganz PA, Adams J, Kahn KL. Arm edema in breast cancer patients. J Natl Cancer Inst. 2001; 93(2):96–111

Földi E. Massage and damage to lymphatics. Lymphology. 1995; 28 (1):1–3

Földi E. Prevention of dermatolymphangioadenitis by combined physiotherapy of the swollen arm after treatment for breast cancer. Lymphology. 1996; 29(2):48–49

Földi E, Földi M, Weissleder H. Conservative treatment of lymphoedema of the limbs. Angiology. 1985; 36(3):171–180

Földi M. Treatment of lymphedema [editorial]. Lymphology. 1994; 27(1):1–5

Getz DH. The primary, secondary, and tertiary nursing interventions of lymphedema. Cancer Nurs. 1985; 8(3):177–184

Greene AK, Borud L, Slavin SA. Blood pressure monitoring and venipuncture in the lymphedematous extremity. Plast Reconstr Surg. 2005; 116(7):2058–2059

Greenlee R, Hoyme H, Witte M, Crowe P, Witte C. Developmental disorders of the lymphatic system. Lymphology. 1993; 26(4):156–168

Herpertz U. Lipedema [in German]. Z Lymphol. 1995; 19(1):1–11

Horsley JS, Styblo T. Lymphedema in the postmastectomy patient. In: Bland KI, Copeland EM, eds. The Breast: Comprehensive Management of Benign and Malignant Diseases. Philadelphia, PA: Saunders; 1991:701–706

Kepics J. Physical therapy treatment of axillary web syndrome. Rehabil Oncol. 2004; 22(1):21–22

Kim DI, Huh S, Hwang JH, Kim YI, Lee BB. Venous dynamics in leg lymphedema. Lymphology. 1999; 32(1):11–14

Koehler L. Axillary web syndrome and lymphedema, a new perspective. LymphLink. 2006; 18(3):9–10

Koehler L. Treatment consideration for axillary web syndrome. Paper presented at the National Lymphedema Network 7th International Conference, Nashville, TN, November 1–5, 2006

Leidenius M, Leppänen E, Krogerus L, von Smitten K. Motion restriction and axillary web syndrome after sentinel node biopsy and axillary clearance in breast cancer. Am J Surg. 2003; 185 (2):127–130

Markowski J, Wilcox JP, Helm PA. Lymphedema incidence after specific postmastectomy therapy. Arch Phys Med Rehabil. 1981; 62 (9):449–452

Mortimer PS, Bates DO, Brassington HD, et al. The prevalence of arm edema following treatment for breast cancer. Q J Med. 1996; 89:377–380

Moskovitz AH, Anderson BO, Yeung RS, Byrd DR, Lawton TJ, Moe RE. Axillary web syndrome after axillary dissection. Am J Surg. 2001; 181(5):434–439

National Cancer Institute (U.S.), Office of Cancer Communications. The Breast Cancer Digest: A Guide to Medical Care, Emotional Support, Educational Programs, and Resources. 2nd ed. Bethesda, MD: U.S. Dept. of Health, Education, and Welfare, Public Health Service, National Institute of Health, National Cancer Institute; 1984:78

NLN. Position Statement of the National Lymphedema Network. Lymphedema risk reduction practices. Available at: http://www.lymphnet.org/pdfDocs/nlnriskreduction.pdf. Accessed June 15, 2012

Petrek JA, Lerner R. Lymphedema: etiology and treatment. In: Harris JR, Lippman ME, Morrow M, Hellman S, eds. Diseases of the Breast. Philadelphia, PA: Lippincott-Raven; 1996:896–901

Petrek JA, Senie RT, Peters M, Rosen PP. Lymphedema in a cohort of breast carcinoma survivors 20 years after diagnosis. Cancer. 2001; 92(6):1368–1377

Ridner SH. Breast cancer lymphedema: pathophysiology and risk reduction guidelines. Oncol Nurs Forum. 2002; 29(9):1285–1293

Rosenfeld RG, Tesch LG, Rodriguez-Rigau LJ, et al. Recommendations for diagnosis, treatment, and management of individuals with Turner syndrome. Endocrinologist. 1994; 4(5):351–358

Shamley DR, Srinaganathan R, Weatherall R, et al. Changes in shoulder muscle size and activity following treatment for breast cancer. Breast Cancer Res Treat. 2007; 106(1):19–27

Stanton AW, Levick JR, Mortimer PS. Cutaneous vascular control in the arms of women with postmastectomy oedema. Exp Physiol. 1996; 81(3):447–464

Winge C, Mattiasson AC, Schultz I. After axillary surgery for breast cancer–is it safe to take blood samples or give intravenous infusions? J Clin Nurs. 2010; 19(9–10):1270–1274

Genetics

Evans AL, Brice G, Sotirova V, et al. Mapping of primary congenital lymphedema to the 5q35.3 region. Am J Hum Genet. 1999; 64 (2):547–555

Ferrell RE, Baty CJ, Kimak MA, et al. GJC2 missense mutations cause human lymphedema. Am J Hum Genet. 2010; 86(6):943–948

Fang J, Dagenais SL, Erickson RP, et al. Mutations in FOXC2 (MFH-1), a forkhead family transcription factor, are responsible for the hereditary lymphedema-distichiasis syndrome. Am J Hum Genet. 2000; 67(6):1382–1388

Alders M, Hogan BM, Gjini E, et al. Mutations in CCBE1 cause generalized lymph vessel dysplasia in humans. Nat Genet. 2009; 41 (12):1272–1274

Irrthum A, Devriendt K, Chitayat D, et al. Mutations in the transcription factor gene SOX18 underlie recessive and dominant forms of hypotrichosis-lymphedema-telangiectasia. Am J Hum Genet. 2003; 72(6):1470–1478

Au AC, Hernandez PA, Lieber E, et al. Protein tyrosine phosphatase PTPN14 is a regulator of lymphatic function and choanal development in humans. Am J Hum Genet. 2010; 87(3):436–444

Ostergaard P, Simpson MA, Brice G, et al. Rapid identification of mutations in GJC2 in primary lymphoedema using whole exome sequencing combined with linkage analysis with delineation of the phenotype. J Med Genet. 2011; 48(4):251–255

Finegold DN, Schacht V, Kimak MA, et al. HGF and MET mutations in primary and secondary lymphedema. Lymphat Res Biol. 2008; 6 (2):65–68

Brice G, Ostergaard P, Jeffery S, Gordon K, Mortimer PS, Mansour S. A novel mutation in GJA1 causing oculodentodigital syndrome and primary lymphoedema in a three generation family. Clin Genet. 2013; 84(4):378–381

McClelland J, Burgess B, Crock P, Goel H. Sotos syndrome: an unusual presentation with intrauterine growth restriction, generalized lymphedema, and intention tremor. Am J Med Genet A. 2016; 170A(4):1064–1069

Joyce S, Gordon K, Brice G, et al. The lymphatic phenotype in Noonan and Cardiofaciocutaneous syndrome. Eur J Hum Genet. 2016; 24(5):690–696

Surgical Procedures

Edwards MJ, Whitworth P, Tafra L, McMasters KM. The details of successful sentinel lymph node staging for breast cancer. Am J Surg. 2000; 180(4):257–261

Hill AD, Tran KN, Akhurst T, et al. Lessons learned from 500 cases of lymphatic mapping for breast cancer. Ann Surg. 1999; 229(4):528–535

Kissin MW, Querci della Rovere G, Easton D, Westbury G. Risk of lymphoedema following the treatment of breast cancer. Br J Surg. 1986; 73(7):580–584

Kwan W, Jackson J, Weir LM, Dingee C, McGregor G, Olivotto IA. Chronic arm morbidity after curative breast cancer treatment: prevalence and impact on quality of life. J Clin Oncol. 2002; 20 (20):4242–4248

Mackay-Wiggan J, Ratner D, Sambandan DR. Suturing techniques. Available at: http://emedicine.medscape.com/article/1824895-overview#showall. Accessed June 15, 2012

National Cancer Institute Website. A collection of material about sentinel lymph node biopsy. Available at: http://www.cancer.gov/cancertopics/factsheet/detection/sentinel-node-biopsy. Accessed August 18, 2004

Filariasis

Fife C, Benavides S, Otto G. Morbid obesity and lymphedema management. National Lymphedema Network. LymphLink. 2007; 19 (3):2–4

Figueredo-Silva J, Dreyer G. Bancroftian filariasis in children and adolescents: clinical-pathological observations in 22 cases from an endemic area. Ann Trop Med Parasitol. 2005; 99(8):759–769

Filariasis.net. Information on filariasis. http://www.filariasis.org/. Accessed October 19, 2012

Mahamaneerat WK, Shyu CR, Stewart BR, Armer JM. Breast cancer treatment, BMI, post-op swelling/lymphoedema. J Lymphoedema. 2008; 3(2):38–44

Molyneux DH. Elimination of transmission of lymphatic filariasis in Egypt. Lancet. 2006; 367(9515):966–968

Ngwira BM, Tambala P, Perez AM, Bowie C, Molyneux DH. The geographical distribution of lymphatic filariasis infection in Malawi. Filaria J. 2007; 6:12

Ottesen EA. The global programme to eliminate lymphatic filariasis. Trop Med Int Health. 2000; 5(9):591–594

Wynd S, Durrheim DN, Carron J, et al. Socio-cultural insights and lymphatic filariasis control–lessons from the Pacific. Filaria J. 2007; 6:3

Axillary Web Syndrome

Bernas MJ. Axillary web syndrome, the lost cord, and lingering questions. Lymphology. 2014; 47(4):153–155

Cheville AL, Tchou J. Barriers to rehabilitation following surgery for primary breast cancer. J Surg Oncol. 2007; 95(5):409–418

Cho Y, Do J, Jung S, Kwon O, Jeon JY. Effects of a physical therapy program combined with manual lymphatic drainage on shoulder function, quality of life, lymphedema incidence, and pain in breast cancer patients with axillary web syndrome following axillary dissection. Support Care Cancer. 2016; 24(5):2047–2057

Josenhans E. Physiotherapeutic treatment for axillary cord formation following breast cancer surgery. Z Physiother. 2007; 59 (9):868–878

Kepics J. Physical therapy treatment of axillary web syndrome. Rehabil Oncol. 2004; 22(1):21–22

Koehler LA, Blaes AH, Haddad TC, Hunter DW, Hirsch AT, Ludewig PM. Movement, function, pain, and postoperative edema in axillary web syndrome. Phys Ther. 2015; 95(10):1345–1353

Koehler LA, Hunter DW, Haddad TC, Blaes AH, Hirsch AT, Ludewig PM. Characterizing axillary web syndrome: ultrasonographic efficacy. Lymphology. 2014; 47(4):156–163

Koehler LA. Axillary web syndrome and lymphedema, a new perspective. LymphLink. 2006; 18(3):9–10

Leduc O, Sichere M, Moreau A, et al. Axillary web syndrome: nature and localization. Lymphology. 2009; 42(4):176–181

Leduc O, Fumière E, Banse S, et al. Identification and description of the axillary web syndrome (AWS) by clinical signs, MRI and US imaging. Lymphology. 2014; 47(4):164–176

Leidenius M, Leppänen E, Krogerus L, von Smitten K. Motion restriction and axillary web syndrome after sentinel node biopsy and axillary clearance in breast cancer. Am J Surg. 2003; 185 (2):127–130

Marsch WC, Haas N, Stüttgen G. 'Mondor's phlebitis'–a lymphovascular process. Light and electron microscopic indications. Dermatologica. 1986; 172(3):133–138

Moskovitz AH, Anderson BO, Yeung RS, Byrd DR, Lawton TJ, Moe RE. Axillary web syndrome after axillary dissection. Am J Surg. 2001; 181(5):434–439

O'Toole J, Miller CL, Specht MC, et al. Cording following treatment for breast cancer. Breast Cancer Res Treat. 2013; 140(1):105–111

Reedijk M, Boerner S, Ghazarian D, McCready D. A case of axillary web syndrome with subcutaneous nodules following axillary surgery. Breast. 2006; 15(3):411–413

Severeid K, Simpson J, Templeton B, York R, Hummel-Berry K, Leiserowitz A. Axillary web syndrome among patients with breast cancer or melanoma referred to physical therapy. Rehabil Oncol. 2007; 25(1):25

Shamley DR, Srinaganathan R, Weatherall R, et al. Changes in shoulder muscle size and activity following treatment for breast cancer. Breast Cancer Res Treat. 2007; 106(1):19–27

Shetty MK, Watson AB. Mondor's disease of the breast: sonographic and mammographic findings. AJR Am J Roentgenol. 2001; 177(4):893–896

Nevola Teixeira LF, Veronesi P, Lohsiriwat V, et al. Axillary web syndrome self-assessment questionnaire: Initial development and validation. Breast. 2014; 23(6):836–843

Torres Lacomba M, Mayoral Del Moral O, Coperias Zazo JL, Yuste Sánchez MJ, Ferrandez JC, Zapico Goñi A. Axillary web syndrome after axillary dissection in breast cancer: a prospective study. Breast Cancer Res Treat. 2009; 117(3):625–630

Winicour J. Axillary web syndrome. Proceedings of the 9th National Lymphedema Network International Conference; Orlando, FL; September 2010

Yeung WM, McPhail SM, Kuys SS. A systematic review of axillary web syndrome (AWS). J Cancer Surviv. 2015; 9(4):576–598

Tissue Dielectric Constant (TDC)

Czerniec SA, Ward LC, Refshauge KM, et al. Assessment of breast cancer-related arm lymphedema–comparison of physical measurement methods and self-report. Cancer Invest. 2010; 28(1):54–62

Mayrovitz HN. Assessing local tissue edema in postmastectomy lymphedema. Lymphology. 2007; 40(2):87–94

Mayrovitz HN, Weingrad DN, Davey S. Local tissue water in at-risk and contralateral forearms of women with and without breast cancer treatment-related lymphedema. Lymphat Res Biol. 2009; 7 (3):153–158

Mayrovitz HN, Bernal M, Brlit F, Desfor R. Biophysical measures of skin tissue water: variations within and among anatomical sites and correlations between measures. Skin Res Technol. 2013; 19 (1):47–54

Lahtinen T, Seppälä J, Viren T, Johansson K. Experimental and analytical comparisons of tissue dielectric constant (TDC) and bioimpedance spectroscopy (BIS) in assessment of early arm lymphedema in breast cancer patients after axillary surgery and radiotherapy. Lymphat Res Biol. 2015; 13(3):176–185

Mayrovitz HN, Weingrad DN, Lopez L. Assessing localized skin-to-fat water in arms of women with breast cancer via tissue dielectric constant measurements in pre- and post-surgery patients. Ann Surg Oncol. 2015; 22(5):1483–1489

Radiation-Induced Brachial Plexopathy

Breast cancer discussion forum. Available at: http://community. breastcancer.org/forum/64/topic/698235. Accessed June 15, 2012

Stephenson RO. Radiation-induced brachial plexopathy. Available at: http://emedicine.medscape.com/article/316497-overview. Accessed June 15, 2012

Senkus-Konefka E. Complications of breast cancer radiotherapy. Available at: http://www.lymphedemapeople.com/wiki/doku.php?id=complications_of_breast_cancer_radiotherapy. Accessed June 15, 2012

Step up, speak out. Available at: http://www.stepup-speakout.org/Radiation_Induced_Brachial_plexopathy.htm. Accessed June 15, 2012

Diagnostic Imaging

Bräutigam P, Földi E, Schaiper I, Krause T, Vanscheidt W, Moser E. Analysis of lymphatic drainage in various forms of leg edema using two compartment lymphoscintigraphy. Lymphology. 1998; 31 (2):43–55

Partsch H, Urbanek A, Wenzel-Hora B. The dermal lymphatics in lymphoedema visualized by indirect lymphography. Br J Dermatol. 1984; 110(4):431–438

Pecking A, et al. In vivo assessment of fluid and fat component in lymphedematous skin. Paper presented at: International Society of Lymphology Congress; Genoa, Italy; 2001

Svensson WE, Mortimer PS, Tohno E, Cosgrove DO. Colour Doppler demonstrates venous flow abnormalities in breast cancer patients with chronic arm swelling. Eur J Cancer. 1994; 30A(5):657–660

Szuba A, Shin WS, Strauss HW, Rockson S. The third circulation: radionuclide lymphoscintigraphy in the evaluation of lymphedema. J Nucl Med. 2003; 44(1):43–57

Complete Decongestive Therapy

Boris M, Weindorf S, Lasinski B, Boris G. Lymphedema reduction by noninvasive complex lymphedema therapy. Oncology (Williston Park). 1994; 8(9):95–106, discussion 109–110

Eliska O, Eliskova M. Are peripheral lymphatics damaged by high pressure manual massage? Lymphology. 1995; 28(1):21–30

Hocutt JE, Jr. Cryotherapy. Am Fam Physician. 1981; 23(3):141–144

Sequential Intermittent Pneumatic Compression

Bernas MJ, Witte CL, Witte MH, International Society of Lymphology Executive Committee. The diagnosis and treatment of peripheral lymphedema: draft revision of the 1995 Consensus Document of the International Society of Lymphology Executive Committee for discussion at the September 3–7, 2001, XVIII International Congress of Lymphology in Genoa, Italy. Lymphology. 2001; 34(2):84–91

Bock AU. Prinzipielle Überlegungen zur Apparativen Inter-mittierenden Kompressionstherapie. LymphForsch. 2003; 7(1):27–29

Dini D, Del Mastro L, Gozza A, et al. The Role of Pneumatic Compression in the Treatment of Postmastectomy Lymphedema: A Randomized Phase III Study. Boston, MA: Kluwer Academic Publishers; 1998

Hammond T, Golla AH. Overcoming barriers in the management of lower extremity lymphedema utilizing advanced pneumatic therapy. Open Rehabil J. 2009; 2:79–85

Lynnworth M. Greater Boston Lymphedema Support Group pump survey. Natl Lymphedema Network Newsletter. 1988; 10:6–7

Richmand DM, O'Donnell TF, Jr, Zelikovski A. Sequential pneumatic compression for lymphedema. A controlled trial. Arch Surg. 1985; 120(10):1116–1119

Ridner SH, McMahon E, Dietrich MS, Hoy S. Home-based lymphedema treatment in patients with cancer-related lymphedema or noncancer-related lymphedema. Oncol Nurs Forum. 2008; 35 (4):671–680

Weissleder H. Stellenwert der Apparativen Intermittieren-den Kompression—Literatureberblick. LymphForsch. 2003; 7(1):15–18

Wilburn O, Wilburn P, Rockson SG. A pilot, prospective evaluation of a novel alternative for maintenance therapy of breast cancer-associated lymphedema [ISRCTN76522412]. BMC Cancer. 2006; 6:84

Nutrition

American Cancer Society. Lymphedema: what every woman with breast cancer should know. Available at: http://www.cancer.org/Treatment/TreatmentsandSideEffects/PhysicalSideEffects/Lymphedema/WhatEveryWomanwithBreastCancerShouldKnow/index. Accessed June 15, 2012

Lymphedema People - Lymphedema Diet. Available at: http://www.lymphedemapeople.com/wiki/doku.php?id=the_lymphedema_diet. Accessed June 15, 2012

Medical News Today. Lymphedema risk for breast cancer survivors increased by obesity. Available at: http://www.medicalnewstoday.com/releases/133691.php. Accessed June 15, 2012

National Cancer Institute. Obesity and lymphedema. Available at: http://www.cancer.gov/cancertopics/pdq/supportivecare/lymphedema/HealthProfessional/page2#Section_29. Accessed June 15, 2012

Medication

Bassett ML, Dahlstrom JE. Liver failure while taking coumarin. Med J Aust. 1995; 163(2):106

Casley-Smith JR, Casley-Smith JR. Lymphedema the poor and benzo-pyrones: proposed amendments to the consensus document. Lymphology. 1996; 29(4):137–140

Casley-Smith JR, Morgan RG, Piller NB. Treatment of lymphedema of the arms and legs with 5,6-benzo-[alpha]-pyrone. N Engl J Med. 1993; 329(16):1158–1163

Cox D, O'Kennedy R, Thornes RD. The rarity of liver toxicity in patients treated with coumarin (1,2-benzopyrone). Hum Toxicol. 1989; 8(6):501–506

Faurschou P. Toxic hepatitis due to benzo-pyrone. Hum Toxicol. 1982; 1(2):149–150

Fentem JH, Fry JR. Species differences in the metabolism and hepatotoxicity of coumarin. Comp Biochem Physiol C. 1993; 104(1):1–8

International Society of Lymphology. The diagnosis and treatment of peripheral lymphedema. Consensus document of the International Society of Lymphology. Lymphology. 2003; 36(2):84–91

International Society of Lymphology. The diagnosis and treatment of peripheral lymphedema. 2009 consensus document of the International Society of Lymphology. http://www.u.arizona.edu/~witte/2009consensus.pdf. Accessed June 15, 2012

Loprinzi CL, Kugler JW, Sloan JA, et al. Lack of effect of coumarin in women with lymphedema after treatment for breast cancer. N Engl J Med. 1999; 340(5):346–350

Loprinzi CL, Sloan J, Kugler J. Coumarin-induced hepatotoxicity. J Clin Oncol. 1997; 15(9):3167–3168

Morrison L, Welsby PD. Side-effects of coumarin. Postgrad Med J. 1995; 71(841):701

NLN. Position Statement of the National Lymphedema Network. The diagnosis and treatment of lymphedema. http://www.lymphnet.org/pdfDocs/nlntreatment.pdf. Accessed June 15, 2012

Surgical Approaches in the Treatment of Lymphedema

Goldsmith HS, De los Santos R. Omental transposition in primary lymphedema. Surg Gynecol Obstet. 1967; 125(3):607–610

International Society of Lymphology. The diagnosis and treatment of peripheral lymphedema. 2009 Consensus Document of the International Society of Lymphology. http://www.u.arizona.edu/~witte/2009consensus.pdf. Accessed June 15, 2012

Miller TA. Surgical approach to lymphedema of the arm after mastectomy. Am J Surg. 1984; 148(1):152–156

NLN. Position Statement of the National Lymphedema Network. The diagnosis and treatment of lymphedema. http://www.lymph-net.org/pdfDocs/nlntreatment.pdf. Accessed June 15, 2012

O'Brien BM, Khazanchi RK, Kumar PA, Dvir E, Pederson WC. Liposuction in the treatment of lymphoedema; a preliminary report. Br J Plast Surg. 1989; 42(5):530–533

Olszewski W. Risk of surgical procedures in limbs with edema (lymphedema). LymphLink. 2003; 15(1):1–2

Chronic Venous Insufficiency

Brand FN, Dannenberg AL, Abbott RD, Kannel WB. The epidemiology of varicose veins: the Framingham Study. Am J Prev Med. 1988; 4(2):96–101

Eliska O, Eliskova M. Morphology of lymphatics in human venous crural ulcers with lipodermatosclerosis. Lymphology. 2001; 34(3):111–123

Földi M, Idiazabal G. The role of operative management of varicose veins in patients with lymphedema and/or lipedema of the legs. Lymphology. 2000; 33(4):167–171

Goldhaber SZ, Morrison RB. Cardiology patient pages. Pulmonary embolism and deep vein thrombosis. Circulation. 2002; 106(12):1436–1438

Griffin JH, Motulsky A, Hirsh J. Diagnosis and treatment of hypercoagulable states. Orlando: Education Program. American Society of Hematology; 1996:106–111

Harris JM, Abramson N. Evaluation of recurrent thrombosis and hypercoagulability. Am Fam Physician. 1997; 56(6):1591–1596, 1601–1602

Hobson J. Venous insufficiency at work. Angiology. 1997; 48(7):577–582

Johnson MT. Treatment and prevention of varicose veins. J Vasc Nurs. 1997; 15(3):97–103

Kim DI, Huh S, Hwang JH, Kim YI, Lee BB. Venous dynamics in leg lymphedema. Lymphology. 1999; 32(1):11–14

Silverstein MD, Heit JA, Mohr DN, Petterson TM, O'Fallon WM, Melton LJ, III. Trends in the incidence of deep vein thrombosis and pulmonary embolism: a 25-year population-based study. Arch Intern Med. 1998; 158(6):585–593

Vanhoutte PM, Corcaud S, de Montrion C. Venous disease: from pathophysiology to quality of life. Angiology. 1997; 48(7):559–567

Wounds and Skin Lesions

Andersson E, Hansson C, Swanbeck G. Leg and foot ulcer prevalence and investigation of the peripheral arterial and venous circulation in a randomised elderly population. An epidemiological survey and clinical investigation. Acta Derm Venereol. 1993; 73(1):57–61

Barton P, Parslow N. Malignant wounds: holistic assessment and management. In: Krasner DL, Rodeheaver GT, Sibbald RG, eds. Chronic Wound Care: A Clinical Source Book for Healthcare Professionals. 3rd ed. Wayne, PA: HMP Communications; 2001:699–710

Bowler PG, Jones SA, Davies BJ, Coyle E. Infection control properties of some wound dressings. J Wound Care. 1999; 8(10):499–502

Bozeman PK. Arterial ulcers. In: Milne CT, Corbett LQ, Dubuc DL, eds. Wound, Ostomy, and Continence Nursing Secrets. Philadelphia, PA: Hanley & Belfast; 2003:168–172

Callam MJ, Harper DR, Dale JJ, Ruckley CV. Arterial disease in chronic leg ulceration: an underestimated hazard? Lothian and Forth Valley leg ulcer study. Br Med J (Clin Res Ed). 1987; 294(6577):929–931

Capeheart JK. Chronic venous insufficiency: a focus on prevention of venous ulceration. J Wound Ostomy Continence Nurs. 1996; 23(4):227–234

Corbett LQ, Burns PE. Venous ulcers. In: Milne CT, Corbett LQ, Dubuc DL, eds. Wound, Ostomy, and Continence Nursing Secrets. Philadelphia, PA: Hanley & Belfast; 2003:163

Kunimoto BT. Management and prevention of venous leg ulcers: a literature-guided approach. Ostomy Wound Manage. 2001; 47(6):36–42, 44–49

Lazzari GB, Monteverdi AM, Adami O, Pezzarossa E. Collagenase for the treatment of torpid ulcerative lesions of the legs [in Italian]. G Ital Dermatol Venereol. 1990; 125(9):XXXVII–XLII

Myers BA. Wound Management: Principles and Practice. Upper Saddle River, NJ: Prentice Hall; 2004:201–228

Naylor W, Laverty D, Mallet J. Handbook of Wound Management in Cancer Care. London: Blackwell Sciences; 2001:73–122

Nelzén O, Bergqvist D, Lindhagen A. Venous and non-venous leg ulcers: clinical history and appearance in a population study. Br J Surg. 1994; 81(2):182–187

Orsted HL, Radke L, Gorst R. The impact of musculoskeletal changes on the dynamics of the calf muscle pump. Ostomy Wound Manage. 2001; 47(10):18–24

Patterson GK. Vascular evaluation. In: Sussman C, Bates-Jensen BM, eds. Wound Care: A Collaborative Practice Manual for Physical Therapists and Nurses. Gaithersburg, MD: Aspen Publications; 2001:177–193

Reichardt LE. Venous ulceration: compression as the mainstay of therapy. J Wound Ostomy Continence Nurs. 1999; 26(1):39–47

Sibbald RG, Williamson D, Orsted HL, et al. Preparing the wound bed–debridement, bacterial balance, and moisture balance. Ostomy Wound Manage. 2000; 46(11):14–22, 24–28, 30–35, quiz 36–37

Slachta PA, Burns PE. Inflammatory ulcerations. In: Milne CT, Corbett LQ, Dubuc DL, eds. Wound, Ostomy, and Continence Nursing Secrets. Philadelphia, PA: Hanley & Belfast; 2003:193–197

Young JR. Differential diagnosis of leg ulcers. Cardiovasc Clin. 1983; 13(2):171–193

Lipedema

Brorson H, Svensson H. Complete reduction of lymphoedema of the arm by liposuction after breast cancer. Scand J Plast Reconstr Surg Hand Surg. 1997; 31(2):137–143

Brorson H, Svensson H. Liposuction combined with controlled compression therapy reduces arm lymphedema more effectively than controlled compression therapy alone. Plast Reconstr Surg. 1998; 102(4):1058–1067, discussion 1068

Brorson H, Svensson H, Norrgren K, Thorsson O. Liposuction reduces arm lymphedema without significantly altering the already impaired lymph transport. Lymphology. 1998; 31(4):156–172

Földi M, Idiazabal G. The role of operative management of varicose veins in patients with lymphedema and/or lipedema of the legs. Lymphology. 2000; 33(4):167–171

Harwood CA, Bull RH, Evans J, Mortimer PS. Lymphatic and venous function in lipoedema. Br J Dermatol. 1996; 134(1):1–6

Klose G, Strössenreuther RHK. Understanding lipedema. LymphLink. 2007; 19(1):1–6

Lehnhardt M, Homann HH, Druecke D, Palka P, Steinau HU. Liposuktion—kein Problem? Majorkomplikationen und Todesfälle im deutschsprachigen Raum zwischen 1998 und 2002. LymphForsch. 2004; 8(2):74–78

Lerner R. Understanding lipedema. LymphLink. 1998; 10(2):1–3

Rudkin GH, Miller TA. Lipedema: a clinical entity distinct from lymphedema. Plast Reconstr Surg. 1994; 94(6):841–847, discussion 848–849

Stroessenreuther RHK. Die Behandlung des Lipoedems. In: Földi M, Kubik S, eds. Lehrbuch der Lymphologie für Mediziner, Masseure und Physiotherapeuten. 6th ed. Munich: Elsevier, Urban und Fischer; 2005

Szolnoky G, Borsos B, Bársony K, Balogh M, Kemény L. Complete decongestive physiotherapy with and without pneumatic compression for treatment of lipedema: a pilot study. Lymphology. 2008; 41(1):40–44

Zelikovski A, Haddad M, Koren A, Avrahami R, Loewinger J. Lipedema complicated by lymphedema of the abdominal wall and lower limbs. Lymphology. 2000; 33(2):43–46

Pediatrics

Browse N, Burnand K, Mortimer P. Diseases of the Lymphatics. London: Arnold; 2003:134–155, 158–166

Kinmonth J. The Lymphatics; Diseases, Lymphography and Surgery. London: Arnold; 1972:114–143, 280–298

Foeldi M, Foeldi E. Foeldi's Textbook of Lymphology for Physicians and Lymphedema Therapsits. 3rd ed. Munich: Elsevier; 2012:438–464

Olszewski W. Lymph Stasis: Pathophysiology, Diagnosis and Treatment. Boca Raton, FL: CRC Press; 1991:387–388

Weissleder H, Schuchhardt C. Lymphedema Diagnosis and Therapy. 4th ed. Essen: Viavital Verlag; 2008:118–129, 341–361

Traumatic Edema

Hutzschenreuther P, Bruemmer H. Die Manuelle Lymphdrainage bei der Wundheilung mit Ecollment—eine experimentelle Studie. Lymphologica Jahresband 1989:97–100

Wingerden BAM. Eistherapie Kontraindiziert bei Sportverletzungen? Leistungssport. 1992; 2:5–8

Rheumatoid Arthritis

Földi M, Földi E. Der rheumatische Formenkreis—allgemeine lymphologische Gesichtspunkte. In: Lehrbuch der Lymphologie. 3rd ed. Stuttgart: Gustav Fischer Verlag; 1993:374

Klippel J, Crofford L, Stone J, et al. Primer on Rheumatic Diseases. 10th ed. New York, NY: Springer; 1993

Schoberth H. Der entzuendliche Rheumatismus. In: Lehrbuch der Lymphologie. 3rd ed. Stuttgart: Gustav Fischer Verlag; 1993:375–378

Reflex Sympathetic Dystrophy

Cantwell-Gab K. Identifying chronic peripheral arterial disease. Am J Nurs. 1996; 96(7):40–46, quiz 47

Clodius L. Das Sudeck Syndrom: lymphologische und funktionelle Aspekte. In: Lehrbuch der Lymphologie. 4th ed. Stuttgart: Gustav Fischer Verlag; 1999:393–395

Kemler MA, Rijks CP, de Vet HC. Which patients with chronic reflex sympathetic dystrophy are most likely to benefit from physical therapy? J Manipulative Physiol Ther. 2001; 24(4):272–278

Mucha C. Ergebnisse einer prospektiven Beobachtungs-reihe zur funktionellen Therapie des Sudeck-Syndroms. Z Phys Therap. 1993; 14(5):329–333

Rockson SG, Cooke JP. Peripheral arterial insufficiency: mechanisms, natural history, and therapeutic options. Adv Intern Med. 1998; 43:253–277

3

Chapter 4

Complete Decongestive Therapy

4 Complete Decongestive Therapy

4.1 Introduction

Complete decongestive therapy (CDT) is a noninvasive, multicomponent approach to treat lymphedema and other conditions related to lymphedema. Numerous studies have proven the scientific basis and effectiveness of this therapy, which has been well established in European countries since the 1970s. CDT has been practiced in the United States in one form or another since the 1980s; it became accepted after definitive guidelines and all components of CDT were included in the teaching curricula of schools providing training in lymphedema management in the 1990s.

4.2 History and Background

The following serves as a selective overview to describe the history of the discovery of the lymphatic system and the development of CDT.

4.2.1 Discovery of the Lymphatic System

Compared with other developments in the history of medicine, the lymphatic system was discovered relatively late. *Hippocrates* (460–377 BC) described vessels containing "white blood," and *Aristotle* (384–322 BC) later spoke of vessels holding "a colorless fluid." Physicians of the Alexandrian school were also aware of the lymphatic system; they described the lymph vessels as ductus lactei (milk-like vessels). This knowledge was forgotten for almost 2,000 years, probably because the Catholic Church considered anatomical studies sinful. The lymphatic system was rediscovered during the European Renaissance.

Gaspare Aselli, also spelled Asellio (1581–1626), an Italian physician, discovered the lacteal vessels during a vivisection of a dog in 1622.

The cisterna chyli was first described by *Jean Pecquet* (1622–1674), a medical student from Dieppe, France, in 1651. He also described the presence of valves within the lymphatics and the communication of the thoracic duct with the left subclavian vein.

Olof Rudbeck (1630–1708) from Sweden, one of Uppsala University's most outstanding figures throughout the centuries, was credited with the first complete description of the lymphatic system in the human body.

Thomas Bartholin (1616–1680), a Danish physician, also claimed to have produced the first complete representation of the lymphatic system, which he published in a book in 1652 (or 1653). He was the first to call the lymph vessels vasa lymphatica and the fluid carried by these vessels lympha (from the Latin *limpidus*, meaning "clear" or "transparent"). Bartholin and Rudbeck had animated discussions about who really delivered the first complete description.

It was because of great improvements in the art of dissection and injection and the invention of new and better instruments that anatomists attained a vast knowledge of the human lymphatic system. *Anton Nuck* (1650–1692), a Dutch anatomist, first employed the technique of intralymphatic injection of mercury in 1692 to outline the lymphatic system. *Mascani* (1787), *Cruikshank* (1789), and *Gerota* (1896) devised modifications of this technique.

Marie P. C. Sappey (1810–1896), a French anatomist, used the injection technique to conduct comprehensive topographical studies of the human lymphatic system to demonstrate the beauty of the vessels; he published his work in 1885. Mercury, or quicksilver, was used as an injection medium on cadavers for filling the lymphatic vessels. The injecting instruments included the lymphatic injecting tube and pipe, which were made of either glass or brass. Sappey's work was continued by another French anatomist named *Henri Rouviere* (1875–1952). Rouviere published a book on the human lymphatic system *(L'anatomie des lymphatiques de l'homme)* in 1932.

Modern technologies (computed tomography, lymphographic imaging techniques, etc.) have made it possible to gain a detailed view and complete understanding of the lymphatic system. Research pioneers such as *M. Földi, A. Gregl, E. Kuhnke* (Germany), *S. Kubik* (Switzerland), and *J. Casley-Smith* (Australia), among others, contributed to the field of lymphology and established the groundwork for current research.

4.2.2 Development of Complete Decongestive Therapy

Many clinicians have used this newly found knowledge and have incorporated it into the treatment of various conditions. *Alexander von Winiwarter* (1848–1917), a surgeon from Austria, successfully treated swollen limbs with elevation, compression, and a special massage technique. After Winiwarter's death, his approach was not developed further.

Emil Vodder (1896–1986), a PhD from Denmark, lived and worked in France between 1928 and 1939. Vodder "intuitively" manipulated the swollen lymph nodes of some of his patients who suffered from chronic colds and sinus infections. He reported that his therapy was successful and that individuals treated with his techniques felt better. He continued to develop his treatment method and moved to Paris to do further research on the lymphatic system. Vodder called his technique "lymph drainage massage" and introduced it during an international health fair as *le drainage lymphatique*. During this time, the medical community did not accept Vodder's technique, and he continued primarily to train cosmetologists throughout Europe.

In 1963, *Johannes Asdonk* (1910–2003), a German physician, learned about Vodder's technique while working in Essen, Germany, and decided to meet personally with Vodder. Asdonk was impressed with the results Vodder achieved and decided to learn his hands-on technique. Asdonk established the first school for manual lymphatic drainage (MLD) in 1969 in Germany, with Emil Vodder and Vodder's wife, Astrid, as instructors.

With a more detailed knowledge about the anatomy and physiology of the lymphatic system and the expanding list of indications for this treatment, it was necessary to add new techniques and to modify Vodder's existing techniques. Vodder and Asdonk had differing opinions regarding the technical aspects of the MLD strokes and subsequently ended their partnership in 1971. Vodder moved to Austria to start his own school, and Asdonk remained in Germany, where he continued his extensive research on the effectiveness of MLD and its effects on the lymphatic system.

Based on Asdonk's work, MLD as a treatment for lymphedema became reimbursable by national health insurance in Germany in 1974. Together with Kuhnke, Földi, Gregl, and others, Asdonk founded the German Society of Lymphology in 1976. The cooperation between these scientists within the society led to the development of a new therapy concept, which enabled the successful treatment of edemas of different geneses with the addition of various and new intervention techniques. The combination of these techniques is known today as CDT. Földi founded his own school for lymphology and phlebology in Freiburg, Germany, in 1981.

Kuhnke's work in the development of limb volume measurement techniques provided evidence of the effectiveness of CDT and helped further establish this therapy in the treatment of lymphedema and other related conditions. Accurate measurement of limb volumes also provided the objective data to prove that the combination of various treatment approaches known as CDT in the treatment of lymphedema is far more effective than the treatment of lymphedema with MLD as the sole therapeutic approach.

Most schools providing lymphedema training throughout the world today teach all components of CDT, which includes the advanced version of Vodder's MLD.

4.3 Goal of Complete Decongestive Therapy

Currently, there is no cure for lymphedema; the main goal of the treatment, therefore, is to return the lymphedema to a stage of latency (see Chapter 3, Stages of Lymphedema), utilizing remaining lymph vessels and other lymphatic pathways. The normal or near normal size of the limb should be maintained, and re-accumulation of lymph fluid should be prevented. Additional goals are prevention and elimination of infections and the reduction and removal of fibrotic tissues.

4.4 Components of Complete Decongestive Therapy

CDT consists of a combination of MLD, compression therapy, decongestive exercises, and skin care. Each component will be discussed individually.

4.4.1 Manual Lymph Drainage

MLD is a gentle manual treatment technique that is based on the four basic Vodder strokes: the "stationary circle," "pump," "rotary," and "scoop." The common denominator in all strokes is the working phase and the resting phase.

In the working phase of a stroke, stretch stimuli are applied to the subcutaneous tissues, resulting in the manipulation of anchoring filaments of lymph capillaries and the smooth musculature in the wall of lymphangions. The light directional pressure in the working phase also serves to move lymph fluid in the appropriate direction. The pressure in this phase should be sufficient to stretch the subcutaneous tissue against the underlying

4

fascia to its elastic capacity. It is not necessary to apply high pressure to achieve this goal. In fact, too much pressure could damage anchoring filaments or other lymphatic structures, or cause lymphangiospasm in lymph collectors. The pressure should also be light enough to avoid vasodilation (active hyperemia). The amount of pressure is sometimes described as the pressure applied while stroking a newborn's head. However, more pressure is needed if fibrotic tissue is present.

The pressure is released during the resting phase, in which the elasticity of the skin moves the therapist's hand passively back to the starting position. In this pressure-free phase, initial lymph vessels absorb tissue fluid from the interstitial spaces.

To achieve maximum results, each working phase should last approximately 1 second and should be repeated five to seven times in the same area in either a stationary or a dynamic pattern.

Massage should not be confused with the techniques of MLD.

The word *massage*, meaning "to knead" (from the Greek *masso/massain*) is used to describe such techniques as effleurage, petrissage, vibration, etc. Massage techniques traditionally are applied to treat ailments in muscle tissues, tendons, and ligaments, and to achieve the desired effect, these techniques are generally applied with considerable pressure.

MLD on the other hand consists of very gentle manual techniques, designed to have an effect on fluid components and lymphatic structures located in superficial tissues, such as the skin and the subcutis. Lymphedema almost exclusively manifests itself in the subcutis, which is a layer of connective tissue between the skin and muscle tissues.

The only commonality between MLD and massage is that both techniques are applied manually. There are significant differences in technique, pressure, and indications for which these two therapeutic measures are used, and it is important to point out the differences between these two techniques because massage should never be used to treat lymphedema. Therefore, the term *massage* should never be used to describe MLD.

One of the main effects of massage is an increase of blood flow in those areas where these techniques are applied. Even if the goal is to have an effect on muscle tissue, massage is always applied to the skin. An increased blood flow in the skin results in more water leaving the blood capillaries into the subcutaneous tissues. This increased

amount of water, for the most part, has to be removed by the lymphatic system, which in the case of lymphedema is not working properly. In case of lymphedema, this not only overloads an already stressed or impaired lymphatic system, but could also seriously worsen the swelling associated with lymphedema.

There are several reasonable explanations why MLD and massage are often confused with each other. One is that there is a tendency to call any hands-on manual therapeutic technique a form of massage; the other is that massage can be very helpful if applied to treat edema. Lymphedema and edema are two very different conditions and it is important to understand these differences. Although both conditions involve swelling, edema and lymphedema have very different causes and are treated differently (see Chapter 2, Edema and Lymphedema at a Glance).

Effects of Manual Lymph Drainage

The most common effects of MLD are the following:

- *Increase in lymph production*: stretching the anchoring filaments of lymph capillaries stimulates the intake of lymphatic loads into the lymphatic system.
- *Increase in lymphangiomotoricity*: (1) mild perpendicular stimuli of the smooth musculature located in the wall of lymph collectors result in an increased contraction frequency of lymphangions and (2) increased lymph production results in an increase of the volume of transported lymph fluid. The subsequently elevated intralymphatic pressure results in increased contraction frequency of lymphangions.
- *Reverse of lymph flow*: in the treatment of lymphedema, MLD moves lymph fluid in superficial lymph vessels against its natural flow patterns. Lymph fluid is rerouted via collateral lymph collectors, anastomoses, or tissue channels.
- *Increase in venous return*: the directional pressure in the working phase of MLD strokes increases the venous return in the superficial venous system. Deeper and more specialized techniques of MLD, especially in the abdominal area, affect the venous return in the deep venous system.
- *Soothing*: the light pressures used in MLD decrease the sympathetic mode and promote the parasympathetic response.
- *Analgesic*: because of accelerated drainage of nociceptive substances from the tissues, the light

pressure used in MLD provides a stimulus for the "gate-control theory" of Melzack and Wall (1996), promoting pain control.

> The goal of MLD in the treatment of lymphedema and related conditions is to reroute the lymph flow around blocked areas into more centrally located healthy lymph vessels, which drain into the venous system.

The techniques of MLD include the manipulation of healthy lymph nodes and lymph vessels, which generally are located adjacent to the area with insufficient lymphatic drainage. The resulting increase in lymphangiomotoricity in the healthy areas creates a "suction effect," which enables accumulated lymph fluid to move from an area with insufficient lymph flow into an area with normal lymphatic drainage. To stimulate the return of lymph fluid into the venous system, the lymph nodes on the neck are manipulated. Depending on the location of the damage to the lymphatic system, the thorax, abdominal area, and ipsilateral and contralateral axillary or inguinal lymph node groups may be included in the treatment. The extremity itself is treated in segments (e.g., the proximal aspect of the affected extremity is decongested prior to expanding the treatment to the more distal aspects).

Basic Strokes

Stationary Circles

This technique consists of an oval-shaped stretching of the skin with the palmar surfaces of the fingers or the entire hand; it may be applied with one hand or bimanually (alternating or simultaneously). Stationary circles are used on the entire body surface, but mainly on the lymph node groups, the neck, and the face.

Working phase: The pressure increases and decreases gradually in the direction of lymph drainage for about half of a circle, using either radial or ulnar deviation in the wrist. In the first portion of the working phase, the stretch is applied perpendicular to the lymph collectors; in the second portion, it is applied parallel to the lymph collectors. The full elasticity of the skin should be used to apply the stretch.

Resting phase: The working hand relaxes and maintains contact with the patient's skin. The pressure is completely released, and the elasticity of the skin moves the therapist's hand passively back to the starting position (▶ Fig. 4.1a).

"Thumb" circles represent a variation of stationary circles. This technique is applied with the palmar surface of the thumb and is used primarily on the hand and foot, in the area of joints, and in the treatment of infants (▶ Fig. 4.1b).

Pump

This stroke applies a circle-shaped pressure operating within almost the full range between ulnar and radial deviation. The entire palm and the proximal phalanges are used in this technique, which is applied primarily on the extremities. Pumps are dynamic strokes (i.e., the working hand moves from distal to proximal), and they can be applied with one hand or bimanually (alternating).

Working phase: The hand is placed on the skin with ulnar deviation and wrist flexion, the fingers are extended, and the thumb is in opposition to the fingers. In this starting position, the radial aspect of the thumb and index finger, as well as the web space between these two phalanges, is in contact with the skin. The pressure increases and

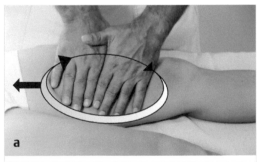

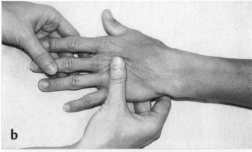

Fig. 4.1 (a) Stationary circles working phase (white half circle) and resting phase of stationary circles. (b) Thumb circles on the dorsum of the hand.

decreases gradually during the transition to radial deviation and wrist extension and reaches its maximum stretch when the entire palm has made contact. Pressure is applied in the drainage direction (▶ Fig. 4.2).

Resting phase: When the skin is stretched to its maximum elasticity and the hand is in radial deviation, the transition to the resting phase begins, in which the elasticity of the skin carries the therapist's hand back to the starting position. To reach the starting point of the next working phase, the hand glides without pressure approximately half a hand width in the proximal direction.

Scoop

Scoops are applied on extremities (mainly the distal parts) and consist of a spiral-shaped movement. A transitional movement from ulnar deviation with forearm pronation, moving into radial deviation with forearm supination, is used in the application of this technique. This dynamic stroke is applied with one hand or bimanually (alternating).

Working phase: The hand is placed in ulnar deviation and pronation onto the skin (perpendicular to the pathway of lymph collectors). The web

space between the index finger and the thumb is in contact with the body surface at this point. The working phase starts with the hand gliding over the skin in a spiral-like movement in the proximal direction. During the gliding phase, the pressure increases gradually, and the palm and the palmar surfaces of the fingers come in contact with the skin. The pressure reaches its maximum value when the palm is in complete contact with the body surface. With the palm in contact, the fingers glide over the skin in a fanlike pattern until they are aligned parallel with the extremity. During this phase, the pressure gradually decreases again (▶ Fig. 4.3).

Resting phase: After the hand and fingers are parallel with the extremity, the hand does not return to the starting position. It returns to ulnar deviation and pronation, approximately one hand width further proximal, where the next working phase starts.

Rotary

This dynamic technique is used on large surface areas—primarily on the trunk, but also on lymphedematous extremities—and can be applied with one hand or bimanually (at the same time or alternating).

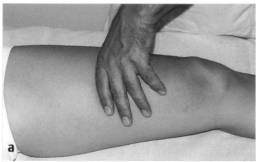
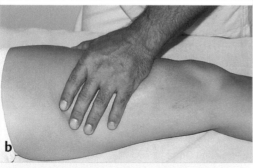

Fig. 4.2 (a) Pump stroke at the beginning of the working phase. (b) Pump stroke at the end of the working phase.

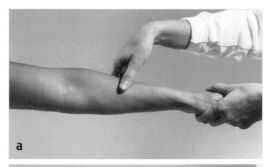
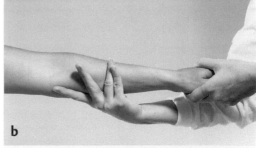

Fig. 4.3 (a) Scoop at the beginning of the working phase. (b) Scoop during the working phase.

Working phase: The hand is placed on the body surface in an elevated position and parallel to the pathway of the lymph collectors. The wrist is in flexion, the finger joints (except the thumb) are in a neutral position, and the thumb is approximately 90 degrees abducted. All fingertips are in contact with the skin. The working phase is initiated as the palm is placed on the skin in an elliptical movement (over the ulnar side). At the same time, the thumb slides to abduction. In this phase, the subcutaneous tissues are stretched against the fascia and perpendicular to the flow of lymph. When contact is established with the full hand and palmar surface, the skin is stretched toward the drainage area with gradually increasing pressure. While the hand stretches, the thumb is adducted until aligned with the hand. The pressure decreases again, the elasticity of the skin moves the hand back to the starting position, and the hand relaxes (▷ Fig. 4.4).

Resting phase: The hand moves back into wrist flexion until it is elevated again. The fingers slide at the same time without pressure (but in skin contact) in the drainage direction, until the thumb reaches approximately 90 degrees of abduction. The sequence continues in this position with the next working phase.

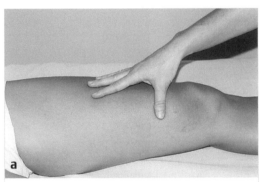
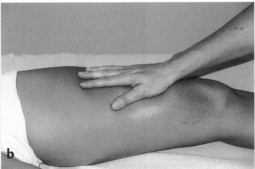

Fig. 4.4 (a) Rotary at the beginning of the working phase. **(b)** Rotary at the end of the working phase.

During the working and the resting phase, the fingers remain in the neutral position.

Additional Techniques

Deep Abdominal Technique

This technique primarily stimulates deep lymphatic structures, such as the cisterna chyli, the abdominal part of the thoracic duct, lumbar trunks and lymph nodes, pelvic lymph nodes, and certain organ systems. Manipulation of these lymphatic structures, particularly the thoracic duct, accelerates lymph transport toward the venous angles. This results in improved lymphatic drainage from structures distal to the thoracic duct, including the lower extremities. The manipulation of deep veins located in the same area also improves the venous return to the heart.

The considerable decongestive effects on the lymphatic and the venous systems make deep abdominal techniques a valuable tool in the treatment of lower extremity swelling.

To reach the deeper structures of the lymphatic system, it is necessary to apply more pressure than with the basic MLD techniques. Therefore, the following cautionary measures must be observed:

- The deep abdominal technique must never cause pain or discomfort.
- Contraindications listed later in this chapter must be observed.
- To reduce the tone and resistance of the abdominal musculature, the head and legs should be elevated during the application.
- To avoid hyperventilation and dizziness, these techniques are not repeated five to seven times, as in basic MLD applications. Instead, the sequence of hand placements is applied only once.

The deep abdominal technique is applied on five different locations (for a total of nine strokes) and combined with diaphragmatic breathing. The different hand placements are discussed in Chapter 5, Abdomen (Superficial and Deep Manipulations). The therapist coordinates the technique with the patient's breathing rhythm. The flat and soft hand follows the patient's exhalation into the abdominal cavity, where it remains until the next inhalation (at this point, it is important to note the patient's response to the pressure). A brief period of moderate resistance is applied during the initial inhalation phase. The resistance is released to allow full inhalation. During this phase, the therapist's hand moves to the next location. The full and soft hand then follows the next exhalation phase; this procedure is repeated for all nine strokes.

Edema Technique

The goal of this specialized technique is to mobilize the free protein-rich and sluggish edema fluid in the extremities toward the drainage area. Edema strokes should be applied only after the drainage area proximal to the application has been previously cleared with basic MLD strokes, the ipsilateral trunk quadrant is free of edema, and the extremity has at least begun to decongest.

Edema techniques are administered with increased pressure and prolonged duration (5–8 seconds) in the working phase, and the hands move dynamically from distal to proximal to cover a certain portion of a limb. Edema techniques are immediately followed by reworking techniques (explained in Chapter 5) and the application of compression bandages.

Two different variations of the edema technique may be used. The less intensive technique consists of bimanual pump techniques, which are applied simultaneously on opposing sides of the extremity. This technique can be used on the entire limb (▶ Fig. 4.5).

The deeper and more effective variation is administered circumferentially with the radial surface of both hands. The hands move simultaneously into the subcutaneous tissue and proceed to move the lymph fluid toward proximal. This technique is applied on the lower leg and foot and the hand and forearm (▶ Fig. 4.6).

This more intense technique cannot be used with the following conditions: painful lipedema or lipolymphedema, pain is present in swellings of other genesis, patients with hemophilia, patients on anticoagulants, and patients with varicose veins or deep venous thrombosis. Other contraindications listed later in this chapter must be observed.

Fibrosis Technique

This modality is used to soften and break up lymphostatic fibrosis and should be used only if the extremity has begun to decongest. Fibrosis techniques are applied directly in the area of lymphostatic fibrosis with more intensity and prolonged duration than the basic techniques of MLD; these techniques may cause local vasodilation. To optimize the fibrinolytic effect, compression bandages (preferably in combination with special foam applications) should be applied directly following fibrosis techniques.

Two different variations of the fibrosis technique may be used. With the "kneading" technique, the fibrotic tissue is lifted softly from the underlying tissue with the flat finger pads. The skinfold is then softly and slowly moved using an S-shaped manipulation between the thumb of one hand and the fingers of the other hand. This treatment can be compared with kneading strokes used in massage techniques (▶ Fig. 4.7).

In the other, more intense technique, the fibrotic tissue fold is lifted softly with the flat fingers of one hand. The flat thumb of the other hand manipulates the skinfold by pressing down on it (▶ Fig. 4.8).

Fibrosis techniques are contraindicated in the area of radiation fibrosis. Other contraindications include the same as discussed for the edema technique.

Vasa Vasorum Technique

This technique uses and optimizes the drainage pathways of the plexuslike lymph vessels in the

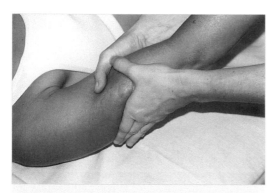

Fig. 4.5 Edema technique (superficial) on the upper arm.

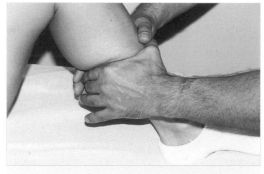

Fig. 4.6 Edema technique (deep) on the lower leg.

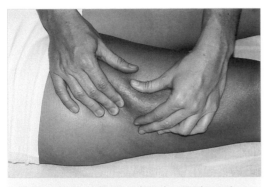
Fig. 4.7 Fibrosis technique ("kneading" technique) on the thigh.

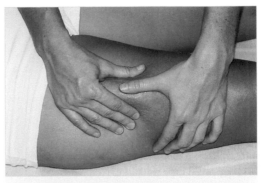
Fig. 4.8 Fibrosis technique ("thumb" technique) on the thigh.

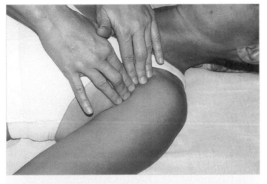
Fig. 4.9 Vasa vasorum technique (cephalic vein).

adventitia of larger blood vessels (veins). These structures serve as additional drainage pathways in the treatment of lymphedema (▶ Fig. 4.9).

Contraindications for Manual Lymph Drainage

General contraindications for MLD include the following:

- *Cardiac edema*: there is no therapeutic benefit of MLD/CDT in the treatment of swellings caused by decompensated cardiac insufficiency. If cardiac edema is combined with lymphedema, MLD may be indicated, but cardiac and pulmonary functions need to be closely monitored by the referring physician.
- Renal failure.
- *Acute infections*: the application of MLD may exacerbate the symptoms.
- *Acute bronchitis*: the parasympathetic effect of MLD may exacerbate the symptoms in the acute phase by producing contractions of the smooth bronchial musculature.

- *Acute deep vein thrombosis*: MLD/CDT is contra-indicated on the affected extremity and the abdominal area.
- *Malignancies*: close cooperation with the referring physician is necessary. MLD/CDT may be indicated as palliative treatment. To date, there is no scientific evidence that the application of MLD (or other manual treatment techniques) would accelerate the spread of malignant cells to other parts of the body or contribute to the growth of malignant tumors.
- *Bronchial asthma*: because of the parasympathetic stimulation, MLD may cause the onset of an asthma attack. In lymphedema patients with a combined diagnosis of bronchial asthma, MLD generally can be applied safely if the treatment time is incrementally increased, starting at approximately 20 minutes of initial treatment time. If no negative reactions are noted during or after the therapy, the treatment time may be increased by 5 to 10 minutes until reaching normal treatment time values.
- *Hypertension*: MLD/CDT may be applied if cardiac functions are monitored.

Local contraindications on the neck include the following:

- *Carotid-sinus syndrome*: hypersensitivity of pressure receptors on the carotid bifurcation may cause cardiac arrhythmia.
- *Hyperthyroidism*: manipulation on the neck may accelerate the release of thyroid hormones and/or medications into the blood.
- *Age*: with patients older than 60 years of age, there may be an increased risk of atherosclerosis in the neck arteries.

Local contraindications for the abdominal area include the following:
- Pregnancy.
- Dysmenorrhea.
- Ileus.
- Diverticulosis.
- Aortic aneurysm (also palpation of strong aortic pulse).
- Recent abdominal surgery.
- Deep vein thrombosis.
- *Inflammatory conditions of the small and large intestines*: Crohn's disease, ulcerative colitis, and diverticulitis.
- Radiation fibrosis, radiation cystitis, and radiation colitis.
- Unexplained pain.

4.5 Compression Therapy

The elastic fibers of the cutaneous tissues are damaged in lymphedema. This is true for lymphedema in its pure appearance (primary and secondary), as well as in lymphedema combined with other pathologies. Although lymphedema may be reduced to a normal or near normal size utilizing proper treatment techniques, the lymphatics are never normal again after lymphedema has been present and the skin elasticity may never be regained completely. The affected body part is always at risk for a re-accumulation of fluid. External support of the affected extremity/body part is therefore an essential component of lymphedema management. The primary goal in compression therapy is to maintain the decongestive effect achieved during the MLD session, that is, to prevent re-accumulation of fluid into the tissues. Without the benefits provided by compression therapy, successful treatment of lymphedema would be impossible.

Based on the phase of the treatment (see 4.8 later in this chapter), compression therapy is applied by specific bandage materials, so-called short-stretch bandages, or by compression garments, or a combination of both modalities.

4.5.1 Effects of Compression Therapy

The following effects are achieved with compression bandages and garments:
- *Increases the pressure in the tissues themselves, as well as on the blood and lymph vessels contained in these tissues*. The tissue pressure plays an essential role in the exchange of fluids between the blood capillaries and the tissues. The beneficial effects of increased tissue pressure are especially important during airplane travel (see Chapter 5, Traveling with Lymphedema).
- *Improves venous and lymphatic return*. External compression forces these fluids in the proximal direction; it also improves the function of the valves contained in these vessels.
- *Reduces net filtration (blood capillary pressure [BCP]—interstitial fluid pressure [IP])*. To determine the fluid value leaving the blood capillary, it is necessary to subtract the inward forces (IP) from the outward forces (BCP) on the capillary (see Chapter 2, Filtration and Reabsorption).
- *Improves the effectiveness of the muscle and joint pumps during activity*. The activity of skeletal musculature is an important factor in the return of fluids within the venous and lymphatic system. Together with other supporting mechanisms, the muscle and joint pump activity propels these fluids back to the heart and ensures an uninterrupted circulation. External compression provides a sufficient counterforce to the working musculature, thus improving its efficiency.
- *Prevents the re-accumulation of evacuated lymph fluid and conserves the results achieved during MLD*. Compression therapy compensates for the elastic insufficiency of the affected tissue.
- *Helps break up and soften deposits of connective tissue and scar tissue*. This effect is especially beneficial in the treatment of lymphostatic fibrosis and can be increased by the use of special foam materials in combination with compression therapy.
- *Provides support for those tissues that have lost elasticity*.
- *Depending on the materials used (compression garments, short-stretch bandages), it provides for a high working pressure and a low resting pressure (see Section 4.5.3 Compression Bandages later in this chapter)*.

4.5.2 Laplace's Law

The value of pressure achieved on a body part by use of external compression is generally measured in millimeters of mercury (mmHg). To achieve the desired effects in compression therapy, it is imperative that the pressure value decreases gradually from distal to proximal. Bandages and compression garments achieve this effect if they are applied correctly. Complications are common if the measurements or compression classes of

4

compression garments are faulty or if short-stretch bandages are applied incorrectly.

> Laplace's law can be used to explain the importance of graded compression using elastic materials. This law states that if the radius (r) of a cylinder (extremity) is increased, the tension (T) needs to be increased to achieve the same pressure (P). This means that if compression is applied on a cylinder using equal tension, the pressure is greatest where the radius (of the cylinder) is the smallest.

A normal extremity can be compared with a cylinder. If compression therapy is applied on a leg, using the same tension (T) between the distal and the proximal end of the extremity, the pressure (P) in the ankle area (smaller radius) would be greater than the pressure on the calf (greater radius), and the pressure on the thigh would be lower than the pressure on the calf.

This law can be applied in a true cylindrical or cone-shaped extremity. In the area of bony prominences (ankles, wrists, or the medial and lateral circumferences of the hand and foot), the pressure is higher due to the smaller radius and the greater tension of the compressive medium, whereas the pressure is lower in concave areas (behind the ankles).

These issues and the fact that swollen extremities generally lose their cone shape make it necessary to use foam materials for padding in combination with compression bandages to "construct" a cylinder.

Padding is usually not necessary in compression garments. Because of the manufacturing process of these materials, a compression gradient is built into the garments.

4.5.3 Compression Bandages

Short-stretch compression bandages are primarily used in the decongestive phase of CDT. These bandages are textile-elastic; the braided cotton fibers used in the production process are woven to achieve a certain degree of elasticity. In newly manufactured short-stretch bandages, this interwoven pattern allows for approximately 60% extensibility of the bandage's original length. To understand the effects of various bandage materials on the tissues and the vascular systems

embedded within the tissues, it is important to discuss the difference between short- and long-stretch bandages.

Two different qualities of pressure can be distinguished in compression therapy: the working pressure and the resting pressure. Relevant in the determination of these pressure qualities are the type of bandage (long stretch or short stretch), the tension used during the application of the bandage, the number of layers, and the condition of the material (age). Bandages lose some of their elasticity over time and with repetitive use and cleaning.

Working pressure: The resistance the bandage sets against the working musculature determines the working pressure. This pressure is temporary, that is, it is active only during muscle expansion, and its value depends on the extent of muscle contraction. The active working pressure results in an increase of tissue pressure (TP), and the venous and lymphatic vessels in the superficial and in the deep systems are compressed. The return of fluids within these vessel systems is improved.

The lower the elasticity of a compression bandage, the higher the working pressure. Short-stretch bandages (up to 60% elasticity) exert a high working pressure on the tissues and form a strong support during muscle contraction.

Long-stretch bandages (commonly known as "ACE" bandages) contain polyurethane and retain a low working pressure. Newly manufactured long-stretch bandages allow for an extensibility of more than 140% of the bandage's original length. This relatively high elasticity exerts a low resistance against the working musculature, and the decongestive effect on the venous and lymphatic system is minimal, especially in the deep systems.

Resting pressure: This is the pressure the bandage exerts on the tissues at rest, that is, without muscle contraction. The resting pressure is a permanent pressure, and its value depends on the amount of tension used during the application of the bandage. The higher the tension (or stretch), the higher the pressure the bandage exerts on the tissues. A bandage with a high extensibility will therefore result in increased pressure on the tissues during rest.

Long-stretch bandages exert a relatively high resting pressure, during which the venous and lymphatic vessels primarily in the skin (above the fascia) are compressed. This permanent compression may cause a tourniquet effect on the bandaged extremity.

Short-stretch bandages employ a very low resting pressure on the tissues and the vascular systems. The risk of a tourniquet effect is therefore relatively low as long as a specially trained individual applies the compression bandages correctly.

The high working and low resting pressure qualities of short-stretch bandages make them the preferred compression bandage in the management of lymphedema and swellings of other geneses.

Long-stretch bandages may constrict veins and lymph vessels at rest and provide minimal support of the tissues during muscle contraction. Long-stretch bandages are therefore not suitable for the treatment of lymphedema.

To avoid constriction of venous and lymphatic vessels and to achieve a compression gradient in the treatment of lymphedema, it is necessary to apply compression bandages in layers. Following the application of a suitable moisturizer on the skin (see 4.7 later in this chapter), a cotton stockinette is applied to absorb sweat and to protect the skin from the padding materials. As discussed earlier, the goal in the use of padding is to protect bony prominences and to bring the extremity into a cylindrical shape. Special soft foam materials or synthetic cotton bandages are used for this purpose. For the padding of concave areas (behind the malleoli, palm) or to increase the pressure over lymphostatic fibrosis or wounds, a more dense foam material is suitable. Short-stretch bandages of various widths are then applied in layers on the extremity. Tape should be used to affix the bandage material, not clips or pins. Sharp bandaging clips or pins may cut into the patient's skin and provide an avenue for infection.

> Only trained therapists or patients and their caregivers who have received instruction in the application of short-stretch bandages from a trained individual should apply compression bandages in the treatment of lymphedema.

Correctly applied compression bandages are safe and effective and represent an indispensable part of CDT. Bandage materials are used primarily during the decongestive phase of CDT and can be bulky. Most patients adjust to and tolerate the compression bandage well after a few applications. Patients should maintain their normal activity level and perform the decongestive exercise program (see "Decongestive Exercises" later in this chapter) while wearing the bandages.

Refer to Chapter 5 for detailed illustrations and guidelines for the application of short-stretch bandages (materials used in compression therapy are listed under "Required Materials").

4.5.4 Compression Garments

Patients with lymphedema graduate from bandages to elastic compression garments once the limb is decongested (phase 2 of CDT). To preserve the treatment success achieved during the decongestion of the edematous limb, compression garments have to be worn throughout the patient's life. Because compression garments will not, by themselves, reduce swelling, they must not be worn on an untreated, swollen extremity.

To ensure the long-term benefits of compression garments described earlier in this chapter, it is important that only trained individuals with a full understanding of the pathology of lymphedema and its related conditions take the appropriate measurements and make an educated choice regarding the garment selection. Compression garments become a part of the patient's life, much like hearing aids or eyeglasses. Ill-fitted and ineffective compression garments not only produce poor results, but also can be dangerous to the patient. Many potential problems and special needs of the individual patient must be addressed and solved to arrive at a comfortable yet supportive garment solution.

Compression garments are available as compression gauntlets, sleeves, and stockings, and are made for specific body parts (e.g., brassieres or vests). They are manufactured in several sizes, variations (circular knit, flat knit), styles, compression levels (or classes), and materials, and they may be ordered in standard sizes or be custom-made.

Compression Levels

Currently an international consensus for compression values in different compression levels for seamless garments is unavailable. The compression levels establish the compression value the garments produce on the skin surface, and are measured in millimeters of mercury (mmHg). To ensure the benefits of compression, a gradient from distal to proximal is necessary. The pressure values within the different levels of compression are measured on the distal circumference of the extremity (on the leg at the ankles), where the pressure is highest.

For seamless (circular-knit) garments, the following values represent the compression ranges most manufacturers in the United States adhere to (► Fig. 4.10):
• Compression level I: 20 to 30 mmHg.
• Compression level II: 30 to 40 mmHg.
• Compression level III: 40 to 50 mmHg.

Compression levels for seamed (flat-knit) garments lean more toward international standards:
• Compression level I: 18 to 21 mmHg.
• Compression level II: 23 to 32 mmHg.
• Compression level III: 34 to 46 mmHg.
• Compression level IV: greater than 50 mmHg.

Values below 20 mmHg are not suitable in the management of lymphedema. These pressures are used in the support-stocking categories, which cover a lower level of compression (~ 8–15 mmHg) or a higher level of compression (~ 15–20 mmHg).

In some cases of lower extremity lymphedema, a compression of more than that available in compression level IV may be used. In these cases, a compression level III knee-high stocking may be worn in addition to a compression level III thigh-high stocking (or pantyhose). It is important to understand that the individual compression values of garments worn on top of each other do not double the values. Two level III stockings, for example, do not add up to a level VI; the resulting pressure would be somewhere between a level IV and a level V.

Physical limitations of the patient could be a rationale for a decision to combine two stockings. For example, an arthritic patient who requires a lower extremity garment of a higher compression level may have less difficulty donning a compression level III thigh-high with a compression level II knee-high stocking.

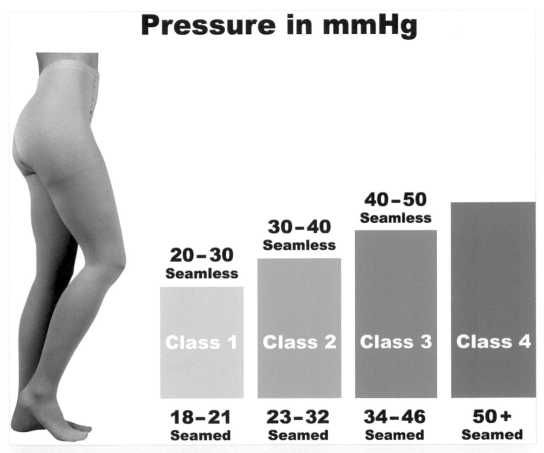

Fig. 4.10 Compression levels. (Reproduced with permission of Juzo USA, Inc.)

The average upper extremity lymphedema patient will use a compression level II arm sleeve, provided there are no contraindications that would require the use of a lower class compression, such as in the case of a partial, completely paralyzed, or flaccid limb. A patient with upper extremity lymphedema may require a compression level III arm sleeve if he or she is involved in a high-intensity and repetitive activity. For example, if a patient wishes to return to playing golf, a level III arm sleeve can be used on the involved extremity during play and a level II arm sleeve for daily activities.

Patients with lower extremity involvement will usually require a compression level III garment. Again, contraindications may be present that may require the use of a lower level of compression, and certain situations may require a higher level of compression.

Many factors must be considered, such as age, activity level, skin integrity, congestive heart failure, partial or complete paralysis, diabetes, and wound care issues, to determine the correct compression level for a patient.

If the patient has tolerated compression well during the decongestive phase, he or she may easily fit into the standard compression levels for the upper and lower extremities. It is important to consider the physical ability of the patient, as well as the patient's home support system, when choosing a compression garment. A 70-year-old patient with lower extremity lymphedema may not be physically able to don a level III garment; thus, a level II garment may better serve the patient's needs.

Circular-Knit (Seamless) and Flat-Knit (Seamed) Garments

Compression garments are manufactured using either a flat-knit (▶ Fig. 4.11) or circular-knit method. Both types are knitted using threads made of some form of rubber (some manufacturers use nonsynthetic rubber). Either cotton or a synthetic material generally covers this elastomer, providing the garment with additional qualities. Covered compression threads are more durable in that they limit or regulate stretch of the elastic fiber and protect it from sweat and skin ointments (▶ Fig. 4.12). The softer cover fibers make the

garments more breathable and easier to apply. The manufacturing process provides compression garments with a two-way elasticity (▶ Fig. 4.13). The more two-way stretch a compression garment provides, the more comfortable it is to wear.

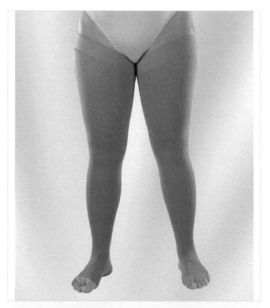

Fig. 4.11 Flat-knit thigh-high compression garment. (Reproduced with permission of Juzo USA, Inc.)

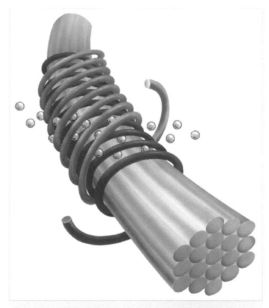

Fig. 4.12 Covered compression threads used in compression garments (Juzo USA Fibersoft). (Reproduced with permission of Juzo USA, Inc.)

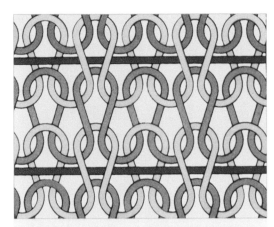
Fig. 4.13 Two-way elasticity in compression garments. (Reproduced with permission of Juzo USA, Inc.)

Circular-knit garments are manufactured on a cylindrical knitting machine, which allows them to be seamless. The same number of needles or meshes is used throughout the length of the garment. The size of the meshes, as well as the degree of prestretch of the inlay elastomer, provides for a smaller circumference on the distal and a larger circumference on the proximal portion of the garment.

In flat-knit garments, the number of needles or meshes varies according to the patient's measurements, which provide these garments with the same density throughout their length. Flat-knit garments can be custom manufactured in any shape or size and are available in various ready-made sizes. Compression levels of more than 50 mmHg are provided only in flat-knit materials; however, flat-knit garments are also available in lower compression levels.

The choice between flat or circular-knit compression garments involves various considerations. Circular-knit materials are less expensive and cosmetically more attractive than flat-knit garments, because they have no seam and are produced using finer and sheerer materials. Because of the manufacturing process of flat-knit garments, these items are usually denser and more costly to produce. However, they produce a more perfect fit because the number of meshes is determined by the patient's circumferential measurements, provided that the measurements are taken correctly. This could be a determining factor for those patients with grossly deformed extremities.

Esthetic considerations are an important aspect in choosing the right compression garment. It is important to understand that compression garments are effective only if they are worn consistently. If the patient is unhappy with the garment and does not want to wear it, the therapeutic benefit is lost. Compression level IV can be provided by a single flat-knit garment, which would be able to provide a constant compression gradient throughout the extremity, or by wearing a compression level III thigh-high (or pantyhose) circular-knit material in combination with a compression level II knee-high (or thigh-high) garment of the same material. Flat-knit stockings can be disguised by wearing a sheer (preferably dark) nylon stocking on top of them.

Custom-Made and Standard Compression Garments

Compression garments with a compression level of more than 50 mmHg are available only in custom-made materials. The high degree of compression requires the garment to be manufactured to the patient's exact circumferential measurements. As discussed earlier, custom-made garments are also a better choice for those individuals with extremely deformed extremities. Some manufacturers provide custom garments with zippers, which could be a choice for patients who may be physically unable to don a closed compression garment.

Standard or ready-made garments are available in compression levels I–III. Ready-made garments can be obtained from most manufacturers and in a large number of premade sizes and styles that can accommodate the vast majority of extremities.

Custom-made garments are very costly, and the production time for these garments is longer. Although some lymphedema patients benefit from custom-made garments, they are certainly not necessary for all lymphedema patients. The availability of a large variety of standard garments helps reduce the cost and allows patients to wear cosmetically more attractive compression garments.

Styles of Compression Garments

Custom-made and standard compression garments are available in different styles and lengths and can be ordered with a variety of fastening systems and integrated pressure pads. Refer to ▶ Fig. 4.14, ▶ Fig. 4.15, ▶ Fig. 4.16 for a summary of available styles and lengths.

Fastening systems are designed to prevent the garments from sliding, which could create a tourniquet effect and thus make the compression

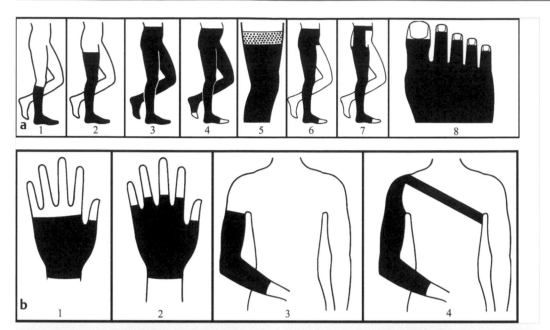

Fig. 4.14 **(a)** Compression styles. 1. Knee-high stocking. 2. Thigh-high stocking. 3. Pantyhose. 4. Pantyhose with highly elastic body part. 5. Thigh-high stocking with fastening border (silicone dots). 6. Thigh-high stocking with hip attachment. 7. Thigh-high stocking with garter belt. 8. Toe caps. **(b)** Compression styles. 1. Compression gauntlet. 2. Compression gauntlet with finger stubs. 3. Arm sleeve. 4. Arm sleeve with shoulder cover and strap. (Reproduced with permission of Juzo USA, Inc.)

garment uncomfortable to wear for the individual. These systems consist of garter belts, hip attachments (▶ Fig. 4.17), or fasteners that attach to shoulder straps or borders made of synthetic polymers (usually silicone dots or stripes) on the inside of the proximal end of the garments (▶ Fig. 4.18).

Some manufacturers provide adhesive lotions, which can be used to prevent the garment from slipping.

Built-in pressure pads constructed of dense foam materials ensure an even distribution of pressure in concave areas, such as behind the malleoli or the palmar surface of the hand.

To ensure maximum therapeutic benefit, it is absolutely necessary that only individuals with a thorough understanding of the pathology of lymphedema, together with the patient, decide on the compression level, style, and length of the garment. Compression garments should be worn daily and applied first thing in the morning. They should be replaced every 6 months or sooner if the garments have lost their elasticity. Refer to Chapter 5, Measurements for Compression Garments, for measuring techniques.

Donning aids can be useful to help in the application of compression garments. Rubber gloves, slip-on/slip-off aids, and nonslip mats are examples of donning systems, which also help protect the garment from damage (▶ Fig. 4.19).

Care of Compression Garments

The primary role of compression garments in lymphedema management is to maintain the reduction of the swelling achieved during the intensive treatment phase of complete decongestive therapy (CDT). A high level of consistency in providing the appropriate compression is crucial to avoid reaccumulation of evacuated lymphedema fluid. This consistency is provided by high-quality compression garments containing inlay threads, which are made of Lycra or rubber. These inlay threads are woven into the material in a continuous manner, thus providing the correct level of compression. It is important to realize that garments of lesser quality, known as off-the-shelf garments do not contain inlay threads and are less suitable for lymphedema management.

Sleeves and stockings are generally worn from first thing in the morning until nighttime, and although compression stockings are constructed of strong elastic and durable materials, they stretch

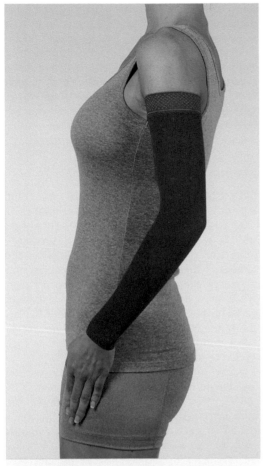

Fig. 4.15 Arm sleeves are available in a variety of colors. (Reproduced with permission of Juzo USA, Inc.)

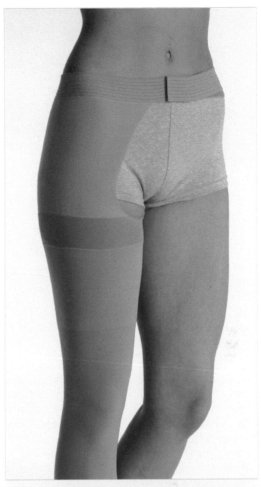

Fig. 4.17 Thigh-high compression stocking with hip attachment. (Reproduced with permission of Juzo USA, Inc.)

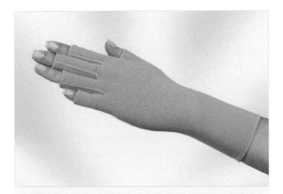

Fig. 4.16 Compression glove with finger stubs. (Reproduced with permission of Juzo USA, Inc.)

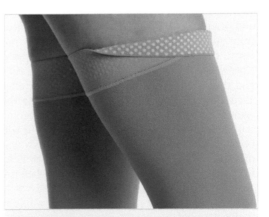

Fig. 4.18 Thigh-high compression stocking with fastening border made of silicone dots. (Reproduced with permission of Juzo USA, Inc.)

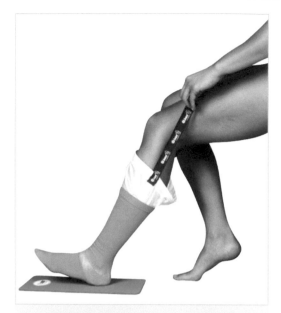

Fig. 4.19 Donning aid for closed-toe compression stockings (Juzo Slippie). (Reproduced with permission of JUZO USA, Inc.)

out after about 12 hours of wearing. This is especially true in regions of increased stretch (knee, elbow) where garments wear out more than in other areas, which may result in pooling of edema fluid in those areas.

Compression garments act as a second layer of skin that provides the resistance the compromised skin no longer can; to maintain color, shape, elasticity, and optimal therapeutic benefits of these garments, proper care is crucial.

Daily washing of compression garments helps them restore and retain their elastic properties as well as removing perspiration, oils, dirt, bacteria, and dead skin that accumulate inside the garment from normal wear. Frequent washing does not harm compression garments if done properly. However, the garments can be damaged easily, and their compressive qualities may be lost after even one tough rinse cycle, or through using the wrong dryer setting or the wrong cleaning agents.

The elastic fibers of a compression garment will break down with wear. While proper care will increase the life span of garments, they will need to be replaced about every 6 months or when the garment shows signs of wear that could adversely affect its compressive properties. As a general rule, if the garment no longer returns to its original shape after washing, has runs or holes in the material, no longer feels compressive, or if the garment becomes easy to put on, it probably needs to be replaced.

Manufacturers include complete care instructions with their compression sleeves and stockings, which should always be followed for optimal care. The points listed below relate to specific guidelines with regard to proper care and washing, reflecting general consensus between various quality compression garment manufacturers.

Machine Wash versus Hand Wash

Garments (sleeves, stockings, pantyhose, gauntlets, face masks, vests, etc.) may be machine or hand washed, depending on the preference of the user. Daily washing is recommended, especially if lotions or creams are being used (moisturizing lotion can break down the fibers in compression garments and should be applied only at night when the garment is removed). When washing garments in a machine, it is recommended to place the garment in a mesh laundry bag to protect the fabric during the washing cycle (the gentle cycle should be utilized).

Water temperature may range between cool and warm, but should not be colder than 30 °C (86 °F), or warmer than 40 °C (104 °F). Darker colored garments should be washed in cool water. It is best to have more than one garment (one to wear, one to wash) and alternate them to allow the elasticity to recover and to prolong their effectiveness. Tips for hand washing procedures are listed below:

1. Start by filling a bowl, bucket, sink, or small tub with water.
2. The compression garment should be dipped gently into the water to dampen it.
3. Add a small amount of washing solution (see below).
4. Let the compression garment soak for a few minutes.
5. For better cleaning, gently rub the fibers of the compression garment together without stretching them excessively.
6. Then, empty the tub and refill with water; dip or rinse the clean compression garment thoroughly especially along the seams to rid the garment of residual salts and oils from perspiration.
7. Gently squeeze the compression garment to remove excess water.
8. Refer to the drying options below.

Washing Solutions

Harsh cleaning agents, solvents, petroleum-based cleaners, etc., can destroy the thin fibers of compression garments. Mild soaps or detergents should be used, free of bleach, chlorine, fabric softeners, or other laundry additives. Some manufacturers offer garment washing solutions, which are formulated to remove oil, body acids, and skin salts quickly and easily without damage to the fabric; using these specially designed solutions is recommended and will help extend the life of elastic garments.

Drying Guidelines

Compression garments may be machine- or air-dried. If using a dryer, the dial should be set on a no-heat (maximum low-heat) air-drying cycle because excessive heat exposure may weaken or even damage the elastic fibers of the garments. If silicone bands are present, the no-heat dryer setting will help protect this material.

When garments are air-dried, it is important not to pull, squeeze, or wring out the residual water from the garment excessively. Rolling up the compression garment in a towel and gently squeezing the towel before laying the garment out to dry speeds up the drying process; garments should never be left rolled up in a towel.

Whether garments are line-dried or laid flat to dry, exposure to direct sunlight should be avoided and the garment should be turned inside out. It is recommended that a towel be placed on a drying rack and that the garment be placed on top to dry. If the garment is hung up directly onto a rack or pole to drip-dry, the weight of the water could stretch the garment, and it may no longer fit properly.

Alternative Materials

In recent years, several adjustable compression devices have been made available for patients with lymphedema and venous disorders. These devices provide gradient compression by use of nonelastic adjustable bands working on the hook-and-loop principle. Some of these devices use foam pads underneath the nonelastic material to provide additional padding; others may be combined with traditional compression garments (▶ Fig. 4.20).

There is a broad consensus between clinicians that these devices should not be used to decongest a swollen limb. The application of short-stretch bandage materials in combination with appropriate padding allows customization of the compression in virtually unlimited variations. Nonelastic, adjustable compression may be used as an alternative to nighttime bandaging in the second phase of CDT, when the extremity has decongested to a normal or near normal size, to balance daytime compression supplied by elastic compression garments. The compression on the limb is safer at night as it approximates the low resting pressure achieved by low-stretch bandaging.

Alternative devices can also be utilized as a supplement to elastic garments in the daytime when elastic compression is insufficient to control edema in a limb with flaccid skin due to massive reduction, or very aggressive edema. Patients who are physically unable (or unwilling) to apply nighttime bandaging may choose this more costly alternative. Most of these garment styles are available ready-made or custom-made for upper and lower extremity, head and neck, truncal and genital applications. The measurement requirements vary more widely in these garment types, and consulting the individual manufacturers' instructions is recommended.

Selecting an Appropriate Garment

Compression garments are a key component in the patient's ability to maintain the reduction achieved during a course of care. Care will not work if the garment chosen is not effective or easily worn by the patient on a daily basis. Garments can be ordered from durable medical equipment providers or from the treating facility if they choose to supply them. The treating therapist is the best person to ascertain the correct garment for a patient given that they are most aware of

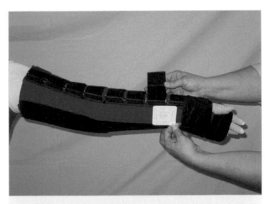

Fig. 4.20 Inelastic padded compression system (circaid graduate arm). (Reproduced with permission of medi USA.)

several important factors in the choice of an appropriate compression garment. These factors include the following:

- How much compression was necessary to achieve the reduction?
- How sensitive is the patient to pressure?
- How difficult will it be for the patient to don/remove the garment?
- What factors in the patient's lifestyle will affect the garment choice?

An understanding of the construction of compression garments is one of the keys to making the appropriate choice for a patient. There are three major techniques used to create a compression garment: circular knitting, flat knitting, or "cut and sew."

Ready-Made Garments

The majority of ready-made garments are circular knit, allowing for two-way stretch and a seamless appearance. The shape of the garment before use is essentially a tube and the two-way stretch is important because it allows the garment to fit properly over the contours of the limb. Garments are available in compression classes I (20–30 mmHg), II (30–40 mmHg), and III (40–50 mmHg), and may be layered to achieve a 50+ mmHg compression though the compression achieved may not be directly additive due to the range of compression achieved in the garment. These garments are usually considerably less expensive than the alternative choice of custom-made garments. An off-the-shelf (also known as ready-made) garment may be the most appropriate choice for a patient if the limb is proportional in shape, not overly long or short and has a relatively firm texture in the portion of the limb to be covered by the garment. A circumferential silicone band is often necessary to allow this type of garment to adequately grip the proximal limb. Circular-knit garments will often roll down at the top when worn on limbs with very soft, loose tissue proximally.

Custom-Made Garments

Custom-made garments are the appropriate choice for patients who have nonproportional and/or irregularly shaped limbs, very short or very long limbs, or very soft tissue or excessively flaccid skin due to a very large reduction during treatment. Both flat-knit and cut-and-sew fabrics are used for custom garments. Custom-made garments are also indicated for patients with deep skinfolds or excessive tenderness at joint lines because they are usually flat-knit garments that will tend not to cut into or bunch at sensitive joint lines or skinfolds. These garments are flat-knit to the appropriate shape or cut from loomed fabric and then each type is seamed to achieve the garment shape. Flat-knit fabrics offer much better containment for the soft tissue as their effect is much closer to that of a short-stretch bandage with greater working pressure and reduced resting pressure due to limited stretch and stiffer fabrics. This is reflected in the reported compression achieved in the various classes. For example, the reported compression rates achieved in the arm are Class 1 (14–18 mmHg), Class 2 (20–25 mmHg), and Class 3 (25–30 mmHg). Less overall pressure is necessary as the fabric offers better working pressure and containment of the tissue. Putting on custom-made garments can be easier because they more closely match the exact profile of the limb, eliminating the need to stretch the garment to fit the contour of the limb. Custom flat-knit garments are available with a variety of knitting adjustments designed to reduce the bunching of garments and improve the fit and comfort of the garment, especially at the joints (▶ Fig. 4.21).

Patient Considerations

Some patient groups offer special challenges as regards fitting. Lipedema patients have very soft tissue, irregularly shaped limbs, and increased sensitivity to pressure. This patient group is best served by flat-knit custom compression garments in compression class I or II depending on the degree of edema noted upon initial evaluation.

Pregnant women require compression garments that are easy to don, provide class II compression to address primarily venous insufficiency (unless there is a prepregnancy diagnosis of lymphedema), with a body part that is adjustable to allow reduced compression over the abdomen. Children with lymphedema generally require custom-made garments, which are replaced with much greater frequency (every 2–3 months) as compared with adults at 4- to 6-month intervals due to their rapid growth from infancy through young adulthood. For small children, an effort should be made to choose softer fabrics for compression and linings at joint lines to protect their more delicate skin.

Patients with very large reductions in volume, or who lead very active lifestyles, will benefit from

lower extremity **solutions**

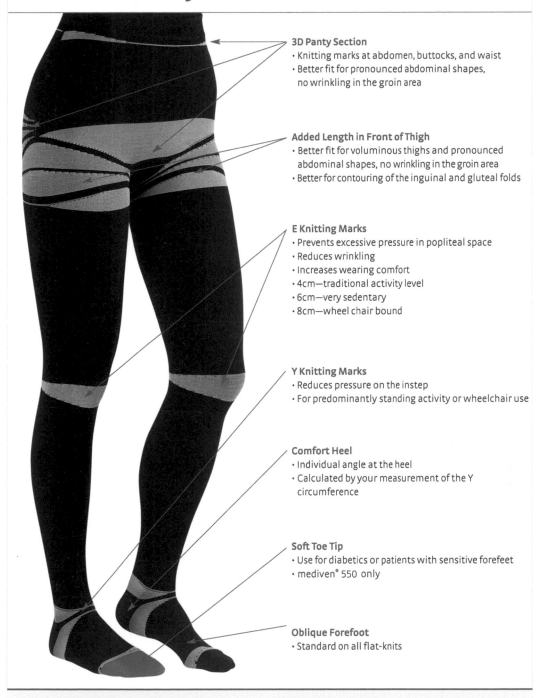

3D Panty Section
- Knitting marks at abdomen, buttocks, and waist
- Better fit for pronounced abdominal shapes, no wrinkling in the groin area

Added Length in Front of Thigh
- Better fit for voluminous thighs and pronounced abdominal shapes, no wrinkling in the groin area
- Better for contouring of the inguinal and gluteal folds

E Knitting Marks
- Prevents excessive pressure in popliteal space
- Reduces wrinkling
- Increases wearing comfort
- 4cm—traditional activity level
- 6cm—very sedentary
- 8cm—wheel chair bound

Y Knitting Marks
- Reduces pressure on the instep
- For predominantly standing activity or wheelchair use

Comfort Heel
- Individual angle at the heel
- Calculated by your measurement of the Y circumference

Soft Toe Tip
- Use for diabetics or patients with sensitive forefeet
- mediven® 550 only

Oblique Forefoot
- Standard on all flat-knits

Fig. 4.21 Lower extremity compression garment solutions. (Reproduced with permission of medi GmbH & Co. KG.)

additional compressive support for the calf. Consider the use of a low-profile bandage alternative (manufacturers, such as CircAid, Farrow Medical, JoviPak, or Sigvaris supply these devices) layered over a thigh-high compression to achieve adequate edema control below the knee. This can be accomplished without excessive pressure on the foot or anterior ankle where the tibialis anterior tendon is prone to excessive pressure with higher compression class garments.

Donning and doffing of compression garments may be a particular challenge for patients who have difficulty reaching their feet or who have a lack of hand strength or who suffer pain because of osteoarthritis. This is most challenging for patients who live alone. Education and practice are key to helping patients or caregivers achieve independence in this skill. It is recommended that an active lymphedema clinic have examples of many of the available donning aids available to allow a patient the opportunity to try different methods prior to purchase of an aid for their own use.

Rubber gloves are an important tool for all patients because they allow for "massaging" of the garment into place, avoiding pinching and pulling of the garment and damage from fingernails or jewelry. Beware of the patient with a latex allergy! Many rubber gloves are made of latex. Some patients despite their best efforts will not be able to reach their feet adequately in order to don elastic garments or will have limited assistance at home.

Bandage alternatives that are low profile are a good choice for full-time usage because they can be removed/replaced on the limb once a day (by an available family member or with the use of a donning/doffing aid) and can safely be worn both day and night due to the nonelastic nature of the compression.

Elastic garments, which offer effective daytime compression, are not appropriate for nighttime use because they can restrict adequate blood flow while the limb is elevated, and they can bunch up when worn in bed. Donning a pantyhose-style garment in a high-compression class is very challenging. A better approach is modular compression by the use of bilateral thigh- or knee-high garments with a layered bike pant ending just above the knee or extending down onto the calf. This allows the patient to don each leg garment separately, and then to add the bike pant to achieve a compression gradient to the waist. This also affords the patient some degree of choice in how much compression to wear throughout the day; they can perhaps remove the waist-high garment when they get home at the end of the day, without losing compression for the legs so they can "breathe" and have a degree of freedom from compression.

The patient with a latex allergy is a special case. Most compression garments today are latex free, but check the stated composition of a garment before ordering. A special circumstance would be a health professional who requires a compression sleeve or glove who is not latex sensitive but who may work closely with a population of patients with a high probability of latex sensitivity (i.e., a pediatric physician or therapist). It is recommended that this patient consider wearing a non-latex upper extremity garment at least during working hours.

Certain garment options appear to be attractive in that they make the donning or wearing of the garment easier, but be wary of these. For example, patients often request zippers for ease of donning. Zippers do not extend past the ankle and since this is the most difficult point to slide the garment past, the zipper is often not as useful as expected. In addition, a zipper has no longitudinal stretch and limits the ability to smooth out a garment over the limb to most accurately fit the length. Zippers are also very difficult to pull together and "zip-up" in garments with high compression, which may lead to injury to the skin. However, zippers are very helpful in donning a garment over a paralyzed limb.

Many patients request an open crotch in a waist-high compression garment because they would prefer to use the toilet without having to pull the garment down. In a patient with lower extremity lymphedema, there is always a risk of genital swelling, and a garment that does not apply compression to the perineum may leave the patient at increased risk of this complication.

Both upper and lower extremity garments are available with a fabric extension for suspension (a sleeve cap or chaps style thigh high). These styles are simply for suspension of the garment; if a patient has swelling in the shoulder region or lateral hip, circumferential compression from a vest or body garment/bike pant is necessary for adequate edema control. Closed-toe garments are not adequate for control of swelling in the toes. As such, toe caps providing circumferential compression for each toe (the fifth toe is usually free of compression) are necessary.

Contraindications for Compression Therapy

The application of compression on an extremity is absolutely contraindicated in the following cases:

- Cardiac edema.
- *Peripheral arterial diseases*: compression therapy is contraindicated with an ankle/brachial index (ABI) of less than 0.8. Normal ABI values are 0.95 to 1.3; mild to moderate arterial disease has values of 0.5 to 0.8. ABI values of less than 0.5 are interpreted as severe arterial insufficiencies (see also Chapter 3).

> The ABI compares the systolic blood pressure of the ankle to that of the arm (brachial). These measurements are useful in the assessment, follow-up, and treatment of patients with peripheral vascular disease.

- Acute infections (cellulitis, erysipelas).

The following is a summary of conditions in which compression therapy may be used with caution (relative contraindications). To determine which level of compression is appropriate, close cooperation with the referring physician is necessary:

- Hypertension.
- Cardiac arrhythmia.
- Decreased or absent sensation in the extremity.
- Partial or complete paralysis, flaccid limbs.
- Age.
- Congestive heart failure.
- Mild to moderate arterial occlusive disease (ABI values 0.8–1.0).
- Diabetes.
- Malignant lymphedema.

4.6 Exercises and Lymphedema

The health benefits of regular exercise cannot be ignored, especially for patients with lymphedema or who are at risk for lymphedema. Exercise has profound benefits for weight reduction and management; improving energy, mood, and immune function; combating chronic health conditions and diseases; and providing socialization and recreation.

Exercise that is performed during the intensive phase of CDT is called "remedial exercise." Remedial exercise has been shown to be effective during the intensive phase and should be done under the supervision of the treating therapist. These specific exercises are performed while the compression bandages are in place to assist the body with remodeling the tissue and decongesting the affected tissue by increasing the return of lymphatic fluid to the circulatory system. There is little controversy regarding remedial exercise. Developing good exercise habits during the intensive phase can help a patient progress to a supervised community-based exercise program as part of their discharge plan. This is where much of the controversy regarding exercise has persisted. What type of exercise is safe for patients with lymphedema? When can they start exercising and how much exercise can they do?

In 2011, researchers published a systematic review of the literature regarding exercise and lymphedema.[1] They found 19 articles that met their criteria for final review. The majority of these studies were specific to breast cancer–related lymphedema (BCRL) and the evidence was strong, supporting the safety of resistance exercise for patients with known lymphedema or those at risk for secondary arm lymphedema after breast cancer treatment.[2] In 2016, two separate systematic reviews were published[3,4] on BCRL and exercise, further supporting the previous findings about the safety and efficacy of exercise for at-risk patients or with known lymphedema following breast cancer treatment, if done in a slowly progressive manner and under initial supervision.

Perhaps the most compelling statements regarding exercise and BCRL comes from Dieli-Conwright and Orozco's 2015 review article that summarized the latest research looking at all different aspects of exercise for breast cancer survivors. They point out that exercise is one of the most important modifiable risk factors for the prevention of primary and recurrent cancers. They go on to report that, "although the scientific knowledge supporting participation in exercise is profound, exercise adherence remains a challenge in breast cancer survivors." If the fear of lymphedema and the ignorance of the current body of evidence we have to support safe exercise for at-risk patients or with known lymphedema prevails, then lives will be at risk. The 2.8 million breast cancer survivors in the United States need improved clinician knowledge to guide them along the path to safe and effective exercise, while we continue to collect data and conduct meta-analysis.[5]

There continues to be a paucity of research in relation to lower extremity lymphedema of any

4

kind. The research group from University of Pennsylvania have published a few new studies since their original 2010 pilot study focused on lower extremity cancer-related lymphedema in uterine cancer survivors.[6] The results are favorable toward increasing physical activity (PA) in uterine cancer survivors. They reported that higher levels of PA or walking was associated with reduced proportions of lower limb lymphedema in dose-response fashion, such that the group who engaged in the highest levels of PA or walking reported the smallest proportion of lower limb lymphedema cases. These were preliminary findings and the need for further research is substantial. Comparable studies are still needed for other cancer-related lymphedema and primary lymphedema. Until further studies are presented, we can rely on a strong background in anatomy, physiology, and pathophysiology of the lymphatic system to guide us with exercise prescription. The benefits of exercise must be available to all patients with lymphedema regardless of the cause.

In 2011, The National Lymphedema Network (NLN) revised their position statement on exercise to reflect much of the above referenced research. These guidelines are very thorough and should be used while developing an individualized exercise plan.[7] A patient must have their lymphedema under good control prior to beginning a new exercise routine. Starting with the supervision of a certified lymphedema therapist (CLT) while in active treatment is optimal. This should be a natural progression from their remedial exercises as the intensive phase transitions to the self-care phase of treatment. A patient who has completed decongestive therapy must have their compression garments prior to starting the exercise program.

All exercises need to be started gradually and to progress at a slow rate; the affected region should be assessed for any changes prior to progression. Particular attention needs to be paid to the form and technique used by the patient while he/she exercises. Modifications may be needed, such as allowing for adequate rest intervals between sets.[7] Garments should be worn and need to be properly fitted. This includes wearing a hand piece with a sleeve for upper extremity lymphedema.

Research is currently under way to examine the need for compression during exercise and alternate types of compression, such as commercially available sports gear. Research also needs to look at the effects of moderate to high-level activities, and activities once considered "high risk" for patients with lymphedema. Patients who want to get back to these higher-level activities and sports need to have specific interventions tailored to the activity. Developing the proper strength, coordination, endurance, power, and flexibility required for the specific sport is vital before returning to the activity. The decision to continue with the activity needs to be made based on the response of the body to the activity. Therapists need to encourage their patients to take the initiative and track their workouts and respective responses to the activity. Subtle changes noted during and after exercise need to be examined. Modifications can be made accordingly.

Exercise should not be avoided in the patient with lymphedema. Sufficient time needs to be invested in the progression of any type of exercise program. Considerations of general safety principles and proper guidance and encouragement toward improving physical fitness should be implemented in the plan of care for every patient with lymphedema or those at risk.

4.6.1 Breathing Exercises

The downward and upward movement of the diaphragm in deep abdominal breathing is an essential component for the sufficient return of lymphatic fluid back to the bloodstream. Patients affected by lymphedema of the leg benefit greatly from an exercise program including diaphragmatic breathing exercises. The movement of the diaphragm, combined with the outward and inward movements of the abdomen, ribcage, and lower back, also promotes general well-being, peristalsis, and return of venous blood to the heart.

4.6.2 Resistive Exercises

Strength exercises improve muscle power, increase the strength in ligaments, tendons, and bones, and positively contribute to weight control. Resistive exercises are typically performed in a repetitive fashion against an opposing load. Gradual progression is imperative and exercise programs should be comparable to the patient's fitness level, while trying to accomplish an improved return of lymphatic fluid without adding further stress to an impaired lymphatic system. Certain strength exercises are beneficial for lymphedema patients and to date, research supports the use of compression garments during these exercises.

> Resistive exercises using weights present possible problems in regard to injury or overuse. However, with appropriate precautions, resistive exercises using weights can be very beneficial.

An improved baseline of strength allows daily tasks to be performed with less effort and possibly prevent muscular or ligament sprain or strain. Improved strength can restore intramuscular balance and normal biomechanics to the involved limb and surrounding joint structures. When beginning a resistance program, weights should be light, with higher repetitions, as opposed to choosing the heaviest weight the patient can only lift one to three times. Negative effects in terms of accumulation of fluid in the affected limb (or the limb at risk) are unlikely if exercises are performed with compression in place on the involved extremity.

An article published in August 2009 in the *New England Journal of Medicine* addressed the topic of weight lifting in women with BCRL.[8] The article summarized an 18-month study performed by Schmitz et al in a controlled trial of biweekly progressive weight lifting involving 141 breast cancer survivors with stable upper extremity lymphedema. While the results of this study suggested that weight lifting not only had no negative effects on the volumes of breast cancer-related lymphedema and increased muscular strength, it also suggested that weight lifting reduced the number and severity of arm and hand symptoms and reduced the incidence of lymphedema exacerbations if proper safety guidelines were followed. In 2014, a systematic review and meta-analysis by Cheema et al indicated that progressive resistive exercise may actually reduce the risk of developing BCRL and does not worsen arm volume or symptom severity.[9]

Weight training should be started in a supervised setting, with an individual who has training as a certified cancer exercise trainer (a certification offered by the American College of Sports Medicine) or training as a CLT. The affected extremity should be in a stable position, that is, the extremity should be decongested and be free of infections for a minimum of 3 months prior to the start of weight exercises. Furthermore, patients should understand and follow the NLN's position papers on risk-reduction practices and exercise.

In some instances, individuals may not tolerate exercises that isolate the involved extremity, and the involved limb may respond adversely to these exercises. In such cases, the patient may benefit from general, systemic activities such as light to moderate walking or biking. Walking and biking will stimulate diaphragmatic breathing, which will promote the return of lymph fluid to the blood circulation.

4.6.3 Aerobic Exercises for Lymphedema

Lymphedema patients can and should be active, and those who never exercised before should consider starting with a daily walk, swim, or spending 20 minutes on a stationary bicycle. The right type of PA helps reduce the swelling by improving the flow of lymph, and presents a vital tool for patients to stay in shape and continue with the normal activities of daily living.

Many patients ask if they can continue their pre-lymphedema activities or if they should adjust or replace them. The answer to that question depends on the activity itself. Tennis and golf, for example, do not rank very high on the list of beneficial activities for individuals with upper extremity lymphedema. For patients with lymphedema of the leg, kickboxing and step aerobics are activities that bear a great risk of injury and therefore should be avoided. But the reality is that for some individuals, exercise plays such a vital role in their daily routine, and is so engrained in their personality, that giving up these so-called high-risk activities would have a serious impact on their well-being.

The simple fact is that nobody knows better than the patient himself/herself what is good for their body and general well-being. As long as the patients are under the care of a trained lymphedema therapist, wear their compression garment during these physical activities, and the exercise regimen does not cause discomfort or pain, it is fine to continue with these activities. However, if the affected limb hurts, feels strained, or increases in volume during and after the activity cannot be easily managed, then the patient should adjust the activity as necessary and consult with their lymphedema therapist or physician. The keywords here are caution and moderation; gradual progression is imperative while trying to accomplish an improved return of lymphatic fluid without adding further stress to an impaired lymphatic system.

Aerobic conditioning is generally performed in a repetitive fashion using large muscle groups. Some long-term benefits include decrease in resting heart rate, improved muscular strength, weight control, and increased return of venous and lymphatic fluids.

It is important to understand that certain aerobic exercises and recreational activities could trigger an increase in swelling, or have higher risks of injury. Ideally, such high-risk activities should be avoided or modified for patients affected by lymphedema. Examples of these high-risk activities include soccer, kickboxing, or step aerobics for lower extremity lymphedema, and tennis, racquetball, or golf for lymphedema affecting the arms.

Beneficial activities for upper and lower extremity lymphedema include (but are not limited to) the following:

- *Swimming or water aerobics*: with the body weight reduced by approximately 90% in chest-deep water, exercises performed in the water improve mobility and enhance strength and muscle tone. In addition, the pressure exerted by the water on the body surface contributes to lymphatic and venous return. Hot water (temperature above 35 °C [94 °F]), usually found in hot tubs and Jacuzzis, must be avoided. High water temperature definitely has a negative impact on lymphedema.
- *Walking*: a 20-minute walk outdoors, or on a treadmill (10–15 minutes, slow walking speed), while wearing the compression garment, will stimulate the circulatory system and contribute greatly to the individual's general well-being. Key points: walk with a normal gait; do not drag the affected leg and avoid limping.
- *Easy biking*: 20 to 25 minutes either outdoors or at the gym, using a comfortable and wide saddle. Legs are placed in a higher position on recumbent bikes, which makes them a better choice for individuals affected by lower extremity lymphedema.
- *Yoga*: the combination of stretching, deep breathing, relaxation, and the positive impact on the venous and lymphatic return makes yoga a perfect choice of exercise. Strenuous yoga practices should be avoided, and if certain poses seem

uncomfortable, they should be altered, or skipped. Many cancer centers and support groups have contacts for yoga classes specifically tailored to cancer survivors and lymphedema patients.
- *Lebed method*: this exercise and movement program is designed for people with lymphedema and cancer survivors. The program incorporates music and dance to focus on overall wellness, range of motion, balance, strength, and endurance.
- *Decongestive exercises*: the exercise program practiced with the lymphedema therapist during the intensive phase of CDT is tailored to each individual patient's needs, abilities, and restrictions. This exercise regimen, which should be performed twice daily, improves circulation, mobility, and well-being.

In general, exercises and activities should always be performed with the compression garment in place; intensity and duration of any exercise should be gradually increased; movements that overstrain or cause discomfort or pain should be avoided; and the extremity should be carefully monitored for any changes in size or shape. The general recommendations that all adults perform a volume of weekly activity of 150 minutes of moderate-intensity aerobic activity should be incorporated into an individualized plan for all patients with lymphedema.

4.7 Skin and Nail Care

Patients affected by lymphedema are susceptible to infections of the skin and nails. Meticulous care of these areas is essential to the success of CDT. Skin is usually impermeable to bacteria and other pathogens, but any defect in the skin, whether from trauma, heat, or other causes, can be an entry site for pathogens or infectious agents. Lymphedematous tissues are saturated with protein-rich fluid, which serves as an ideal breeding ground for pathogens. In addition, the local immune defense is low due to the increased diffusion distance, which hinders a timely response of the defense cells in the affected area. Lymphedematous skin can also become thickened and scaly, which increases the risk of skin cracks and fissures.

Streptococcus bacteria most commonly cause infections in patients with lymphedema. At a local level, *Streptococcus* is not highly toxic, and the body's defenses react slowly initially; therefore, the infectious bacteria can reproduce and migrate to other parts of the body. The process of inflammation may develop into a serious medical crisis and can make lymphedema much worse by accelerating the progression through its stages. The basic consideration in skin and nail care is therefore the prevention and control of infection.

Patients are instructed in proper cleansing and moisturizing techniques to maintain the health and integrity of the skin. This educational process includes how to inspect the skin for any wounds or signs of infection or inflammation. A checklist of precautions should be presented to the patient in the early stages of treatment. This list increases compliance and helps the patient avoid situations and activities that may worsen the lymphedema or cause infections. A list of precautions and high- and medium-risk activities is provided in Chapter 5, Precautions.

Suitable ointments or lotions formulated for sensitive skin, radiation dermatitis, and lymphedema should be applied before lymphedema bandages while the patient is in the decongestive phase of the treatment. After the limb is decongested and the patient wears compression garments, moisturizing ointments should be applied twice daily. Ointments, as well as soaps or other skin cleansers used in lymphedema management, should have good moisturizing qualities, contain no fragrances, be hypoallergenic, and be formulated to be in either the neutral or acidic range of the pH scale (around pH 5.0). The acidity or alkalinity of the skin is measured on the pH scale, which ranges from 0 (extremely acidic, as in lemon juice) to 14 (extremely alkaline, as in lye). Level 7 on the pH scale represents a neutral value (as in water). Normal skin pH is around 5.0.

To identify possible allergic reactions to skin care products, they should be first tested on healthy skin before the initial application on lymphedematous skin.

Tight-fitting compression sleeves or stockings, as well as materials used in compression bandaging, may cause skin irritation. Some patients may be allergic to a certain material used for compression therapy. This situation usually can be remedied easily by switching to other materials.

In mosquito-infested areas, it is necessary to apply insect repellents to the affected extremity (some moisturizers contain natural repellents) to avoid bites, which could cause infections.

4.8 The Two-Phase Approach in Lymphedema Management

Successful lymphedema management is performed in two phases. In phase 1, also known as the intensive or decongestive phase, the patient is seen on a daily basis, and treatments are given until the limb is decongested. It is imperative for the success of the treatment that treatments are given daily and that the patient is thoroughly informed about all components of CDT before treatment is initiated (see Chapter 3, Evaluation of Lymphedema). Patients unable or unwilling to present for daily treatments should not be admitted.

The duration of the intensive phase varies with the severity of the condition and averages 2 to 3 weeks for patients with upper extremity lymphedema and 2 to 4 weeks for patients with lymphedema of the leg. In extreme cases, the decongestive phase may last up to 6 to 8 weeks and may have to be repeated several times.

> The end of the first phase of treatment is determined by the results of circumferential or volumetric measurements on the affected extremity.

When the measurements approach a plateau, the end of phase 1 is reached, and the patient progresses seamlessly into phase 2 of CDT, also known as the self-management phase.

Depending on the stage of lymphedema, the involved extremity or body part may have reached a normal size at the end of the intensive phase, or there may still be a circumferential difference between the involved and the uninvolved limb. If treatment is initiated in the early stage 1 of lymphedema, which is characterized by a soft-tissue consistency without any fibrotic alterations, limb reduction can be expected to a normal size (compared with the uninvolved limb). If intervention starts in the later stages of lymphedema, where lymphostatic fibrosis in the subcutaneous tissues exists, the edematous fluid will recede, and fibrotic areas may soften. However, in most cases the indurated tissue will not completely regress during the intensive phase of CDT. Reduction in fibrotic tissue is a slow process, which can take several months or longer, and is achieved mainly in the second phase of CDT.

In phase 2 of CDT, the patient assumes responsibility for managing, improving, and maintaining the results achieved in phase 1. To reverse the symptoms associated with later stages of lymphedema, good patient compliance is indispensable. Compression garments have to be worn daily, and bandages have to be applied during the night. This self-management phase is a lifelong process; regular check-ups with the physician and the lymphedema therapist are necessary.

4.8.1 Intensive Phase

Components of this phase are skin and nail care, manual lymph drainage (MLD), compression therapy, and decongestive exercises.

Skin and Nail Care

Before compression bandages are applied, appropriate moisturizers or lotions are used to cover the lymphedematous limb. During the intensive phase of CDT, patients are continuously instructed in proper cleansing and moisturizing techniques to maintain the health and integrity of the skin and to prevent infections (refer to Chapter 3, "Wounds and Skin Lesions" and "Lower Extremity Wound Considerations").

Manual Lymph Drainage

In the first phase of therapy, MLD is applied at least once a day, 5 days a week. The MLD portion of the treatment generally requires 30 to 60 minutes. The duration of individual treatments depends on the number of involved limbs and body parts, as well as on the severity of the symptoms.

The most important aspect of MLD in phase 1 is to identify drainage areas with sufficient and healthy lymphatics. These pathways and lymph nodes are used to reroute the accumulated protein-rich lymph fluid around the blocked areas from the swollen extremity or body part back to the venous system.

To discuss the basic procedural pattern of treatment, the example of a unilateral secondary upper extremity lymphedema shall be used (detailed treatment sequences for this and other pathologies are found in Chapter 5). The swelling in upper extremity lymphedema usually involves the ipsilateral truncal quadrant. Healthy lymphatics are generally found in adjacent truncal territories (e.g., the contralateral upper quadrant and the ipsilateral lower quadrant), as well as the lymph vessels and lymph nodes in the supraclavicular area of the same side. To maximize the therapeutic effect of MLD, the method of procedure can be broken down into the following steps.

Manipulation of lymph nodes and collectors located in the healthy adjacent quadrants as well as in the supraclavicular area on the ipsilateral side will increase lymph angiomotoricity and result in a "suction effect" on the protein-rich lymph fluid in the congested area. Following this initial preparation, the congested body quadrant is included in the treatment. The protein-rich lymph fluid located in this area is carefully moved across the watersheds toward the previously manipulated adjacent territories, using primarily the appropriate anastomoses (in this case, the anterior and posterior axillo-axillary and the ipsilateral axillo-inguinal anastomoses). Even though MLD is not directly applied to the swollen extremity during this period of the treatment, a volume reduction occurs, which can be noted in a decrease of circumferential measurements in the affected extremity. This volume reduction is generally observed following a series of two to four treatments.

When the extremity starts to decongest, the initial preparation is reduced to the relevant lymph nodes (in this case, axillary lymph nodes on the contralateral side and inguinal lymph nodes on the ipsilateral side) and anastomoses. The treatment area is now expanded to include the affected extremity on a step-by-step basis. To avoid stress (e.g., overload of the healthy lymphatics in the drainage areas), it is suggested initially to include only the upper arm in the treatment protocol. In severe cases of lymphedema, it may be necessary to treat only parts of the upper arm. In the following treatments, the forearm, then the hand and fingers are carefully included.

Patients should be instructed early in the course of treatment how to perform simple self-MLD techniques (see Chapter 5). These techniques are used to stimulate lymph drainage during the weekends in the intensive phase as well as in the self-management phase.

Compression Therapy

In the intensive phase of the treatment, compression therapy is administered using short-stretch bandages in combination with appropriate padding materials. Bandages are applied following MLD and skin care measures and worn by the patient until the next treatment session, 23 hours a day. Patients should be instructed not to remove the bandages at home. It is important that the bandages are taken off in the treatment facility prior to the next treatment session for the following reasons: skin marks left by the bandages and padding materials give the clinician important clues as to where to apply more padding if necessary, or if bandage tension needs to be adjusted in specific areas. If bandages are removed several hours before the scheduled treatment time, lymph fluid will re-accumulate in the extremity, forcing the clinician to spend part of the treatment time removing this fluid again.

Patients cover the bandaged extremity with cast covers, garbage bags, or the like during showers at home. The extremity is cleaned in the facility after the removal of the compression bandages using either a shower (if available) or a washcloth.

Time management is essential in the intensive phase of the therapy. Depending on the number of bandages and padding materials used, it may take experienced lymphedema therapists 10 to 20 minutes (in extreme cases, even longer) to apply a compression bandage. Novices in the field should set aside ample time for this essential part of the therapy.

An important aspect in this stage of the treatment is to instruct the patient, and preferably a family member, in self-bandaging techniques. This requires a lot of practice, which makes it necessary to initiate the patient instruction early on in the intensive phase. It is also necessary to reserve sufficient time during the treatment session to allow the patient to learn and practice the bandaging techniques under the supervision of the clinician. To preserve and improve the treatment success following the intensive phase, it is essential that patients and/or family members are proficient in the application of compression bandages. Self-bandaging techniques should therefore be monitored and critiqued regularly during the intensive phase.

Self-bandaging during the decongestive phase is necessary on weekends should the bandages slide. Many patients also require compression bandages during the night during the self-management phase.

Decongestive Exercises

The goal of the exercise program is to improve lymph circulation and to maximize functional ability. Exercises are performed at least twice a day for approximately 10 to 15 minutes wearing the compression bandages. To promote patient compliance, it is important to create an exercise protocol that is easy to learn and perform. Short protocols should be taught and tailored to the individual needs and limitations of the patient. The patient should assume the primary responsibility for the exercise portion as early as possible in the treatment program. A specific time should be set aside for the exercise sessions so that the patient can establish a daily routine. The therapist should monitor the exercise program regularly.

In addition to the decongestive exercise program, beneficial recreational activities should be discussed with the patient. High-risk activities (see Chapter 5, Patient Education) that could trigger a further decrease in lymphatic transport capacity should be avoided or kept at a minimum. A balanced program of recreational activities supports general well-being, improves lymph drainage, and controls weight.

The vast majority of lymphedema patients will benefit from CDT, provided that a clinician thoroughly trained in all components of CDT administers the treatment. Patient adherence to the treatment program and compliance are also indispensable components to ensure treatment success.

A lack of progress during treatment may be caused by the following:
- *Improper treatment techniques:* if CDT is applied only in part (MLD as the only form of intervention, no MLD, or improper bandaging), there is inappropriate use of pneumatic compression pumps, or the therapist is poorly trained, the treatment is prone to failure.
- Poor patient compliance.
- *The patient suffers from malignant lymphedema*: the referring physician decides if CDT (or parts of this intervention) is suitable for palliative care.
- *The patient has self-induced lymphedema*: this form of lymphedema is caused by self-mutilation. In most cases, a tourniquet is applied to an extremity, which causes reduced lymphatic and venous return and the onset of swelling. If a diagnosis of self-induced (artificial) lymphedema is established by the physician, a cast may be applied to the affected extremity to prevent further strangulation.
- The severity of the symptoms, especially lymphostatic fibrosis, may have an impact on the

treatment progress. The results in these cases generally are less dramatic and take a longer time to establish.

- *Associated conditions*: certain pathologies (see Chapter 3, Complications in Lymphedema) may slow treatment progress.

4.8.2 Self-Management Phase

With proper compliance and thorough instruction by the clinician, the majority of patients are able to maintain and improve the treatment results achieved during the intensive phase of therapy. Self-management is only effective if it is performed properly and adherence to the self-care regimen designed for each individual patient is crucial to maintaining treatment results and preventing the progression of lymphedema. It is important to understand that the symptoms associated with lymphedema may have a negative psychological and psychosocial impact on some patients affected by this condition, which may create barriers to the adherence to self-management of lymphedema.[10] Positive patient reinforcement, motivation in taking an active role in their health and self-care plan, and education about lymphedema, its treatment components and risk reduction guidelines (see Chapter 5, Patient Education) are of great value to further patient compliance with self-management protocols.

Many patients report that changes in body weight and climate can cause their symptoms to fluctuate. Female patients commonly report that the swelling tends to increase during the menstrual cycle. Usually, these situations can be remedied by following the self-management protocol more closely.

For those patients who are unable to maintain decongestion, or who experience an increase in swelling during the second phase of CDT, it is necessary to follow up with additional CDT sessions in the clinic. Individual circumstances determine if follow-up treatments are applied in weekly, biweekly, or monthly sessions or if another shortened intensive phase is necessary (see Chapter 3, Therapeutic Approach to Lymphedema).

The components in phase 2 of CDT are similar to those in phase 1. The emphasis in phase 2 is self-improvement and self-management.

Skin and Nail Care

Patients apply proper cleansing and moisturizing techniques learned during the intensive phase of the treatment. Appropriate skin moisturizers should be applied twice daily to maintain the health and integrity of the skin.

Self-Manual Lymph Drainage

To stimulate lymph drainage, the patient performs simple self-MLD techniques and breathing exercises at least twice daily (refer to Chapter 5, Self-Manual Lymph Drainage).

Compression Therapy

Compression in this phase of the treatment is applied by compression garments, which have to be worn during the daytime hours. Measurements for compression garments are taken at the end of the decongestive phase, when the maximum level of decongestion is achieved. Measurement techniques for medical compression garments are documented in Chapter 5, Measurements for Compression Garments. At this time, the patient should be thoroughly instructed in donning techniques and garment care. The condition of the compression garment is evaluated during regular check-ups (at least every 6 months), and the patient's measurements are taken again to ensure proper fit. Compression garments should be replaced every 6 months or sooner if the material is damaged or has lost its elasticity. Patients should have at least two sets of compression garments—one to wear and one to wash.

As a general rule, the highest possible and most tolerable compression level should be used for lymphedema garments. In some cases of lower extremity lymphedema, it may be necessary to wear two compression garments, one on top of the other. As discussed earlier, the most important aspect is the patient's comfort level. In some cases, it may be necessary to select a compression garment of a lower pressure level to improve patient compliance. A compression garment that is worn inconsistently or not at all has no beneficial effect.

The severity and chronicity of the symptoms determine whether a lymphedema patient should continue to apply compression bandages during the night in this phase. Self-bandaging techniques are explained and illustrated in Chapter 5, Self-Bandaging.

Bandages may be applied on top of the compression garment during times with increased swelling or activities that may trigger the onset of swelling (airplane travel, standing over long periods of time, high-risk activities).

Decongestive Exercises

Patients should continue the exercise program to maintain and improve the treatment success. For maximum benefit, the compression garment or compression bandages should be worn during the exercise protocol. Patients are also encouraged to maintain the level of recreational activities discussed with the clinician during the intensive phase of the treatment. The exercise program and any recreational activities should be discussed and re-evaluated during regular check-ups with the physician and the lymphedema therapist.

Most patients are able to maintain and improve the results achieved during the intensive phase. The volume may continue to decrease and/or the tissue may continue to soften. A lack of progress, frequent relapses, or a permanent increase in limb volume during the second phase of CDT may be caused by the following:

- Lack of compliance, lack of hygiene.
- Recurrence of cancer.
- The severity of the symptoms (as discussed earlier, treatment progress may be slower in those patients with extreme lymphostatic fibrosis and sclerosis).
- Associated conditions (see Chapter 3, Complications in Lymphedema).

4.9 Documentation Techniques for Lymphedema

Documentation is necessary for several reasons. It serves as proof of the effectiveness of the therapy, which may be required by some insurance carriers for reimbursement, and it records the patient's progress. A reduction in limb volume not only indicates that the treatment is successful, but also encourages patient compliance.

Documentation values also determine the end of the decongestive phase and the beginning of the self-management phase.

Measures to use to determine the end of phase 1 and the beginning of phase 2 include photographic documentation and simple circumferential and volumetric measurements. Photographic documentation has the advantage of providing visual evidence of before and after effects of treatment, in addition to providing evidence of wound healing and changes in skin color. Simple circumferential measurements taken on defined areas of the extremity reflect a change in circumferential values of these areas. These values can be compared

with the uninvolved extremity (in unilateral involvement) but do not provide limb volume values. Circumferential measurements are also used to determine the appropriate size of the compression garment.

A variety of methods have been used over the years to determine limb volume, ranging from sophisticated imaging techniques (magnetic resonance imaging), bioelectrical impedance analysis, computed tomography, and the infrared photoelectronic perometer technique, tissue dielectric constant, to simple water displacement methods and geometrical calculations from limb circumference measurements using the truncated cone formula (see also Chapter 3, Measurement Issues in Lymphedema).

Each of these procedures has its advantages and disadvantages. Imaging techniques are costly and time-consuming and generally require equipment not available in lymphedema treatment centers. Perometers are more commonly used by treatment centers throughout the United States (▶ Fig. 4.22, **3.33**). These devices use infrared light transmitters to determine circumferential measurements, which are then used to calculate the volume of the limb using the truncated cone formula. The advantage of this device is that the measurements can be compared with built-in sizing charts of different compression garment manufacturers for upper and lower extremity garments. The sizing charts can also be customized to correlate with sizing charts of other garment manufacturers.

The water displacement method uses volumeters filled with water and equipped with an overflow spout and a beaker. The extremity is then partially or completely immersed in the water, and the displaced water is collected in the beaker. The amount of displaced water represents the extremity volume. Though theoretically an accurate and precise technique, the water displacement method cannot be used if wounds are present; furthermore, it is cumbersome to perform and provides no information on the shape of the extremity. However, the water displacement method provides a reliable modus to include hand and foot measurements in the total limb volume measurement.

Volume calculations using the truncated cone formula from girth measurements is a common and relatively precise method employed in lymphedema treatment centers. A swollen extremity can be viewed as a series of cones or cylinders.

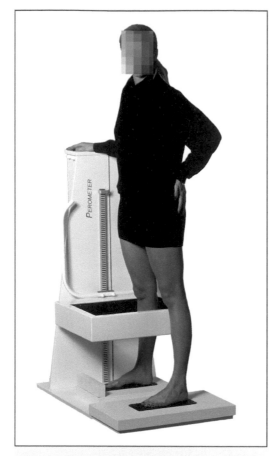

Fig. 4.22 Perometer. (Reproduced with permission of Juzo USA, Inc.)

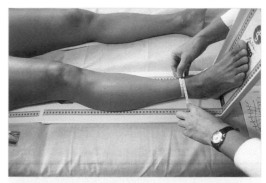

Fig. 4.23 Measuring board.

Circumferential measurements are made in intervals of typically 4 to 6 cm along the extremity (generally, the smaller the segments, the more accurate the geometrical values). The volume of each segment (or cone) is determined, and the total volume is calculated by summing the volumes of each individual segment. User-friendly computer programs for volumetric measurements are available from various sources.

General considerations: Accurate measurements are necessary to determine circumferential and volumetric values. If girth measurements are taken manually, the same examiner should take them each time. If several examiners are involved in measurements, a spring-loaded measuring tape should be used to maximize accuracy. Measurements should be taken on a measuring board (▶ Fig. 4.23) to ensure the same body position between different measuring sessions.

Measurements are taken on the exact same points each time; it is therefore necessary to document each measuring point on the patient's chart.

Measuring levels for simple circumferential measurements: Seven measuring points are recommended for the upper extremity—one on the hand, one on the wrist, two points on the forearm, one measurement on the cubital fossa, and two measurements on the upper arm (▶ Table 4.1). Similar number of measuring points are recommended for the lower extremity: one point on the foot, one at the ankle area, two on the lower leg, one measurement in the popliteal fossa, and two on the thigh are recommended (▶ Table 4.2). The location of the different measuring points should be determined by length measurements from the longest finger (in arm measurements) or from the heel/sole of the foot (in leg measurements) to ensure accuracy between measuring sessions.

Circumferential measurements to determine extremity volume: Incremental measurements of 3 cm should be used on the hand and foot (the water displacement method is usually a more reliable and easier to use method to determine hand or foot volumes). If hand or foot volumes are not included in the calculation, the circumferential measurements start at the wrist or ankle area and continue in increments of 4 cm along the extremity. The location of the initial measuring level is noted on the patient's chart.

Circumferential and/or volumetric measurements should be taken at least once a week to document treatment progress. Both techniques can be used for unilateral or bilateral involvement. In some cases, the uninvolved extremity shows some level of involvement in the swelling; in these cases, a reduction of the uninvolved extremity can be expected.

Table 4.1 Circumferential measurement chart for the upper extremity (UE) patient: Jane Doe, diagnosis: secondary UE lymphedema. Affected limb, right (), left (X), both ()

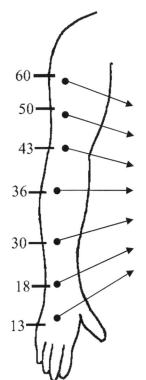

1/19		1/23	1/30	2/6
Measurements				
Right	Left	L	L	L
37	44	40.5	39.5	38
36	42.5	38	37	37
32	37	35	33.5	33
30	34.5	31.5	31	31
23	28.5	25	24.5	23.5
19	24	21.5	20.5	20
21	25.5	22.5	22	22

Measurements are taken in centimeters (2.54 cm = 1 in)
Weight
Date weight

	1/23	1/30	2/6
198 lb (90 kg)	196	193	193
Date measured			

Table 4.2 Circumferential measurement chart for the lower extremity (LE) patient: Jane Doe, diagnosis: primary LE lymphedema. Affected limb, right (X), left (), both ()

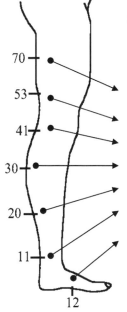

	11/10	11/14	11/17	11/21	11/24	11/28	12/1	12/4
Measurements								
Right	Left	R	R	R	R	R	R	R
127	59	110	116.5	86	89	81	79	79
129	51	109.5	112	84	87	79	77	75.5
82	38	71	68	53	51.5	47	47	46
81.5	38	70.5	68.5	59	59	47.5	43.5	43
69	30	59.5	58	49.5	47	40.5	39	38
34.5	25	31.5	30.5	28.5	27.5	27	27.5	27
33	25	30	30	30	30	27.5	27	27

Measurements are taken in centimeters (2.54 cm = 1 in)
Weight
Date weight

	11/14	11/17	11/21	11/24	11/28	12/1	12/4
305 lb (138.6 kg)	294	298	290	292	288	284	287
Date measured							

4.10 Complete Decongestive Therapy for Cancer Survivors

4.10.1 Introduction

CLTs treat persons with a current diagnosis or past history of cancer on a daily basis. It is imperative that lymphedema therapists are familiar with the disease of cancer and its comorbidities. Cancer interventions, including surgery, systemic therapy, and radiation must be documented in detail. Knowledge concerning specific cancer diagnoses, cancer therapies administered, and treatment side effects will improve safety and result in effective complete decongestive therapy (CDT).

According to the National Cancer Institute, cancer occurs as a result of unregulated growth and spread of abnormal cells.[11] Cancer can occur anywhere in the body, and is caused by environmental, behavioral, and genetic factors. A total of 1,685,210 new cancer cases and 595,690 cancer deaths are projected to occur in the United States in 2016. The lifetime probability of being diagnosed with cancer is 43% for men and 38% for women.[12] A cancer survivor is defined as a person who has been diagnosed as having cancer. This distinction lasts through treatment, recovery, and if the cancer recurs at a later date.

The incidence of lymphedema causing disruption of the inguinal or axillary lymph node beds is reported from 15 to 30%.[13] Women who had 10 or more lymph nodes removed from the axillary lymph node bed were more likely than women who had fewer lymph nodes resected to develop arm symptoms and subsequent lymphedema. Medical comorbidities, increasing age, weight gain, increase in BMI (body mass index), history of cellulitic infection in the effected limb, history of radiation therapy, axillary seroma, axillary web syndrome, chemotherapy, genetic predisposition, and axillary dissection are believed to contribute toward increasing a female breast cancer survivor's risk for lymphedema.[14]

It is becoming standard of care that breast cancer survivors undergo a lymphedema bioimpedance (Impedimed) and surveillance program at set intervals postoperatively. This gives the clinician a chance to evaluate the person, not only for lymphedema, but also for other comorbidities of cancer treatment. Pain (30–50% present), chemotherapy-induced peripheral neuropathy (average of 50–60% present), cancer-related fatigue (up to 80% present), and shoulder morbidity, balance, and the effects on strength/cardiorespiratory/

boney changes can be investigated as well as the swelling.[15] Other causes of lymphedema, such as melanomas are being evaluated as well. Bilateral involvement is not evaluated as of yet with the bioimpedance unit.

Another common complication of axillary surgery is axillary web syndrome (lymphatic cording), defined as a congestion of the lymphatic collectors. In 2009, axillary web syndrome was reported by Lacomba in 48.3% of women breast cancer survivors investigated.[16] According to earlier studies, lymphatic cording is often self-limiting and may spontaneously resolve.[17,18] This condition is variable but may appear as visible prominence of local lymphatic collectors originating in the proximal lateral trunk (named Mondor's syndrome) and extending through the axilla, the cubital fossa to the lateral thumb. Range of motion (especially shoulder abduction) and functional use of the involved extremity may be limited and interfere with effective delivery of radiation therapy and daily functional activities. The CLT may discover an axillary web as early as 1 week postoperatively. Lymphatic cording can persist and become chronic.[19] Axillary webbing is illustrated in ▶ Fig. 4.24.

Most commonly cancer-related lower extremity lymphedema occurs with uterine cancer, prostate cancer, lymphoma, or melanoma.[20] Following gynecological cancer, the prevalence of lymphedema is reported as high as 36% among vulvar cancer survivors and as low as 5% among ovarian cancer survivors. The onset of lower quadrant lymphedema is dependent upon the extent of surgery including lymph node resections (abdominal, pelvic, and inguinal), a history of abdominal or pelvic radiation, and presence of tumor burden in the pelvis or abdomen.[20] The at-risk quadrant is often bilateral lower extremities due to cancer therapies

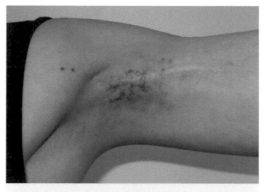

Fig. 4.24 Axillary web syndrome.

proximally with gynecological cancer. Early referral and CDT will decrease patient morbidity due to lower extremity and/or genital lymphedema.

There is a negative correlation between the presence of lymphedema and physical functioning, financial status and participation in social activities.

Appropriate cancer treatment is dependent upon the site of cancer, the tumor characteristics (hormone receptive), individual factors (age, medical comorbidities), and the cancer stage. Oncologists routinely use the TNM system of staging cancer where T represents the Tumor extent, N describes involvement of regional lymph nodes, and M defines the presence of distant metastasis.[21] Symbols following each of the above letters represent the extent of involvement, if known. These include X (unknown), 0 (no evidence of involvement), IS (pre-invasive), and 1 through 4 (describing the extent of involvement). Refer to ▶ Table 4.3 for details concerning the TNM classification system.

The cancer stage is determined considering the site of the primary tumor, the extent/size and number of tumors involved, the presence of lymph node involvement, the pathology report defining the tumor cells specifically, and the presence of distant metastasis. Cancer staging is generally 0 to IV, representing increasing involvement. Stage III cancer often indicates regional lymph node involvement.[21] Cancer prognosis is determined, allowing the CLT to develop an appropriate plan of care and developing treatment goals.

A condition related to cancer stage is cancer-related fatigue. It is present in up to 80% of all cancer survivors and is defined as a distressing, persistent, subjective sense of physical, emotional and/or cognitive tiredness or exhaustion related to cancer or its treatments, not proportional to recent activity and interrupts the persons' usual functioning. It occurs with other symptoms, such as pain,

distress, anemia, and sleep disturbances, and occurs in symptom clusters. It is therefore important that patients are screened for multiple symptoms that change according to location of cancer, type of treatment administered, and the stage of cancer. Rehabilitation for cancer-related fatigue should begin upon cancer diagnosis according to the National Comprehensive Cancer Network's recent publication, Version 2.2015.[22] Strategies such as interval aerobic training during peak energy times and gradually increasing the work time and decreasing the rest may help combat fatigue. Energy conservation is helpful. Decreasing the daytime rest to less than 1 hour helps decrease the nighttime disturbance of sleep. A person referred for lymphedema treatment must be questioned if they have cancer-related fatigue.

A number of studies have shown that aerobic and resistance exercises are safe and beneficial for people with lymphedema or at risk of lymphedema. The person needs to progress slowly, use recommended compression if indicated, and report any adverse effects to a professional, who will modify their exercise regimen.[23]

As stated previously, there is a direct relationship between BMI greater than 30 and the occurrence of lymphedema. Therefore, an increase in lean tissue is indicated. Exercise also combats cancer-related fatigue. Weight bearing exercises help prevent demineralization of bone. Exercise will help increase the ipsilateral weakness and range of motion/strength deficits seen as a result of disruption of the normal scapular humeral rhythm in those undergoing surgery and cancer therapies.

The CLT will need to access the client's written or electronic medical record. This may require written client permission. Persons undergoing cancer treatments currently or in the past may have difficulty recalling the details of their cancer treatments due to multiple appointments or a mild cognitive impairment. The CLT will need to

Table 4.3 TNM cancer classification

T = primary tumor	TX = primary tumor not identified T0 = absence of primary tumor Tis = preinvasive cancer. Abnormal cells locally. Cancer in situ T1, 2, 3, 4 = Tumor size and extent of involvement
N = regional lymph node	NX = regional nodes unable to be evaluated N0 = absence of regional lymph node involvement N1, 2, 3 = extent of regional lymph node involvement
M = distant metastasis	MX = metastasis unable to be evaluated M0 = absence of metastasis M1 = presence of metastasis

investigate the medical findings, past and present, in order to deliver safe and appropriate intervention. This is especially true for a person as the stage of cancer increases.

Treatments for cancer including surgery, radiation, and systemic therapy are reviewed in greater detail. All of these interventions have side effects that will affect CDT. Guidelines to improve the safety of CDT in persons with cancer are reviewed.

4.10.2 Surgery

According to the National Cancer Institute's Dictionary of Cancer Terms, surgery is described as a procedure in which affected areas are excised or repaired. Surgery may also be diagnostic.[24] Surgical interventions vary according to the site of cancer, the stage of cancer, and the surgeon's individual approach.

Surgery may follow clinical evaluation, diagnostic imaging, and laboratory testing that confirm the diagnosis of cancer. The primary goals of cancer surgery are to prevent cancer, assist in delivery of cancer therapies (port insertion), or to remove tumor burden. Individuals at high risk for developing cancer may undergo prophylactic surgery, even in the absence of cancer. If present, tumor may be removed and the appropriate at-risk areas treated with cancer therapies to prevent recurrence. Alternately, no distinct borders may be defined or larger/multiple tumors may be identified, leading to the diagnosis of later-stage cancer.

Subsequent surgery may be indicated in order to remove the remaining tumor and achieve cancer-free tissue margins adjacent to the tumor. In some cases, the entire tumor burden cannot be removed due to invasion of surrounding structures; the surgeon must decide if debulking the tumor is indicated. This is done to alleviate pain or

address disability, resulting in improved function, decrease pain, and/or increase survival.[25]

Breast surgery may consist of removal of the tumor while sparing the remaining healthy breast tissue. This type of surgery is often referred to as a lumpectomy or segmental mastectomy. Breast-conserving surgery is routinely followed by radiation therapy, often resulting in a firmer involved breast and asymmetrical breast tissue.[25] Whole breast irradiation, even with newer radiation techniques will deliver a dose of radiation to level I and level II lymph nodes, with resultant impairment in lymphatic function. Breast asymmetry following radiation therapy is depicted in ▶ Fig. 4.25.

Breast surgery may conserve the uninvolved part of the breast; however, if the lesion is large, the breast is small, there are multiple lesions in the breast, or the contralateral breast is at risk for cancer, mastectomy is often suggested.[25,26] Some women opt for an external prosthesis following removal of the entire breast or decide not to use any prosthetic device. An example of a simple mastectomy without reconstruction is illustrated in ▶ Fig. 4.26.

Surgery may also be performed in order to reconstruct a removed body part. This is an option often offered to women following breast cancer–related mastectomy. Some women opt for breast reconstruction in order to achieve symmetrical breasts, change their breast shape/size, or to avoid the use of an external prosthetic breast. Appropriate candidates for reconstructive surgery include younger nonsmokers with relatively little medical comorbidity. Persons with a tendency to scar, clotting disorders, diabetes mellitus, or a history of delayed healing may not be good candidates for these procedures.[25,26,27,28] Reconstruction can be immediate, at the time of initial surgery, with the

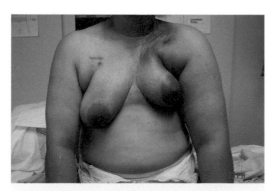

Fig. 4.25 Asymmetrical breasts following irradiation.

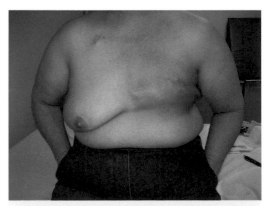

Fig. 4.26 Mastectomy in the absence of reconstruction.

breast surgeon and plastic surgeon working during the same surgical procedure. If radiation is planned following surgery, complications such as radiation fibrosis, encapsulated breast tissue, fat necrosis, or ipsilateral shoulder morbidity may present. Consequently, reconstruction is delayed until a later date.[27,28] ▶ Fig. 4.27 demonstrates reconstruction following radiation. The woman is offered choices concerning the type of reconstruction and the size of the replacement breast. ▶ Table 4.4 outlines some of the more common breast reconstructive procedures, including complications that the CLT may observe. In order to undergo any of the abdominal procedures, candidates must have adequate abdominal adipose.

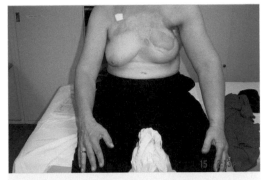

Fig. 4.27 Breast reconstruction with expander placement following radiation therapy. Note the presence of lymphedema in the left upper extremity.

Table 4.4 Breast reconstruction

Reconstructive approach	Procedure	Possible rehabilitation considerations
TRAM • Tissue flap • Transverse rectus abdominis muscle flap	• Pedicle flap = reflecting a portion of the rectus abdominis muscle and lower abdominal adipose with its blood supply and skin upward to create a breast mound. • Free flap = muscle and tissue create a breast mound through microvascular surgery.	• Areas of fat necrosis in the breast mound. • Residual weakness of rectus abdominis. • Hip flexor tightness and ipsilateral shoulder deficits. • Early posture abnormalities important, often flexed. • Low back pain.
Latissimus flap • Tissue flap • Latissimus dorsi	• Tunneling of a portion of the latissimus dorsi with its blood supply, adipose, and skin to create a breast mound.	• Residual weakness in the ipsilateral latissimus. • Ipsilateral shoulder deficits. • Asymmetry of back musculature—back pain. • Fat necrosis in the breast.
DIEP/SIEP • Deep inferior epigastric perforator/superficial inferior epigastric perforator • Microvascular surgery	• Tissue from the lower abdominal area with little rectus abdominis muscle creates a breast mound.	• Reduction in overall morbidity versus TRAM. • Fat necrosis in the breast mound. • Temporary weakness of rectus abdominis. • Hip flexor tightness and ipsilateral shoulder deficits. • Early posture abnormalities important—often flexed. • Low back pain.
SGAP • Microvascular surgery • Superior gluteal artery perforator	• Tissue including gluteus maximus, skin, blood supply, and adipose create a breast mound.	• Adherence to postoperative restrictions imperative. • Asymmetry of back resulting in low back pain. • Ipsilateral hip weakness. • Ipsilateral shoulder deficits.
Implant • Silicone or saline • Replacement necessary	• Immediate = definitive implant inserted at time of mastectomy. • Delayed = expander placed deep to the pectoralis major muscle. Gradually filled to stretch tissue. Definitive implant inserted at a later date.	• Breast capsular tightness. • Ipsilateral shoulder deficits. • Pectoralis major tightness. • Pressure or pain with filling. • Infection.

4

Adherence to all postoperative physical limitations is imperative. These limitations vary among surgeons. All women undergoing breast reconstruction have sensory deficits secondary to surgery. Lymphatic territories are often altered due to surgery, modifying manual lymph drainage (MLD) sequences.

4.10.3 Radiation Therapy

According to the National Cancer Institute's Dictionary of Cancer Terms, radiation (irradiation, radiotherapy) is defined as the use of high-energy radiation from X-rays, gamma rays, neutrons, protons, or other sources with the purpose of destroying cancer cells or reducing tumor burden. The source of radiation can be external, internal, or systemic.[24] Side effects of radiation can be early (acute) or late (chronic) and depend on the site of irradiation. Early effects depending on where the radiation is performed include involvement of rapidly dividing cells and may include alopecia, skin irritation (erythema, local disruptions, edema, mouth lesions), xerostomia (dry mouth that may

be permanent), bowel and/or bladder dysfunction, cancer-related fatigue, nausea, and perhaps vomiting. Early side effects of radiation therapy are illustrated in ▶ Fig. 4.28. Some late effects of local radiation therapy can include local tissue fibrosis, vital organ damage, bowel and bladder dysfunctions, changes in sexuality and fertility, skin fibrosis, bone demineralization, memory loss, muscle fibrosis, and lymphedema. ▶ Fig. 4.29 illustrates some of the late effects of radiation. A secondary cancer can occur following radiation, especially if treatment occurs when the patient is a child or adolescent.[29] The CLT must consider structures that have been included in the radiation field, usually surrounded by tattoos. Deep structures may be affected, which could include local vital organ compromise. Monitoring vital signs is important in persons undergoing radiation therapy.[30,31] The CLT avoids areas of painful or nonintact skin. The radiation oncologist must agree to MLD during radiation therapy.

The CLT will evaluate the radiation field and assess skin condition. In persons undergoing recent radiation, the skin may become reddened and friable. Although the reddened area fades, tissue changes from radiation therapy continue for years and result in decreased skin elasticity and hydration in the treated areas.[31] The amount of scar tissue that forms and the depth of involvement vary among cancer survivors, as does the radiation type and dose. Adherence of the skin and incisions within the radiation field impede superficial lymphatic flow, and may compromise CDT outcomes.

Local compression therapy is contraindicated in the radiation field during active treatment in order to preserve the prescribed dose and absorption. When compression is ordered by the radiation oncologist be prepared to discuss the rationale for

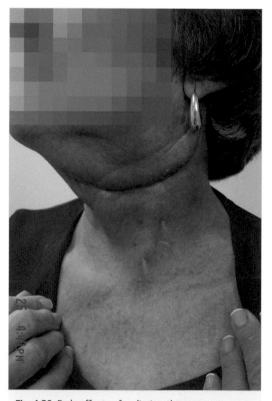

Fig. 4.28 Early effects of radiation therapy.

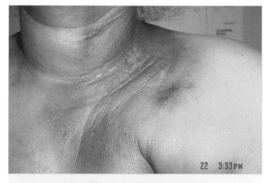

Fig. 4.29 Later effects of radiation therapy.

this contraindication. Care must be taken with manual therapy to avoid injury to irradiated tissue by friction or pulling, especially at the borders of adherent tissue. The tissues along the border of the radiation site may become hypermobile. Manual techniques are contraindicated in the presence of friable tissue, avoiding local trauma. Your radiation oncologist will guide you in safe treatment of persons undergoing radiation therapy.

4.10.4 Breast Radiation

Breast Conservation

Breast conservation is removal of a portion of the breast including the abnormal tissue and some surrounding healthy tissue in an effort to spare the residual breast. Whole breast radiation therapy is considered current standard of care in persons undergoing breast conservation. In 2014, the American Society for Radiation Oncology (ASTRO) guideline was developed for stage 1 and II breast cancer and use of radiation treatment including whole breast radiation. This is helping with mitigation of cancer in persons with positive margins, and therefore decreasing the need for surgery in this group.[32] In 2009, the ASTRO developed a guideline in early breast cancer including partial breast irradiation, focusing on local radiation to the tumor site, therefore shortening the treatment course to 1 week or less. The ASTRO recommends specific candidates be considered for partial breast irradiation including women with breast cancer who are 50 years or older, with a single tumor size less than 2 cm, identifiable margins, estrogen receptive positive, and lymph node negative disease.[33]

Mastectomy

A mastectomy includes removal of all ipsilateral breast tissue.[24] Radiation therapy is currently performed only in the presence of four or more positive lymph nodes or/and large or high-grade primary tumors.[25] Radiation therapy following mastectomy results in a decrease in locoregional recurrence.

New Breast Cancer Treatment Approaches

A systemic review performed in JAMA suggests that axillary node dissection is more harmful than beneficial in women undergoing breast-conserving

therapy who do not have palpable, suspicious lymph nodes, who have tumors 3.0 cm or smaller, and who have three or fewer positive nodes on sentinel node biopsy.[34]

The CLT knowledgeable about these new findings, as well as the current standard of care, in their referring medical facility will gain client confidence and improve CDT intervention. This information will assist the CLT in predicting current and future client needs for CDT.

4.10.5 Chemotherapy

Chemotherapy is the use of systemic antineoplastic agents with the goal of cancer cure, control of its progression, or palliation by interfering with the replication of deoxyribonucleic acid (DNA).[24] Adjuvant chemotherapy is administered following surgery or radiation in order to prevent recurrence from remaining microscopic cancer cells. Neoadjuvant chemotherapy is dispensed prior to surgery or radiation therapy with the goals of decreasing tumor burden, preventing morbidity, or improving the effect of subsequent cancer therapies.

Systemic treatment is often administered in combinations that have been proven by medical research to be most effective in eliminating cancer or improving duration of survival. Chemotherapy is given in cycles that coincide with the phase of DNA cell replication.

Persons undergoing current chemotherapy may experience several side effects. These side effects are agent dependent, with a direct relationship between side effect and administered dose. Possible side effects of chemotherapy can include alopecia, anemia, appetite changes, cognitive dysfunction, constipation, diarrhea, cancer-related fatigue, edema, infection, mucosal inflammation/openings, nausea and vomiting, peripheral neuropathy, pain, sexual and fertility issues, and urinary changes.[31]

Another side effect of chemotherapy may be chemotherapy-induced peripheral neuropathy (CIPN). This may be due to cytotoxic effects of the chemotherapy medications administered. The person may have a preexisting peripheral neuropathy from other medical comorbidities. Differing medical evidence document the incidence of CIPN as low as 30% and as high as 80% present. The cancer survivor may have sensory problems and motor problems as a result of administration of certain drugs. Platinum compounds, vincristine, taxanes, epothilones, bortezomib, thalidomides, lenalidome, and others are documented as leading to

CIPN. It usually begins in lower or upper extremities and proceeds up the extremities in a stocking and glove fashion. CPIN may start as sensory changes. Other times it may result in trouble with fine or gross motor dexterity. There are various medications including steroids, topical analgesics, antidepressants, antiseizure, opioids, and narcotics for treatment of CIPN. Physical and occupational or alternative therapies may be employed if function is disrupted and the problem becomes chronic.

It is imperative that the CLT familiarize himself/herself with possible side effects of each specific chemotherapeutic agent. Daily monitoring of the patient's medical status will allow safe and effective administration of CDT. This includes daily medical record review and current laboratory values with close monitoring of vital signs. Persons undergoing chemotherapy must be monitored due to rapid changes in medical status.[31] Refer to ▶ Table 4.5 for details.

4.10.6 Targeted Therapy

Targeted agents are used in cancer therapy in order to interrupt the cancer cell growth on a molecular level. Targeted therapy has fewer side effects than traditional chemotherapy due to reduced toxicity to normal tissue. Examples of targeted agents include small molecule tyrosine kinase and multikinase inhibitors, differentiating agents, angiogenesis inhibitors, monoclonal antibodies, proteosome inhibitors, histone deacetylase inhibitors, gene therapy strategies, and vaccines.

Resistance is problematic with kinase inhibitors, angiogenesis inhibitors, and monoclonal antibodies.

These agents are also generally considered not curative.

Currently, combining these agents with more conventional chemotherapy agents improves effective outcomes.

The CLT will need to become familiar with specific targeted therapy drugs, including side effects and treatment duration. Examples of more commonly administered targeted therapies for receptor-positive breast cancer survivors include the chemotherapeutic agent Herceptin and adjuvant hormone therapies of either tamoxifen (for premenopausal women) or aromatase inhibitors (for postmenopausal women).

4.10.7 Guidelines for Safe Complete Decongestive Therapy Intervention

A physician orders CDT after the cancer survivor has been medically cleared for participation. The CLT is a licensed professional and must work within the guidelines of their individual professional practice act.

Persons with cancer are medically fragile. The person's medical status is rapidly changeable, especially while undergoing cancer therapies. The physician should be contacted immediately if the patient has any new onset or increase in symptoms including fever, cardiac abnormalities, weakness or fatigue, leg pain or cramps, unusual joint pain, bruising, nausea, rapid weight loss, diarrhea or vomiting, changes in mental status, dizziness, blurred vision, fainting, gray or pale skin appearance, or night pain without a history of an injury.

Table 4.5 Chemotherapy daily certified lymphedema therapist checklist

Monitor	Daily questions	Observe
Pain	Cognition	Fluid retention/edema
Vital signs	Cancer-related fatigue	Skin/nails
Body weight	Appetite/diet	Hair loss
Body temperature Signs of infection	Constipation/diarrhea	
Chemotherapy-induced peripheral neuropathy		
Laboratory values INR Anemia Neutropenia		

Table 4.6 Frequent adverse medical findings in persons undergoing cancer therapies

Category	Finding	Cancer diagnosis	Signs and symptoms
Metabolic	Increase in calcium	Lung Esophageal Head and neck Cervical	Onset • Gastrointestinal (GI) symptoms Progression • Central nervous system symptoms Late • Renal symptoms
	Tumor lysis syndrome	Blood cancers with fast growing tumors Acute leukemia High-grade lymphoma Presents very infrequently with medical monitoring	Onset • Polyuria • Nausea/vomiting Progression • Muscle weakness • Joint pain Late • Fatigue, lethargic • Cardiac arrhythmias • Seizures • Cloudy urine
Hematologic	Febrile neutropenia	Active chemotherapy Fungal infections	Onset • Neutropenia Progression • Single oral body temp > 101 °F • 100.4 °F for > 1 h Late • Signs of local infection often absent • Septic shock
Structural	Spinal cord compression	Metastasis to spine Breast Lung Kidney Prostate Myeloma	Onset • Local back pain escalates while supine Progression • Paralysis • Numbness Late • Loss of bowel and bladder control
	Malignant pericardial effusion	Metastatic lung/breast Melanoma Leukemia Lymphoma Chemo to chest wall	Onset • Dyspnea • Cyanosis Progression • Venous distention in neck • Orthopnea
	Superior vena cava syndrome	Lung Lymphoma Central venous catheter	Onset • Facial swelling • Tight shirt collar • Ruddy complexion • Protruding eyes Progression • Upper extremity fullness/edema Late findings • Cardiopulmonary • central nervous system • GI

4

4

CDT may be interrupted for medical reasons. The CLT must call the medical team in order to apprise them of the cancer survivor's change in medical status. In cases of severe respiratory, cardiac, bleeding emergencies, sepsis, and hemodynamic findings, the cancer survivor is transferred to a hospital for emergent medical care.[35]

A worsening or rapidly progressing lymphedema is a sign of a local mass that may result in local vascular or neurologic compromise and must be reported to the referring physician.

Local pain, associated with distal progressive weakness and sensory changes may later present as a change in continence. This may indicate the presence of compression of neurologic tissue by tumor or unstable vertebral fracture and also must be reported to the physician.

The CLT may discover a recurrence of cancer while treating a cancer survivor. These suspicions may be best discussed with the referring medical professional in order to minimize patient anxiety. The CLT may palpate an area of fat necrosis or other tissue abnormalities that mimic a recurrence or new cancer.

Venous thromboembolic events occur four to seven times more frequently in persons with malignancies than in those without any.[36] Early symptoms of a deep venous thrombosis include swelling/pain and tenderness while standing or walking/heat as well as erythema of the affected extremity. Persons with pulmonary emboli present with dyspnea, tachycardia, a cough, hemoptysis, chest pain, increase in respiratory rate, and anxiety.[37]

The CLT monitors subjective and objective data daily and is familiar with the cancer survivor's medical status. As a result, the lymphedema therapist arrives at an appropriate and safe clinical decision concerning the interruption of CDT and level of appropriate medical care. ▶ Table 4.6 reviews the most frequent cancer, medical findings, and signs and symptoms in detail.

4.10.8 Summary

Cancer survivors will consistently seek the expertise of the CLT for evaluation and treatment of lymphedema. The CLT knowledgeable about cancer and its comorbidities will be able to safely and effectively intervene at any time during cancer survivorship.

References

[1] Kwan ML, Cohn JC, Armer JM, Stewart BR, Cormier JN. Exercise in patients with lymphedema: a systematic review of the contemporary literature. J Cancer Surviv. 2011; 5(4):320–336

[2] Schmitz KH, Ahmed RL, Troxel AB, et al. Weight lifting for women at risk for breast cancer-related lymphedema: a randomized trial. JAMA. 2010; 304(24):2699–2705

[3] Keilani M, Hasenoehrl T, Neubauer M, Crevenna R. Resistance exercise and secondary lymphedema in breast cancer survivors-a systematic review. Support Care Cancer. 2016; 24 (4):1907–1916

[4] Nelson NL. Breast cancer-related lymphedema and resistance exercise: a systematic review. J Strength Cond Res. 2016; 30 (9):2656–2665

[5] Dieli-Conwright CM, Orozco BZ. Exercise after breast cancer treatment: current perspectives. Breast Cancer (Dove Med Press). 2015; 7:353–362

[6] Katz E, Dugan NL, Cohn JC, Chu C, Smith RG, Schmitz KH. Weight lifting in patients with lower-extremity lymphedema secondary to cancer: a pilot and feasibility study. Arch Phys Med Rehabil. 2010; 91(7):1070–1076

[7] NLN. Position Statement of the National Lymphedema Network. Exercise 2011. http://www.lymphnet.org/pdfDocs/nl-nexercise.pdf. Accessed June 20, 2012

[8] Schmitz KH, Ahmed RL, Troxel A, et al. Weight lifting in women with breast-cancer-related lymphedema. N Engl J Med. 2009; 361(7):664–673

[9] Cheema BS, Kilbreath SL, Fahey PP, Delaney GP, Atlantis E. Safety and efficacy of progressive resistance training in breast cancer: a systematic review and meta-analysis. Breast Cancer Res Treat. 2014; 148(2):249–268

[10] Ostby PL, Armer JM. Complexities of adherence and post-cancer lymphedema management. J Pers Med. 2015; 5(4):370–388

[11] National Cancer Institute. http://www.cancer.gov/publications/dictionaries/cancer- terms?expand=C. Published May 15, 2015. Accessed October 30, 2015

[12] Siegel RL, Miller KD, Jemal A. Cancer statistics, 2016. CA Cancer J Clin. 2016; 66:7–30

[13] Silver JK, Baima J, Mayer RS. Impairment-driven cancer rehabilitation: an essential component of quality care and survivorship. CA Cancer J Clin. 2013; 63(5):295–317

[14] Drouin JS, Morris GS. Oncology Section EDGE Task Force breast cancer outcomes: a systemic review of clinical measures of cardiorespiratory fitness tests. Rehabilitation Oncology.. 2015; 33(2):24–36

[15] Schmitz KH, DiSipio T, Gordon LG, Hayes SC. Adverse breast cancer treatment effects: the economic case for making rehabilitative programs standard of care. Support Care Cancer. 2015; 23(6):1807–1817

[16] Torres Lacomba M, Mayoral Del Moral O, Coperias Zazo JL, Yuste Sánchez MJ, Ferrandez JC, Zapico Goñi A. Axillary web syndrome after axillary dissection in breast cancer: a prospective study. Breast Cancer Res Treat. 2009; 117(3):625–630

[17] Leidenius M, Leppänen E, Krogerus L, von Smitten K. Motion restriction and axillary web syndrome after sentinel node biopsy and axillary clearance in breast cancer. Am J Surg. 2003; 185(2):127–130

[18] Moskovitz AH, Anderson BO, Yeung RS, Byrd DR, Lawton TJ, Moe RE. Axillary web syndrome after axillary dissection. Am J Surg. 2001; 181(5):434–439

[19] Black J, Green D, McKenna C, Squadrito J, Taylor S, Palombaro KM. Therapists' perspectives and interventions in the

management of axillary web syndrome: an exploratory study. Rehabil Oncol. 2014; 32(4):16–22

[20] Kim JH, Choi JH, Ki EY, et al. Incidence and risk factors of lower-extremity lymphedema after radical surgery with or without adjuvant radiotherapy in patients with FIGO stage I to stage IIA cervical cancer. Int J Gynecol Cancer. 2012; 22 (4):686–691

[21] American Joint Committee on Cancer. www.cancerstaging. org. Accessed October 31, 2015

[22] National Comprehensive Cancer Network. NCCN Clinical Practice Guidelines in Oncology: Cancer-Related Fatigue. Version 2.2015. Fort Washington, PA: National Comprehensive Cancer Network, 2015

[23] Schmitz KH. Exercise for secondary prevention of breast cancer: moving from evidence to changing clinical practice. Cancer Prev Res (Phila). 2011; 4(4):476–480

[24] National Cancer Institute. Dictionary of cancer terms. http:// www.cancer.gov/dictionary?CdrID=45570. Accessed October 31, 2015

[25] Moran MS, Schnitt SJ, Giuliano AE, et al. Society of Surgical Oncology-American Society for Radiation Oncology consensus guideline on margins for breast-conserving surgery with whole-breast irradiation in stages I and II invasive breast cancer. Int J Radiat Oncol Biol Phys. 2014; 88(3):553–564

[26] Paul H, Jr, Prendergast TI, Nicholson B, White S, Frederick WA. Breast reconstruction: current and future options. Breast Cancer (Dove Med Press). 2011; 3:93–99

[27] Ogunleye AA, de Blacam C, Curtis MS, Colakoglu S, Tobias AM, Lee BT. An analysis of delayed breast reconstruction outcomes as recorded in the American College of Surgeons National Surgical Quality Improvement Program. J Plast Reconstr Aesthet Surg. 2012; 65(3):289–294

[28] Hirsch EM, Seth AK, Dumanian GA, et al. Outcomes of tissue expander/implant breast reconstruction in the setting of pre-reconstruction radiation. Plast Reconstr Surg. 2012; 129 (2):354–361

[29] Tukenova M, Diallo I, Anderson H, et al. Second malignant neoplasms in digestive organs after childhood cancer: a cohort-nested case-control study. Int J Radiat Oncol Biol Phys. 2012; 82(3):e383–e390

[30] McGale P, Darby SC, Hall P, et al. Incidence of heart disease in 35,000 women treated with radiotherapy for breast cancer in Denmark and Sweden. Radiother Oncol. 2011; 100(2):167–175

[31] Miller KD, Triano LR. Medical issues in cancer survivors–a review. Cancer J. 2008; 14(6):375–387

[32] Jin J. JAMA PATIENT PAGE. Breast Cancer Screening Guidelines in the United States. JAMA. 2015; 314(15):1658

[33] Smith BD, Arthur DW, Buchholz TA, et al. Accelerated partial breast irradiation consensus statement from the American Society for Radiation Oncology (ASTRO). Int J Radiat Oncol Biol Phys. 2009; 74(4):987–1001

[34] Rao R, Euhus D, Mayo HG, Balch C. Axillary node interventions in breast cancer: a systematic review. JAMA. 2013; 310 (13):1385–1394

[35] Demshar R, Vanek R, Mazanec P. Oncologic emergencies: new decade, new perspectives. AACN Adv Crit Care. 2011; 22 (4):337–348

[36] Morris GS, Brueilly KE, Paddison NV. Oncologic emergencies: implications for rehabilitation. Top Geriatr Rehabil. 2011; 27 (3):176–183

[37] Foulkes M. Nursing management of common oncological emergencies. Nurs Stand. 2010; 24(41):49–56, quiz 58

Recommended Reading

Bringezu G, Schreiner O. Die Therapieform Manuelle Lymphdrainage. Lübeck: Verlag Otto Haase; 1987

Camrath J. Physiotherapie—Technik und Verfahrensweise. Stuttgart: Thieme Verlag; 1983

Chikly B. Who discovered the lymphatic system. Lymphology. 1997; 30(4):186–193

Despopoulos A, Silbernagel P. Color Atlas of Physiology. 5th ed. New York: Thieme; 2003

Eliska O, Eliskova M. Are peripheral lymphatics damaged by high pressure manual massage? Lymphology. 1995; 28(1):21–30

Földi E. Massage and damage to lymphatics. Lymphology. 1995; 28 (1):1–3

Földi E, Földi M, Weissleder H. Conservative treatment of lymphoedema of the limbs. Angiology. 1985; 36(3):171–180

Guyton A, Hall J. Textbook of Medical Physiology. 9th ed. Philadelphia, PA: WB Saunders; 1996

Hutzschenreuther P, Bruemmer H, Silberschneider K. Die Vagotone Wirkung der Manuellen Lymphdrainage nach Dr. Vodder. Lymph-Forsch. 2005; 7(1):7–14

Hutzschenreuter P, Ehlers R. Effect of manual lymph drainage on the autonomic nervous system [in German]. Z Lymphol. 1986; 10 (2):58–60

International Society of Lymphology. The diagnosis and treatment of peripheral lymphedema. Consensus document of the International Society of Lymphology. Lymphology. 2003; 36(2):84–91

Kuhnke E. Die Volumenbestimmung entrundeter Extremitäten aus Umfangsmessung. Eine Analyse der Fehler und die Möglichkeiten zu ihrer Beseitigung. Z Lymphol. 1978; 02(1):35

Kuhnke E. Wirkung und Wirksamkeit – Nachweismöglichkeiten unter besonderer Berücksichtigung manueller Behandlungsverfahren. Z Lymphol. 1978; 02(1):15: (Fortbildungsteil)

Kurz I. Einführung in die manuelle Lymphdrainage nach Dr. Vodder: Therapie I/II. 3rd ed. Stuttgart: Haug Verlag; 1984

Position Statement of the National Lymphedema Network on Exercises. http://www.lymphnet.org/pdfDocs/nlexercise.pdf

Melzack R, Wall PD. The Challenge of Pain. 2nd ed. London: Penguin Books; 1996

NLN. Position paper of the National Lymphedema Network. Lymphedema risk reduction practices. http://www.lymphnet.org/ pdfDocs/nlnriskreduction.pdf. Accessed June 27, 2012

Sander AP, Hajer NM, Hemenway K, Miller AC. Upper-extremity volume measurements in women with lymphedema: a comparison of measurements obtained via water displacement with geometrically determined volume. Phys Ther. 2002; 82(12):1201–1212

Schmitz KH, Ahmed RL, Troxel A, et al. Weight lifting in women with breast-cancer-related lymphedema. N Engl J Med. 2009; 361 (7):664–673

Tierney S, Aslam M, Rennie K, Grace P. Infrared optoelectronic volumetry, the ideal way to measure limb volume. Eur J Vasc Endovasc Surg. 1996; 12(4):412–417

Vodder E. Die technischen Grundlagen der manuellen Lymphdrainage. Phys Ther. 1983; 4(1):16–23

4

Chapter 5

Treatment

5 Treatment

5.1 General Considerations

The techniques outlined in this chapter should not be substituted for the thorough instructions provided in comprehensive lymphedema management courses offered by qualified training centers. As with many manual techniques, the skills required to deliver adequate intervention using all components of complete decongestive therapy (CDT) cannot be learned from reading a book, watching videos, or attending weekend classes. A high level of competency and skill is needed to master all components of CDT and to provide patients with a proper degree of intervention. The quality of training will have a great impact on the level of care the patients receive or do not receive. CDT and its components have been practiced safely and effectively in Europe for many decades and became the standard of treatment for lymphedema in the 1970s, when the National Health Insurance System in Germany started to reimburse for lymphedema treatment. To ensure proper teaching standards, training centers in Germany have to comply with strict guidelines specified by professional organizations in the training and certification of lymphedema instructors as well as therapists. Certain organizations in the United States have acknowledged the need for certification programs in lymphedema management to ensure a base of knowledge considered fundamental in the treatment of lymphedema and related conditions.

5.2 Application of Basic MLD Techniques on Different Parts of the Body

The four basic techniques of Dr. Vodder's manual lymph drainage (MLD)—stationary circle, pump, scoop, and rotary—their effects on the lymphatic system, and the contraindications for MLD are discussed in Chapter 4. Additional techniques incorporated into MLD sequences are soft and rhythmic strokes known as *effleurage*. This method is adopted from more traditional massage techniques and is used to stimulate local sympathetic activity and to promote directional flow of lymph.

The techniques and sequences outlined in the following sections are applied in conditions where edema is present, but the lymph nodes are not removed or treated with irradiation. Examples include posttraumatic and postoperative swelling, lower extremity edema caused by pregnancy, swellings caused by partial or complete loss of mobility (pareses, paralysis), reflex sympathetic dystrophy (when swelling is present), migraine headache (swelling is present in the perivascular areas of intracranial blood vessels), cyclic idiopathic edema, and rheumatoid arthritis. Selected indications are cited in the appropriate sections.

Basic treatment sequences may also be used to accomplish a general increase in lymph circulation or to achieve a common soothing effect by decreasing sympathetic activity.

In the treatment of lymphedema, these techniques are used to improve lymph production and lymph angiomotoricity, as well as to promote the lymphatic return from the drainage areas described in Chapter 4 (Intensive Phase) to the venous system. In the lymphedematous extremity and/or body part, the treatment sequences are modified accordingly, as outlined later in this chapter.

Common denominators to all techniques and sequences are the following:

- Hand positions of all basic strokes are adapted to the anatomy and physiology of the lymphatic system.
- *Central pretreatment*: Areas closest to the venous angles and regional groups of lymph nodes are stimulated first. This allows for drainage of the peripheral areas. At extremities, the stimulation begins proximal and is continued toward distal, in accordance with the direction of the lymph drainage.
- *Stroke intensity*: The applied pressure in individual strokes should be enough to utilize full elasticity of the skin and subcutaneous tissues, and to promote lymph formation and lymph angiomotoricity. Too much pressure may cause unwanted vasodilation and lymphangiospasm.
- *Stroke sequence*: Each technique consists of a working and resting phase, during which the manual pressure increases and decreases gradually. The goal in the working phase is to promote lymph formation, lymph angiomotoricity, and directional flow by stretching the anchoring filaments and smooth musculature located in the wall of lymph angions. The suction effect created in the resting phase results in a refilling of lymph collectors with lymph fluid from more distal areas.

- *Stroke duration*: The relatively high viscosity of lymph fluid requires the working phase to last approximately 1 second. To ensure adequate reaction of the lymph collectors to the manual stimuli, the strokes should be repeated five to seven times in one area.
- *Working direction of the strokes*: The direction of the strokes depends on the anatomical actualities and generally follows the physiological patterns of lymphatic drainage. If surgery, radiation, or trauma results in an interruption of regular drainage pathways, it will become necessary to redirect the lymph flow around the blocked areas and toward regions with sufficient lymph flow patterns.

5.2.1 Lateral Neck and Submandibular Area

Selected indications: Pretreatment for other drainage areas; postsurgical (oral, dental, plastic surgery, etc.) and posttraumatic swellings (whiplash injury, others); migraine headache; partial treatment for primary head and neck lymphedema; general increase in lymph circulation, or to achieve a common soothing effect by decreasing sympathetic activity.

An abbreviated sequence is used if the lateral neck serves as a pretreatment for other drainage areas. This shorter sequence consists of the first three techniques used in the complete sequence (see the following).

Patient in supine position; therapist on the patient's side:
1. Effleurage, two or three times from the sternum to the acromion.

2. Manipulation of the inferior cervical lymph nodes; stationary circles in the supraclavicular fossa (horizontal plane).
3. Manipulation of the deep lateral cervical lymph nodes (▶ Fig. 5.1).
4. Stationary circles from the earlobe to the supraclavicular fossa in two hand placements, if necessary (sagittal plane).
5. Manipulation of the parotid and retroauricular lymph nodes (▶ Fig. 5.2).
6. Stationary circles with fingers in front of and behind the ear, followed by reworking the deep lateral cervical lymph nodes as in step 3 (both placements in sagittal plane).

Patient in supine position; therapist at the head-end of the patient:
1. Manipulation of submandibular lymph nodes (▶ Fig. 5.3). Stationary circles with distal phalanges (2–5) from the tip of the chin in the direction of the angle of the jaw (superior cervical lymph nodes). Two hand placements if necessary (phalanges in horizontal plane). This technique is followed by reworking the deep lateral cervical lymph nodes as in step 3.

Patient in supine position; therapist on the patient's side:
1. Manipulation of the shoulder collectors. Stationary circles in two hand placements, which should cover the area located cranial to the anterior and posterior upper horizontal watershed. First hand placement on the acromion and second hand placement on the medial shoulder (both placements in horizontal plane).
2. Effleurage (as in step 1).

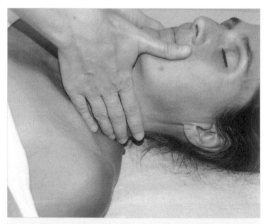

Fig. 5.1 Stationary circles on the lateral cervical lymph nodes.

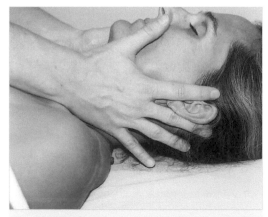

Fig. 5.2 Stationary circles on the lymph nodes in front of and behind the ear.

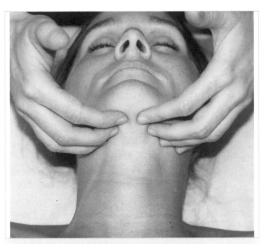

Fig. 5.3 Stationary circles on the submandibular lymph nodes.

5.2.2 Abbreviated Neck Sequence

Review ▶ Fig. 5.4 for drainage areas on the lateral neck.

1. Effleurage, two or three times from the sternum to the acromion.
2. Manipulation of the inferior cervical lymph nodes. Stationary circles in the supraclavicular fossa (horizontal plane).
3. Manipulation of the deep lateral cervical lymph nodes (▶ Fig. 5.1).
   a) Stationary circles from the earlobe to the supraclavicular fossa in two hand placements, if necessary (sagittal plane).

5.2.3 Posterior Neck and Occipital Area

Selected indications: postsurgical (oral, dental, plastic surgery, etc.) and posttraumatic swellings (whiplash injury, others); migraine headache; partial treatment for primary head and neck lymphedema; general increase in lymph circulation, or to achieve a common soothing effect by decreasing sympathetic activity (▶ Fig. 5.5).

   Pretreatment: Lateral neck.

   Patient in prone position; therapist at the head-end of the patient:

1. Effleurage, two or three times starting at the back of the head and following the descending trapezius muscle to the acromion.
2. Manipulation of the deep lateral cervical lymph nodes. Stationary circles starting at the angle of

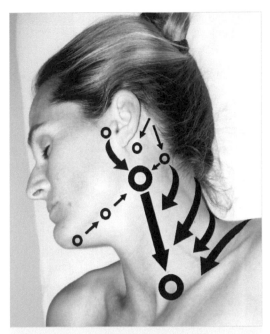

Fig. 5.4 Drainage areas for the lateral neck.

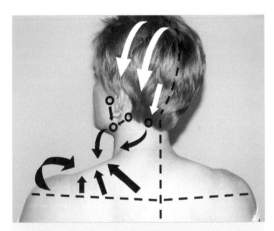

Fig. 5.5 Drainage areas for the posterior neck and occipital area.

the jaw in the direction of the supraclavicular fossa (sagittal plane). Two hand placements if necessary.
3. Manipulation of the occipital and parietal region. Alternating stationary circles in several tracks, starting on the posterior head toward the parietal area (frontal plane). Working phase in the direction of the occipital and retroauricular lymph nodes.

5

4. Manipulation of the parotid and retroauricular lymph nodes.
   a) Stationary circles with fingers in front of and behind the ear, followed by reworking the deep lateral cervical lymph nodes as in step 2 (both placements in sagittal plane).
5. Manipulation of the shoulder collectors. Alternating pump techniques on both shoulders, starting at the acromion, following the upper trapezius muscle in the direction of the supraclavicular fossa. Both hands in horizontal plane.
6. Manipulation of the inferior cervical lymph nodes. Bimanual thumb circles in the supraclavicular fossa (horizontal plane).

Patient in prone position; therapist on the patient's side:
1. Manipulation of the paravertebral lymph nodes and vessels.
   a) Stationary circles paravertebrally with the finger pads (working deep).
2. Effleurage (as in step 1).

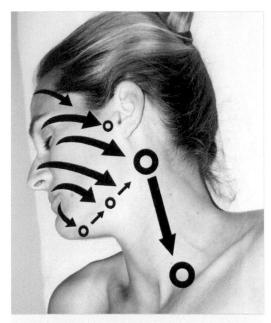

Fig. 5.6 Drainage areas for the face.

5.2.4 Face

Selected indications: postsurgical (oral, dental, plastic surgery, etc.) and posttraumatic swellings (whiplash injury, etc.); migraine headache; partial treatment for primary head and neck lymphedema; general increase in lymph circulation, or to achieve a common soothing effect by decreasing sympathetic activity (▶ Fig. 5.6).

Pretreatment: Lateral neck (posterior neck if necessary).

Patient in supine position; therapist at the head-end of the patient:
1. Effleurage, two or three times along lower jaw, upper jaw, the cheek, and the forehead in the direction of the angle of the jaw (following the pathway of the collectors).
2. Manipulation of the submental and submandibular lymph nodes (▶ Fig. 5.3).
3. Stationary circles with distal phalanges (2–5) from the tip of the chin in the direction of the angle of the jaw (superior cervical lymph nodes). Two hand placements if necessary (phalanges in horizontal plane). This technique is followed by stationary circles along the deep lateral cervical lymph nodes (sagittal plane).
4. Manipulation of the lower and upper jaw. Alternating stationary circles working toward the submandibular lymph nodes. This

technique is followed by stationary circles in the direction of the angle of the jaw and the supraclavicular fossa as described in step 2.
5. Manipulation of the lymph vessels in the area of the bridge of the nose and cheek.
6. Alternating stationary circles starting at the bridge of the nose, to include the lower eyelid, toward the cheeks. This technique is followed by the technique described in step 2, with the purpose of manipulating the lymph fluid toward the supraclavicular fossa.
7. Manipulation of the upper eyelid and eyebrows. Alternating stationary circles (one or more fingers) in the direction of the preauricular lymph nodes (option: eyebrow roll).
8. Manipulation of the forehead and temporal area. Stationary circles starting at the middle of the forehead, traveling to the temple with the working phase directed toward the preauricular lymph nodes.
9. Manipulation of the parotid and retroauricular lymph nodes.
10. Stationary circles with fingers in front of and behind the ear, followed by stationary circles along the deep lateral cervical lymph nodes (sagittal plane).
11. Effleurage (as in step 1).

5

5.2.5 Posterior Thorax

The treatment area is outlined by the lower horizontal watershed (caudal limitation), the upper horizontal watershed (cranial limitation), and the sagittal watershed (medial limitation) (▶ Fig. 5.7).

Selected indications: Pretreatment for unilateral secondary upper extremity lymphedema (this sequence is applied on the healthy quadrant); postsurgical and posttraumatic swellings; general increase in lymph circulation, or to achieve a common soothing effect by decreasing sympathetic activity.

Pretreatment: Lateral neck (abbreviated; see lateral neck sequence, steps 1–3).

Patient in prone position; therapist contralateral to the healthy quadrant:

1. Manipulation of the axillary lymph nodes. Stationary circles bimanually with flat hands between the latissimus dorsi and pectoral muscles (sagittal plane), with the working direction toward the apex of the axilla (subclavian trunk).
2. Effleurage, two or three times in several pathways, starting at the posterior sagittal watershed in the direction of the axillary lymph nodes (following the pathway of the collectors).
3. Manipulation of the lateral thorax.
   a) Stationary circles alternating and dynamic from the horizontal watershed toward the axillary lymph nodes (sagittal plane). This sequence follows the thoracic portion of the inguinal axillary (IA) anastomosis.
4. Manipulation of the posterior thorax (▶ Fig. 5.8). Rotary techniques in several tracks starting at the sagittal watershed in the direction of the axillary lymph nodes (following the

pathway of the collectors). This technique should cover the entire treatment area as outlined previously (▶ Fig. 5.7).
5. Manipulation of the posterior and lateral thorax. Combination of alternating rotary techniques (upper and lower hands) starting at the sagittal watershed (lower hand is parallel to and just above the lower horizontal watershed). The rotary techniques travel alternating toward the lateral direction until the thoracic portion of the IA anastomosis is reached. Dynamic stationary circles follow this technique as outlined in step 3.
6. Manipulation of the posterior axillo-axillary (PAA) anastomosis.
   a) Bimanual stationary circles, with the working phase directed toward the axillary lymph nodes. The hands are aligned parallel with the sagittal watershed (frontal plane).
7. Manipulation of the paravertebral lymph nodes and vessels (if necessary).
   a) Stationary circles paravertebrally with the finger pads (working deep).
8. Manipulation of intercostal lymph vessels. Stationary circles, with the finger pads working from lateral placements to medial placements, using wavelike movements, with pressure working deep (perforating precollectors).
9. Effleurage (as in step 1).

5.2.6 Lumbar Area

The treatment area is outlined by the lower horizontal watershed (cranial limitation), the horizontal gluteal fold (caudal limitation), and the sagittal watershed (medial limitation; ▶ Fig. 5.8).

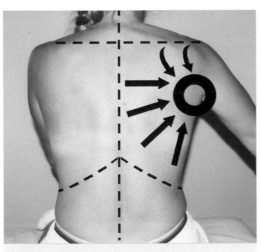

Fig. 5.7 Drainage areas for the posterior thorax.

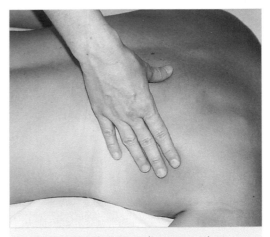

Fig. 5.8 Rotary technique on the posterior thorax.

Selected indications: Pretreatment for unilateral secondary and primary lower extremity lymphedema (this sequence is applied on the healthy quadrant); phlebolymphostatic edema; lipedema and lipolymphedema; postsurgical and posttraumatic swellings; general increase in lymph circulation, or to achieve a common soothing effect by decreasing sympathetic activity.

Pretreatment: Lateral neck (abbreviated; see lateral neck sequence, steps 1–3), abdomen, inguinal lymph nodes.

Patient in prone position; therapist contralateral to the healthy quadrant:

1. Effleurage, two or three times in several pathways, starting at the posterior sagittal watershed toward the inguinal lymph nodes (remaining in the lumbar quadrant).
2. Manipulation of the lumbar area.
   a) Alternating rotary techniques from the sagittal watershed toward the hip (ASIS, anterior superior iliac spine). The upper hand is parallel to and just below the lower horizontal watershed; the lower hand follows the collectors of the posterior interinguinal (PII) anastomosis.
3. Manipulation of the PII anastomosis.
   a) Bimanual stationary circles simultaneously on the PII anastomosis, with working direction toward the inguinal lymph nodes. Both hands are parallel to the sagittal watershed (frontal plane).
4. Manipulation of the paravertebral lymph nodes and vessels (if necessary).
   a) Stationary circles paravertebrally with the finger pads (working deep).
5. Effleurage (as in step 1).

5.2.7 Anterior Thorax

The treatment area is outlined by the lower horizontal watershed (caudal limitation), the upper horizontal watershed (cranial limitation), and the sagittal watershed (medial limitation; ▶ Fig. 5.10).

Selected indications: Pretreatment for unilateral secondary and primary upper extremity lymphedema (this sequence is applied on the healthy quadrant); postsurgical and posttraumatic swellings; general increase in lymph circulation, or to achieve a common soothing effect by decreasing sympathetic activity.

Pretreatment: Lateral neck (abbreviated; see lateral neck sequence, steps 1–3).

Patient in supine position; therapist contralateral to the healthy quadrant:

1. Manipulation of the axillary lymph nodes. Bimanual stationary circles, with flat hands between the latissimus dorsi and pectoral muscles (sagittal plane), with the working direction toward the apex of the axilla (subclavian trunk).
2. Effleurage, two or three times in several pathways (following the collectors), starting at the anterior sagittal watershed in the direction of the axillary lymph nodes (not over the nipple).
3. Manipulation of the lymph vessels in the healthy mammary gland.
4. This technique is performed with a combination of alternating and dynamic pump and rotary techniques. The lower hand starts with dynamic pump techniques in three placements in the direction of the axillary lymph nodes: the first placement is on the mammary fold, the second placement in the glandular tissue, and the third placement below the nipple. The

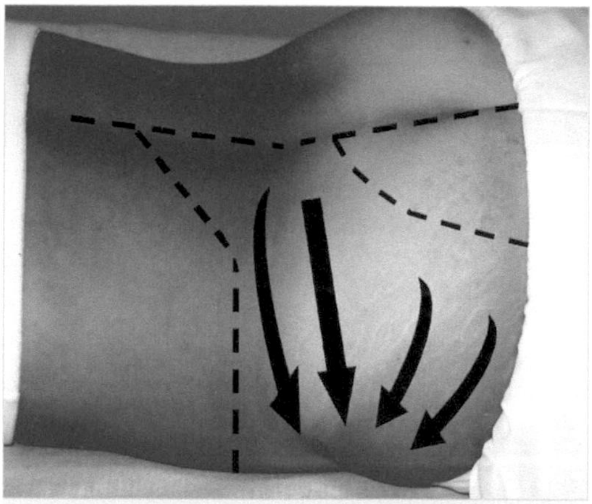

![Fig. 5.9 Drainage areas for the lumbar area.]

Fig. 5.9 Drainage areas for the lumbar area.

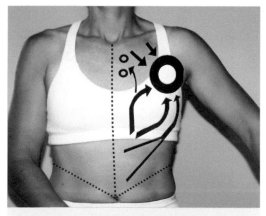

Fig. 5.10 Drainage areas for the anterior thorax. Arrows indicate direction of lymph drainage.

upper hand uses rotary techniques starting at the anterior sagittal watershed, following a line below the upper horizontal watershed in three hand placements toward the axillary lymph nodes.

5. Manipulation of the lateral thorax.
6. Dynamic and alternating stationary circles from the lower horizontal watershed toward the axillary lymph nodes (sagittal plane). This sequence follows the thoracic portion of the IA anastomosis.
   a) Manipulation of the anterior and lateral thorax. Combination of alternating rotary techniques (upper and lower hands) starting at the anterior sagittal watershed (lower hand is parallel to and just above the lower horizontal watershed). The rotary techniques travel alternating in the lateral direction until the thoracic portion of the IA anastomosis is reached. The technique is then followed by dynamic stationary circles, which follow the IA anastomosis toward the axillary lymph nodes (as outlined in step 4).
7. Manipulation of the anterior axillo-axillary (AAA) anastomosis.
8. Bimanual stationary circles, with the working phase directed toward the axillary lymph nodes. The hands are aligned parallel with the anterior sagittal watershed (frontal plane).
9. Manipulation of the parasternal lymph nodes and vessels (if necessary).
10. Stationary circles parasternally with finger pads (working deep).
11. Manipulation of intercostal lymph vessels (▶ Fig. 5.11). Stationary circles with three or four finger pads working from lateral placements to medial placements, using wavelike movements with pressure working deep (perforating precollectors).
12. Effleurage (as in step 2).

5.2.8 Abdomen (Superficial and Deep Manipulations)

Refer to the list of local contraindications for the abdominal area in Chapter 4, Contraindications for Manual Lymph Drainage. Abdominal techniques should not be applied if they cause pain or discomfort, or directly following meals. Patients should empty their bladder before treatment starts.

Abdominal sequences can be separated into superficial and deep techniques. The skillful manipulation of the intra-abdominal areas, especially

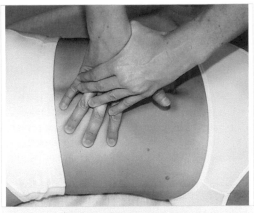

Fig. 5.11 Intercostal technique on the anterior thorax.

when combined with diaphragmatic breathing, results in increased lymph transport within the thoracic duct and larger lymphatic trunks. A decongestive effect on organ structures located within the abdominal and pelvic cavities, as well as on lymphatic drainage areas located more distally (the lower extremities), is additionally realized when performing abdominal techniques.

Selected indications: part of the treatment sequence for lower extremity lymphedema (primary and secondary) as well as lymphedema involving the external genitalia; chronic venous insufficiency (CVI) stages II and III (phlebolymphostatic edema); lipedema and lipolymphedema; part of the treatment sequence for primary lymphedema of the genitalia; part of the treatment sequence for upper extremity lymphedema (particularly with removal or irradiation of both axillary lymph node groups); part of the treatment for cyclic idiopathic edema; general increase in lymph circulation.

Superficial Abdominal Treatment (Modified)

Pretreatment: Lateral neck (abbreviated; see lateral neck sequence, steps 1–3).

Patient in supine position; with the legs and the head elevated and the arms resting on the patient's side; therapist on patient's right side (next to pelvis):

1. Effleurage.
   a) Two or three times starting at the pubic bone, following the rectus abdominis muscle to the xiphoid process, then along the thoracic cage and the iliac crest back to the pubic bone.

b) Two or three times following the ascending, transverse, and descending part of the colon.
2. Manipulation of the colon.
   a) *Descending colon:* The right hand is placed on the descending colon, with the fingertips on the thoracic cage and the fingers pointing up toward the midclavicular point. This is a two-handed technique; the bottom hand (right hand) is in contact with the skin and remains passive; pressure is applied with the left hand, which rests on top of the right hand. *Working phase:* Moderate (but soft) pressure is applied down into the abdomen (deep), then along and in the direction of the descending colon (caudal), ending in a partial supination directed toward the cisterna chyli. The hand relaxes in the resting phase, and the tissue elasticity carries the hand back to the starting position. This sequence is repeated two or three times.
   b) *Ascending colon:* The therapist is on the patient's right side (next to the thorax, facing the direction of the patient's feet). The right hand is placed on the ascending colon, with the fingertips near the inguinal ligament and the fingers pointing downward toward the pubic bone. The right hand, which is in contact with the skin, remains passive; pressure is applied with the left hand, which rests on top of the right hand. *Working phase:* Moderate (but soft) pressure is applied down into the abdomen (deep), then along and in the direction of the ascending colon (cranial), ending in a partial supination directed toward the cisterna chyli. The hand relaxes in the resting phase, and the tissue elasticity carries the hand back to the beginning position. This sequence is repeated two or three times.
   c) Effleurage (as in step 1).

Deep Abdominal Treatment (Modified)

With this technique, the caudal part of the thoracic duct, the cisterna chyli, the larger lymphatic trunks, the pelvic and lumbar lymph nodes, and the organ structures with their lymphatic system are stimulated. Deep abdominal sequences are applied on five different hand placements on the abdominal area and are combined with the patient's diaphragmatic breathing (▶ Fig. 5.12). To avoid hyperventilation, the therapist performs only one sequence per placement. Ideally, the placements on the thoracic cage and in the center of the abdomen are repeated during the full sequence, resulting in a total of nine manipulations (depending on the patient's reaction). During each manipulation, the therapist's hand follows the patient's exhalation into the abdominal area and offers moderate (but soft) resistance to the initial subsequent inhalation phase. The therapist then releases the resistance and stays in skin contact until the end of the inhalation phase. The hand is moved to the next placement on the abdomen during the pause between inhalation and the next exhalation phase. To avoid discomfort, the hand, which is in contact with the patient's skin, remains soft and passive. Pressure is applied with the top hand, which rests on top of the working hand.

Pretreatment: Lateral neck (abbreviated; see lateral neck sequence, steps 1–3).

Patient in supine position, with the legs and the head elevated and the arms resting on the patient's side; therapist on the patient's side, with the hand placements as follows:
1. Center of the abdomen, over the umbilicus (this placement should be avoided if a pulsating aorta is felt with the soft and passive hand).

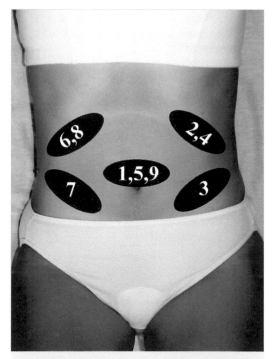

Fig. 5.12 Hand placements for the deep abdominal technique.

2. Below and parallel with the thoracic cage on the contralateral side.
3. Above and parallel with the inguinal ligament on the contralateral side.
4. Repeat step 2.
5. Repeat step 1.
6. Below and parallel with the thoracic cage on the ipsilateral side.
7. Above and parallel with the inguinal ligament on the ipsilateral side.
8. Repeat step 6.
9. Repeat step 1.

5.2.9 Upper Extremity

Selected indications: Postsurgical and posttraumatic swellings (including edema caused by immobility due to partial or complete paralysis); reflex sympathetic dystrophy; rheumatoid arthritis; lipedema; general increase in lymph circulation, or to achieve a common soothing effect by decreasing sympathetic activity.

Pretreatment: Lateral neck (abbreviated; see lateral neck sequence, steps 1–3 and shoulder collectors).

Patient in supine position; therapist on the patient's side ipsilateral to the involved quadrant (in sequences 1–3, the therapist stands next to the patient's head):

1. Manipulation of the axillary lymph nodes. Stationary circles on the axillary lymph nodes in two hand placements; the hand closer to the patient's head is working, the other hand holds the arm in proper elevated position.
2. Effleurage, two or three times covering the entire arm.
3. Manipulation of the medial aspect of the upper arm. Stationary circles with the hand closer to the patient's head, beginning on the medial epicondyle. Several hand placements are applied to cover the medial upper arm, with the working phase direction toward the axillary lymph nodes. The other hand holds the patient's arm in a comfortable and elevated position.
4. Manipulation of the tissues covering the anterior and posterior portion of the deltoid muscle. Stationary circles bimanually and alternating on the anterior and posterior portion of the deltoid muscle; the working phase is directed toward the axillary lymph nodes.
   Note: In the treatment of upper extremity lymphedema, the working phase of this sequence is directed toward the AAA and PAA anastomoses (► Fig. 5.13).

5. Manipulation of the lateral aspect of the upper arm. Pump technique, with the hand closer to the patient's head on the lateral upper arm in several placements from the lateral epicondyle toward the acromion. The other hand holds the patient's arm in a comfortable and elevated position.
   a) Combination of pump technique and stationary circle (alternating hands) on the lateral aspect of the upper arm, beginning at the lateral epicondyle in several hand placements toward the olecranon.
6. Manipulation of the antecubital fossa.
   a) Thumb circles (one hand or alternating) covering the antecubital fossa from ~5 cm below to ~5 cm above. Several pathways are applied to cover the antecubital fossa from distal to proximal. This area can also be treated using stationary circles with the palmar surfaces of the fingers.
7. Manipulation of the forearm.
   a) Scoop techniques with one hand on the anterior and posterior aspect of the forearm between the wrist and the elbow. To manipulate both aspects with the same

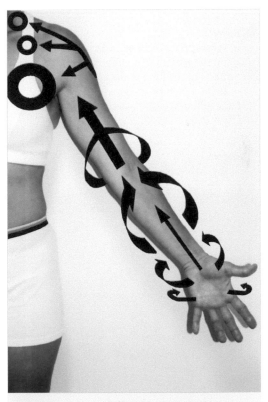

Fig. 5.13 Drainage areas for the upper extremity.

hand, the patient's forearm is rotated in pronation and supination, respectively. The other hand holds the patient's arm at the wrist in a comfortable and elevated position.

b) Combination of pump technique and stationary circles between the wrist and the elbow to cover the patient's anterior and posterior aspects of the forearm. The patient's forearm is rotated in pronation and supination, respectively, to cover both surfaces.

8. Manipulation of the dorsum of the hand and wrist. Thumb circles (one thumb or alternating) over dorsum of the hand and posterior wrist, starting on the metacarpophalangeal (MP) joints, ending at the styloid processes.

9. Manipulation of the palmar aspect of the hand and the anterior wrist (▶ Fig. 5.14).

a) Thumb circles (one thumb or alternating) in the palm, following the ulnar and radial bundle from the center of the palm toward the ulnar and radial edges of the hand (following the path of the collectors).

10. Manipulation of the fingers.

a) Combination of thumb/finger circles on each individual finger from the distal to the proximal ends.

11. Rework.

a) Appropriate techniques are used (depending on the patient's condition) covering specific parts of the limb or the entire extremity to increase lymph angiomotoricity.

12. Final effleurage (as in step 2).

5.2.10 Lower Extremity

Selected indications: Postsurgical (joint replacement, etc.) and posttraumatic swellings (including edema caused by immobility due to partial or complete paralysis); CVI stages II and III (phlebolymphostatic edema); lipedema; part of the treatment sequence for primary lymphedema of the genitalia; part of the treatment for cyclic idiopathic edema; general increase in lymph circulation, or to achieve a common soothing effect by decreasing sympathetic activity.

Pretreatment: Lateral neck (abbreviated; see lateral neck sequence, steps 1–3), abdomen.

Anterior Leg

Patient in supine position, with the leg slightly abducted and externally rotated; therapist on the patient's involved side:

1. Manipulation of the inguinal lymph nodes. Stationary circles with both hands at the same time, with the working phase directed toward the inguinal ligament; three hand placements in the medial femoral triangle (▶ Fig. 5.15).

a) *First hand placement:* The upper hand lies parallel to the inguinal ligament (the fifth metacarpophalangeal joint is aligned with the patient's ASIS), and the lower hand is positioned diagonally to the upper hand (with the fingertips touching the inguinal ligament).

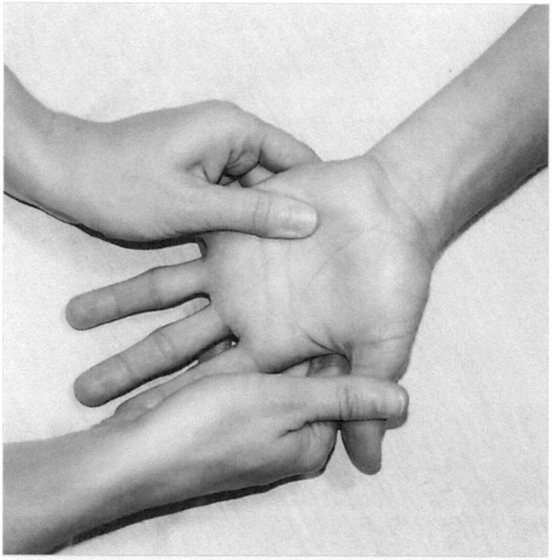

Fig. 5.14 Thumb circles on the palm (ulnar bundle).

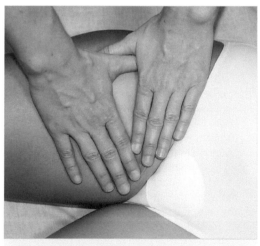

Fig. 5.15 Stationary circles on the inguinal lymph nodes (second hand placement).

b) *Second hand placement*: The same hand positions are applied on the medial thigh (medial aspect of the femoral triangle).

c) *Third hand placement*: Both hands lie parallel on the medial aspect of the thigh (sagittal plane) to address the lymph nodes located in the distal apex of the medial femoral triangle.

2. Effleurage, two or three times covering the entire leg.

3. Manipulation of the anterior thigh.
   a) Alternating pump techniques following the rectus femoris muscle between the base of the patella and the ASIS.

4. Manipulation of the anterior and lateral thigh. Combinations of pump techniques and stationary circles with alternating hands, beginning at the knee to proximal. The lateral pathway follows the iliotibial tract; the anterior pathway follows the rectus femoris muscle.

5. Manipulation of the medial thigh.
   a) Stationary circles alternating and dynamic at the medial thigh, beginning at the medial aspect of the knee to the groin (sagittal plane).

6. Manipulation of the knee.
   a) Pump technique in several hand placements (three or four) covering the anterior knee.
   b) Stationary circles (dynamic and simultaneously) on the medial and lateral knee, covering the knee from distal to proximal.
   c) Stationary circles in several hand placements covering the popliteal fossa from distal to proximal.
   d) Stationary circles (bimanual and simultaneous) below the medial aspect of the knee ("bottleneck" area).

7. Manipulation of the lower leg.
   a) Scoop technique alternating at the calf between the malleoli and the popliteal fossa (patient's knee is flexed). Either hand can be used by the therapist. Pump technique on the anterior aspect of the lower leg, scoop technique on the calf (alternating and dynamic), between the malleoli and the knee.

8. Manipulation on the foot.
   a) Stationary circles (simultaneous and dynamic) between the malleoli and the Achilles tendon in several hand placements.
   b) Thumb circles (one thumb or alternating) covering the dorsum of the foot and the ankle. Thumb circles may start on the toes or the metatarsophalangeal (MTP) joints.

9. Rework.
   a) Appropriate techniques are used (depending on the patient's condition), covering specific parts of the limb, or the entire extremity to increase lymph angiomotoricity.

10. Final effleurage (as in step 2).

Posterior Leg

The treatment of the posterior leg with the patient in the prone position is recommended in those cases where the decongestion of the limb does not advance as expected ("stubborn legs") with the treatment in supine, or if the swelling is more distally emphasized (e.g., larger swelling on the lower leg). The techniques on the posterior leg are similar to the sequences for the anterior leg (▶ Fig. 5.16, ▶ Fig. 5.17). Manipulation of the inguinal lymph nodes in the supine position precedes the treatment of the posterior leg (▶ Fig. 5.15).

Patient in prone position, with the leg slightly abducted; therapist on the patient's same side:

1. Effleurage, two or three times covering the entire leg.

2. Manipulation of the posterior thigh.

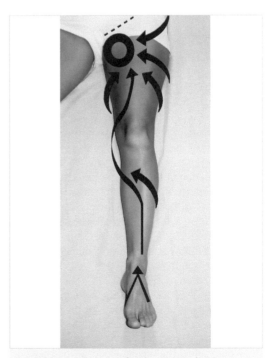

Fig. 5.16 Drainage areas for the anterior lower extremity.

5

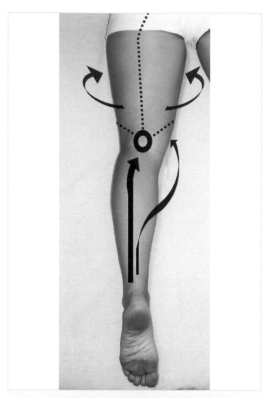

Fig. 5.17 Drainage areas for the posterior lower extremity.

3. Alternating pump techniques between the popliteal fossa and the horizontal gluteal fold (frontal plane).
4. Manipulation of the medial thigh.
   a) Stationary circles alternating and dynamic at the medial thigh, beginning at the medial aspect of the knee to the groin (sagittal plane).
5. Manipulation of the posterior and lateral thigh. Combinations of pump techniques and stationary circles with alternating hands, beginning at the popliteal fossa to proximal. The lateral pathway follows the iliotibial tract; the posterior pathway follows the posterior thigh musculature in a frontal plane.
6. Manipulation of the knee.
   a) Stationary circles or pump techniques covering the popliteal fossa from distal to proximal (three or four hand placements).
   b) Stationary circles (bimanual and simultaneous) below the medial aspect of the knee ("bottleneck" area).
7. Manipulation of the lower leg.

a) Alternating pump techniques in several hand placements covering the calf musculature between the heel and the popliteal fossa.
   b) Combination of pump techniques and stationary circles covering the calf musculature between the heel and the popliteal fossa in several hand placements. Thumb circles (one thumb or alternating) between the malleoli and the Achilles tendon. To include joint and muscle pump functions, this technique can be combined with passive ankle movements.
8. Rework.
   a) Appropriate techniques are used (depending on the patient's condition) covering specific parts of the limb, or the entire extremity to increase lymph angiomotoricity.
9. Final effleurage (as in step 1).

5.3 Treatment Sequences

In the treatment of lymphedema, in particular in those cases where lymph node groups are removed and/or irradiated, some of the sequences outlined earlier in section "Application of Basic MLD Techniques on Different Parts of the Body" are modified. These modifications are noted in the appropriate sections in the text.

In many cases of extremity lymphedema, the ipsilateral truncal quadrant (this may include the external genitalia) is also congested.

5.3.1 Truncal Lymphedema

Lymphedema affecting the chest, breast, and posterior thorax, also known as truncal lymphedema, is a common problem following breast cancer surgery, but it is often difficult to diagnose, especially if the patient does not also present with lymphedema of the arm, or it may be dismissed as a side effect of breast cancer surgery, which will resolve by itself over time.

While truncal lymphedema is often not reported or is poorly documented, and available studies are not easy to compare, the literature suggests an incidence of up to 70% of lymphedema affecting the trunk and/or breast following breast cancer treatment.

Given the fact that the breast, anterior and posterior thorax, and the upper extremity share the axillary nodes as regional lymph nodes (**Fig. 1.7**, **Fig. 1.8**, **Fig. 1.17**), it is predictable that disruption of lymphatic drainage pathways by partial or complete removal of axillary lymph nodes, with or without radiation therapy, can cause the onset of swelling in the chest wall and breast on the same side. The swelling can either be subtle or quite obvious in presentation and may be present with or without swelling in the arm.

The disruption of the natural lymphatic drainage pattern is further complicated by scars on the upper trunk wall following lumpectomy, mastectomy, and reconstructive breast surgery, biopsies, or drain sites. Fibrotic tissues in the chest wall or armpit following radiation treatments may further inhibit sufficient lymphatic drainage.

Certain breast reconstructive procedures, such as the TRAM-flap reconstruction, also disrupt lymphatic drainage in the abdominal area, which may cause the onset of additional swelling in the lower truncal (abdominal) area.

Like lymphedema in the extremities, swelling affecting the breast, chest, and posterior thorax is typically asymmetrical in appearance if compared with the other side (▶ Fig. 5.18). However, there are often other symptoms present prior to the onset of visible swelling, which can include altered sensation (numbness, tingling, diffuse fullness and pressure, and heat), pain, and decreased shoulder mobility. Once lymphedema is visibly present, the swelling can include the entire thorax wall, or it can be localized to the armpit, the scapula, the area over the clavicle or around mastectomy or lumpectomy scar lines, around the reconstructed breast or implants, or it may be limited to the breast tissue only.

The breast in patients who have undergone lumpectomy or reconstructive surgery may be larger and heavier, or the shape and height of the breast tissue may change due to fibrotic tissue, resulting in added psychological distress due to problems involving clothing, bra fitting, and body image issues.

Postoperative swelling following breast cancer surgery is to be expected and generally lasts up to about 3 months; it appears almost immediately following surgery and places additional stress on the lymphatic system by contributing to the lymphatic workload. The difference between "normal" postoperative edema and lymphedema is its perseverance following the completion of treatment, and the presence of changes in tissue texture, such as lymphostatic fibrosis.

While several methods are available to assess truncal and breast edema (skinfold calipers, bioimpedance), subjective examination of the anterior and posterior aspect of the thorax and breast focused on the observation of signs of swelling (asymmetry, bra strap and seam indentations, orange peel phenomenon, changes in skin color), palpation of the tissue texture, and comparison of skinfolds between the affected and unaffected sides, remain the most practical means for assessment of lymphedema affecting the trunk. Serial photographs depicting the anterior and posterior view are helpful tools in assessing changes before and after treatment.

Most of the symptoms associated with truncal lymphedema can be treated successfully with CDT. Treatment may be necessary only during the initial period following breast cancer treatment to facilitate edema removal and wound healing, or it may be applied at a later point; truncal lymphedema with or without the involvement of the arm may appear at any time following surgery for breast cancer.

MLD: Due to the fact that truncal involvement is difficult to identify, particularly if obesity is a factor, it is recommended to generally assume truncal involvement in extremity lymphedema, in which case the decongestion of the involved trunk has priority over the treatment of the swollen extremity, and the truncal preparation is more complex. MLD techniques concentrate on the neck, the anterior and posterior aspects of the upper trunk, as well as the inguinal lymph nodes, followed by techniques focused to redirect lymphatic fluid from congested areas into areas with sufficient lymphatic drainage. If necessary, additional techniques aimed to soften fibrotic tissues may also be

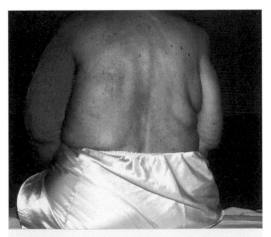

Fig. 5.18 Truncal lymphedema on the left side.

applied. The treatment sequences listed in section "Unilateral Secondary Upper Extremity Lymphedema" are based on this assumption.

Once the adjacent truncal quadrant is successfully decongested (this is generally the case if volume reduction in the involved extremity is noted), the treatment of the lymphedematous extremity becomes the priority, and the truncal preparation may be abbreviated.

For patients who have undergone TRAM-flap procedures, careful attention should be given to address scar tissue that could lead to trapping of lymphatic fluid.

During the initial stages of the treatment, patients should be instructed for self-MLD (see 5.20.4) and encouraged to perform self-treatment for at least 20 to 30 minutes daily.

Skin Care

Areas between skinfolds on the trunk and the underside of the breast are particularly prone to skin damage and infections. Edematous areas should be kept clean and dry and suitable ointments or lotions formulated for sensitive skin, radiation dermatitis, and lymphedema should be applied (refer to section "Skin and Nail Care" in Chapter 4 for more information on skin care).

Exercises

Truncal lymphedema is often associated with restrictions in thorax and shoulder movements, which should be evaluated by a physical therapist. Specific exercises addressing these issues and to increase range of motion and function with daily activities should be performed.

Depending on the location and quality of scars, mobilization of adherent scar tissue by a qualified therapist may be necessary to improve range of motion. Breathing and aerobic exercises further facilitate decongestion by improving drainage in superficial and deep lymphatic pathways.

Compression Therapy

Frequently, compression of the affected area may be challenging due to tenderness of the tissue, or irritated skin secondary to radiation therapy. However, to address fluid accumulation and to avoid worsening of the swelling, the application of compression bandages and/or compression bras or

vests is very important. Compression bandages are applied circumferentially around the chest with special care not to impair blood supply to grafts and/or healing scars.

Owing to the lack of muscle pump activity in the truncal area, the use of wide-width (15–20 cm), medium, and long-stretch bandages is preferable over the normally used short-stretch bandages for lymphedema affecting the extremities.

Custom-cut or commercially manufactured foam pads (▶ Fig. 5.19) or foam chips may be inserted underneath the bandages or compression bra or vest to increase localized pressure in areas of excess fluid pooling, or to soften localized fibrotic tissue. Flat foam pieces can be used to shape and stabilize the compression bandages and to distribute the pressure evenly over a greater surface area.

The patient should be fitted with a specially designed lymphedema bra (▶ Fig. 5.19) or compression vest following decongestion of the trunk to assist with maintaining the positive results of CDT. Compression bras and vests have minimal seams and wide straps, are available as off-the-shelf or custom-made garments, and ensure that the trunk and breast tissues are properly supported. Compression bras and vests should fit comfortably, provide sufficient support around the trunk, and not squeeze breast tissue; pockets to accommodate a prosthesis can be sewn into these garments.

Patients using regular bras or sports bras should make sure to avoid narrow bra straps and obtain bra strap pads or wideners, if necessary, to avoid restriction of lymphatic pathways on the shoulder.

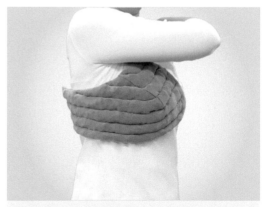

Fig. 5.19 Compression foam pad (with permission from Solaris, WI).

5.3.2 Unilateral Secondary Upper Extremity Lymphedema

This condition is most often the result of mastectomy or lumpectomy with the removal and/or irradiation of the axillary lymph nodes in breast cancer surgery.

The following sequence should be used until the truncal quadrant is decongested (▶ Fig. 5.20).

Patient in supine position:
1. Abbreviated manipulation of the lateral neck lymph nodes, including the shoulder collectors (observe contraindications).
2. Activation of the axillary lymph nodes on the contralateral side. Anterior thorax on the contralateral side (omit intercostal and parasternal techniques).
3. Activation and utilization of the AAA anastomosis to move lymph fluid from the affected to the unaffected side.
4. Manipulation of the inguinal lymph nodes on the ipsilateral, affected side.

Therapist moves to the other side of the treatment table:
1. Activation and utilization of the AI anastomosis on the affected side.
2. Manipulation of lymph fluid from the congested upper quadrant in the direction of the inguinal lymph nodes on the same side, utilizing the AI anastomosis. Rotary techniques and stationary circles should be used.

3. Intercostal and parasternal techniques on the affected trunk quadrant to utilize deep drainage pathways.

Patient on the side (or prone position), with the affected extremity on top:
1. Rework of the AI anastomosis and shoulder collectors.

Patient in prone position (or on the side):
1. Posterior thorax on the unaffected side (omit intercostal and paravertebral techniques).
2. Activation and utilization of the PAA anastomosis to move lymph fluid from the affected to the unaffected side. Stationary circles should be used.

Therapist moves to the other side of the table:
1. Manipulation of lymph fluid from the congested posterior upper quadrant in the direction of the inguinal lymph nodes on the same side, utilizing the AI anastomosis. Rotary techniques and stationary circles should be used.
2. Intercostal and paravertebral techniques on the affected trunk quadrant to utilize deep drainage pathways.

Patient on the side (or prone position), with the affected extremity on top:
1. Rework of PAA anastomosis, AI anastomosis, and shoulder collectors.

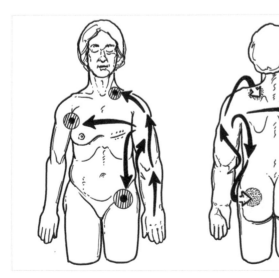

Fig. 5.20 Drainage directions for unilateral lymphedema on the upper extremity.

Patient in supine position:

1. Rework of AAA anastomosis, axillary lymph nodes on the contralateral side, and inguinal lymph nodes on the ipsilateral side.
2. Application of compression bandages on the involved extremity.

The following sequence should be used if the truncal quadrant is decongested and the treatment of the upper extremity is the primary focus:

Patient in supine position. Abbreviated trunk preparation (pretreatment):

1. Abbreviated manipulation of the lateral neck lymph nodes, including the shoulder collectors (observe contraindications).
2. Manipulation of the axillary lymph nodes on the contralateral side.
3. Activation and utilization of the AAA anastomosis to stimulate lymph flow from the affected to the unaffected side.
4. Manipulation of the inguinal lymph nodes on the ipsilateral (affected) side.

Therapist moves to the other side of the table:

1. Activation and utilization of the AI anastomosis on the affected side to stimulate lymph flow toward the drainage area.

Patient on the side (or prone position), with the affected extremity on top:

1. Rework of AI anastomosis and shoulder collectors.
2. Activation and utilization of the PAA anastomosis to stimulate lymph flow from the affected to the unaffected side.

> If the upper extremity is considerably swollen, it is not recommended to treat the entire extremity during a single session. The treatment should proceed in steps; for example, only the upper arm (or parts of it) may be treated, which prevents overload of the healthy lymphatics in the drainage areas.

3. Manipulation of the lateral upper arm between the lateral epicondyle and the acromion, using basic techniques ("bulk flow" techniques).
4. Rework of shoulder collectors, AI, and PAA anastomosis.

Patient in supine position:

1. Rework of AAA anastomosis.
2. Manipulation of the lateral upper arm between the lateral epicondyle and the acromion. Modified effleurage as well as pump techniques and combination of pump and stationary circles should be used (see techniques lateral upper arm). This sequence should be followed up with rework techniques across the watershed into pretreated drainage areas.
3. Manipulation of the medial aspect of the upper arm toward the lateral aspect, using stationary circles (dynamic technique). This technique should be followed up with rework techniques of drainage areas as in step 11. The entire length of the upper arm is treated in this manner.
4. Vasa vasorum technique in the area of the cephalic vein (**Fig. 4.9**).
5. Manipulation of elbow, forearm, and hand as outlined in the basic sequence techniques.
6. If necessary, edema or fibrosis techniques should be incorporated at this point.
7. Rework of upper extremity, AAA anastomosis, axillary lymph nodes on contralateral side, inguinal lymph nodes on ipsilateral side, and shoulder collectors.

Patient on the side (or prone position), with the affected extremity on top:

1. Rework of the PAA and AI anastomoses (on the same side).
2. Application of compression bandages on involved extremity.

5.3.3 Bilateral Secondary Upper Extremity Lymphedema

This condition is most often the result of mastectomy or lumpectomy with the removal and/or irradiation of the axillary lymph nodes in breast cancer surgery. Ideally, bandages should be applied on both upper extremities. If this is not possible, compression bandages should be applied to the more involved extremity.

The following sequence should be used until the truncal quadrant(s) is/are decongested (▶ Fig. 5.21).

Patient in supine position:

1. Abbreviated manipulation of the lateral neck lymph nodes, including the shoulder collectors (observe contraindications).
2. *Abdominal treatment*: Superficial and deep (modified) techniques as outlined in the basic

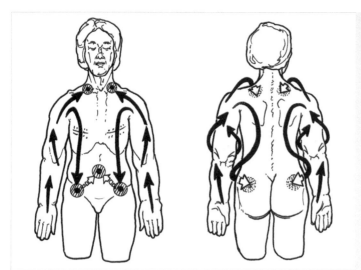

Fig. 5.21 Drainage directions for bilateral lymphedema on the upper extremities.

sequences (observe contraindications). If abdominal techniques are contraindicated, diaphragmatic breathing should be used to substitute.

3. Manipulation of the inguinal lymph nodes on both sides.
4. Activation and utilization of the AI anastomoses on both sides to promote lymph flow from the congested quadrants to the drainage areas.
5. Manipulation of lymph fluid from the congested upper quadrants in the direction of the inguinal lymph nodes, utilizing the AI anastomoses. Rotary techniques and stationary circles should be used.
6. Intercostal and parasternal techniques on both affected trunk quadrants to utilize deep drainage pathways.

Patient in prone position (or on side):
1. Rework of both AI anastomoses.
2. Manipulation of lymph fluid from the congested posterior upper quadrants in the direction of the inguinal lymph nodes, utilizing the AI anastomoses. Dynamic rotary techniques and stationary circles should be used.
3. Intercostal and paravertebral techniques on both affected trunk quadrants to utilize deep drainage pathways.

Patient in supine position:
1. Rework of AI anastomoses on both sides, deep abdominal technique (modified), inguinal lymph nodes on both sides, and shoulder collectors.
2. Application of compression bandages on both, or the more involved extremity.

The following sequence should be used if the truncal quadrant(s) is/are decongested and the treatment of the upper extremities becomes the primary focus.

> It is not recommended to treat both extremities in the same session. The more involved extremity should be treated first until decongested, then fitted with a compression sleeve. If the extremity is considerably swollen, it should be treated in steps; for example, only the upper arm (or parts of it) should be treated, which prevents overload of the healthy lymphatics in the drainage areas.

Therapy proceeds with the other arm, once the more involved extremity is decongested. Patient in supine position:
1. Abbreviated manipulation of the lateral neck lymph nodes, including the shoulder collectors (observe contraindications).
2. Deep abdominal technique (modified) as outlined in the basic sequence (observe contraindications). If abdominal techniques are contraindicated, diaphragmatic breathing should be used to substitute.
3. Manipulation of the inguinal lymph nodes on both sides.
4. Activation and utilization of the AI anastomoses on both sides to promote lymph flow across the watersheds into the drainage areas.

Patient on the side (or prone position), with the more involved extremity on top:

1. Rework of AI anastomosis on the more involved side, and the shoulder collectors.
2. Manipulation of the lateral upper arm between the lateral epicondyle and the acromion, using basic techniques ("bulk flow" techniques).
3. Rework of shoulder collectors and AI anastomosis on more involved side.

Patient in supine position:

1. Manipulation of the lateral upper arm (more involved extremity) between the lateral epicondyle and the acromion. Modified effleurage as well as pump techniques and combination of pump and stationary circles should be used (see sequences 4–5, upper arm). This sequence should be followed up with rework techniques across the watershed into pretreated drainage areas.
2. Manipulation of the medial aspect of the upper arm toward the lateral aspect, using stationary circles (dynamic technique). This technique should be followed up with rework techniques of drainage areas. The entire length of the upper arm is treated in this manner.

3. Vasa vasorum technique in the area of the cephalic vein.
4. Manipulation of elbow, forearm, and hand as outlined in the basic sequence techniques.
5. If necessary, edema or fibrosis techniques should be incorporated at this point.
6. Rework of upper extremity, inguinal lymph nodes on both sides, AI anastomoses on both sides, shoulder collectors, and deep abdominal technique (modified).
7. Application of compression bandages on both, or the more involved extremity.

5.3.4 Unilateral Secondary Lower Extremity Lymphedema

This condition is most often the result of the removal and/or irradiation of the inguinal and/or pelvic lymph nodes in cancer surgery (prostate, bladder, female reproductive organs, melanoma). Secondary lower extremity lymphedema may also occur as a result of trauma and may be combined with swelling of the lower truncal quadrant on the same side, and/or the external genitalia.

The following sequence should be used until the truncal quadrant is decongested (▶ Fig. 5.22).

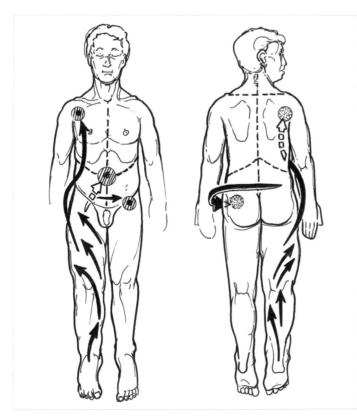

Fig. 5.22 Drainage directions for unilateral lymphedema on the lower extremity.

Patient in supine position:
1. Abbreviated manipulation of the lateral neck lymph nodes (observe contraindications).
2. Manipulation of the axillary lymph nodes on the ipsilateral side.
3. Activation and utilization of the IA anastomosis to move lymph fluid from the swollen lower quadrant toward the drainage area.
4. Manipulation of the inguinal lymph nodes on the contralateral side.
5. Activation and utilization of the AII anastomosis to move lymph fluid from the swollen lower quadrant toward the drainage area on the opposite side.
6. *Abdominal treatment*: Superficial and deep (modified) techniques as outlined in the basic sequences (observe contraindications). If abdominal techniques are contraindicated, diaphragmatic breathing should be substituted.

Patient on the side (or prone position), with the affected extremity on top:
1. Rework of the IA anastomosis on the affected side.

Patient in prone position (or on side):
1. Manipulation of the lumbar area on the unaffected side (omit step 4).
2. Activation and utilization of the PII anastomosis to move lymph fluid from the swollen lower quadrant toward the drainage area on the opposite side.
3. Paravertebral techniques on the affected lumbar area to promote deep lymphatic pathways.
4. Rework of the PII anastomosis.

Patient in supine position:
1. Rework of AII anastomosis, IA anastomosis on the affected side, inguinal lymph nodes on contralateral and axillary lymph nodes on ipsilateral sides, and deep abdominal techniques (modified).
2. Application of compression bandages on the affected extremity.
   a) The following sequence should be used if the truncal quadrant is decongested and the treatment of the lymphedematous leg is the primary focus.

Patient in supine position. Abbreviated trunk preparation (pretreatment):
1. Abbreviated manipulation of the lateral neck lymph nodes (observe contraindications).

2. Manipulation of the axillary lymph nodes on the ipsilateral side.
3. Activation and utilization of the IA anastomosis to promote lymph flow across the watershed toward the drainage area.
4. Manipulation of the inguinal lymph nodes on the contralateral side.
5. Activation and utilization of the AII anastomosis to promote lymph flow across the watershed toward the drainage area on the opposite side.
6. Deep abdominal technique (modified) as outlined in the basic sequences (observe contraindications). If abdominal techniques are contraindicated, diaphragmatic breathing should be substituted.

Patient on the side (or prone position), with the affected extremity on top:
1. Rework of the IA anastomosis on the affected side.
2. Activation and utilization of the PII anastomosis to promote lymph flow across the watershed toward the drainage area on the opposite side.
3. Manipulation of the lateral thigh between the lateral knee and the iliac crest, using basic techniques ("bulk flow" techniques).
4. Rework of the PII and IA anastomoses (on the affected side).

Patient in supine position:
1. Rework of the AII anastomosis.

If the lower extremity is considerably swollen, it is not recommended to treat the entire extremity in a single session. The treatment should proceed in steps; for example, only the thigh (or parts of it) should be treated, which prevents overload of the healthy lymphatics in the drainage areas.

2. Manipulation of the lateral thigh between the knee and the iliac crest. Modified effleurage as well as pump techniques, combination of pump and stationary circles, and rotary techniques should be used. This sequence should be followed up with rework techniques across the watersheds into pretreated drainage areas.
3. Manipulation of the medial aspect of the thigh toward the lateral aspect, using stationary circles (dynamic technique). This technique should be repeated over the entire length of the thigh and followed up with rework techniques toward the drainage areas.

4. Vasa vasorum technique in the area of the femoral vein.
5. Manipulation of the knee, the lower leg, and the foot as outlined in the basic sequence techniques.
6. If necessary, edema or fibrosis techniques should be incorporated at this point. It may also be necessary to turn the patient into the prone position for the treatment of the posterior leg.
7. Rework of lower extremity, AII anastomosis, IA anastomosis on the affected side, axillary lymph nodes on ipsilateral side, inguinal lymph nodes on contralateral side, and deep abdominal techniques (modified).

Patient on the side (or prone position), with the affected extremity on top:
1. Rework of the PII anastomosis.
2. Application of compression bandages on the affected extremity.

5.3.5 Bilateral Secondary Lower Extremity Lymphedema

This condition is most often the result of the removal and/or irradiation of the inguinal and/or pelvic lymph nodes in cancer surgery (prostate, bladder, female reproductive organs, melanoma). Secondary lower extremity lymphedema may also occur as a result of trauma and may be combined with swelling of the lower truncal quadrant on the same side, and/or the external genitalia. Ideally, bandages should be applied on both lower extremities. If this is not possible, compression bandages should be applied to the more involved extremity.

The following sequence should be used until the truncal quadrant(s) is/are decongested (▶ Fig. 5.23).

Patient in supine position:
1. Abbreviated manipulation of the lateral neck lymph nodes (observe contraindications).
2. Manipulation of the axillary lymph nodes on both sides.
3. Activation and utilization of the IA anastomoses on both sides to promote lymph flow from the congested quadrants to the drainage areas.
4. *Abdominal treatment*: Superficial and deep (modified) techniques as outlined in the basic sequences (observe contraindications). If abdominal techniques are contraindicated, diaphragmatic breathing should be substituted.

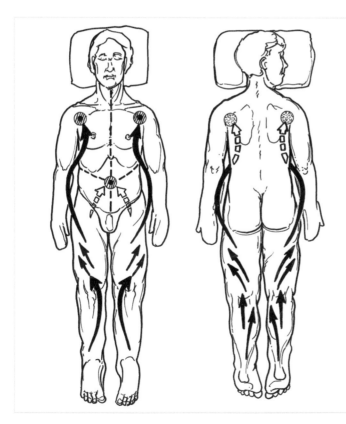

Fig. 5.23 Drainage directions for bilateral lymphedema on the lower extremities.

Patient in prone position (or on side):
1. Rework of IA anastomoses on both sides.
2. Decongestion of the swollen lower truncal quadrants on both sides toward the axillary lymph nodes, using modified lumbar techniques: modified effleurage; rotary techniques starting at the sagittal watershed to the side, followed by stationary circles (dynamic technique) toward the axilla using the IA anastomosis; paravertebral techniques to utilize deep drainage pathways.

Patient in supine position:
1. Rework of IA anastomoses and axillary lymph nodes on both sides.
2. *Rework of abdominal area:* Superficial and deep (modified) techniques.
3. Application of compression bandages on both or the more involved extremity.

The following sequence should be used if the truncal quadrant(s) is/are decongested and the treatment of the lower extremities becomes the primary focus.

> It is not recommended to treat both extremities in the same session. The more involved extremity should be treated first until decongested. If the extremity is considerably swollen, it should be treated in steps; for example, only the thigh (or parts of it) should be treated, which prevents overload of the healthy lymphatics in the drainage areas.

Therapy proceeds with the other leg, once the more involved extremity is decongested. Generally, a pantyhose-style compression garment is ideal for this condition once both extremities are decongested. To preserve the results in the leg that was treated first, compression bandages should be applied. If this is not possible, the patient should be fitted with a thigh-high compression garment (preferably a relatively inexpensive standard-size garment) while the other extremity receives treatment, then he or she should be fitted with a pantyhose-style garment.

Patient in supine position. Abbreviated trunk preparation (pretreatment):
1. Abbreviated manipulation of the lateral neck lymph nodes (observe contraindications).

2. Manipulation of the axillary lymph nodes on both sides.
3. Activation and utilization of the IA anastomoses on both sides to promote lymph flow across the watersheds into the drainage areas.
4. *Abdominal treatment*: Superficial and deep (modified) techniques as outlined in the basic sequences (observe contraindications). If abdominal techniques are contraindicated, diaphragmatic breathing should be substituted.

Patient on the side (or prone position), with the more involved extremity on top:
1. Rework of the IA anastomosis on the more involved side.
2. Manipulation of the lateral thigh between the lateral knee and the iliac crest, using basic techniques ("bulk flow" techniques).

Patient in supine position:
1. Rework of IA anastomoses on both sides.

Treatment of the lower extremity:
1. Manipulation of the lateral thigh between the knee and the iliac crest. Modified effleurage as well as pump techniques, combination of pump and stationary circles, and rotary techniques should be used. This sequence should be followed up with rework techniques across the watersheds into pretreated drainage areas.
2. Manipulation of the medial aspect of the thigh toward the lateral aspect, using stationary circles (dynamic technique). This technique should be repeated over the entire length of the thigh and followed up with rework techniques toward the drainage areas.
3. Vasa vasorum technique in the area of the femoral vein.
4. Manipulation of the knee, the lower leg, and the foot as outlined in the basic sequence techniques.
5. If necessary, edema or fibrosis techniques should be incorporated at this point. It may also be necessary to turn the patient into the prone position for the treatment of the posterior leg.
6. Rework of lower extremity, IA anastomoses on both sides, axillary lymph nodes on both sides, and abdominal techniques.
7. Application of compression bandages on both, or the more involved extremity.

5

5.3.6 Unilateral Primary Lower Extremity Lymphedema

This condition is the result of developmental abnormalities (see Chapter 3, Primary Lymphedema) of the lymphatic system, which are either congenital or hereditary. Primary lower extremity lymphedema may be combined with swelling of the adjacent truncal quadrant and/or the external genitalia.

Congenital malformations of the lymphatic system may also be present in the contralateral leg. If the volume of the unaffected leg increases, or if any changes in tissue consistency are noted during the treatment, the use of inter-inguinal anastomoses (AII and PII) should be discontinued.

Treatment sequences for this condition are very similar to the treatment of secondary lymphedema of the lower extremity. The inguinal lymph nodes in primary lymphedema are still present and should be stimulated. The goal of intervention, however, is to relieve these lymph nodes; lymph fluid is therefore rerouted around the inguinal lymph nodes toward sufficient drainage areas located in the adjacent trunk territories.

The following sequence should be used until the truncal quadrant is decongested (▶ Fig. 5.22).

Patient in supine position:
1. Abbreviated manipulation of the lateral neck lymph nodes (observe contraindications).
2. Manipulation of the axillary lymph nodes on the ipsilateral side.
3. Activation and utilization of the IA anastomosis to move lymph fluid from the swollen lower quadrant toward the drainage area.
4. Manipulation of the inguinal lymph nodes on the contralateral side.
5. Activation and utilization of the AII anastomosis to move lymph fluid from the swollen lower quadrant toward the drainage area on the opposite side.
6. *Abdominal treatment*: Superficial and deep (modified) techniques as outlined in the basic sequences (observe contraindications). If abdominal techniques are contraindicated, diaphragmatic breathing should be substituted.

Therapist moves to the other side of the treatment table:
1. Manipulation of the inguinal lymph nodes on the affected side.

Patient in prone position (or on side):
1. Manipulation of the lumbar area on the unaffected side (omit manipulation of the inguinal lymph nodes).
2. Activation and utilization of the PII anastomosis to move lymph fluid from the swollen lower quadrant toward the drainage area on the opposite side.
3. Paravertebral techniques on the affected lumbar area to promote deep lymphatic pathways.
4. Rework of the PII anastomosis.

Patient in supine position:
1. Rework of AII anastomosis, IA anastomosis on the affected side, axillary lymph nodes on the ipsilateral side, inguinal lymph nodes on both sides, and deep abdominal techniques (modified).
2. Application of compression bandages on the affected extremity.

The following sequence should be used if the truncal quadrant is decongested and the treatment of the lymphedematous leg is the primary focus.

Patient in supine position. Abbreviated trunk preparation (pretreatment):
1. Abbreviated manipulation of the lateral neck lymph nodes (observe contraindications).
2. Manipulation of the axillary lymph nodes on the ipsilateral side.
3. Activation and utilization of the IA anastomosis to promote lymph flow across the watershed toward the drainage area.
4. Manipulation of the inguinal lymph nodes on the contralateral side.
5. Activation and utilization of the AII anastomosis to promote lymph flow across the watershed toward the drainage area on the opposite side.
6. Deep abdominal technique (modified) as outlined in the basic sequences (observe contraindications). If abdominal techniques are contraindicated, diaphragmatic breathing should be substituted.

Patient on the side (or prone position), with the affected extremity on top:
1. Rework of the IA anastomosis on the affected side.
2. Activation and utilization of the PII anastomosis to promote lymph flow across the watershed toward the drainage area on the opposite side.
3. Manipulation of the lateral thigh between the lateral knee and the iliac crest, using basic techniques ("bulk flow" techniques).

4. Rework of the PII and IA anastomoses (on the affected side).

Patient in supine position:
1. Rework of the AII anastomosis.

> If the lower extremity is considerably swollen, it is not recommended to treat the entire extremity in one session. The treatment should proceed in steps; for example, only the thigh (or parts of it) may be treated, which prevents overload of the healthy lymphatics in the drainage areas. If the swelling is more distally pronounced (as is often the case in primary lymphedema), more time should be spent treating the areas below the knee.

2. Manipulation of the inguinal lymph nodes on the affected leg.
   a) As discussed earlier, inguinal lymph nodes in primary lymphedema are used as additional drainage areas. Lymph fluid from more distal sections of the leg should not be manipulated toward the inguinal nodes but rerouted around them as in the treatment of secondary lymphedema.
3. Manipulation of the lateral thigh between the knee and the iliac crest.
   a) Modified effleurage as well as pump techniques, combination of pump and stationary circles, and rotary techniques should be used. This sequence should be followed up with rework techniques across the watersheds into pretreated drainage areas.
4. Manipulation of the medial aspect of the thigh toward the lateral aspect, using stationary circles (dynamic technique). This technique should be repeated over the entire length of the thigh and followed up with rework techniques toward the drainage areas.
5. Vasa vasorum technique in the area of the femoral vein.
6. Manipulation of the knee, the lower leg, and the foot as outlined in the basic sequence techniques.
7. If necessary, edema or fibrosis techniques should be incorporated at this point. It may also be necessary to turn the patient into the prone position for the treatment of the posterior leg.
8. Rework of lower extremity, including the inguinal lymph nodes; rework of the anterior AII

anastomosis, IA anastomosis on the affected side, axillary lymph nodes on the ipsilateral side, inguinal lymph nodes on the contralateral side, and deep abdominal techniques (modified).

Patient on the side (or prone position), with the affected extremity on top:
1. Rework of the PII anastomosis.
2. Application of compression bandages on the affected extremity.

5.3.7 Bilateral Primary Lower Extremity Lymphedema

This condition is the result of developmental abnormalities (see Chapter 3, Primary Lymphedema) of the lymphatic system, which are either congenital or hereditary. Primary lower extremity lymphedema may be combined with swelling of the adjacent truncal quadrant and/or the external genitalia.

Treatment sequences for this condition are very similar to the treatment of bilateral secondary lymphedema of the lower extremities. The inguinal lymph nodes in primary lymphedema are still present and should be stimulated. The goal of intervention, however, is to relieve these lymph nodes; lymph fluid is therefore rerouted around the inguinal lymph nodes toward sufficient drainage areas located in the upper truncal territories (axillary lymph nodes).

The following sequence should be used until the truncal quadrant(s) is/are decongested (▶ Fig. 5.23).
Patient in supine position:
1. Abbreviated manipulation of the lateral neck lymph nodes (observe contraindications).
2. Manipulation of the axillary lymph nodes on both sides.
3. Manipulation of the inguinal lymph nodes on both sides.
4. Activation and utilization of the IA anastomoses on both sides to promote lymph flow from the congested quadrants to the drainage areas.
5. *Abdominal treatment*: Superficial and deep (modified) techniques as outlined in the basic sequences (observe contraindications). If abdominal techniques are contraindicated, diaphragmatic breathing should be substituted.

Patient in prone position (or on side):
1. Rework of IA anastomoses on both sides.
2. Decongestion of the swollen lower truncal quadrants on both sides toward the axillary

lymph nodes, using modified lumbar techniques: modified effleurage; rotary techniques starting at the sagittal watershed to the side, followed by stationary circles (dynamic technique) toward the axilla using the IA anastomosis; paravertebral techniques to utilize deep drainage pathways.

Patient in supine position:
1. Rework of IA anastomoses and axillary lymph nodes on both sides.
2. *Rework abdominal area:* Superficial and deep (modified) techniques.
3. Application of compression bandages on both or the more involved extremity.

The following sequence should be used if the truncal quadrant(s) is/are decongested and the treatment of the lower extremities becomes the primary focus.

> It is not recommended to treat both extremities in the same session. The more involved extremity should be treated first until decongested. If the extremity is considerably swollen, it should be treated in steps; for example, only the thigh (or parts of it) may be treated, which prevents overload of the healthy lymphatics in the drainage areas.

Therapy proceeds with the other leg, once the more involved extremity is decongested. In general, a pantyhose-style compression garment is ideal for this condition, once both extremities are decongested. To preserve the results in the leg that was treated first, compression bandages should be applied. If this is not possible, the patient should be fitted with a thigh-high compression garment (preferably a relatively inexpensive standard-size garment) while the other extremity receives treatment, and then be fitted with a pantyhose-style garment.

Patient in supine position. Abbreviated trunk preparation (pretreatment):
1. Abbreviated manipulation of the lateral neck lymph nodes (observe contraindications).
2. Manipulation of the axillary lymph nodes on both sides.
3. Activation and utilization of the IA anastomoses on both sides to promote lymph flow across the watersheds into the drainage areas.

4. Manipulation of the inguinal lymph nodes on both sides.
5. As discussed earlier, inguinal lymph nodes in primary lymphedema are used as additional drainage areas. Lymph fluid from more distal sections of the leg should not be manipulated toward the inguinal nodes, but rerouted around them, as in the treatment of secondary lymphedema (see secondary lower extremity lymphedema).
6. *Abdominal treatment:* Superficial and deep (modified) techniques as outlined in the basic sequences (observe contraindications). If abdominal techniques are contraindicated, diaphragmatic breathing should be substituted.

Patient on the side (or prone position), with the more involved extremity on top:
1. Rework of the IA anastomosis on the more involved side.
2. Manipulation of the lateral thigh between the lateral knee and the iliac crest, using basic techniques ("bulk flow" techniques).

Patient in supine position:
1. Rework of IA anastomoses on both sides.

Treatment of the lower extremity:
1. Rework of the inguinal lymph nodes on the more involved leg.
2. Manipulation of the lateral thigh between the knee and the iliac crest.
3. Modified effleurage as well as pump techniques, combination of pump and stationary circles, and rotary techniques should be used.
4. This sequence should be followed up with rework techniques across the watersheds into pretreated drainage areas.
5. Manipulation of the medial aspect of the thigh toward the lateral aspect, using stationary circles (dynamic technique). This technique should be repeated over the entire length of the thigh and followed up with rework techniques toward the drainage areas.
6. Vasa vasorum technique in the area of the femoral vein.
7. Manipulation of the knee, the lower leg, and the foot as outlined in the basic sequence techniques.
8. If necessary, edema or fibrosis techniques should be incorporated at this point. It may also be necessary to turn the patient into the prone position for the treatment of the posterior leg.

9. Rework of the lower extremity, including the inguinal lymph nodes; rework of the IA anastomoses on both sides, axillary lymph nodes on both sides, inguinal lymph nodes on the less swollen leg, and abdominal techniques.
10. Application of compression bandages on both, or the more involved extremity.

5.3.8 Genital Lymphedema

Genital lymphedema is a challenging condition that very often causes real and long-lasting physical, emotional, and social problems for the affected patients. This condition can affect both males and females; however, it is more common in males due to the greater tissue elasticity of the scrotum and penis, combined with the effects of gravity (▶ Fig. 5.24).

Reliable numbers on the incidence of genital swelling are unavailable because this condition often remains undiagnosed; genital edema is generally not a topic of conversation, unlike swelling of an extremity following surgery.

Genital lymphedema is usually irreversible without treatment, and once it develops, it tends to become more fibrotic and increases in size. It can be effectively controlled and maintained with CDT. In some cases, genital swelling may occur acutely following surgery or trauma and may resolve completely by itself.

In most cases, genital lymphedema is combined with lower extremity lymphedema.

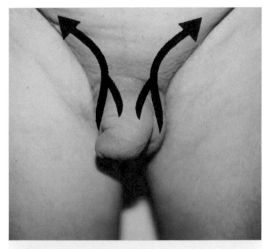

Fig. 5.24 Genital lymphedema with involvement of the penis in an uncircumcised patient. Arrows indicate drainage directions.

Classification

Genital swelling can be classified as malignant, benign, primary, and secondary.

Malignant Conditions

Advanced pelvic and/or abdominal malignancies may block or reduce the lymphatic and venous return from the genital area.

The onset of genital swelling without apparent reason, the presence of a clear vaginal discharge, or lymphorrhea, may be a symptom of an active malignant process and needs to be thoroughly examined by a physician.

Primary Conditions

Primary genital swelling is usually the result of congenital malformations (dysplasia) of lymph vessels and/or lymph nodes in the region. As with all primary forms, the swelling may be present at birth (rare) or develop later in life with or without obvious cause. Minor surgical interventions, such as a circumcision, may trigger the onset of pediatric genital swelling if congenital malformations of the lymphatic system are present.

Isolated swelling of the genital region is not common. In many cases, other parts of the body are involved in the swelling as well, such as the lower quadrant(s) and/or one or both of the lower extremities.

It was also reported that obese patients with lower extremity lymphedema have an increased risk of developing genital swelling due to greater pressure on the lymphatic system in the groin from the enlarged abdomen.

Secondary Conditions

Trauma or surgical interventions in combination with the removal and/or irradiation of lymph vessels and/or lymph nodes (especially pelvic lymph nodes) to remove gynecological, testicular, penile, urological, abdominal, intestinal, or prostatic cancers are a common cause.

The incidence of genital swelling tends to increase with the combination of surgery and radiation, and if the patient has a history of recurrent episodes of cellulitis.

The swelling may occur immediately postsurgery or years later as with other forms of lymphedema. Reports suggest that genital swelling in combination with lower extremity lymphedema occurs in approximately 10% of patients.

The incidence of genital swelling in females has been estimated at 10 to 20% of patients following surgery.

In males, the incidence of genital edema following oncological surgery (prostatectomy, bladder cancer) and/or irradiation seems to be considerably higher.

Filariasis is another common cause of genital swelling in endemic regions (see Chapter 3, Pathology, and **Fig. 3.4a, b**).

A very common reason for the onset of genital swelling is the use of pneumatic compression pumps for the treatment of lower extremity lymphedema. Boris et al published an article in the March 1998 edition of *Lymphology* and concluded that the use of external pneumatic compression pumps in the treatment of lower extremity lymphedema produces an unacceptable high incidence of genital edema[1] (See Chapter 3, Therapeutic Approach to Lymphedema).

Clinical Picture

Various combinations of genital anatomy swelling may occur. In males, isolated penile swelling is rare. Combined penile and scrotal swelling is a more common presentation. The scrotum may swell to such an extent that ambulation becomes difficult. The lower quadrants and/or lower extremities often accompany genital swelling. Additional involvement of the pubic area frequently causes the penis to retract into the scrotum.

In females, the labia minora and the labia majora may be included in the swelling. These areas could project several centimeters out of the vagina. Clear labial/vaginal discharge (lymphorrhea), the appearances of papillomas or warty growths are often symptoms indicating genital involvement, especially if the patient had pelvic or gynecological procedures. Vaginal discharge for other reasons is often a curdish, white, thick discharge.

Genital swelling frequently causes problems in urination and sexual activity, depending on the extent of the involvement.

Evaluation

Other conditions, such as active malignancies or renal, liver, cardiac, or venous problems, can cause genital edema. A thorough evaluation with a clear diagnostic picture is necessary before MLD/CDT can be initiated.

History

- What kind of surgery (if any) was performed and how many lymph nodes were excised?
- Were there any cellulitis attacks in the past? Where did they start?
- Pain? Some patients describe bursting sensation or an ache around the genital area (pain generally recedes with treatment). Males often complain about painful erections.
- Were/are there any problems with bowel or bladder function following surgery or radiation?
- Are appropriate hygienic measures possible?
- Is the patient circumcised?

Inspection

- Check for any moist areas, lymphatic cysts, lymphatic fistulas (▶ Fig. 5.25), and lymphorrhea (patients often use sanitary or incontinence pads)
- Check for extent of the swelling: Penis/scrotum, external/internal labia, pubic area, lower quadrant, and/or lower extremity (unilateral/bilateral).
- Check for scars.
- Check for skinfolds in the genital region.
- Check for Papillomas, warts.
- Check for Bacterial or mycotic infections. (Patients with discharge from the area often complain about malodor; lymph itself has no odor, but is very high in protein content, which presents an excellent breeding ground for bacteria, causing malodor.)

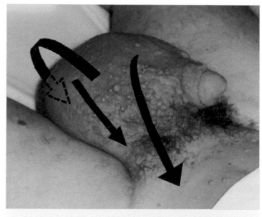

Fig. 5.25 Genital lymphedema with lymphatic cysts and fistulas. Arrows indicate drainage directions.

Palpation

- Tissue quality—fibrosis, scars.
- Tissue quality in other involved areas.
- Can the foreskin be pulled back in uncircumcised male patients?

Treatment

As discussed earlier, genital swelling is often associated with lower extremity lymphedema. The treatment of the genital swelling may be included in the treatment sequence or it may be performed as a stand-alone treatment. If lower extremity swelling (or truncal edema) is present, the treatment of the genital swelling should precede the sequence for leg lymphedema.

Lymphatic cysts and/or fistulas, lymphorrhea, and bacterial and mycotic infections are common complicating factors found in combination with this condition. Meticulous hygiene is therefore imperative. If fistulas are present, the area must be cleaned and disinfected with proper agents, and the treatment should be performed wearing sterile gloves.

To maximize the therapeutic effect, genital bandaging may be performed prior to the application of hands-on techniques for the pretreatment of the drainage areas. Following the treatment sequence, the bandages are removed and the MLD techniques in the swollen genital area are performed (see Compression Bandaging for Male Genital Lymphedema). The therapist then proceeds with the application of the final compression bandage. The application of compression bandages on the genital area is discussed later in this chapter.

Patient in supine position:

1. Abbreviated manipulation of the lateral neck lymph nodes (observe contraindications).
2. Manipulation of the axillary lymph nodes on both sides.
3. Activation and utilization of the IA anastomoses on both sides to promote lymph flow across the watershed into the drainage areas.
4. If inguinal lymph nodes are present, manipulation of the inguinal lymph nodes on both sides.
5. *Abdominal treatment*: Superficial and deep (modified) techniques as outlined in the basic sequences (observe contraindications). If abdominal techniques are contraindicated, diaphragmatic breathing should be substituted.

If the lower truncal quadrants are congested, the patient is turned into the prone position at this point, and the lumbar areas are decongested in the following manner. Decongestion of the swollen lower truncal quadrants on both sides toward the axillary lymph nodes, using modified lumbar techniques; modified effleurage; rotary techniques starting at the sagittal watershed to the side, followed by stationary circles (dynamic techniques) toward the axilla using the IA anastomosis; paravertebral techniques to utilize deep drainage pathways. The patient is then turned back into the supine position.

1. *Treatment of the scrotum*: Stationary circles on both sides of the scrotum to manipulate the lymph fluid toward the pubic area, and from here toward the axillary lymph nodes on the respective side, utilizing the IA anastomoses.
2. Application of bandages (see Section 5.11.5 and subsection Compression Bandaging for Male Genital Lymphedema later in this chapter).

5.3.9 Phlebolymphostatic Edema

This condition is a result of a venous insufficiency (for pathology, refer to Chapter 3, Chronic Venous and Lympho-Venous Insufficiency). The deficient venous valves in CVI fail to prevent retrograde flow of venous blood during muscle pump activity, which in turn directly affects the lymphatic system.

Over time, and if CVI is left without treatment, damage to the lymphatic system combined with reduction in transport capacity is unavoidable. The presence of lymphedema in stages II and III of CVI necessitates the application of the complete spectrum of CDT. If venous ulcerations are present, appropriate wound dressings and skin care products, prescribed by the physician, are applied before CDT starts (refer to Chapter 3, Complete Decongestive Therapy). The wound remains covered during the treatment, and MLD techniques are directed away from and around the ulcer bed. Treatment in and around the wound area is performed wearing sterile gloves. Decongestion of the extremity greatly increases the tendency of venous stasis ulcerations to heal.

The treatment protocol for lymphedema associated with CVI corresponds with the protocol for primary lymphedema; fibrosis and edema techniques are contraindicated.

Should any signs or symptoms of thrombophlebitis in deep veins or symptoms of pulmonary embolism develop (see Chapter 3, Thrombophlebitis in Deep Veins), the patient must see a doctor immediately, and any treatment must be interrupted until the condition is cleared up.

Patient in supine position. Abbreviated trunk preparation (pretreatment):
1. Abbreviated manipulation of the lateral neck lymph nodes (observe contraindications).
2. Manipulation of the axillary lymph nodes on the ipsilateral side.
3. Activation and utilization of the IA anastomosis to promote lymph flow across the watershed toward the drainage area.
4. Manipulation of the inguinal lymph nodes on the contralateral side.
5. Activation and utilization of the AII anastomosis to promote lymph flow across the watershed toward the drainage area on the opposite side.
6. Deep abdominal technique (modified) as outlined in the basic sequences (observe contraindications). If abdominal techniques are contraindicated, diaphragmatic breathing should be substituted.

Patient on the side (or prone position), with the affected extremity on top:
1. Rework of the IA anastomosis on the affected side.
2. Activation and utilization of the PII anastomosis to promote lymph flow across the watershed toward the drainage area on the opposite side.
3. Manipulation of the lateral thigh between the lateral knee and the iliac crest, using basic techniques ("bulk flow" techniques).
4. Rework of the PII and IA anastomosis (on the affected side).

Patient in supine position:
1. Rework of the AII anastomosis.
   a) Treatment of the lower extremity (experience shows that the swelling in phlebolymphostatic edema is generally pronounced more distally; in these cases, more time should be spent treating the tissues distal to the knee joint).
2. Manipulation of the inguinal lymph nodes on the affected leg.

3. Manipulation of the lateral thigh between the knee and the iliac crest.
   a) Modified effleurage as well as pump techniques, combination of pump and stationary circles, and rotary techniques should be used.
   b) This sequence should be followed up with rework techniques across the watersheds into pretreated drainage areas.
4. Manipulation of the medial aspect of the thigh toward the lateral aspect, using stationary circles (dynamic technique). This technique should be repeated over the entire length of the thigh and followed up with rework techniques toward the drainage areas.
5. Manipulation of the knee, the lower leg, and the foot as outlined in the basic sequence techniques.
   1. To maximize the decongestive effect, it is often beneficial to turn the patient into the prone position at this point for the treatment of the posterior lower leg.
6. Rework of lower extremity, including the inguinal lymph nodes. Rework of the AII anastomosis, IA anastomosis on the affected side, axillary lymph nodes on the ipsilateral side, inguinal lymph nodes on the contralateral side, and deep abdominal techniques (modified).
   1. Patient on the side (or prone position), with the affected extremity on top:
7. Rework of the PII anastomosis.
8. Application of compression bandages on the affected extremity. In many cases of phlebolymphostatic insufficiency, compression bandages need to be applied only up to the knee; this depends on the severity of the swelling and is determined by the physician.

5.3.10 Lipolymphedema

Lipolymphedema generally involves both lower extremities, and the treatment protocol of this condition corresponds with that of primary lymphedema. The lymphedematous component responds well and relatively fast to CDT; the lipedema itself responds more slowly, sometimes not at all. Lighter pressures in manual and compression bandage techniques during the initial treatment sessions may be necessary because lipedema and lipolymphedema are often associated with hypersensitivity and pain, which typically diminish after several treatments. Patients often require more padding under the compression bandages, particularly in the anterior tibial area. In some cases, it may be necessary not to apply a bandage at all during the first few treatments. Edema and fibrosis techniques are contraindicated in the treatment of this condition.

The following sequence should be used until the truncal quadrant(s) is/are decongested.

Patient in supine position:

1. Abbreviated manipulation of the lateral neck lymph nodes (observe contraindications).
2. Manipulation of the axillary lymph nodes on both sides.
3. Manipulation of the inguinal lymph nodes on both sides.
4. Activation and utilization of the IA anastomoses on both sides to promote lymph flow from the congested quadrants to the drainage areas.
5. *Abdominal treatment*: Superficial and deep (modified) techniques as outlined in the basic sequences (observe contraindications). If abdominal techniques are contraindicated, diaphragmatic breathing should be substituted.

Patient in prone position (or on side):

1. Rework of IA anastomoses on both sides.
2. Decongestion of the swollen lower truncal quadrants on both sides toward the axillary lymph nodes, using modified lumbar techniques: modified effleurage; rotary techniques starting at the sagittal watershed to the side, followed by stationary circles toward the axilla using the IA anastomosis; paravertebral techniques to utilize deep drainage pathways.

Patient in supine position:

1. Rework of IA anastomoses and axillary lymph nodes on both sides.
2. Rework of abdominal area: Superficial and deep (modified) techniques.
3. Application of compression bandages on both, or the more involved extremity.

The following sequence should be used if the truncal quadrant(s) is/are decongested and the treatment of the lower extremities becomes the primary focus.

> It is not recommended to treat both extremities in the same session. The more involved extremity should be treated first until decongested. If the extremity is considerably swollen, it should be treated in steps; for example, only the thigh (or parts of it) may be treated, which prevents overload of the healthy lymphatics in the drainage areas.

Therapy proceeds with the less involved leg, once the more involved extremity is decongested. In general, a pantyhose-style compression garment is ideal for this condition, once both extremities are decongested. To preserve the results in the leg that was treated first, compression bandages should be applied. If this is not possible, the patient should be fitted with a thigh-high compression garment (preferably a relatively inexpensive standard-size garment) while the other extremity receives treatment, and then he/she can be fitted with a pantyhose-style garment.

Patient in supine position. Abbreviated trunk preparation (pretreatment):

1. Abbreviated manipulation of the lateral neck lymph nodes (observe contraindications).
2. Manipulation of the axillary lymph nodes on both sides.
3. Activation and utilization of the IA anastomoses on both sides to promote lymph flow across the watersheds into the drainage areas.
4. Manipulation of the inguinal lymph nodes on both sides.
5. Deep abdominal techniques (modified) as outlined in the basic sequences (observe contraindications). If abdominal techniques are contraindicated, diaphragmatic breathing should be substituted.

Patient on the side (or in prone position), with the more involved extremity on top:

1. Rework of the IA anastomosis on the more involved side.
2. Manipulation of the lateral thigh between the lateral knee and the iliac crest, using basic techniques ("bulk flow" techniques).

Patient in supine position:

1. Rework of IA anastomoses on both sides.

Treatment of the lower extremity:

1. Rework of the inguinal lymph nodes on the more involved leg.
2. Manipulation of the lateral thigh between the knee and the iliac crest. Modified effleurage as well as pump techniques, combination of pump and stationary circles, and rotary techniques should be used. This sequence should be followed up with rework techniques across the watersheds into pretreated drainage areas.
3. Manipulation of the medial aspect of the thigh toward the lateral aspect, using stationary circles. This technique should be repeated over the entire length of the thigh and followed up

5

with rework techniques toward the drainage areas.

4. Vasa vasorum technique in the area of the femoral vein.
5. Manipulation of the knee, the lower leg, and the foot as outlined in the basic sequence techniques.
6. Rework of lower extremity, including the inguinal lymph nodes.

If necessary, patient in prone position:
1. Manipulation of the posterior knee and lower leg as outlined in the basic sequence techniques.

Patient in supine position:
1. Rework of the IA anastomoses on both sides, axillary lymph nodes on both sides, inguinal lymph nodes on the less swollen leg, and abdominal techniques.
2. Application of compression bandages on both, or the more involved extremity.

5.4 Head and Neck Lymphedema

5.4.1 Introduction

Head and neck lymphedema (HNL) is much less common than edema of the extremities, but HNL is a particularly concerning complication for patients and their families, especially when severe, as in the case shown in ▶ Fig. 5.26**a,b**. When HNL causes eyelid swelling, tasks involving vision, such as reading, writing, walking, and driving, may be affected. When the lips and tongue are edematous, articulation, chewing, swallowing, and even respiration can be impaired, possibly requiring a tracheotomy. Breathing can also be affected in patients who have undergone a total laryngectomy when severe submental and anterior neck edema occludes the tracheostoma, requiring the use of a device such as a laryngectomy tube or a laryngectomy button to maintain a patent airway, as in ▶ Fig. 5.26**b**. Even when the edema is relatively minor and does not create a functional impairment, cosmetic concerns can arise that create psychosocial and emotional issues, as neck and facial edema cannot be easily hidden. HNL is often overlooked, misdiagnosed, or minimized as an inevitable and untreatable outcome of cancer treatment. At other times, a clinician may identify HNL but be ill prepared to treat the patient because of a lack of experience with the condition. The ability

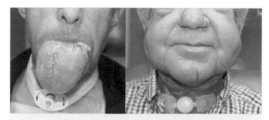

Fig. 5.26 Severe lingual and facial edema. **(a)** 16 days after base of tongue resection. **(b)** 11 months after total laryngectomy.

to effectively evaluate and treat HNL is crucial to maximizing the patient's quality of life. The information presented in this chapter is intended to reduce clinician concerns and assist in the evaluation, treatment planning, and management of HNL.

5.4.2 Etiology

HNL may be present with primary lymphedema, either in isolation or as part of a syndrome, and is a characteristic of Hennekam's syndrome, Turner's syndrome, Milroy's disease, Apert's syndrome, and other disorders.[2] Primary lymphedema of the head and neck, however, is less common than primary lymphedema of the extremities and will not be addressed in this chapter.

Inflammatory causes of facial lymphedema include severe rosacea (including rhinophyma and otophyma), acne vulgaris, Melkersson–Rosenthal syndrome, and other dermatologic conditions.[2] While the most common cause of lymphedema worldwide is filariasis,[3,4] this author is unaware of any articles documenting filarial lymphedema of the head and neck. More commonly, HNL presents as a secondary lymphedema due to injury of the lymphatic tissues from chronic infections, blunt force trauma, surgery, radiotherapy, or vascular obstruction by a mass (malignant lymphedema)[2] as shown in ▶ Fig. 5.27. Facial edema is a potential complication of certain cosmetic and dermatologic procedures, though chronic HNL after cosmetic procedures is not commonly reported. MLD following facelift procedures has been used to reduce postoperative edema. Variations of traditional facial drainage pathways are implemented according to surgically altered tissue orientation.[5] HNL is not common after surgery for noncancerous maladies of the head and neck, though with any

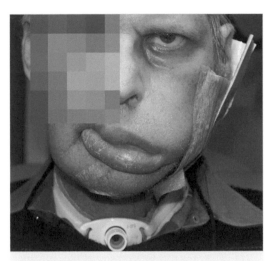

Fig. 5.27 Edema from tumor recurrence.

surgery the potential exists for drainage impairment and edema due to scarring. One possible explanation for the higher incidence of HNL after the removal of malignant lesions compared with nonmalignant lesions is that the lymphatics are typically not removed in head and neck surgeries for patients not undergoing cancer treatment.[6,7,8,9]

5.4.3 HNL after Cancer Treatment

HNL occurs most frequently in patients who have undergone surgery and/or radiotherapy for cancer[3] and seems to be most severe when multimodality treatment is provided, though the role of chemotherapy in the development of HNL is not known. Taxane-based chemotherapy has been linked to lymphedema of the extremities,[10] and HNL has been reported in patients treated with cisplatin[10,11] combined with radiotherapy. There are no published accounts of HNL following chemotherapy in isolation for head and neck cancer, though pemetrexed-induced edema of the eyelid and periorbital region has been reported with lung cancer treatment.[12] Currently, there are no sufficient data to suggest a causative relationship between most current chemotherapy regimens and chronic HNL.

HNL has been documented in 48 to 75%[13] of patients who received radiotherapy to the head and neck.[14] The insult to the lymphatic system that occurs from radiotherapy can be widespread, as the primary tumor, adjacent soft tissues, bony structures, and relevant lymphatic drainage pathways may all be irradiated in an effort to shrink existing tumors, treat persistent microscopic disease, and prevent metastasis. Tissue fibrosis is a common complication of radiotherapy and can inhibit lymphangiomotoricity and effective tissue drainage. Patients who receive radiation to the head and neck often develop chronic edema of tissues within the irradiated field, which commonly encompasses the lower face, neck, and supraclavicular fossa. When re-irradiation is required to treat cancer recurrence, further tissue damage occurs, increasing the severity of tissue fibrosis and associated HNL.[15]

Surgery to address head and neck cancer commonly requires the removal of the tumor and the surrounding soft tissues. Removal of bone may also be required if there is tumor invasion or if there is severe damage to the bone from radiotherapy (osteoradionecrosis).[16] Depending on the extent of the surgery, reconstruction may be required with pedicled flaps such as pectoralis and rotational flaps, which retain their native venous, arterial, and lymphatic vessels. In more complex cases, free tissue transfers from one part of the body to another may be required. For example, tissue from the forearm or thigh may be used to replace a portion of the tongue or pharynx or to cover the surgical defect after removal of a portion of the face, as shown in ▶ Fig. 5.28. These "free flaps" require

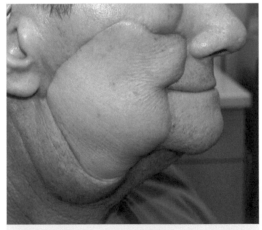

Fig. 5.28 Facial reconstruction with a free flap from the thigh.

microvascular surgery to reattach blood vessels for flap viability. Lymphatic vessels are not commonly reconnected in these procedures, however, leaving only the venous system to drain the free flap, which can swell substantially at times. Lymphadenectomy is a common surgical procedure in the treatment of head and neck cancer, often requiring removal of more than 30 cervical, facial, mediastinal, paratracheal, or supraclavicular lymph nodes.[17,18,19] When sacrifice of jugular veins is required due to tumor involvement or severe radiation scarring, the disruption of the venous drainage system in the head and neck increases the risk of HNL. This lymphatic and venous disruption results in a lympho-venous or "mixed edema," which is typically less responsive to treatment than a pure lymphedema. Additionally, surgical scarring can directly impact the development of HNL due to a "trapdoor effect,"[20] in which a scar prevents drainage through the lymphatic channels of the skin, resulting in edema above the scar but not below. Multimodality cancer treatment creates a unique environment for the development of both mild and severe lymphedemas in the face and neck that can be challenging to evaluate and treat.

5.4.4 Evaluation

Piso et al published a reliable assessment protocol for facial edema in 2001,[21] yet HNL evaluations vary from facility to facility and often from clinician to clinician. Inconsistency in evaluation methodology hinders objective data acquisition and analysis to determine best treatment practices, forcing reliance on subjective data such as visual assessment, patient questionnaires, and clinician-scored rating scales. Development of high-tech solutions to evaluate HNL has been limited, though ultrasound and magnetic resonance imaging have been reported as diagnostic tools for edema assessment in the head and neck.[2,22,23] Efforts are being made, however, to implement standard evaluation protocols for HNL.[13,24] Components of a basic HNL evaluation are suggested below.

Clinical Assessment

Clinical assessment of the patient is the most important aspect of any lymphedema evaluation, but there are specific concerns when evaluating a patient with HNL. The traditional assessment of tissue integrity, warmth, color, firmness, pitting, and tissue changes must be included. An accurate, thorough medical history is crucial, as intraoral,

facial, or neck edema may result from infection, hypothyroidism, allergic reactions, postoperative seroma, hematoma, angioedema, lymphatic metastasis, or other causes.[2,25] When the presentation and history do not support the diagnosis of lymphedema, referral to the patient's physician for further evaluation is appropriate. For example, distended jugular veins in the presence of facial edema suggests superior vena cava syndrome, which is often caused by a mass compressing the superior vena cava and can constitute a medical emergency.[26]

A significant history of upper-quadrant deep vein thrombosis (DVT), cerebrovascular accident (CVA), transient ischemic attack (TIA), carotid artery compromise, congestive heart failure (CHF), renal disease, hyperthyroidism, tissue breakdown, or other medical concerns may be sufficient to withhold lymphedema treatment, despite the severity of the swelling.[25] Lymphedema treatment may result in a CVA or increased edema if provided inappropriately and could cause death if there is tumor invasion of the carotid artery and manipulation results in rupture of the vessel (carotid blow-out). Lymphedema management may be requested as a palliative treatment to temporarily alleviate discomfort or reduce functional impairments that result from massive facial edema. Palliative treatment can improve the patient's quality of life and should be provided if it appears that treatment can be effective and there is no immediate risk of harm; however, treatment is not appropriate in all cases. If you have concerns about the patient's safety, further discussion with the patient's physician may be warranted, as physician approval is essential before initiating any HNL treatment.

Tape Measurement

Tape measurements are an essential tool for documenting change over time and assessing the effectiveness of treatment. Consistent tape placement and tightness are required for the most accurate measurements possible, though the potential for error exists with all manual tape measurement practices. For consistency, the following guidelines should be observed. If possible, obtain measurements while the patient is sitting upright with the head in a neutral position to assess edema in a natural posture. Mark the measurement landmarks on the skin to ensure consistent tape placement. Measurements should be obtained in centimeters and recorded on a tracking form or in a database

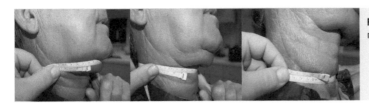

Fig. 5.29 Superior, medial, and inferior neck measurements.

for future comparison. The patient's trunk and head positions should be replicated in each evaluation to ensure consistent data acquisition. The measurement protocol published by Smith and Lewin[24] includes a combination of neck circumferences, head circumferences, and point-to-point facial measures to provide a comprehensive assessment of the face and neck. These are described later.

The superior, middle, and inferior neck circumferences, shown in ▶ Fig. 5.29, can be combined to obtain a composite neck measurement that reflects change throughout the entire neck rather than in just one area. The superior circumference should be obtained by placing the tape measure horizontally around the upper portion of the neck, just below the mandible and chin. The inferior neck circumference is obtained in a similar fashion at the base of the neck. The medial neck circumference is obtained at the midpoint between the superior and inferior neck measurement sites. Adding these three circumferences creates a composite neck score that can then be used for comparison over time. A difference of 2% or more between the baseline and follow-up composite scores has been considered significant.[27] Changes of less than 2% are not considered clinically significant because of the potential for errors in tape placement, positional inconsistencies, and other variables. Only composite scores, and not individual measurements, can be assessed using the 2% rule.

Obtaining a Composite Neck Measurement

1. Superior neck: immediately beneath mandible.
2. Medial neck: midway point between 1 and 3.
3. Inferior neck: lowest circumferential level.

Source: Adapted from Smith and Lewin (2010).[24]

Facial Composite

A composite facial score can be achieved by combining seven point-to-point facial measurements, as shown in ▶ Fig. 5.30. These measurements are

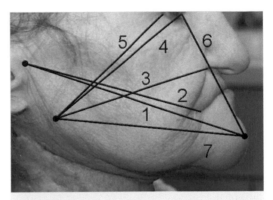

Fig. 5.30 Facial composite measurements. 1. Tragus to mental protuberance; 2. Tragus to mouth angle; 3. Mandibular angle to nasal wing; 4. Mandibular angle to internal eye corner; 5. Mandibular angle to external eye corner; 6. Mental protuberance to internal eye corner; 7. Mandibular angle to mental protuberance. (Adapted from Smith and Lewin [2010].)[24]

totaled on each side of the face to create left and right hemifacial scores. The hemifacial scores are then combined to create the total facial composite score, which can be compared with facial composite scores over time to assess facial changes using the 2% rule. The hemifacial scores cannot be compared with each other to determine the presence of edema in one side of the face, unlike comparisons made between right and left limbs. Treatment of head and neck cancer is often provided bilaterally, but even when provided unilaterally, bilateral edema is common. There are no published data specifying a percentage of swelling to distinguish between edematous and normal facial tissues. Therefore, measurements of facial edema should be reported as a total facial composite.

Indicators of Change

While treatment effectiveness can be demonstrated by a 2% change in composite scores, a reduction of less than 2% may not be indicative of a lack of improvement overall. Other clinical indicators of improvement should also be considered, including but not limited to reductions in tissue firmness, reductions in edema duration and fluctuation, and obvious visual changes over time. The clinician should be aware of weight gain or loss between evaluations, which can minimize or exaggerate the percentage of edema reduction demonstrated by measurements.

Other Measurements

Additional measurements as shown in ▶ Fig. 5.31 can be used to assess submental or lateral facial and mandibular edema. Distances between the right and left tragus or between the right and left mandibular angles can be helpful, as can vertical and diagonal circumferences of the head. These measurements are not included in the neck or facial composite scores and are not subject to the 2% rule, but they can provide valuable feedback regarding treatment changes. Additional circumferential measures can be obtained when there is substantial edema in the forehead, eyebrows, eyelids, or lips. Measures of lip or tongue protrusion and swelling of the nose or ear can also be obtained if necessary, but these are not commonly utilized.

Facial Irregularities

Sometimes a total facial composite cannot be obtained because a facial landmark cannot be identified. This may result from surgical removal of the landmark, tissue breakdown, tumor eruption, nonremovable dressings, or excessive edema that prevents palpation. Comparison of partial composites or hemifacial scores may be helpful when only certain measurements can be obtained, though the 2% rule cannot be applied if the total facial composite is unavailable. However, composite scores can be obtained if the correlate of the missing landmark can be used to replicate its position. For example, if the right mandibular angle cannot be identified, the vertical distance between the unaffected left tragus and the left mandibular angle can be measured. If this distance is 5 cm, a mark can be placed 5 cm below the tragus on the right side, providing a usable landmark for the affected side. Likewise, if the right tragus is not present, the clinician should first obtain a horizontal measurement from the existing tragus to the tip of the nose. If this distance is 13.5 cm, a mark can be made 13.5 cm from the tip of the nose to the approximate location of the left ear, providing an alternative tragus landmark that can be used to complete the facial composite score. If both landmarks are missing, as in ▶ Fig. 5.32, first re-create the tragus landmark, and then the mandibular angle location can be determined. Photographic documentation featuring the locations of the replicated landmarks and the distances between each

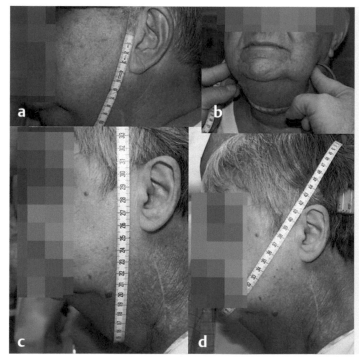

Fig. 5.31 Additional measurements for assessing edema. **(a)** Tragus to tragus. **(b)** Distance between mandibular angles. **(c)** Vertical circumference. **(d)** Diagonal circumference.

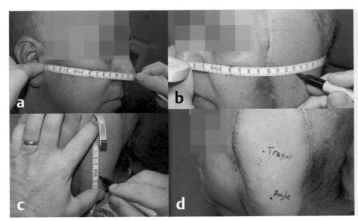

Fig. 5.32 Re-creating missing tragus and mandible landmarks. **(a)** Measure from existing tragus to existing mandibular angle (not shown) and from tragus to nose. **(b)** Re-create the measurement on the other side from nose to alternative tragus. **(c)** Re-create the measurement from alternative tragus to alternative mandibular angle. **(d)** Alternatives marked.

5

anchoring point are helpful for re-creating the landmarks in future evaluations.

Neck Irregularities

On occasion, a patient may present with an irregular neck shape that interferes with the determination of superior, medial, or inferior marking points for circumferential measures. Neck irregularities may be the result of scarring, the slope of the neck, skinfolds, edema, or other causes and can require the use of nontraditional tape placements. It may be possible to use these irregular landmarks as measuring points if they are stable. Surprisingly, when a slender patient has a very prominent mandible, the absence of submental edema can make it difficult to obtain separate medial and superior neck measures. It may be necessary to request assistance to hold the tape at the proper location on the upper neck or submandibular region to obtain the appropriate circumference.

Photography

Basic photographic documentation is an excellent source of data and should be used to evaluate a patient's appearance before, during, and after treatment. Digital photography provides immediate access to high-resolution images, allowing for instant comparison of baseline and follow-up photos and even for assessment of changes that occur during a single treatment. While detailed photographs of particular areas of concern may be helpful, a standard series of three portrait-style photos featuring the face and neck from the front, right, and left are typically the most beneficial. It is important to maintain a consistent camera angle, patient body alignment, and distance between the photographer and the patient during each photo session so that images can be compared reliably. Side-by-side photographic comparisons can be very powerful tools, providing feedback to patients, physicians, and third-party payers who may require proof of improvement to continue funding lymphedema rehabilitation services.

Three-Dimensional Imaging

Although seldom used outside of large facilities because of their cost, three-dimensional (3D) imaging systems offer the potential to provide more advanced head and neck measurement data. Surface area, volumetric measures, and both linear and contoured point-to-point measurements are purported as benefits of this technology. Current systems are able to instantly capture a 3D image of the face and neck without requiring the patient to remain still for long periods of time, as is required with 3D scanning technology. The ability to superimpose baseline and follow-up images for volumetric assessment promises to be one of the technology's most beneficial applications for HNL assessment. Currently, 3D imaging provides excellent feedback for visual comparison of changes in facial edema, but there remain concerns with consistency of patient alignment from session to session, making comparisons of combined face and neck images difficult. Measurement templates and landmark capabilities appear to offer great promise for point-to-point measurement without the variances that can occur with manual placement of a tape measure on the skin. The increased precision of measurement offered by this technology would improve the reliability of the data collected and the quality of future HNL research.

Lymphedema Rating Scales

The severity of lymphedema has traditionally been classified according to clinician-graded rating scales. The most well-known is the Földi's scale,[3] which was developed on more than 100,000 patients and features stages 0, 1, 2, and 3, ranging from nonvisible but perceptible edema to irreversible swelling with severe fibrosis and tissue changes including hyperkeratosis and papillomatosis. Most lymphedema rating scales, including the Földi's scale, were developed for assessment of limbs and have been applied to the head and neck by default. Unfortunately, these scales do not capture subtle differences that often exist with HNL, resulting in a forced classification that does not completely describe the HNL patient's presentation. The Patterson's scale[13,28] has been used to assess internal edema of the pharynx, larynx, and base of the tongue, but it is limited to visual assessment via endoscopy and does not address "external lymphedema" in the neck or face. In 2010, the MD Anderson Cancer Center Head and Neck Lymphedema (MDACC HNL) Rating Scale was published.[24] The MDACC HNL scale is a nonvalidated tool developed to document lymphedema presentations common among patients with HNL, but not identified by Földi's scale. It offers a stage 1a classification to identify patients with visible but nonpitting edema and stage 1b for patients presenting with pitting, reversible edema. Criteria for stages 0, 2, and 3 reflect the original descriptions by Földi. ▶ Table 5.1 compares these two scales. It should be noted that all clinician-rating scales are subjective assessment tools, and clinician judgment can vary according to training and experience. Further investigation and development of a comprehensive, standardized, user-friendly scale that accurately depicts the characteristics of HNL would enable more consistent data comparison for future clinical research.

5.4.5 Treatment of HNL

HNL has historically been perceived as a difficult condition to manage. This perception may be due to limited experience with head and neck cancer and its treatment, unfamiliarity with the anatomy of the head and neck, the various presentations of HNL, or uncertainty regarding treatment techniques, which can differ from traditional treatment of lymphedema in the extremities. Techniques used to manage HNL are often taught in advanced courses and are not typically addressed during training for certification in MLD or CDT, most likely due to the relatively low incidence of head and neck cancer compared with that of breast cancer and other conditions. Clinicians who do not practice in a tertiary-care center[29] with an emphasis on head and neck cancer, which comprises only 3 to 5% of all cancers,[30] may rarely encounter a patient with HNL.

HNL should be treated using a standard CDT approach, though MLD and compression are typically the two primary CDT components used to address the head and neck.[31] Exercises and stretches for the neck, face, and shoulder region are commonly applied as part of posttreatment rehabilitation to address speech and swallowing function, as well as cervical and upper extremity range of motion. These rehabilitation techniques are generally appropriate for HNL as well, especially while the patient is wearing compression. Skin and wound care is extremely important for patients recovering from surgery and for those undergoing radiotherapy. Skin and wound care

Table 5.1 Comparison of the MDACC HNL and Földi's scales

MDACC HNL scale	Földi's scale
0. No visible edema, patient reports heaviness	0. No visible edema, patient reports heaviness
1a. Soft, visible edema, no pitting, reversible	1. Clinical swelling, pitting edema, reduced swelling with elevation
1b. Soft pitting edema, reversible	
2. Firm, irreversible edema without tissue changes	2. Hard swelling, does not recede during the day, no tissue change
3. Hard, nonpitting, irreversible edema, tissue changes	3. Clinical symptoms of elephantiasis, tissue changes

Abbreviation: MDACC HNL, MD Anderson Cancer Center Head and Neck Lymphedema.

Source: Adapted from Smith and Lewin (2010)[24]

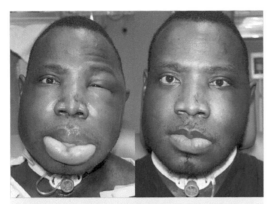

Fig. 5.33 A patient before and after 10 sessions of manual lymph drainage.

should be performed under the guidance of the patient's medical team when required, but once the skin is healed, persistent care is not commonly required for patients with HNL. Variations of MLD and compression techniques may be needed to treat HNL. Irradiated tissues should be addressed with caution, and certain precautions must be observed when applying compression to the head and neck region. While the differences between treating HNL and lymphedema of the extremities may be considered challenging, HNL can be treated very effectively with appropriate intervention, as shown in ▶ Fig. 5.33. Additional treatment considerations are outlined below.

Outpatient versus Self-Administered Treatment

Traditionally, lymphedema has been treated on an outpatient basis so that skilled MLD treatment, compression wrapping, and wound care can be provided by a certified lymphedema therapist (CLT) several times a week for a period of weeks or months. When possible, it is recommended that HNL be treated on an outpatient basis by a CLT, though the frequency and duration of treatment is often less than that required for lymphedema of the extremities. While extended therapy may be required in some cases, it is not uncommon for HNL treatment plans to feature two to three visits per week for 1 to 2 weeks, after which patients are discharged to perform their home program. Patients should always be trained in a home program during the early stages of rehabilitation to enhance carryover. After treatment, follow-up evaluations at 1, 3, and 6 months are recommended to ensure adequate home program

follow-through and continued progress. However, treatment modifications are common and more frequent reassessments or prolonged treatment may be required depending on the patient's progress. Naturally, severe cases may require intensive treatment of greater frequency per week and longer duration overall.

Although outpatient treatment is preferred, patients with HNL have also been shown to benefit from training in the use of a "self-CDT" approach, primarily featuring self-administered MLD and compression.[27,32] The self-administered therapy approach is most appropriate when the patient presents with mild edema and is physically and mentally capable of self-treatment or has good caregiver support. It can also be implemented when consistent access to a qualified lymphedema therapist is not available as a result of the patient's illness, issues with finances, transportation, or because health care resources are limited in the patient's home locale. Once the patient and caregiver are trained, the treatment is implemented at home, with follow-up evaluations to evaluate progress and address any changes required in the treatment plan.

Of course, treatment effectiveness is of utmost importance, and self-CDT does have limitations. These may be related to the physical or cognitive abilities of the patient or caregiver, inconsistent or inaccurate performance of MLD routines, or lack of caregiver support. The absence of a CLT is a disadvantage, as well. However, Smith et al[27,32] reported compliance as the primary factor influencing successful edema reduction in patients primarily treated with a self-administered lymphedema management protocol. Significant edema reductions were observed at the first follow-up visit in 74% of patients who were compliant in their home management program and in 56% who were partially compliant. The noncompliant group did not demonstrate improvement as a whole.

Whether a self-administered home lymphedema management protocol is appropriate for a particular patient depends on the ability and willingness of the patient or caregiver to perform the prescribed routine independently. For example, when a patient requires posterior drainage due to significant neck scarring, it is preferable that the anterior and posterior trunk be decongested for maximum benefit. MLD of the back cannot typically be performed by the patient, mandating caregiver's assistance. If a caregiver is unavailable and the patient must perform self-MLD, only anterior trunk decongestion can be achieved, which is less

5

efficient and may not be as effective for posterior drainage. However, a capable caregiver may be able to perform the prescribed routine proficiently, so caregiver's availability and willingness to assist should always be addressed in the evaluation. Simultaneous training of the patient and caregiver is preferred, and individual responsibilities should be clearly identified to ensure acceptable levels of involvement by both parties.

When outpatient treatment for HNL is recommended but is not convenient, the use of a self-CDT home program often becomes the primary intervention. While success has been achieved with some severe cases using a home management approach, many cases are simply too complex for self-administered treatment and require intensive outpatient treatment by a skilled, experienced clinician to achieve significant improvement. If it is clear during re-evaluation that the home program has been ineffective and reasonable treatment modifications are not possible, further discussion may be required to determine additional options to obtain treatment from a qualified lymphedema therapist.

MLD Treatment Sequences for HNL

In theory, MLD sequences for HNL are not vastly different from standard MLD protocols for limbs. Anterior and posterior MLD sequences for HNL are intended to mobilize lymph from the head and neck to the bilateral axillae, with sequence selection dependent on scarring or other obstructions. Stationary circles can be used as the primary MLD technique in almost all locations, making these routines easy to teach for self-MLD treatment. Other techniques may be substituted by CLTs as appropriate. Standard Vodder technique[25] tempo (once per second) and frequency (7–10 repetitions per location) apply until the edematous region is reached, where a minimum of 20 to 30 repetitions should be performed in each location. Progression to the next adjacent area is based on tactile changes identified by the clinician.

Positioning

Patient positioning during treatment can vary with HNL management. While a supine or reclined sitting position is preferred for posterior facial and neck drainage in patients with significant scarring or severe edema, many patients with HNL do not tolerate lying in a supine, prone, or even reclined position because of respiratory difficulties,

kyphosis, neck fibrosis, or other conditions. In these cases, MLD should be performed with the patient lying on his or her side or sitting in an upright position. The most important benefit of seated treatment is that the patient can breathe more easily and remain comfortable during treatment. Although seated treatment may reduce the effectiveness of posterior drainage in severe HNL, seated MLD is very effective for most posterior, anterior, and trunk decongestion routines.

Trunk Decongestion

For maximum effectiveness, trunk decongestion must be performed to open lymphatic channels and promote lymph flow from congested areas to functional drainage basins. Many clinicians have started treatment for patients with HNL in the edematous face and neck without first decongesting the trunk. This is not recommended. Likewise, it is common to perform a neck decongestion routine in a "normal" neck before addressing the trunk as part of upper extremity treatment.[25] This is not appropriate when HNL is present. Decongestion of the terminus, abdomen, axillae, and trunk should be addressed before the edematous head or neck is treated. An exception to this recommendation is when the patient has very mild edema and has not received radiotherapy to the neck or supraclavicular fossa. If the supraclavicular region is not damaged, it may be possible to treat with an abbreviated MLD routine that begins at the terminus and progresses directly to the neck and face, without the need to decongest the trunk or axillary lymph node beds. Otherwise, trunk decongestion is essential prior to addressing edema in the head and neck.

Strossenreuther and Klose previously described posterior trunk decongestion for HNL in a seated position.[31] However, a standard trunk decongestion sequence featuring anterior and posterior trunk decongestion is preferred for maximum drainage. If the patient is in an upright seated position, a clinician or caregiver can decongest the anterior and posterior trunk simultaneously via the "sandwich technique" shown in ▶ Fig. 5.34. To perform the sandwich technique, the clinician or caregiver is positioned to the side of the patient. In steps 1, 5, 6, 7, and 8 in the sequence outlined below, hands are placed on the chest and back simultaneously, sandwiching the patient between them. Performing simultaneous stationary circles, pulling laterally toward the axilla, the clinician can simultaneously decongest the anterior and

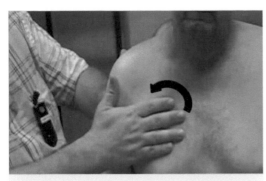

Fig. 5.34 The "sandwich technique" for simultaneous decongestion of the anterior and posterior trunk.

posterior trunk on one side. The clinician or caregiver can then move to the opposite side of the patient or reposition the patient's chair so that the remainder of the trunk can be addressed, allowing for a complete trunk decongestion in 5 to 8 minutes, typically. This is a more efficient means of addressing the trunk, providing much more time to address the edematous regions of the face and neck during the treatment session.

Trunk Decongestion Manual Lymph Drainage Sequence

A standard trunk decongestion sequence is shown below. If pitting edema is present, the patient should wear a softening pad 30 minutes prior to and during the trunk decongestion sequence (steps 1–8). The softening pad should be removed at step 9 and a flattening pad applied after MLD is complete. Additional information regarding compression padding is outlined in Section 5.11.2 in this chapter. This sequence can be performed with the patient in any position, although it is recommended in a seated position.

Deep System

1. Stationary circles in supraclavicular fossa.
2. Abdominal decongestion routine/diaphragmatic breathing.

Surface System Trunk (Target: Axillary Nodes)

1. *Axillary node decongestion*: Fingers in the axilla. Stationary circles up and inward.
2. *Pectoral node decongestion*: Flat hand beneath axilla, on side of the chest. Stationary circles vertical to axilla.

3. *Inferior anterior chest*: Flat hand, little finger above nipple. Overhand stationary circles out to axilla.
4. *Mid-chest*: Move hand up one hand width. Repeat overhand stationary circles out to axilla.
5. *Upper chest*: Move hand beneath clavicle. Repeat overhand stationary circles out to axilla.
6. *Supraclavicular fossa*: Repeat stationary circles as in step 1.

Repeat trunk sequence steps 1 to 8 on opposite side.
1. "Softening pad" should be removed after trunk decongestion to allow access to the head and neck region.

Anterior Face and Neck Drainage for HNL

Once the trunk is decongested, MLD should be applied to the head and neck. Anterior drainage is appropriate when no significant scarring is present in the face or neck to prevent drainage through the lateral and anterior neck to the axillary lymph nodes. Patients who have undergone radiotherapy without surgery or who have minor surgical scars are most likely to benefit from this approach. Although simultaneous bilateral facial MLD is typically preferred, unilateral self-MLD of the lateral and anterior neck is recommended to avoid simultaneous carotid sinus stimulation. The direction of MLD should be toward the lateral neck and jugular lymph node chains.

HNL Anterior MLD Routine

1–8. Bilateral trunk decongestion, as described earlier.

9. *Posterior neck:* Overhand anterior stationary circles toward the ear. (If the posterior trunk has been decongested, the posterior neck circles can be directed posteriorly rather than anteriorly.)

10. *Lateral neck*: Move hand anteriorly, fingertips beneath the ear. Overhand posterior stationary circles toward ear. (For unilateral approach, patients may elect to use opposite hand.)

11. *Anterior neck*: Move hand to midline of anterior neck, second knuckle beneath chin. Overhand posterior stationary circles toward ear. (Opposite hand preferred for patients.)

12. *Preauricular and postauricular region*: Bilateral. Two fingers on either side of ear. Stationary circles down and posteriorly.

5

13. *Lateral face*: Bilateral. Flat hands on lateral cheeks and mandible, posterior stationary circles toward ear.

14. *Anterior face*: Bilateral. Flat hands to anterior cheeks, posterior stationary circles toward ear. Avoid upward movement toward eyes to prevent filling of lower eyelids.

If applicable, relevant areas of edema, including the intraoral region, nose, eyelids, and forehead, can now be addressed as described in section "Intraoral MLD" below.

If no additional sequences are required, reverse the sequence and perform steps 14, 13, 12, 11, 10, 9, 8, 7, 6, and 5 to mobilize fluid from the face through the neck to the bilateral axillae.

After completion of this MLD sequence, compression should be applied as directed.

Scarring and Other Obstructions

In some cases, significant scars exist that prevent anterior drainage. Scars can frequently be softened and reduced with the use of scar massage, scar reduction creams, silicone sheeting, elastic therapeutic tape, myofascial release, and other techniques. Scar reduction can improve the ability to mobilize lymph through the scarred area, allowing a more direct drainage pathway. Reestablishment of drainage across scars in the head and neck has been documented,[33] supporting long-standing clinical beliefs that with proper intervention, the effects of scarring can be overcome to some degree. However, thick scars, tissue breakdown, or erupted tumors may force a redirection of lymph from the preferred drainage channels, requiring posterior drainage.

Posterior Neck and Facial Drainage for HNL

The HNL posterior MLD sequence is designed to mobilize lymph away from significant scarring in the face or neck as discussed earlier. Stationary circles can be used as the primary technique in almost all locations. Before this sequence is performed, posterior trunk decongestion is required. This sequence should be performed by a caregiver or clinician. If self-MLD is required, please refer to the sequences in Combined Self-Manual Lymph Drainage for Head and Neck Lymphedema later in this chapter.

HNL Posterior MLD Routine

1–8. Bilateral trunk decongestion, as described earlier.

9. *Posterior neck*: Flat hands, perform MLD downward into upper back.

10. Repeat inferior MLD movements, progressing up to the posterior neck into the lower posterior scalp, mobilizing fluid into the neck and back.

11. Progressively moving across the lateral scalp, perform posterior MLD techniques to mobilize fluid to the posterior head and upper neck.

12. Move hands to the preauricular region, mobilizing upward and posteriorly to the lateral scalp using MLD techniques.

13. Move hands to the anterior face, performing downward stationary circles away from midline toward the preauricular region, avoiding upward pressure that can fill the eyelids.

14. Move hands inferiorly to address the lateral jowls and mandibular regions. Perform MLD techniques upward to the preauricular region and primary drainage channel over the ear and into the lateral scalp.

15. If intraoral edema is present, perform intraoral techniques at this time.

16. Move hands to the submandibular and submental regions, performing MLD techniques upward to the lateral face.

17. Continue in this fashion in the upper neck, mobilizing away from midline and upward, away from the neck scar. Begin posteriorly, then advance anteriorly until the midline is reached.

18. Once the neck and face have been decongested, reverse the sequence and perform steps 17, 16, 15, 14, 13, 12, 11, 10, 9, 8, 7, 6, and 5 to mobilize the fluid to the axillary nodes.

After completion, apply compression as directed.

Intraoral MLD

Intraoral edema may range from mild to severe and can impair articulation, chewing, swallowing, and respiration, depending on the structures involved. MLD can usually be performed to reduce intraoral swelling but should be avoided in patients with mucositis (▸ Fig. 5.35), open surgical wounds, and other tissue injuries.[25] Depending on hand size, the presence of trismus, and the severity of the edema, the patient, caregiver, or clinician may only be able to use one or two fingers to address intraoral edema. Caution should be observed with loose or jagged teeth, stitches, and hypersensitive gag or bite reflexes to avoid injury. Owing to the moisture in the mouth, fingers tend to slide along the mucosa. Water-based lubricants that are safe for intraoral use can be beneficial if the mouth and lips are excessively dry. In most

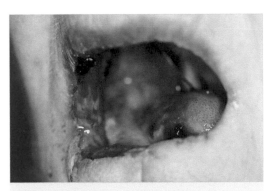

Fig. 5.35 Mucositis as a result of radiotherapy.

cases, bilateral intraoral MLD is recommended due to the extensive contralateral drainage in this region.[34] Occasionally, an oral free flap will be present and may also appear edematous. MLD is generally not recommended for free flaps due to the lack of lymphatic re-anastomosis, but MLD can be performed on the flap if trials prove effective. Free flaps atrophy over time, and MLD to this tissue does not typically affect the speed of flap reduction. As a result, intraoral MLD should address native tissues in most cases. A description of intraoral MLD is provided below.

MLD techniques for the tongue, floor of the mouth, and palate follow a similar pattern of lateral and posterior drainage. Decongestion should begin as far posterior as tolerated, with posterior and lateral stationary circles away from the midline.[25] Move anteriorly to the next adjacent area once judged appropriate. Repeat the sequence until the entire region is decongested. MLD of the tongue requires caution, as MLD without cushioning the underside of the tongue may result in tissue injury from friction against the teeth. If swelling is not too severe, it may be possible to position the tongue lower in the mouth between the teeth before treating. If the tongue is protruding from the mouth or lying against sharp teeth, the clinician should protect the underside of the tongue by using a finger, tongue depressor, gauze pad, or by grasping and supporting it during MLD. Protection of the tissue is of utmost importance to avoid infection, and MLD in this region should be avoided if there is potential for injury as a result of tissue manipulation.

Decongestion of the lips also begins laterally, near the oral commissure. Place the lip between the thumb and forefinger, with the thumb inside the mouth, and stabilize with the outer finger. Finger and thumb placement can be reversed if necessary. Perform stationary circles laterally to the mouth corner. After the appropriate number of repetitions, move medially and repeat the sequence until reaching the midline. Reverse the sequence and drain laterally from the midline until the oral commissure is reached and the entire half of the lip is decongested. Repeat the sequences on the other half of the lip. In severely swollen lips, this sequence may need to be repeated multiple times in one session, but immediate reductions can often be obtained. Pressing the lips together for 10 to 20 seconds during brief stoppages of MLD can also help prevent the rapid refilling of tissues during treatment.

MLD for the cheek and buccal mucosa should address the inner and outer tissues. Place one or two fingers against the swollen buccal mucosa. Support the outer cheek with the opposite hand.[25] Begin as far posteriorly as possible and perform posterior overhand stationary circles. Repeat the sequence in the anterior, superior, and inferior portions of the buccal mucosa until the entire cheek is addressed. The exterior cheek can also be addressed in this fashion, with the internal fingers providing support. Patients can perform a one-handed approach using the thumb inside the opposite side of the mouth and using the remaining fingers to support the cheek. Again, posterior overhand stationary circles can be applied. This method is usually less efficient because less tissue is being manipulated during MLD, but may be beneficial in some cases.

"Internal Lymphedema"

Intraoral MLD can be a very effective tool for reducing edema of the oral cavity. Unfortunately, MLD has not been proven effective in the reduction of edema that is present in the pharynx or larynx, sometimes called internal lymphedema,[13] which can affect swallowing and pose airway concerns. While the presence of edema in these regions for 3 to 6 months is not uncommon and edema around the internal carotid artery has been identified 2 years after completion of radiotherapy,[15,23,35,36] there remains debate whether persistent swelling in the pharynx and larynx is edema or lymphedema. The inability to assess tissue characteristics with techniques other than endoscopic examination currently limits clinical evaluation of edema in the upper aerodigestive tract. Regardless of etiology, treatment options available to address internal lymphedema have been limited to medical management with steroids or other anti-inflammatory regimens. Traditional approaches for direct lymphedema management, such as MLD, are impractical for addressing internal structures such as the pharynx and larynx. No studies that demonstrate the effectiveness of CDT for reducing internal edema of the larynx and pharynx are available, though anatomic connections suggest that MLD to the external tissues of the neck should reduce edema internally.[34] Additional research is warranted.

5.4.6 Compression for HNL

The use of compression garments and wrapping for the head and neck is a controversial subject, with proponents utilizing a wide variety of compression techniques and opponents using no compression at all. The primary concern related to compression in this region is the potential for compression of major blood vessels in the neck and complications from resultant vascular events, such as hypoxia, thrombosis, and CVA/TIA.[37,38] This risk is markedly increased in patients with blockages of the carotid artery, significant cerebrovascular disease, history of CVA, or other vascular abnormalities such as tumor invasion of a major blood vessel in the neck. These contraindications should have been identified during the initial evaluation, but their absence must be verified before the application of compression. Excessive anterior neck compression is also problematic, often creating respiratory distress in patients with a compromised airway or other pre-existing respiratory conditions.

A secondary effect of excessive compression is the blockage of lymphatic drainage in the neck, creating increased facial edema. This is a common finding during reevaluations when neck measurements have decreased with treatment but facial measures have increased. Proper fit must be assessed by the clinician to ensure that garments or wraps are not too tight. Chinstraps worn too tightly can increase fullness throughout the cheeks and anterior face. Excessive tightness of a facial compression mask can result in swelling of tissues through eye or mouth openings, worsening the edema in those regions. The increased edema can often be reversed by decreasing the tightness of the compression device, though sometimes complete garment revisions are required if edema is too great or the patient has gained a substantial amount of weight. However, increasing edema or a sudden plateau in progress during treatment may be related to a recurrent mass impeding lymphatic

flow and should be evaluated by the patient's physician if the pattern does not reverse when garment adjustments have been made.

Compression of the head and neck is not without risk, and not all patients with HNL are candidates for its use, though modifications can sometimes allow treatment despite the area of concern. For example, if severe submental edema is compromising the airway of a laryngectomized patient with one blocked carotid artery, it may be possible to modify the compression and MLD regimens sufficiently to avoid the area of concern and still apply appropriate pressure to the remainder of the neck and face. When in doubt regarding medical contraindications for use of compression for HNL, the therapist should contact the patient's physician to determine the patient's risk for adverse effects. If excessive risk exists, compression may be completely contraindicated. In most cases, however, compression can be applied safely and effectively. The proper use of compression has been shown to be an effective and essential component of CDT for HNL[32,39,40] and should be implemented when appropriate. However, specific instructions and training must be provided to ensure patient safety. Use of excessive compression by a patient may be accidental or intentional, to increase the effect of treatment. If repeated instances of misuse occur, modifications must be made or the compression garment/wrap should be discontinued for the patient's safety, despite the potential impact the loss of compression will have on treatment effectiveness.

Compression Padding

Historically, lymphedema therapists may or may not have elected to use foam padding as a component of compression treatment. The use of foam padding as an adjunct to compression wrapping has been reported to improve uniform pressure distribution to the tissues, provide structure for wrapping irregular surfaces, and soften fibrotic tissues.[39] Many padding options can either be fabricated or purchased, but in general, HNL treatment benefits from softening pads and flattening pads, such as those shown in ▶ Fig. 5.36. These pads are held in place by either a short-stretch bandage or an off-the-shelf compression garment.

Softening pads, also known as "chip bags" or "Schneider packs,"[39,41] are used prior to MLD when pitting edema is present. The pad softens the edematous tissue, increasing skin pliability and responsiveness to treatment. In most cases,

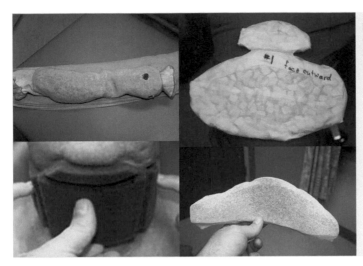

Fig. 5.36 Types of compression padding. **(a)** Chip bag. **(b)** Custom Schneider pack. **(c)** Custom flattening pad. **(d)** Beveled flattening pad.

softening pads should be worn for a minimum of 30 minutes before beginning MLD and throughout the trunk decongestion portion of the routine. After trunk decongestion is complete, the pad and compression garment should be removed as the neck and face are addressed. Softening pads are typically not used after MLD except in cases of very hard, fibrotic tissues.

Softening pads can be constructed from open or closed cell foam, depending on the firmness of the tissues being addressed. Chip bags are most appropriate for soft pitting edema and are constructed by filling a length of tubular gauze or stockinette with small (about 6–12 mm) blocks of 12-mm gray open cell foam. The spongy, resilient texture of the gray foam makes it an excellent choice for this application. Advantages of the chip bag include flexible positioning for irregular surfaces and the ability to reach crevices and skin contours when necessary. Disadvantages of the chip bag are its lack of durability and the need to redistribute the foam blocks within the stockinette to ensure even coverage with each application. Closed cell foam blocks do not stay evenly distributed within chip bags and are better suited for Schneider packs.

Schneider pack-style pads can be constructed by placing foam blocks between two sheets of soft cloth surgical tape, moleskin, or other flexible adhesive-backed material to create a flat, flexible pad with an uneven surface that can be used to soften firm edema and enhance the pliability of even somewhat fibrotic skin. To increase durability and decrease skin irritation, these pads should be covered by a stockinette or similar material before use. A pad made with small blocks of 12-mm gray open cell foam usually is sufficient to address a soft pitting edema, though there are concerns with foam expansion, resulting in separation of the tape layers over time, resulting in a less stable pad. However, firm edema typically requires the use of closed cell foam cut into 6-mm blocks. The author now uses only this style of pad due to long-term success with its use. Advantages of Schneider packs include their low profile, flexibility, and effectiveness on both soft and firm edemas. Another advantage is the fact that the foam blocks are held in position, providing a consistent application of pressure with each application. Also, Schneider pack pads can be cut into various shapes or modified to add an extended pad where additional coverage is required, as shown in ▶ Fig. 5.36**b**. Disadvantages are lengthier time for fabrication, difficulty with coverage of concave surfaces, increased product cost, and the potential for tissue damage from the closed cell foam if not used properly.

Additional options for softening tissue include smaller, textured closed cell foam sheets that are available in various styles featuring fine nap for softening fibrotic tissue or narrow drainage channels designed to improve directionality of lymphatic flow. These products are much thinner than the 12-mm closed cell sheeting or the coarse nap products used for larger surfaces and can be appropriate for HNL use, but skin integrity should be monitored carefully.

Finally, quilted pads featuring various levels of firmness are also available for compression of the head and neck. As the foam padding or other items are sewn into soft fabric, quilted pads can be used directly against the skin and can be laundered, unlike homemade pads. Another advantage of quilted pads is their durability and the wide variety of shapes, sizes, and textures, which range from very soft to very hard to address severely fibrotic tissue. Great caution must be exercised, however, when using extremely hard products due to the risk of tissue breakdown. Use of a very hard product on severely fibrotic tissue may soften the skin within 3 minutes and cause breakdown if left in place for longer periods of time, so careful monitoring is required. Quilted pads can be used by themselves or with compression bandaging, non-quilted off-the-shelf garments, or custom-quilted compression garments to achieve the desired coverage and pressure.

Once MLD is complete, immediate compression with a flattening pad under a wrap or garment is recommended, regardless of the edema stage. Flattening pads are intended for use with all patients receiving compression to reshape and flatten tissues after MLD, prevent refilling of edematous tissues, and promote continued lymph flow to the axilla. Flattening pads are typically cut from 12-mm open cell foam sheets into various shapes dictated by the area to be compressed. A typical shape for a flattening pad for the neck is a rectangle with a rounded top, shown in ▶ Fig. 5.36**d**. This allows the pad to fit well beneath the chin and curve along the top of the neck, staying below the mandible. The pad should cover the entire anterior and bilateral neck, extending back to the mandibular angles if bilateral edema is present, but can be customized as needed or constructed for unilateral use. The edges of the flattening pad should be beveled to lay flat against the skin, preventing creases that can occur if the edge is unbeveled. Modifications can be made if the pad is needed to compress the lower face or chin, and often, slots or vents can be cut into the exterior surface of the foam to enhance flexibility, as shown in ▶ Fig. 5.36**c**. The smooth side of the pad should always be against the skin. The flattening pad should be comfortable and should not restrict range of motion when in place.

Flattening pads should only be constructed of open cell foam to avoid tissue breakdown, which is possible if a closed cell pad is used. A pad constructed from 12-mm gray foam provides adequate pressure to the tissues without collapsing under the garment, which can occur with 6-mm foam. However, when a patient is very petite or supplemental padding is needed near the eyes, 6-mm foam is more appropriate. Also available are smaller open cell products with drainage channels to help direct lymph flow, as well as Velfoam,

which connects directly to Velcro and is soft enough to use for padding in areas of increased sensitivity.

Anecdotally, there appears to be a positive correlation between the length of time the flattening pad is worn after MLD and the refilling of the tissues. However, it is often difficult for patients with HNL to wear a compression garment or wrap for extended periods of time for a variety of reasons. Some report feeling claustrophobic if they wear the compression garment or wrap for more than 1 hour, while others may be able to wear a compression mask all night while sleeping. The minimum recommended wear time is 3 to 4 hours immediately after MLD, but more time is encouraged if tolerated by the patient, as longer wear time will generally enhance the effect of the treatment.

Short-Stretch Bandages

Compression bandaging for HNL can be very difficult, especially when one attempts to apply an entire bandage using a traditional multilayer wrap. Pressure application to the neck must be light to avoid vascular constriction, so circumferential neck wrapping should be avoided if possible. Because of the need to drain each side of the face away from the midline, compression of the face is quite difficult using bandages. While it is possible, facial wrapping can be impractical and typically will result in coverage of one eye, the mouth, and/or the nose, creating additional functional impairments. It is typically easier to achieve a functional degree of facial compression using a compression garment. However, short-stretch bandages can be especially effective for submental compression when the patient's neck circumference is greater than 50 cm or the diagonal head circumference is greater than 70 cm, based on anecdotal experience. These patients typically cannot wear off-the-shelf facial compression garments, even with Velcro strap extensions, because the improper fit would decrease effectiveness. There are two primary techniques for using bandages to address submental edema.

The first technique uses a complete short-stretch bandage. First, place the appropriate foam pad against the neck or submental area as necessary. Anchor the bandage against the pad as appropriate, and wrap the bandage diagonally from the neck around the crown of the head, adjusting each layer with a 50 to 75% overlap to ensure adequate coverage of the neck and relevant facial structures. The pad should be held securely in place and the bandage secured with tape or the clips that come with the bandage. If clips are used, careful bandage placement is required so that the clips can be placed on the foam pad rather than the skin. Bandaging is often difficult for patients to perform independently, so caregiver's assistance may be required.

An easier way of using a bandage for compression of the anterior neck and submental region is to cut the bandage and create a shorter compression wrap that can be directly connected to the compression pad. Depending on the portion of the neck to be compressed, the alignment may be more vertical than horizontal, as shown in ► Fig. 5.37. To create this type of wrap, hold the pad in place and wrap the bandage vertically or diagonally, as appropriate, until one circumference has been achieved with a single layer of the compression bandage. Mark the distance where the bandage overlaps. If the distance is 70 cm, double the length of that segment and cut the bandage at 140 cm. In most cases, the remaining bandage can be used to create a second compression wrap. Fold the bandage in half so that the two loose edges of the cut bandage meet, and then secure them to the foam pad with a safety pin, tape, or by sewing. Hold the pad against the neck and wrap the folded bandage around the top or crown of the head; the

end of the bandage should terminate in the middle of the foam pad. After ensuring proper tightness, secure the end to the pad with the bandage clips. Adjust the wrap alignment if necessary to ensure that the patient's skin is not touched by any of the retention clips or pins. This technique features a double layer of bandaging with padding to provide adequate pressure to the edematous tissues. Once the bandage is attached to the pad, it is easily placed and removed by the patient in most cases, increasing patient independence.

Off-the-Shelf HNL Compression Garments

Non-custom or off-the-shelf garments are commercially available and can be used without detailed neck or facial measurements. They may be offered as "one-size-fits-all" garments or in small, medium, and large sizes based on measurements of head or neck circumference. These are appropriate for the neck and lower face only because they do not provide coverage for the upper or midface. Some chinstraps compress only the submental region, while others address the neck as well. Two styles are shown with pads in ► Fig. 5.38. Other chinstraps are hybrids of these two styles and feature variations in neck length as well as general size options. These garments are generally less expensive than custom garments, though prices vary widely by manufacturer. Owing to their lower cost and immediate availability, these garments are sometimes stocked by lymphedema clinics to be issued at the onset of treatment, whether for home program use or as an interim device to be used while awaiting a custom garment. These off-the-shelf chinstraps are generally considered appropriate for lymphedema management but must be used under the supervision of a CLT to ensure patient safety.

Non-custom full-facial compression masks are also available but should be approached with caution; most are inappropriate for HNL use due to several concerns. Primarily, an off-the-shelf full-face mask cannot properly fit the specific facial features of every individual with HNL. Improper fit can result in misalignment of eye, ear, or mouth openings, creating improper distribution of edema due to excessive tightness in some areas and insufficient compression in others. Generic facial masks often do not feature adequate adjustment capabilities, preventing appropriate pressure adjustments to prevent tissue damage and worsening edema. Low-cost fleece or neoprene facemasks and

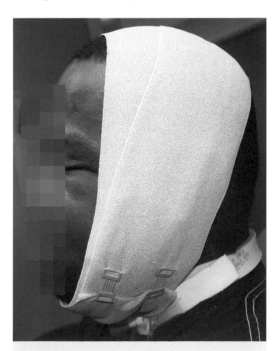

Fig. 5.37 A compression bandage for head and neck lymphedema.

5

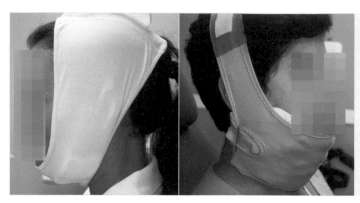

Fig. 5.38 Noncustom garments with padding. (a) Jobst facioplasty. (b) Epstein facioplasty by Jobst.

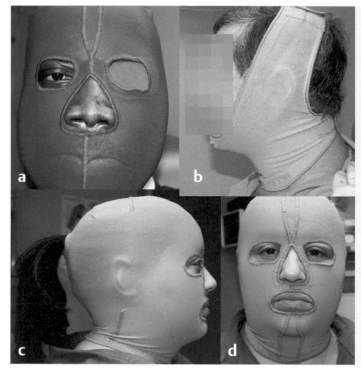

Fig. 5.39 Custom facial garments. (a) No mouth, eye patch. (b) Chinstrap. (c) Ponytail opening. (d) Standard facemask.

spandex turtleneck shirts that are not designed for HNL have also been used as inexpensive alternatives. Appropriate evaluation and supervision by a qualified therapist is essential before implementing these types of garments.

Custom Compression Garments for HNL

Custom-fit, made-to-measure chinstraps and full-facial compression masks are almost always preferred if available. Custom face and neck measurements are required to fabricate these garments and may be obtained by a vendor representative or by clinicians using the manufacturer's measurement templates. These measurements make it possible to accommodate the patient's individual physical characteristics, and a proper fit is usually guaranteed by the manufacturer. Revisions are typically available for little or no charge, depending on the vendor. Another benefit of custom garments is the availability of options such as eye or mouth patches, closure of ear or mouth openings, ponytail openings, etc., as shown in ▶ Fig. 5.39. Quilted custom garments are also available, providing bulkier material to help soften tissues after MLD if necessary. The cost of custom garments varies widely and usually reflects differences in the materials used and the manufacturing process. These garments can cost several hundred dollars, which may delay or prevent their acquisition for some patients. The lower cost custom garments are functional, appropriate, and especially advantageous when finances are limited, but there is often a difference in quality and comfort. An additional disadvantage of custom garments is the delay in acquisition due to the need to fabricate the garment. Although some vendors can deliver a custom garment in a few days for rush orders, others require weeks for delivery. In some cases, immediate compression is necessary while awaiting the arrival of the custom garment; therefore, consideration of all compression options is essential for each patient.

5.4.7 Elastic Therapeutic Tape

An adjunct to compression is the use of tape (such as K tape, Kinesio tape, muscle tape, etc.). Its ability to stimulate lymphatic drainage by opening lymphatic channels during natural skin movement makes it a very appealing option for some patients. With proper application, elastic therapeutic tape can be a very effective tool to facilitate drainage outside of outpatient or home-based therapy sessions. It can also be used effectively for musculoskeletal support and scar management, though caution must be exercised due to concerns with skin irritation from the adhesive. Of particular concern is previously irradiated skin, though each patient should be considered individually and carefully monitored for adverse effects. For patients with HNL, the use of this product may meet with some resistance because of its high

visibility when placed on the face or neck, but this is not true in all cases.

In general, the application of elastic tape is consistent with its use to facilitate lymphatic drainage in other parts of the body, anchoring with a solid piece of tape near the drainage destination, and radiating with "fingers" to drain the edematous region. As seen in ▶ Fig. 5.40, common anchor points for HNL use are the anterior chest near the axilla, the supraclavicular fossa, and the scapular region, depending on the location of the edema. The tape can be placed bilaterally or unilaterally and in certain cases may be applied to create contralateral drainage if significant scarring prevents drainage ipsilaterally. Adequate skin pliability can be achieved by placing the tape with "zero stretch," as the patient looks up and away from the clinician, resulting in tape contraction when the patient returns to the neutral position. The tape may be left in place for 2 to 3 days before removal in most cases. Again, careful observation of the skin is required to prevent adverse skin reactions, especially with irradiated tissue. Excessive wear time has been noted to cause significant skin irritation in some patients, even with no previous history of tape allergy. Elastic tape, when used appropriately, is an excellent option for HNL management.

5.4.8 Supplemental MLD Sequences

Alternative HNL MLD Sequence for Unilateral Axilla

Appropriate when one axilla is unavailable due to previous treatment.

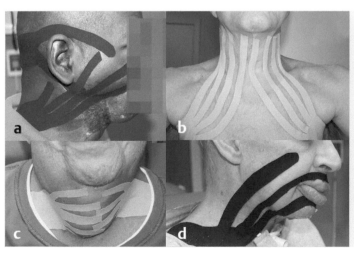

Fig. 5.40 Elastic therapeutic tape for head and neck lymphedema. **(a)** Unilateral face. **(b)** Bilateral to axilla. **(c)** Bilateral neck to supraclavicular fossa. **(d)** Contralateral face.

1–8. Unilateral trunk decongestion on available side, as described earlier (see Trunk Decongestion routine).

9. Sequentially decongest upper chest of impaired side, MLD toward available axilla.

10. Stationary circles in supraclavicular fossa, medially, away from impaired axilla.

11. Proceed with anterior or posterior drainage of the neck and face, as appropriate.

12. Reverse head, neck, and trunk sequence to available axilla.

Combined Self-Manual Lymph Drainage for Head and Neck Lymphedema

Appropriate for self-MLD when posterior facial drainage is needed without a caregiver.

1–8. Bilateral anterior trunk decongestion with self-MLD to axillae, as described earlier (see Trunk Decongestion routine).

9. *Posterior neck*: Overhand anterior stationary circles toward the ear and lateral neck. Can use one or both hands, depending on the patient's physical abilities.

10. *Lateral neck*: Using opposite hand, move anteriorly on one side of the neck only. Place fingertips beneath the ear. Overhand posterior stationary circles toward ear.

11. *Anterior neck*: Move hand to midline of anterior neck, second knuckle beneath chin. Overhand posterior stationary circles toward ear.

12. Repeat on opposite neck with opposite hand.

13. *Pre- and postauricular region*: Bilateral. Two fingers on either side of ear. Stationary circles down and posterior.

14. *Lateral face*: Bilateral. Flat hands on lateral cheeks and mandible, posterior stationary circles toward ear.

15. *Anterior face*: Bilateral. Flat hands to anterior cheeks, posterior stationary circles toward ear. Avoid upward movement toward eyes to prevent filling of lower eyelids.

If applicable, relevant areas of edema, including the intraoral region, nose, eyelids, and forehead, can now be addressed.

16. Reverse the sequence and perform steps 14, 13, 12, 11, 10, 9, 8, 7, 6, and 5 to mobilize fluid from the face through the neck to the bilateral axillae.

Manual Lymph Drainage for the Forehead, Eyelid, Nose, and Ear

Forehead and Eyebrows

1–8. Bilateral trunk decongestion.

9. Standard neck and facial decongestion as described in other routines.

Address before moving into anterior face.

10. Posterior decongestion of temples and central scalp into posterior head.

11. Proceed with posterior and lateral MLD away from midline toward posterior head, first addressing the superior aspect of the forehead, then moving inferiorly to the lower forehead and eyebrows as appropriate.

12. Once the forehead is decongested, the rest of the face can be addressed.

13. Reverse sequence and mobilize fluid to posterior head and neck.

Eyelids

1–8. Bilateral trunk decongestion.

9. Standard neck and facial decongestion as described in other routines.

Address once lateral face and forehead (if necessary) are decongested.

10. Using fingertips with very light pressure, begin at the lateral edge of the eyelid.

11. Perform stationary circles outward, away from midline.

12. Move medially and repeat until the entire eyelid has been decongested.

13. Reverse sequence and mobilize fluid to lateral face.

Nose

1–8. Bilateral trunk decongestion.

9. Standard neck and facial decongestion as described in other routines.

Address once lateral and anterior face has been addressed.

If a scar divides the nose, direct to adjacent drainage areas, even if it requires crossing midline. If there are no significant scars on the nose,

10. Begin at the lateral edge of the lower part of the nose.

11. Perform stationary circles away from midline, moving medially to address the entire lower nose.

12. Move superiorly up the nose, repeating lateral to medial decongestion.

13. Exercise caution near the top of the nose so that fluid is not moved into the eyelid.

14. Once the entire nose has been decongested, reverse sequence and mobilize fluid to lateral face.

Ear

1–8. Bilateral trunk decongestion.

9. Standard neck and facial decongestion as described in other routines.

Depending on scarring, drainage may be limited. Address after the neck and adjacent facial regions have been decongested.

10. Grasp the ear between your fingers in the area closest to a functional drainage pathway.

11. Stationary circles between your fingers toward the target pathway, moving sequentially around the ear. If a scar is present, begin away from it and move toward the scar as MLD progresses.

12. Once the entire ear has been addressed, reverse sequence until the fluid has been mobilized to the face.

5.4.9 Summary

HNL management can be straightforward or complex. As outlined in this chapter, proper evaluation is key to identifying proper treatment candidates and establishing effective treatment plans. Documentation of progress with tape measurement and photography allows clinicians to gather reliable data to support treatment and perhaps perform clinical research that will contribute to improved treatment methods over time. With proper use of the CDT methods described earlier, facial and neck edema after cancer treatment can be effectively managed, improving the quality of life for patients affected by HNL.

5.5 Elastic Taping for Lymphedema

5.5.1 General Information and Effectiveness

Therapeutic elastic taping originated with the work of Japanese chiropractor, Kenzo Kase, in the early 1970s with introduction into European practice developing over the following 30 years. Elastic taping has continued to gain mainstream popularity since its introduction to the United States during the 2008 summer Olympics. Growing evidence is developing and remains contradictory; however, many different techniques have been adopted in common clinical practice with several product manufacturers in the current market. In recent years, applications for edema techniques have evolved to include specialty methods for patients with lymphedema, demonstrating positive anecdotal clinical outcomes. Influence upon lymphatic taping technique evolution and research resulted from Shim's foundational study showing a 24 to 37% increase of lymphatic flow rates when elastic taping and passive range of motion were combined.[42] Additional research is clearly needed to support efficacy of this treatment modality.[43,44]

Elastic taping for lymphedema is utilized to encourage uptake of lymphatic loads, improve blood and lymphatic circulation, reroute fluid congestion, reduce fibrosis, increase tissue mobility, reduce pain, and facilitate muscle activation. Lymphangiomotoricity is influenced by deformation of the integument through movement, breathing, exercise, MLD, vessel pulsation, and pressure changes. As the patient performs respirations, general daily movements, and therapeutic exercise, the addition of elastic tape facilitates a slight tug on the superficial integument, which replicates the effect of MLD. Taking up the elasticity of the skin through rhythmical movements results in stimulatory mechanical stresses on the anchoring filaments and a resultant "open junction" of the initial lymphatic vessels allowing for uptake of lymphatic loads. Although the exact mechanism of action remains unknown, elastic taping most likely influences fluid dynamics and lymphatic transport through cyclic tissue changes within the soft tissues and allows for continuous effect beyond the clinical setting when worn.[45]

When applied with convolutions, elastic taping for edema conditions has been proposed to create variations in pressure with resultant tissue deformation. A negative pressure effect under the superficial integument is also thought to lift the skin from the fascia and subcutaneous tissues below, which allows for increased lymphatic pathway flow[46] (▶ Fig. 5.41). Two recent studies challenge the convolution concept and propose that patients can be taped in any position with no change in outcomes.[47,48]

Similar to MLD treatment effectiveness, elastic taping techniques are most beneficial in early stages of lymphedema. As the disease process progresses, subcutaneous tissues proliferate with pathological adipose tissues, fibrosis, and reduced elasticity.[49] When treating stage 1 and early stage 2 lymphedema breast cancer patients, researchers were able to demonstrate a significant reduction in circumferential measurements with various elastic taping techniques.[45,50] However, when taping is applied in more advanced stages 2 and 3 lymphedema, clinically significant results are

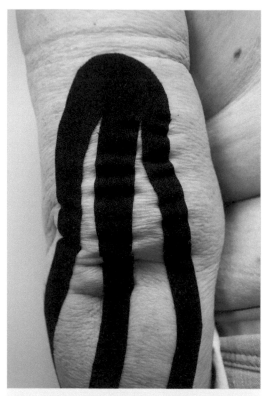

Fig. 5.41 Demonstration of the general fan cut and application over the elbow in a patient with stage 2 left upper extremity lymphedema. The base of the tape is placed proximal to the desired lymphatic flow route with the tails following distally to cover the desired treatment area. Notice the tape was applied with the elbow in flexion to allow full range of motion and visible convolutions upon recoil to neutral position (pictured).

contradictory, as demonstrated in several studies.[49,51,52,53] Inconsistent outcomes with this advanced population may be due to increased fibrosis and reduction of effect on fluid dynamics.

An early pilot study questioned whether elastic taping could replace bandaging and has shown therapeutic elastic taping to have better patient comfort, satisfaction, and quality-of-life indicators and was as effective as bandaging in the control group.[54,55] Sensations of heaviness and pain are also shown to decrease with taping.[52] In addition to edema reduction, elastic taping application has also been shown to improve range of motion, strength, and function of edematous upper extremities.[50]

Although lymphedema results from a mechanical insufficiency, elastic taping has also been advocated for utilization in dynamic insufficiencies such as

edema, seroma after surgical interventions, and posttraumatic/postoperative conditions.[56,57,58,59]

The majority of recently published research includes articles focused specifically on secondary lymphedema after breast cancer.[45,49,50,51,52,54,55,60,61] However, additional support exists and a body of literature is consistently growing regarding utilization of taping with primary lymphedema, head/neck, and lower extremities.[53,62,63]

Current sentiment among researchers and practitioners supports utilizing elastic taping as an adjunct to all components of CDT whenever possible. Efficacy of taping at this time does not support utilizing taping as a stand-alone treatment or to replace any component of CDT, but instead to enhance current treatment standards. In the case of contraindications/complications to MLD or compression bandaging, elastic taping could be utilized as a viable alternative.[64]

5.5.2 Safety/Complications

Extreme care must be taken to apply the base and tails of the application without tension to avoid potential skin tears and minimize irritation. The practitioner should also avoid wrinkles, folds, and creases, as well as utilize caution in areas with fragile integument. Commonly, practitioners recommend a small test strip application to an uninvolved area to assess for any type of adverse reaction 1 day prior to widespread treatment.

An increase in integumentary impairment has been documented with elastic taping, which puts the lymphatic patient at risk for complications.[54,65] Taping patients demonstrated occurrence ranges of 5 to 20% for experiencing inflammatory and allergic reactions and many were forced to withdraw from the associated studies.[49,51] A study specifically evaluating safety and tolerability of taping with arm lymphedema patients demonstrated no instances of serious integumentary effect or wounds; however, more than 40% of the participants experienced mild rash.[55]

It is recommended that practitioners utilizing elastic taping for lymphedema populations are certified in both CDT and elastic taping, to reduce risk of harm to this vulnerable population.[64]

5.5.3 Indications and Contraindications

With lymphedema patients, indications for elastic taping treatment include activation of anastomoses (▶ Fig. 5.42, ▶ Fig. 5.43, ▶ Fig. 5.44, ▶ Fig. 5.45), generalized and focal areas of edema (▶ Fig. 5.46, ▶ Fig. 5.47), truncal and head/neck edema where bandaging is difficult (▶ Fig. 5.48, ▶ Fig. 5.49, ▶ Fig. 5.50, ▶ Fig. 5.51, ▶ Fig. 5.52), scar management, traditional and alternative drainage pathways (▶ Fig. 5.50), ecchymosis (▶ Fig. 5.46), and pain relief. As previously discussed, elastic taping could be used as an alternative to bandaging when this technique is not possible or preferred due to compression contraindications, cost, environmental temperature tolerance, allergy, and quality of life.[60,65]

Contraindications/precautions include the following: direct use over new scars/incision sites,

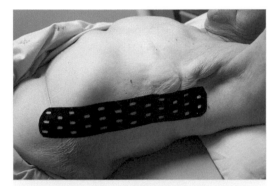

Fig. 5.42 Punch tape is applied to the axillo-inguinal anastomosis from the impaired axilla crossing the lower horizontal watershed.

radiation fibrosis, wound sites, cysts, and fistulas; skin sensitivities; skin insensitivity such as neuropathy; fragile skin; allergy; sunburn; and DVT. Use caution with systemic causes of edema such as cardiac and renal conditions.

5.5.4 Preparation and Materials

Elastic tape properties vary slightly between manufacturers; however, tape is generally 100% cotton with acrylic heat-activated adhesive, has a 5-day wear schedule, is able to be worn in water and with activities, and is hypoallergenic. Elastic taping was designed originally to replicate "normal" skin properties of epidermal thickness and longitudinal extensibility of 140%. Tape is applied to the backing with approximately 10% pre-stretch. The tape can be purchased in 1-, 2-, and 3-inch-width rolls as well as precut versions. A new taping concept, with precut holes allowing additional extensibility horizontally across the width of the tape, is also gaining popularity (**Fig. 5.42**). The goal of edema taping is to cover and stimulate a wide skin surface area in which the 3-inch roll is typically preferred.

Additional materials include high-quality scissors with carbon-coated stainless steel for preventing adhesive buildup and dulling. An electric razor may be needed for hair removal and is typically

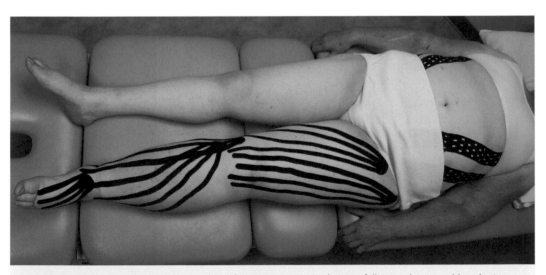

Fig. 5.43 This application demonstrates traditional anatomic taping techniques following the manual lymphatic drainage route for a patient with stage 3 primary lymphedema. Punch tape is applied bilaterally along the IA anastomoses. The limb is taped with fan cuts covering the treatment areas in a successive series over specific zones. Taping toward ipsilateral (involved), inguinal nodes may be utilized in general edema techniques or primary lymphedema; however, rerouting laterally may also be an appropriate strategy as shown in the photograph. Secondary lymphedema should be treated with lateral rerouting and taping toward involved lymph nodes should be avoided.

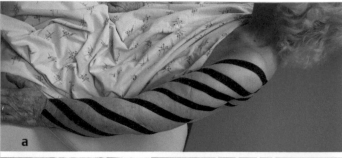

Fig. 5.44 Coverage taping is performed on a patient with secondary left upper extremity lymphedema to facilitate activation of the initial lymphatic plexus on the arm. The strips are applied individually and extend in a wave pattern over the poster axillo-axillary anastomosis.

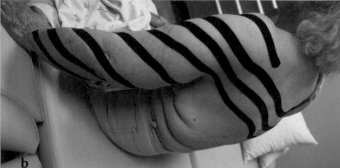

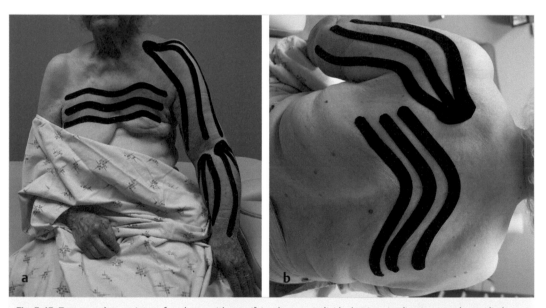

Fig. 5.45 Tape may be cut into a fan shape with a unifying base or individual strips. Application may be applied following the anatomical lymphatic drainage pathways or in a wave form to increase integumentary surface area coverage and intensity effect.

recommended over a straight razor due to micro-trauma that can occur to the skin surface with close shaving when combined with possible tape irritation. Athletic adhesive spray or skin preparation pads (typically utilized in wound care) can also be incorporated in treatment to form a protective barrier film on the skin surface for prevention of trauma and irritation with wearing and removal of elastic tape. Adhesive removal preparation pads are also helpful for removing the tape; however,

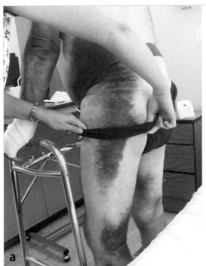

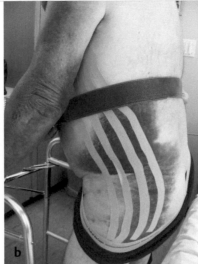

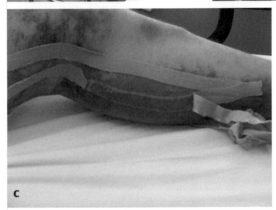

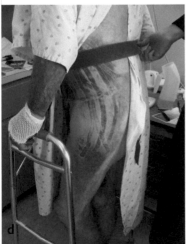

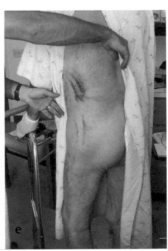

Fig. 5.46 The patient in this case study was taped for ecchymosis and facilitation of lymphatic load uptake. The patient was elderly; thus, a less intensive anatomical lymphatic strategy was utilized with clearance toward decongested axillary lymph nodes. Photos are 8/30, 9/4, and 9/10 respectively. Notice light coloration under tape tails indicating negative pressure under the strips, resultant uptake, and overall speed of recovery.

5

5

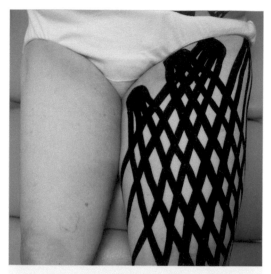

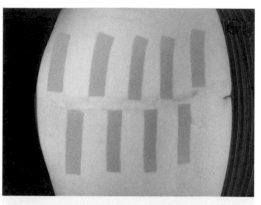

Fig. 5.48 The stable scar is treated after assessing for restrictions. The tape is cut into tabs for alternating application of mechanical stress to the tissues. The bases on each end of the tab are applied without stretch, while the central portion of each strip is stretched to ~ 50%. With subsequent applications, the orientation and stress to the tissue should be altered depending on patient-specific mobility restrictions.

Fig. 5.47 Intensity can be increased over an area of focal edema or ecchymosis by overlapping tape strips in a crisscrossed grid pattern. The closer together the tape tails are applied, the more intensive the effect.

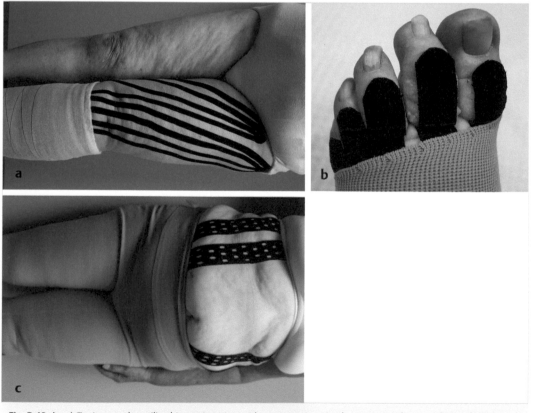

Fig. 5.49 (a–c) Taping can be utilized in conjunction with compression. Applications may be worn beneath garments and bandages or proximal/distal to compression. Care must be taken to avoid dislodging the tape when applying and removing compression.

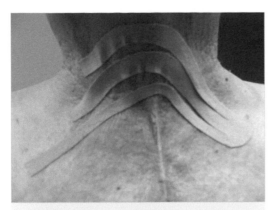

Fig. 5.50 Rerouting technique: Elastic taping can be applied with the goal of rerouting lymphatic loads around barriers to lymphatic flow. Since the tape affects the anchoring filaments and initial lymphatics, the plexus can be utilized for altering the pathway of flow in any direction. In this example, the patient has a fibrotic and restricting scar from the base of the neck distally to the umbilicus. To facilitate flow from the right upper quadrant to the left upper quadrant, taping was applied proximal to the scar in the general direction manual lymph drainage would also be applied for rerouting.

most oil-based products (olive, mineral, baby, etc.) could also be utilized.

5.5.5 Application

As with MLD, the goal of elastic taping is to direct lymphatic fluids toward areas of a less congested lymphatic pathway or lymph node grouping. The patient is assessed for the optimal route of clearance. This may include taping across an anastomosis for activation, along a bundle in the limbs, global stimulation of the initial lymph plexus, an alternative route to decongested lymph nodes, around scars or other barriers, etc. The taping application should enhance and follow the patient's individualized lymphatic drainage treatment strategy.

Two main lymphatic treatment strategies have evolved. The first and most common follows lymphatic anatomy, generally is congruent with MLD pathways, and is known as "directional" or "anatomic" taping. The base of the tape is applied in the uncongested target area with the tails trailing and covering the congested treatment area (▶ Fig. 5.43). The second aims to cover large amounts of skin surface area to maximize activation of the initial lymphatic plexus and is known as "coverage" or "zone" taping. This can be achieved by spiraling on a limb, crisscrossing or creating waves in the treatment

zone[9] (▶ Fig. 5.44). When utilizing the initial lymph plexus, tape orientation may occur in any direction toward a less congested area. Pop et al found that spiral wrapping resulted in greater reductions than traditional directional applications.[50]

Additionally, two tape cutting techniques have also emerged. The original "fan" cut application is prepared by estimating the length of tape needed to cover the treatment area. A 2-inch or longer base is reserved with cutting the remainder of the strip into tails. The fan-shaped cut allows for spreading of the tails to cover a larger surface area. Tail numbers can range from three to eight typically, depending on the skin properties, experience of the practitioner, surface area to be treated, and width of the tape. Tails are usually one-quarter to one-half inch width, with variability in this recommendation as well depending on specific circumstances. The second technique advocates for all strips to be independent without a unifying base. The strips are cut and applied individually to improve treatment area coverage, increase versatility, allow for easy access and removal of one strip without disturbing other strips, and decrease potential irritation under the base portion of the application[50,64] (▶ Fig. 5.45).

Lymphedema and Generalized Edema Technique

Preparation
- On the roll, the tape strip is placed over the patient's treatment zone to allow an estimation of the length needed for application. The goal of the treatment can be achieved in one long application (typically 6 to 8 inches), or in several smaller length applications placed in succession to one another (▶ Fig. 5.43).
- The tape is then cut into a fan shape or individualized strips to the estimated lengths. It is recommended that all squared corners are rounded off with the scissors to decrease unintentional tape nonadherence, but is not required. The paper backing is then torn to allow for the separation of the base from each individual tail for ease of precise application. Once the skin has been prepared and is free of oils, lotions, perspiration, and hair, the tape is ready to be applied.

Skin Application

- Place the patient's skin into a position of full stretch through positioning if possible, or the skin may be stretched manually if desired. Upon

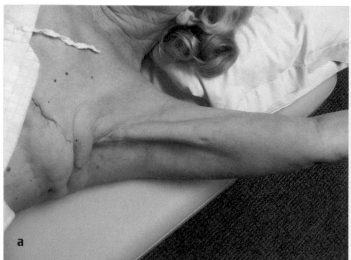

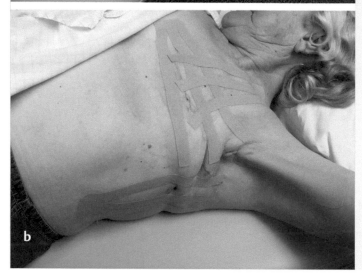

Fig. 5.51 (a,b) Secondary left upper extremity lymphedema with axillary webbing strategy: Complete decongestive therapy is enhanced by applying fan cuts to anastomoses including anterior and posterior axillo-axillary toward the right upper quadrant, left axillo-inguinal toward left lower quadrant, and above the upper horizontal watershed toward the left supraclavicular nodes. An additional strip of tape is applied over the axillary web syndrome cording presenting in this patient from the mastectomy scar distally toward the elbow. Tape is applied from distal point of cording adhesion toward proximal adhesion with off the paper tension or no stretch.

application in the stretched position, return to the natural resting state allows the skin and tape recoil with convolutions. Skin may also be taped in neutral, as the efficacy of convolutions has been contested in the literature.[47,48] Consideration for joint/skin position when taping to allow for full range of motion during wear and decrease in excessive tension during end ranges must be incorporated (▶ Fig. 5.41).

- The base of the tape is adhered at the "end point" where flow is directed with the tails following over the treatment area.
- Each tail strip is then adhered by removing the paper backing and placing the strip over the skin with no stretch or "off the paper stretch" applied to the tape. Repeat tail application individually

until all strips have been placed over the treatment coverage area. Tape tails are allowed to overlap or cross one another, with resultant increase in intensity.

- Once the tape is in place, the practitioner gently rubs over the tape longitudinally to adhere and warm the acrylic adhesive. Maximal adherence is achieved in 30 to 60 minutes due to body heat activation. Tape removal should be avoided during the first 24 hours secondary to risk of skin damage upon removal.

Ecchymosis/Focal Edema Specialty Technique (▶ Fig. 5.46, ▶ Fig. 5.47)

- The skin and tape are prepared in the same manner as described previously.

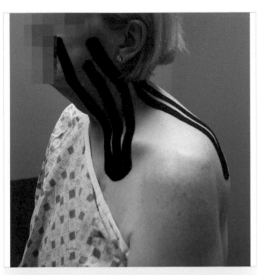

Fig. 5.52 Taping for head and neck lymphedema presentations are a useful treatment strategy as constant compression is often difficult to achieve. Careful consideration for scars and radiation fibrosis must be observed. This patient is taped with anatomical taping following manual lymph drainage patterns toward the left axilla. The base of the fan application is below the anterior and posterior upper horizontal watershed with tails covering the treatment zone. In general, taping can be applied unilaterally or bilaterally depending on patient presentation and treatment strategy.

- Application of the focal area is in a less intense anatomical or crisscross pattern for increased intensity and stimulation of the tissues. If indicated, the clinician may create a grid over the involved area. The base and tails of one strip are nearly perpendicular to the other strip with an overlapping checkered pattern covering the area of involvement. In an area of normal lymphatics, the orientation of the base and tails is unimportant as the goal of application is to move lymphatic loads to a functional surrounding area to be carried away by intra-territorial lymphatic anastomoses.

Taping Strategies for Increased Intensity (▶ Fig. 5.45, ▶ Fig. 5.47)

- The skin and tape are prepared in the same manner as described previously.
- Therapists may choose to increase the intensity of the taping effect via several different strategies, including the following: increasing the number of strips utilized in a treatment area, applying the strips closer together, overlapping

the strips, and applying in a wave pattern as opposed to straight lines in order to increase affected surface area. Tape strips may overlap or crisscross into a herringbone-like pattern over an area of focal edema as described previously. When applying waves, the concave and convex sides of the tape alter mechanical stresses to the integument and a greater surface area is covered to maximize stimulation. Reducing space between the strips increases the intensity, and increasing the width allows a more conservative approach.[66] Maximal intensity is achieved when the width between the strips is equal to the width of the tape strip itself.[66]

Stable Scar Technique (▶ Fig. 5.48)

- An additional specialty technique can be utilized for stable scars that demonstrate hypertrophy, decreased mobility, pain, and adherence issues. This technique is most typically utilized for surgical incision sites, but can be adapted to other scarring as well. Scarring over large body surface areas, such as burns, wide range radiation fibrosis, etc., is not an ideal population for this technique.
- Skin is prepared as previously described. The tape is cut into several 1 × 1.4-inch tab-like strips, making sure that the stretch of the tape remains longitudinal.
- The base of the first tiny strip is placed near the edge and perpendicular to the scar. The backing paper is torn away and the base adhered with no stretch on the tape. The central portion of the tape is then pulled to a 50% stretch on the tape and applied. The second base of the tape is then laid down with no stretch applied.
- The second strip is applied in the same manner and placed the width of one tape strip distally along the scar, but pulling to the opposite direction. This continues to alternate in pull direction as the strips are placed along the length of the scar. With subsequent applications, the direction of pull can be alternated for increased mobilization of the tissues in all directions.

Combined with Compression (▶ Fig. 5.49)

- Elastic taping can be very effective when applied under compression bandaging and can also be advantageous when applied as an alternative to bandaging.[52] Elastic tape may also be applied in areas that bandaging is not capable, such as across anastomoses; around scarring; or on the head, neck, and trunk. As an adjunct, tape can also be applied proximal or distal to bandages and garments.

Punch Tape (▶ Fig. 5.42, ▶ Fig. 5.43)

- A unique product new to the market allows longitudinal and perpendicular stretch through small precut holes in the tape and does not require cutting into strips or tails, which can save valuable clinical time. The holes allow for improved airflow and less adhesives contacting the integument. The positive and negative pressure differences create alternative mechanical stressors and stimulation of the lymphatics.[64] The tape is applied in one continuous strip over the predetermined treatment zone.

5.5.6 Patient Education

As with all aspects of CDT, the elastic therapeutic taping component requires extensive patient education. With initial applications, patients are instructed to avoid high level activity for 60 minutes before and after application to allow for improved adherence. Removal of the tape is discouraged in the first 24 hours, except in the case of adverse reaction, because it can cause epithelial damage during this time period of maximal bonding. Patients are allowed to swim and shower, but should pat the tape dry and expect a sensation of moisture for up to 1 hour. In the case of areas that begin to loosen or peel, patients or caregivers are encouraged to carefully cut the tape back to the level of the skin to avoid further premature removal. In case of emergency, patients also need to be instructed safe removal techniques, which are explained below.

Patients are encouraged to perform muscle pumping exercise and stretches, as well as general daily activities to facilitate maximal tape effectiveness and lymphatic uptake. Taping can be utilized with or without bandages, with combination of both techniques found to be highly effective in the clinic. Utilization of elastic taping and MLD are also complementary and can be beneficial in conjunction with one another. The elastic properties of the tape pull on anchoring filaments and create a slow, smooth stretch on the lymph collectors with resultant angion contraction, which are the same effects as MLD. When taping is used in combination with manual techniques, the resultant effects are enhanced.

Although elastic taping should not be clinically performed by untrained professionals, in time patients can be instructed correct usage for long-term therapeutic effects. Elastic taping is readily available via public vendors and internet resources. If using a traditional fan cut, an easy-to-understand patient analogy is that the tape is shaped like and behaves like an octopus. The head of the octopus (base) should be placed where you want the fluid to flow toward, with the tentacles (tails) following behind. Remind the patient that the "octopus swims where you want the fluid to go."

5.5.7 Removal

After several days of wear, the tape is usually easily removed due to shedding of the superficial epithelium. Ease of removal is enhanced when the tape is moistened and is removed in the direction of the body hair. As mentioned earlier, commercial adhesive removers, as well as oils, will also reduce the adhesive bond. During removal, fixate the proximal integument and separate the tape from the skin by utilizing your finger to push the skin down and away from the tape, rather than pulling up on the tape itself. Inspect the integument for any adverse effect. It is recommended that the tape be altered in application site or given 1 day between applications to the same area to allow for recovery of the integument.

5.6 Treatment Strategies for Common Complications of Lymphedema

The so-called typical lymphedema patient routinely presents with a complex medical history and clinical picture resulting in significant and sometimes numerous additional complicating concerns. Secondary lymphedema by definition involves trauma and or removal of lymphatic tissue, often at the demise of surrounding structures. Primary lymphedema is often neglected due to misdiagnosis and or poorly designed plans of care, making advancement of severity and subsequent tissue changes common. With more advanced stage 2 or 3 limbs, a far more extensive clinical intervention (intensive phase CDT) and long-term comprehensive care plan are mandatory to achieve adequate results.

In both possible classifications (primary, secondary), the underlying cause is a mechanical insufficiency of the lymphatic system. Inherited dysplasia or secondary tissue damage result in the same treatment challenges with predictable advancement through stages of severity. As the lymphedema therapist is working with a less robust lymphatic transport system, it is of great importance that treatment be adjusted to preserve the remaining integrity and status of lymphatic tissues and surrounding structures. In so doing a more generalized improvement in residual lymphatic drainage and the reversal of lymphostatic fibrosis and its sequelae can be achieved. If the immune system is severely compromised, infections may be frequent, acute, and life threatening. Regarding complications to therapy, it should be noted that poorly administered therapy could have lasting negative impact tarnishing the appeal of the gold standard of care CDT which should be avoided at all costs. The following complications are considered common in the lymphedema patient population and require a heightened awareness of negative consequences and vigilant tailoring of CDT protocols to deliver safe and effective care.

5.6.1 Surgical Scars

Surgical scars disrupt the superficial vessels in many patients especially where consideration of the superficial lymphatic collector anatomy has been disregarded. Lymphatic vessels are capable of repair and will, if undisturbed, re-anastomose via lymphangiogenesis. Upon close inspection, vessels repair in a less structured fashion, often missing valves or smooth muscle; however, this repair process is crucial to avoid secondary lymphedema in tissues distal to the node beds.[67] When nodes are removed, lymphedema is more likely because these represent the terminal point for a whole network of vessels. Without this inherent vessel repair process, simple cuts and lacerations during a person's lifetime would cause significant loss of lymphatic transport.

Assess Scars to Discern the Impact on Lymphatic Transport

With an understanding of the normal superficial anatomy of limb and truncal areas, assess the potential for interrupted flow within a territory. A poorly healed, disturbed, thickened, inflamed, or keloid scar may entrap fluid on the distal side of the skin region. If so a palpable tissue change (fibrosis) and or pitting quality (congestion) of the edematous tissues will be present.

Treatment Strategy

The MLD sequence should relate to any collateral pathways around the scar rather than through the scar when possible. In general, MLD should strive to utilize the most efficient intact pathways and substantiate the lion's share of the session. Scar tissue mobilization techniques or other specialized scar work should only be administered during secondary treatment sessions to avoid inefficient use of valuable MLD session time. Remember the overarching treatment goal is improvement of collateral drainage pathways via intact and patent collectors rather than local scar improvement.

5.6.2 Debulking Scars

Surgical treatment of lymphedema occurs by default when patients are not informed of CDT as the prevailing noninvasive therapy. Primary lymphedema patients are the most common recipients of surgical treatments due to the lack of appropriate diagnostic resources available to most physicians, insufficient physician knowledge about primary lymphedema pathophysiology, and the lack of a clear external cause (idiopathic edema).

Primary lymphedema patients may also receive less radical procedures such as collector transplantation, microvascular bridging, lymphovenous anastomosis, or liposuction. Others, however, receive the most radical procedures which "debulk" the limb of much or all of the involved tissues with the foremost goal of limb girth reduction (▶ Fig. 5.53). These radical procedures effectively remove the entire superficial lymphatic network leaving the therapist with little viable tissue with which to recruit efficient alternative drainage.

Debulking Procedures

- Staged excision techniques (Sistrunk, Homans, Thompson).
- Radical excision techniques (Charles).

Staged Excision Techniques

These procedures involve removal of the subcutaneous tissues (fat, lymphostatic fibrosis) down to the deep fascia via a large longitudinal incision. These incisions may extend along the medial and lateral calf and thigh and are usually planned as staged operations. The reduction involves more than the local incision area encompassing several centimeters of margin on either side, effectively removing large strips of subcutaneous tissue.

5

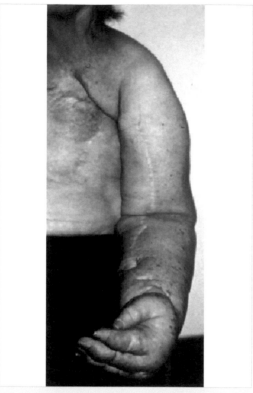

Fig. 5.53 A patient following a debulking scar procedure.

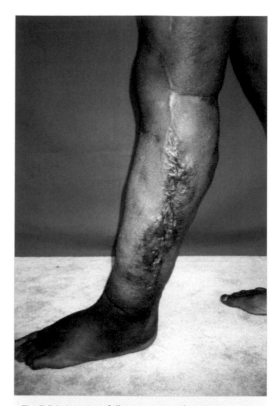

Fig. 5.54 A patient following a staged excision.

Strong tourniquets are applied and remain in place for as long as 2 hours. An Esmarch bandage, essentially a wide rubber band, is applied in spiral fashion to squeeze venous blood from the limb under great pressure in preparation for the surgery. Steinman's pins are drilled into the calcaneus and proximal tibia to suspend the leg for circumferential access to all involved surfaces (▶ Fig. 5.54).

Radical Excision Techniques

These procedures involve complete removal of all skin from the surgical area. The deep fascia is exposed and split-thickness skin grafts are harvested from the excision tissue to be sutured in strips back onto the muscle fascia. Similar presurgical preparation techniques are used to minimize blood loss and improve access to all sites. The removal of all tissues leaves an extremely altered and unsightly appearance in all patients. Commonly the calf region is excised using the Charles' procedure.[68] Thigh areas may more commonly employ Homans' or Sistrunk' procedures.[69]

Treatment Strategy

Status Post-Radical Charles Procedure

As the entire superficial lymph vessel network has been removed, MLD treatment of the grafted tissues has no apparent impact or rationale. With skin grafted directly to the deep fascia, no true subcutaneous space exists where swelling can occur. Furthermore, skin grafts quickly scar down adhering to the fascia and lose normal elasticity, rendering manual traction (MLD) impossible. Distal nonexcised tissues on the foot, ankle, and toes (a typical occurrence) tend to worsen, progressing toward elephantiasis more rapidly than they would as a natural course (▶ Fig. 5.55). Effective long-term drainage of these tissues relies on perforating collectors interfacing with the deep spared lymphatics of the limb. As such, treatment should encompass the following:

- Focus on proximal, spared areas and the deep lymphatic anatomy with MLD.
- Moisturize the grafted skin areas liberally to improve hydration status and elasticity (slow improvement can be expected).

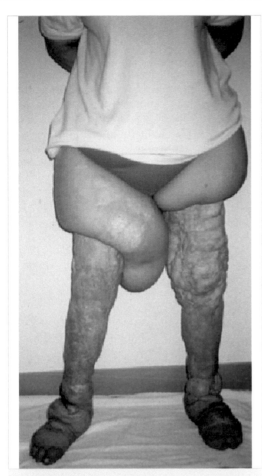

Fig. 5.55 A patient following radical Charles' procedure.

- Compress all tissues (edematous and scarred) from toes to proximal edema margins. Include grafted areas (although not swollen).
- Use foam padding generously to fill the defect areas and assist in creating a more conical limb contour for gradient flow of blood and lymph.
- Expect distal nonexcised areas to remain chronic and largely treatment resistant. These patients typically require more intensive follow-up and home care protocols.

Status Post "Staged Excision" (Homans, Sistrunk, Thompson) Procedures

Cosmetic results are far better in these cases, leaving the epidermis more elastic and less altered. As described, the subcutaneous space has still been radically altered and as such superficial lymph

vessels are far less numerous. Coupled with hypoplasia, the most common underlying dysplasia in primary lymphedema patient cases, a far less treatment-responsive limb can be expected. All postsurgical patients are candidates for CDT, but individual outcomes may be more difficult to predict. Considerations include the following:

- Assume surgical scars are effective barriers to drainage (will entrap fluid).
- Plan MLD to maximize collateral flow around scars.
- Expect slow improvement as compared with nondebulked limbs.
- Expect compression garment to be stronger compression class.
- Expect bandaging pressures to be higher to achieve softening and volume reduction.
- Compression strategy is normal regarding padding (no alterations are necessary).

5.6.3 Hyperkeratosis

Hyperkeratosis can be described as an epidermal hyperplasia due to lymph stasis, which appears as a local overabundant thickening of the skin with rough calluses,[70] wartlike formations, or papillomas (▶ Fig. 5.56). Hyperkeratosis is one of the key descriptors of stage 3 lymphedema (elephantiasis), which is a common consequence of chronic lymph stasis, which always involves secondary connective tissue disease. These skin changes are most commonly seen in the toes, but may encompass larger regions that are directly associated with the most chronic areas of static lymph. Sometimes, the term "lichenization" is used to describe odd presentations of hyperkeratosis due to the mosslike appearance seeming to grow on the skin surface. It is important to note that the presentation of

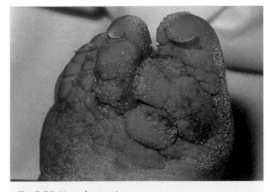

Fig. 5.56 Hyperkeratosis.

hyperkeratosis in venous disease (venous edema) changes the diagnosis more accurately to phlebo-lymphostatic edema.

Treatment Strategy

Hyperkeratosis may be extreme, imparting a resistant quality due to extensive overgrowth of hardened, calloused tissue. Surgical excision should be avoided due to local immune deficiency and delayed healing of edematous tissues. The presence of hyperkeratosis, especially on the toes, usually corresponds with a loss of normal shape or cross-sectional contour, making toes appear square. This leads to a loss of normal air circulation and the accumulation of moisture and fungal colonies. Maceration, tissue fragility, and recurrent infections are frequently associated with this clinical picture. Some suggestions include the following:

Compress Using Closed Cell Foam (Komprex) and Short-Stretch Materials

Fibrosis will soften, although initially it will be stubborn. Continued compression will allow some tissues to be restored over time and toes can become remodeled from square to round in cross-section.

Manual Tissue Manipulation

Self-administered gentle skin rolling and focused digital pressure can decongest underlying swelling, allowing hardened epidermal skin to become more pliable and slowly be restored to a more normal texture.

Lotions

Amlactin is an ammonium lactase lotion, which gently softens and erodes calloused tissue. Prescription grade: 12% concentration is available, or over-the-counter (OTC) 9% solution is available. Apply daily to regions of hyperkeratosis only and monitor for improvement while avoiding adverse tissue affects.

Meticulous Hygiene

Keep the interdigital spaces dry and all skin clean. Identify tissue erosion early from treatment elements that may be too intensive. Protect fragile areas from further breakdown because avoidance of infection is of paramount importance.

5.6.4 Abnormal Folds

As severity of lymphedema progresses, skin creases develop due to edema filling forces, gravity, limb position, elasticity of the skin, and even genetic traits (▶ Fig. 5.57). In some cases, a limb enlarges without contour changes, in others the distortions can be remarkable and alarming. When abnormal limb contours exist, the lymphedema therapist must adapt the compression strategy accordingly. Therapist's considerations should include the following before commencing treatment:

- Is the current limb shape counterproductive to the laws of LaPlace? (reverse cone shape, areas of narrowing, lobular outgrowths).
- Will the folds/creases entrap the fluid or allow for accumulations of bandages that are counterproductive to therapy?
- Are the folds/creases sites of recurrent infections?
- Are the areas within the skinfolds clean and dry or macerated and colonized with bacteria or fungus?

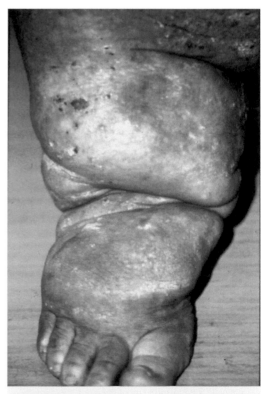

Fig. 5.57 Abnormal folds.

Treatment Strategy

During the pretreatment presentation, lymphedema will appear in its most advanced and treatment-resistant form. Lobular outgrowths and distorted tissues typically exhibit a pitting-resistant texture due to extensive fibrosis, hyperkeratosis, and fluid pressure. It is important to adapt treatment with sensible, thoughtful approaches such as the following:

- Cleaning and inspecting folds and skin creases.
- Treating with antibacterial preparations as necessary.
- Drying and protecting skin-on-skin areas thoroughly; tissue fragility is likely in protected, unstimulated skin areas.
- Packing the region with synthetic cotton and/or soft foam strips.
- Building out valleys (with padding) to create a continuous, smooth plane.
- Building out narrow girths (with padding) to avoid entrapment of fluid (Law of LaPlace).

In all cases, a correctly bandaged limb will improve texturally each session, allowing odd contours to become progressively more supple and compliant for each subsequent bandage application. In brief, the limb will transform rapidly from day to day so that even the most strikingly abnormal shapes will return toward normalcy again. Although cases involving abnormal lobes and folds are generally categorized as elephantiasis limbs, they should not be viewed as untreatable. However, commonsense modifications can be made to accommodate the abnormal contours. Bandage suggestions include the following:

- Modifying the directions of bandage turns (e.g., omit heel–ankle–sole [HAS] pattern, use the figure-eight pattern only, omit toe wraps if impossible, etc.)
- *Bandage first*: Bandage distal limb areas prior to performing MLD, and then nonbandaged regions (thigh); finish with proximal limb bandaging to complete the limb coverage).
- Use generous amounts of padding to offset defects and deformed tissue contours.
- Leave distal (more advanced areas) limb wrapped longer to focus on proximal decongestion (e.g., rewrap every 2 days).
- Use adhesive tape generously to secure regions that slip or seem unsecured.
- Alter bandage turns creatively. Depart from basics and use many more layers to create necessary structure and adherence.

5.6.5 Odors and Odor Control

Lymph Leakage (Lymphorrhea)

With advancement through the stages, lymphedema tissues become more prone to leaking lymph fluid. This stagnant lymph has a characteristic, malodorous smell that is difficult to describe but is largely consistent from one patient to the next. Usually with thorough hygiene and decongestion, this problem can be managed and if small wound areas exist closure can be expected as the limb decongests. Sometimes, lymph will encrust on regions around superficial wounds (cysts, abrasions, punctures) creating a scablike feature of yellow, dried exudate (▶ Fig. 5.58).

Treatment Strategy

- Clean meticulously with normal soap and water.
- Protect fragile skin with soft materials or wound dressings.
- Avoid maceration (use absorbent dressings).
- Watch for evidence of cellulitis (occurrence is common).

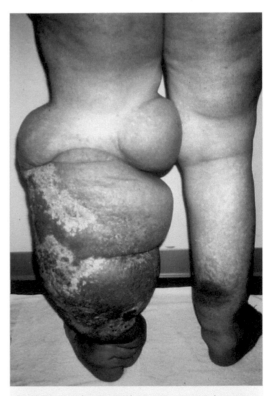

Fig. 5.58 Lymph encrusted on regions around superficial wounds can form malodorous exudate.

- Expect spontaneous closure of lesions with decongestive therapy.
- Avoid active debridement of lymph crust. As with a scab, fragile underlying skin loses protection. Allow sloughing to occur naturally.
- Hyperhydrate crust areas with petroleum jelly to soften and promote sloughing.

Bacterial Skin Colonies

Another source of odor may be related to the presence of bacterial colonies on the surface of the skin or those harbored in creased skinfolds. Some emit distinctive odors that can be specifically described and treated. Regardless of type, bacterial colonies must be controlled with meticulous hygiene and antibiotic ointments or other topical preparations to avoid potential cellulitis.

Treatment Strategy

- Triple antibiotic ointment.
- Atomized Flagyl spray (requires prescription and preparation).
- Regular soap and water (antibacterial soaps may create resistance).
- Corn starch (for moist skin areas).
- Towel dry after showering.

Odor Absorbers

- Activated charcoal pads (use external to wound dressings, not against skin).
- Stoma powder (use as indicated).
- Atomized Flagyl spray (requires prescription and preparation).
- Shaving cream (use generously on malodorous, intact skin areas).

Fungal Odor

Fungal infections produce a characteristic sweet or yeastlike odor and generally reside on the feet, or in skin creases, where moisture, warmth, and darkness prevail. Sometimes the groin or abdominal pannus become involved or areas where limbs are so enlarged that skin-to-skin contact cannot be avoided.

Treatment Strategy

OTC antifungal preparations may be adequate to arrest infections. However, a physician should be consulted to accurately assess the severity and type of infection to determine if special intraoral medication is necessary. Odors should resolve with treatment.

Fistulas

A fistula is an abnormal connection between two epithelial-lined organs or, as is the case in lymphatic abnormalities, lymphatic vessels and the surface of the skin creates a lymphocutaneous fistula. In lymphedema patients, fistulas may be present in a variety of anatomical places, such as the genital and rectal regions, within irradiated tissue, between arteries and veins as in complex vascular syndromes, or, in some cases of primary lymphedema, fistulas may occur between lymphatic vessels and the skin surface. In such cases, leakage of body fluids directly from these openings can create strong malodorous and infectious complications.

Treatment

If surgical repair can be performed, fistulas may be corrected or closed. However, when active disease such as cancer is causal, fistulas can remain persistent and untreatable. Activated charcoal pads as a palliative treatment perform well in these situations to control odor, increase the patient's sense of dignity, and make treatment progress more comfortable for both therapist and patient.

5.6.6 Fungal Infections

Patients with lymphedema of the legs and feet often encounter fungal infections due to several factors such as the following:
- Loss of normal contour of toes (square instead of round): decreases air flow and increases moisture, darkness, and warmth (▶ Fig. 5.59).

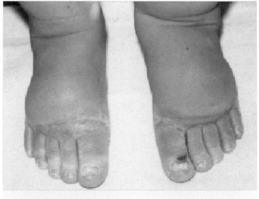

Fig. 5.59 Fungal infections.

- Loss of footwear choices due to abnormal size and shape of foot: causes recontamination within same pair of shoes.
- Decreased local immune function.

Although fungal infections may be acute, they are usually not regarded as strict contraindications to therapy unless the tissues are fragile or open. A normal plan of care would dictate that fungal infections be arrested prior to commencement of therapy to reduce the avoidable complication of spread to other skin regions. However, should treatment begin during an active fungal infection of lesser severity, with caution, the therapist may carry out CDT bearing in mind the following suggestions:

Treatment Strategy

- Apply topical antifungal preparations, stockinette, and toe bandages with hands gloved.
- Wrap to the knees first (prior to MLD) to cover distal involvement and avoiding contamination of other areas.
- Administer MLD to proximal, truncal areas (above bandage) only to avoid contact and spread. MLD is not required in the infected areas temporarily.
- Discard all materials that are intimate with skin to avoid recontamination, daily.
- Discard contaminated footwear and instruct patient as to how to avoid future problems.

5.6.7 Radiation Trauma

When considering lymphedema patients, the single largest group comprised cancer therapy recipients (in the western hemisphere north of the equator).

As radiation therapy is a mainstay of gold-standard care for many types of cancer, lymphedema therapists must carefully consider the secondary effects of this therapy on tissues within the field. MLD and compression, although approached with care, skill, and a low level of intensity, can have harsh effects on irradiated tissue. Radiation causes a slow retreat of microcirculation (dieback) in soft tissues leading to ischemia and scar-tissue formation. Soft tissues may become palpably altered and exhibit a loss of elasticity, supple texture, and normal color. When assessing radiation effects, lymphedema therapists should familiarize themselves with the conditions in the following sections.[71]

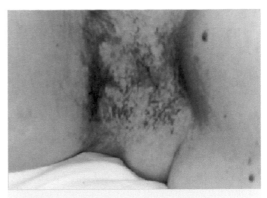
Fig. 5.60 Telangiectasia.

Telangiectasia

Upon close inspection in some cases, a visual, palpably undetectable yet permanent change occurs in the superficial skin of the area of irradiation. Telangiectasia is a spider-vein–like presentation, where the capillary plexus of blood vessels is distinctly visible, engorged or even varicose in appearance (▶ Fig. 5.60). Although the presentation may, at first glance, be alarming, it is generally not an indication of severe radiation trauma. Tissues remain elastic and normal to the touch. The cause of telangiectasia is related to the loss of sympathetic motor control of the precapillary arteriole's ring of smooth muscle. This sphincter muscle controls the arterial inflow within the blood capillary plexus and when paralyzed relaxes to allow an excess of pressure locally. This increased blood capillary pressure dilates and enlarges the capillary bed, making it more visibly apparent.

Treatment Strategy

- Avoid forceful stretch and pull on the local area—even normal MLD traction force may be excessive.
- Further assess the status of the underlying tissues in the region as they may indicate or raise suspicion of further radiation damage necessitating strong caution. Is radiation fibrosis present?
- Moisturize skin thoroughly and instruct the patient in careful self-management.

Radiation Fibrosis

Tolerance of radiation therapy is highly variable and some patients do not suffer secondary effects. In others, however, with the development of ischemia, connective tissue slowly impregnates the region of irradiation. As it becomes more extensive, tissue texture, elasticity, and skin tension continue to worsen. As time passes and without physical therapy, fibrosis may become irreversible causing many additional concerns.

Superficial and Deep Radiation Fibrosis

Upon palpation, superficial textural changes may be apparent. The skin and subcutaneous tissue may feel like a continuous, solid sheet with a loss of normal elasticity. In some cases, the margins of this connective tissue may define and correspond precisely to the field of irradiation. If the skin is still pliable and nonadherent to underlying structures (mobile), it is generally considered a less advanced presentation. Regardless of this, superficial radiation fibrosis may still present challenges, indicating a significant reduction in local lymphatic collector transport capacity due to mechanical entrapment. Superficial nerve and/or blood vessel entrapment is also possible, causing collateral vein formation and numbness or other neurological changes.

With extensive radiation damage, soft tissues become chronically and severely altered, exhibiting signs of color change (rusty red, brown) with a complete loss of elasticity and further adherence to the underlying structures (bone, soft tissues; ▶ Fig. 5.61).

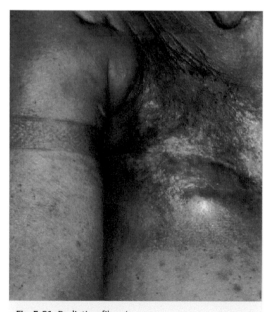

Fig. 5.61 Radiation fibrosis.

Complications from Deep Radiation Fibrosis

These include the following:
- *Osteonecrosis*: Damage to the periosteum causes bone necrosis, decalcification, and possible bone reabsorption. This condition is irreversible.
- *Limb paralysis*: Motor and sensory nerve entrapment from direct damage to nerve plexuses with demyelination. Secondary connective tissue entrapment resulting in total loss of function and sensation. This condition is irreversible.
- *Collateral vein formation*: Fibrosis can slowly entrap veins and arteries. Deep vein strangulation results in collateralization of the venous blood, causing visibly apparent vein formations in the skin.
- *Skin fragility*: Superficial skin may become extensively dry, brittle, atrophic, and prone to ulceration. Tearing is possible if overstretched.

Treatment Strategy: Superficial Radiation Fibrosis (Nonadherent)

Significant improvement of tissue affected by radiation therapy is slow and should not detract from the overarching aim of therapy, which addresses total limb edema reduction. A separate session with new goals may be advisable if a special focus on fibrotic tissue release is desired or planned.
- Avoid deep techniques (MLD or other) in the field regardless of severity.
- Liberally apply moisturizer to maintain hydration and avoid fragility or dryness.
- Study the radiation zone to see how it impedes the known anatomical vessel drainage and then strategize to redirect the flow toward collateral vessels and anastomoses.
- *Time permitting*: Using very light pressure, stretch the tissue using only MLD techniques (stationary circles with finger pads) to soften and reorganize the connective tissue (collagen matrix).
- Palpate the region daily to detect improvements and adjust the intensity of manual techniques with special caution at all times. Ask for patient feedback.
- Gentle compression with foam padding (either smooth or contoured surface) may soften tissues depending on the severity of induration. A careful study of the outcome of each treatment is required to further moderate intensity and avoid tissue injury.

5

Treatment Strategy: Deep Radiation Fibrosis (Adherent)

When damage is so extensive that a "glued down" or adherent quality is clearly present, the lymphedema specialist's chief concern must be avoidance of secondary tissue injury during therapy. Skin tears, hemorrhage, unremitting pain, and spontaneous bone fracture are real concerns while positioning patients during therapy. Flaccid paralysis of the edematous limb is not uncommon when significant radiation has been administered in the regions of major nerves and nerve plexuses.

Additional Considerations

- Position the patient with consideration for the inextensibility (frozen state) of irradiated tissue and underlying structures. The supine or prone position may not be possible.
- Bolster flaccid or insensate limbs to avoid loss of limb position control (slippage).
- Do not attempt to reorganize or soften irradiated tissues with manual therapy because it may create significant, irreversible damage or pain.
- Hydrate tissues often to offset dryness and brittle skin. Consider special skin products.
- Do not attempt to improve lymph drainage through tissues severely affected by irradiation. Use treatment time wisely recruiting neighboring healthy regions.
- Look out for minor skin tears at the edge of radiation field tissues. Stretching of adjacent normal skin (with MLD) can extend backward into the atrophic, adherent skin region causing chafing and small tears.
- Instruct the patient in sensible lifestyle adjustments to avoid injury and preserve or improve the current tissue status. Do not employ aggressive strategies.
- Avoid direct compression over severely irradiated tissue. Irritation or allergy caused by compression materials can be slow to heal. Softening with compression may be too aggressive to warrant application. Risks may be too high.
- Deep MLD techniques are strictly contraindicated. Superficial MLD must be extremely light if used at all. Strict avoidance may be the safest plan.

5.6.8 Papillomas

A papilloma is defined as an overgrowth of the papillae of the skin or mucous membrane and is

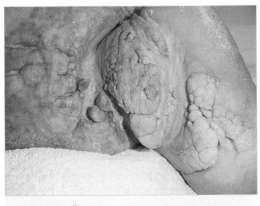

Fig. 5.62 Papillomas.

one of the key descriptors of stage 3 lymphedema.[72] This benign formation could be characterized as a skin tag that has become inflated with fluid and is therefore a bulbous, balloon-like feature attached with a highly vascularized stem of tissue (▸ Fig. 5.62). When lymphedema becomes chronic, a direct relationship exists between the level of inflammation and the formation of hyperkeratosis and papillomatosis in certain individuals. Typically, papillomas form at the most chronic distal tissue regions or along scar formations following debulking procedures. Other papillomas form in thin pliable tissues such as those found in the genitalia. Notably, if regional decongestion is achieved through treatment and before the papilloma becomes impregnated with fibrosis, a dramatic shrinking and even complete disappearance of these formations can occur in many cases.

Owing to the fragile nature of the papilloma, injury is common due to mechanical stresses, such as toweling, donning and removing of garments, application of lotions, etc. For this reason, they can often be cited as the entry point for pathogens and may be responsible for recurrent episodes of cellulitis. Leaking and bleeding are common and lead to great patient frustration. Lymph exudate is commonly malodorous and affects a patient's sense of dignity, compounds quality-of-life constraints, and, in particular, affects his or her enjoyment of socialization.

Treatment Strategy: Considerations

- Many papillomas will soften and shrink away if not yet fibrotic. Injury and leakage may cease and further improvement may occur with continued compression.

- Chronic fibrotic papillomas are prone to injury and infection, warranting surgical removal. Decongest the territory first so that postoperative healing will be enhanced.

> Although surgical interventions are not embraced as treatment for lymphedema, and protection of the skin barrier is of paramount importance, a suggestion for surgical removal of chronic papillomas is viewed as a minor, low risk procedure aimed at correcting a defect that is responsible for cellulitis.

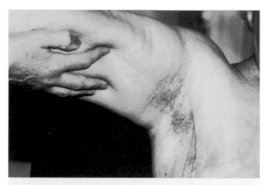

Fig. 5.63 Lymph cysts and varicosities.

5.6.9 Lymph Cysts and Varicosities

Lymph cysts occur due to congestion and dilatation of lymph vessels (▶ Fig. 5.63). Cysts mostly occur due to congenital malformation; however, a local surgical interruption of lymph drainage can also create sufficient collector hypertension and reflux to cause cyst formation.[73] This is more commonly evident in areas where skin is thin and extensible such as the axillae and genital regions. Depending on the tissue structure related to the cyst (collector, capillary), a distinction can be made as to the level of congestion of surrounding tissues and origin of the problem. If caused by primary malformation, cysts may be less correctable by decongestive therapy because the underlying cause may involve valvular incompetence or hyperplasia of the deep lymphatic system. In some cases, chylous fluid is seen weeping from the skin.

White cysts rather than clear cysts indicate chylous reflux from deep intestinal lymphatics or the thoracic duct itself.[72] A lymph varicosity is similar to a varicose vein and involves a collector (▶ Fig. 5.63). In thin-skinned (geriatric) patients, visualization of hypertensive, engorged, or varicosed lymphatics may be possible. This presentation is not common, however, where subcutaneous adipose is more substantial.

Treatment Strategy

- Cysts are extremely fragile and are likely to rupture when exposed to any mechanical stressors (bandages, garment, MLD, exercise). Apply a sterile, highly absorbent dressing over cysts prior to compression bandage application.
- Assess patients' risk level for infection based on history or level of concern. Always identify antibiotic of choice and attain full prescription as a precaution.
- Discuss signs and symptoms of cellulitis with the patient and a sensible plan for antibiotic administration (physician directed) if required.
- Expect most cysts to resolve (shrink or disappear) once the involved territory is thoroughly decongested.
- If chylous reflux is present, consider imaging studies to determine if a surgical solution is required. Recurrent cellulitis is life threatening with pathogens gaining direct access to the deep lymphatic system via chylous cysts.

5.6.10 Collateral Veins

During an initial physical examination, close inspection of the involved quadrant should be thoroughly documented. When lymphedema is caused by surgical intervention, secondary trauma may be apparent. Upon close inspection, certain asymmetries may require further investigation, such as comparative status of nonirradiated skin to irradiated skin, atrophic or hypertrophic tissues, palpable or visual masses, abnormally prominent or altered vein formations, etc. It is always important to recall the causes of swelling to differentiate between various presentations. Venous obstruction alone may cause swelling (venous edema).

Causes of venous obstruction include the following:
- Superficial or deep vein thrombus.
- Tumor obstruction.
- Mechanical entrapment due to radiation fibrosis, scar tissue formation, bone fracture, etc.

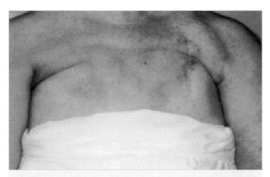

Fig. 5.64 Collateral veins.

As lymphedema is a diagnosis of exclusion, patients with complicated medical histories must be thoroughly scrutinized to avoid atypical findings being overlooked or dismissed. Collateral veins are not typical features of benign secondary lymphedema. A collateral vein indicates an altered pathway of venous return when a primary vein is not functioning properly. Unless a definitive recent medical assessment of the cause of collateral vein formation is provided, the lymphedema therapist must regard collateral veins as evidence of current obstruction requiring physician examination (see ▶ Fig. 5.64).

Once cleared, permission to commence or resume treatment should be granted. If collateral veins are directly associated with the field of irradiation, there is a high suspicion of entrapment of veins due to the slow development of radiation fibrosis. During evaluation and interview, the patient should be familiar with the onset and physical presence of these collateral veins and report a history of slow and gradual onset inconsistent with the therapist's grave suspicions. However, if the veins are a rapid new development and have escaped the patient's notice or appear in an unrelated area (not in the radiation therapy field), a high suspicion of obstruction (DVT, tumor) must be investigated especially when there is a history of cancer.

Treatment Strategy

- Collateral veins from the above causes are chronic and will not resolve or disappear with treatment.
- When collateral veins are caused by a DVT, follow guidelines for postthrombotic syndromes (PTSs) as outlined by vascular medicine, before commencing treatment.

- If collateral veins appear within the radiation field, refer to "Treatment Strategy: Superficial Radiation Fibrosis (Nonadherent)" previously in this chapter. Collateral veins are not the focus of treatment.
- When collateral veins are clearly caused by tumor obstruction, cancer management takes priority. The physician will clear the patient for CDT if appropriate. Palliative care may be the goal.

5.6.11 Limb Paralysis

Lymphedema patients with extensive underlying trauma due to accidental injury, cancer therapy (e.g., Cobalt radiation), or other disease processes (post-polio, spina bifida, multiple sclerosis, etc.) may present with functionless, insensate, and dependent edematous limbs. Although these patients are suitable candidates for CDT, they must be categorized separately as "special needs individuals," given the mechanical nature of therapy will place them at considerable risk of additional injury if not employed with a high degree of care and skill. Tissue fragility leading to wound formation is a chief concern.

Treatment Strategy: Considerations

- Before bandaging, analyze the cross-sectional shape of the area receiving compression:
  - Oval, bony, conical, cylindrical?
  - The Law of LaPlace dictates smaller radii will receive more pressure ($P = Tc/R$). The Law of LaPlace guides the compression strategy (overall gradient and local pressure distribution).
  - Employ padding strategy appropriate to shape.
- Observe that tissue atrophy and lack of sensory feedback set the stage for compression-related wounds.
- Realize that patients rely entirely on the therapist's skill because feedback related to comfort is not possible to assess pressure and intensity.
- Always err on the side of "too light" rather than "too tight" when bandaging.
- Thoroughly inspect the treated area each day and look for erythema or "hot spots." Buffer against excessive pressure in these areas. Daily cumulative pressure effects may cause irreversible tissue injury.
- If blistering or lesions occur, healing will be greatly delayed. Special wound care administration may be required and CDT may be postponed or coordinated with wound dressings.

- Assess the impact of additional bandaging on limb weight and the patient's ability to move without danger.

Compression Tips

The hands and feet are oval in cross section unless extremely swollen. To comply with La-Place's law, oval-shaped areas must be padded toward a more circular cross section to modify the distribution of pressure. Ample padding applied to the dorsum and palm, for instance, will reduce pressure on small radii (radial/ulnar surfaces) and increase pressure on larger radii (dorsum/palm) avoiding predictable "hot spots" and tissue injury.

5.6.12 Self-Induced Lymphedema (Artificial, Factitious)

Although rare in the United States, cases of self-induced lymphedema are reported. In some countries where social services are more generous, self-induced lymphedema is more common and may be viewed as a means of disabling oneself in order to receive government-administered benefits.

The clinical appearance of artificial lymphedema shows a distinct margin between the edematous and uninvolved tissues (▶ Fig. 5.65). This stark demarcation is associated with subcutaneous atrophy and discoloration at the site of applied tourniquets proving that a constriction method has been employed to block lymphatic flow causing the appearance of a chronic, enlarged, or "painful swelling." When treatment is initiated, the patient may be motivated to sabotage the results, tying off the proximal limb with a tourniquet to obstruct drainage. Failure of conservative treatment (CDT) must be expected unless the patient's motivations are addressed and corrected.[74] Direct confrontation or accusations of self-mutilation may be counterproductive and referral for psychiatric evaluation is imperative.

5.6.13 Malignant Lymphedema

The lymphedema treatment specialist is commonly viewed as an important resource for terminal cancer patients by providing end-stage edema and pain management. Malignant lymphedema by definition involves proximal tumor masses which physically obstruct the outflow of lymph and venous blood, affect arterial inflow, and compromise nerve structures eliciting intense pain, numbness, or limb paralysis (▶ Fig. 5.66).[75]

A patient with malignant lymphedema requires considerable modification in the plan of care but should still be viewed as an ideal candidate for CDT, tailored sensibly and with appropriately adjusted end goals. Although malignancy is regarded as a relative contraindication to CDT, this is due to the suspected complexity of the entire medical history. Physician clearance is required before proceeding in order to address any grave concerns related to possible adverse effects of the modalities of CDT.

Depending on the disease, an adapted CDT approach will eventually follow a palliative care model. However, if energy is still high, and pain levels are managed, activities of daily living may

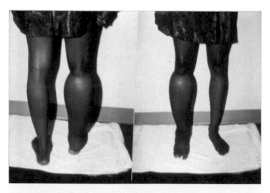

Fig. 5.65 Self-induced lymphedema.

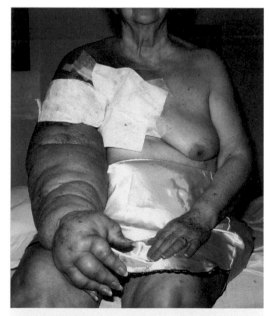

Fig. 5.66 Malignant lymphedema.

be greatly enriching to the patient. As such, a minimal adjustment in the treatment approach (as compared with uncomplicated CDT) may be very productive for some time, bringing great relief from discomfort. As the disease progresses, typical modifications include the following:

Treatment Strategy: Considerations

- Greater reliance on MLD for pain and fluid management.
- Less intense bandage pressures (very low resting pressures).
- Greater reliance on compression bandage due to high containment (working pressure) and low resting pressures.
- Less reliance on elastic compression. High resting pressures are poorly tolerated and do little to control edema.
- Relax the treatment schedule requirements of the "intensive phase." Expect appointment cancellations due to loss of energy, conflicting medical appointments, and failing health. Patient should feel no psychological pressure to comply with a daily CDT regime if health conditions worsen.

It should be noted that MLD employed as a pain management modality is quite beneficial and has proven extremely productive as a complementary tool with no adverse effects. Even when the general health condition becomes grave, patients remain highly receptive to MLD above all other therapies. For this reason. MLD should be offered frequently for as long as possible and will be prized by the patient and family as a loving extension of compassion during hospice care.

5.6.14 Cellulitis

A troubling side effect of a mechanically compromised lymphatic system is the immune deficit leading to the development of infections (cellulitis, erysipelas). Interestingly, there does not seem to be a direct correlation between extent of swelling (volume, severity) and the frequency or severity of cellulitis. Many mildly involved limbs may be severely prone to cellulitis, while a massively swollen extremity may be surprisingly resistant and resilient to skin injury or poor hygiene. Regardless of clinical presentation, all patients must be educated and familiarized with the signs, symptoms, precautions, and treatment of cellulitis to arrest the progression immediately (▸ Fig. 5.67). Early

antibiotic intervention not only avoids critical complications (toxic shock, death) but also protects the involved tissues from secondary inflammatory processes. Inflammation involves the production of free radicals, which if not removed via a functional lymphatic system create a toxic interstitial environment, accelerating reactive fibrosis of the skin and the staged progression toward elephantiasis. The cause of cellulitis is the invasion of resident skin bacteria such as group A streptococci and *Staphylococcus aureus*.[76]

The clinical picture of cellulitis includes the following:
- Chills, followed by high fever.
- Severe malaise.
- Nausea, headache.
- Local pain.
- Warm/hot skin, redness.
- Maplike borders.
- Rapid progression (within hours).

Treatment Strategy: Suggestions

- Immediate antibiotic administration.
- Stop treatment if CDT is under way.
- Watch for stabilization and fever reduction on schedule.
- Expect skin to remain red and warm for several days.
- Sloughing may occur.
- Resume CDT once the core temperature returns to normal.

As a temporary combined insufficiency (dynamic and mechanical) occurs during infections, resume CDT as soon as the core body temperature returns to normal so that compression and MLD can offset the swelling and promote more efficient lymphatic transport. Long-term precautionary measures

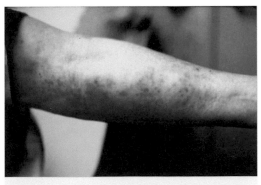

Fig. 5.67 Cellulitis.

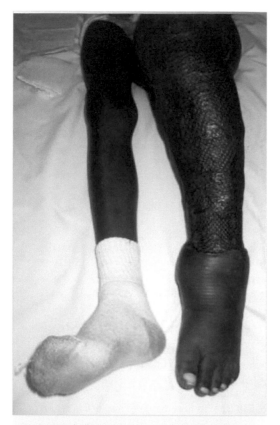

Fig. 5.68 Debulking procedure performed at major academic hospital in 2005.

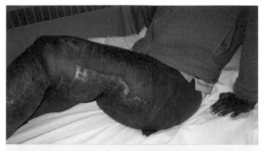

Fig. 5.69 Radical Charles' procedure (1912) performed on a patient with primary lymphedema, 8 years of age.

center around hygiene and avoidance of injury to the skin while hydration is maintained to avoid chapped, scaly skin. Low-pH lotions focus on creating an intact acid mantle that is less penetrable to resident microbes while reducing the bacterial count on the surface of the skin.

5.7 Adapting CDT to the Pediatric Patient

5.7.1 Avoiding High-Risk Treatment

At present, there is no cure for lymphedema. Alarmed and distraught parents not aligned with generally conservative lymphedema specialists have commonly undertaken radical surgeries as a form of treatment. Although many well-intentioned surgeons have undertaken and continue to attempt a myriad of ingenious techniques, it

remains a fact that no reliable benefits have come from these procedures. More often, surgery results in significant additional cosmetic disfigurement or lymphatic impairment, and further delays access to the gold-standard techniques of CDT.

Surgery

The most common type of surgery can be categorized as a "debulking procedure." It defies logic to believe that the removal of substantial amounts of subcutaneous tissue, containing functional lymphatic vessels, will result in an improvement of the overall condition. Furthermore, primary lymphedema is caused in the majority of cases by hypoplasia of vessels and nodes. Removal of what remains simply renders the limb more disabled (▶ Fig. 5.68, ▶ Fig. 5.69).

In some, the Radical Charles Procedure is performed (as seen in the photo). This technique involves total removal of the skin down to the muscle fascia, followed by split-thickness skin grafts applied over the fascia. Other excisional techniques like (Thompson's or Homans') involve long incisions that spare the epidermis but effectively amputate the subcutaneous tissues by stripping from either side of the flaps. Excisional surgery is not indicated for primary lymphedema, especially in children.

Complications include the following:
• Clinical depression due to body image and disfigurement issues.
• Nonhealing wounds, risk of limb loss.
• Loss of sensation.
• Impaired function.
• Severe worsening of lymphedema in areas distal to excision.

Currently refined surgical procedures such as lymphovenous anastomosis, vascularized lymph node transfers (VLNTs). and lipo-lympho-suction (suction-assisted protein lipectomy [SAPL]) are becoming popularized for some adult candidates. These techniques are still investigational but show promise in some instances. At present, such procedures are not recommended for pediatric patients. Primary lymphedema typically involves hypoplasia, so autologous donor sites are predisposed to develop lymphedema with greater likelihood than individuals with normal transport capacity. Furthermore, risk of infection is high in those with immune deficiency that usually accompanies primary lymphedema.

5.7.2 Moderate-Risk Treatments

Pumps

Another common treatment for lymphedema is the intermittent pneumatic compression (IPC) pump. Although pumps provide some relief and may temporarily halt the advancement of swelling, the benefits are nearly always temporary, and may result in abnormally large accumulations of lymph at the root of the limbs and within the trunk. A significant number of patients with lower extremity lymphedema treated by pumps report genital lymphedema following daily use. This very serious consequence is always avoided by comprehensive treatment with CDT. As with surgical intervention, pediatric patients should be spared IPC with its risks and complications so that appropriate therapy can be initiated immediately.

Concerns with pump use include the following:
- Provide temporary, diminishing relief.
- Risk to ipsilateral trunk congestion.
  - Genitals in lower extremity cases.
  - Chest/back in upper extremity cases.
- Do not remove proteins.
  - Hasten fibrosis formation.
  - Dehydrate the pumps region.
- Unsafe pressures if unmonitored.
  - Common when effect diminishes.
- Act to delay effective therapy which should commence immediately.
- Consume allocated resources away from conservative therapy.
- Fit of pump may be poor for pediatric sizes.
- Promote inactivity.

Compression Garments and Bandages (Ill-Fitting or Unskilled Applications)

It is not uncommon for pediatric patients to acquire compression tools for independent use at home by caregivers. Without proper training or education, parents can blindly administer compression without consideration for the potential risk of injury to the child. Children younger than 1 year may be too small for safe compression bandaging or garment application. Limb girths are so small that relative pressures are higher than in adult limbs due to LaPlace's law. Intertarsal and intercarpal spaces between bones are very susceptible to pressures due to the tenderness of ligaments and other connective tissues. Bones move spontaneously under pressure in very young children.

Elastic bandages are strictly contraindicated. If compression is appropriate, these materials should be replaced with standard short-stretch bandaging. Short-stretch materials should only be administered case by case (dependent on age and other concerns) with ample lymphedema specialist-guided training and review with responsible caregivers. Similar to elastic bandages, compression garments possess high resting pressures, so may be inappropriate for children less than 1 year old or if very petite. It is the responsibility of the CLT to identify high-risk modalities or compression tools that can be discontinued and replaced with medically correct and safe compression therapy.

Identifiers for compression contraindications:
- Deep, red pressure marks or blisters at key areas along the limb.
  - Legs: Base of toes, instep, heel, popliteal crease, proximal margin of garment.
  - Arms: Web-spaces, wrist, cubital crease, proximal margin of garment.
- Rolling, cutting, or doubled-over garment edges.
- Compression class is either not identifiable or too high (CCLs 2, 3, 4) for pediatric applications.
- Misshapen limb areas due to strangulation, excessively high pressures (i.e., foot narrowing) or prolonged duration of wear.
- Bargain brands without proper medical clearance.
- Coverage is too extensive for the involved area (impeding distal limb drainage).
- Coverage is insufficient (ignoring an area that requires support).

5

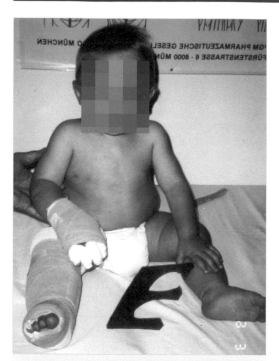

Fig. 5.70 Milroy's disease, right upper and lower quadrant involvement. Short-stretch bandaging over open–cell foam and synthetic cotton.

5.7.3 Complete Decongestive Therapy for the Child

Even when lymphedema is apparent in infancy, implementing a course of conservative treatment early is advisable. By initiating a sensible treatment strategy early on, it is hoped that the chronic and progressive consequences of the disease can be significantly lessened (▶ Fig. 5.70).

CDT liberates the patient from surgery and encumbrances such as pneumatic compression pumps, limb elevation, and forced inactivity; and it encourages healthy activity levels with proactive child involvement. The four components of CDT—MLD, compression bandaging, remedial exercise, and infection prevention with meticulous skin and nail care—can be coordinated into a seamless strategy for adult patients. However, in the pediatric population, education for autonomous home care therapy involves selecting any CDT components appropriate to the child's tolerance, with the goal of optimizing a typically abbreviated clinical (intensive phase) treatment. This implies that, dependent on age, compression therapy (either elastic or inelastic) may be premature.

Activity and Lifestyle

Owing to the chronic and lifelong nature of lymphedema, parents are encouraged to permit their child to engage in normal activities such as sports, arts and crafts, and outdoor play. It is valid to consider the fact that with lymphedema comes an increased risk of acute infection and cellulitis, especially when the skin is injured. However, to disallow normal play may bring about significant and more troubling psychological or emotional consequences.

Interestingly, as with adults, many children with lymphedema are spared infections following numerous traumas, and are therefore considered at lower risk than others regarding the consequences of normal activity. For each child, his or her unique immune robustness will be learned in time. If infections occur, some activities may require modification if they appear directly causal to the event. Lymphedema in the majority of cases is not a disabling condition; however, children who have been raised to feel disabled are truly at a disadvantage, and may not experience the joy and freedom of childhood.

5.7.4 Practical Guidelines for Pediatric Patients

As noted, the typical approach to treatment must be significantly modified for the pediatric patient, especially in the case of infantile lymphedema. The following suggestions arise from clinical experiences gathered from treatment involving dozens of children.

General Adaptations of CDT

Treat the Parents First

All parents of children with lymphedema must be educated about the condition so that a realistic picture of the chronic attributes can be digested and appreciated. No surgical cure or pharmaceutical therapy is available. It is unfortunate that lymphedema remains an incurable condition; however, with early, competent guidance, the secondary tissue changes associated with lymphedema (lymphostatic fibrosis) can be greatly reduced. Optimally, limb girth can be maintained at nearly normal size. As a goal, immune function and systemic and regional lymph drainage are enhanced with increasingly intensive MLD treatments as the child grows. These benefits cannot be underestimated because the long-term impact is quite positive and rewarding. By addressing parent's fears first, which often mitigate overreactions, despair, and frustration, the therapist can build a relaxed and trusting family partnership to the child's benefit. Limb function without limitation allows for normal physical and psychosocial activity and is an achievable goal in most cases of well-managed lymphedema. For all parents, this goal is of paramount importance and helps address their strong concerns related to lymphedema as a permanent "handicap."

If parents strongly believe nothing better exists than CDT, they will look no further and ultimately protect their child from desperate, high-risk, and unproven alternative therapies.

Therapist's objectives include the following:
- Argue against high-risk procedures.
  - *Suggest imaging*: Lymphangioscintigraphy (LAS), although considered optional and typically not impacting the CDT treatment plan, may be helpful for managing some parents' anxiety, ensuring better overall compliance with the CDT program. The LAS proves a deficiency exists, which is a strong argument against surgical procedures.
- Instill confidence in CDT.
  - The body of literature is vast and support CDT as the gold standard in all cases. All other approaches to care are ancillary and do not constitute comprehensive care.
  - Provide education about CDT before initiating therapy so that parents are comfortable with moving forward and committed.
- Provide clinical perspective.
  - Although absolute predictions cannot be made to address extent, severity, infection risk, or outcome to therapy, therapists can provide sound answers to questions.
  - Become the parents' ongoing lymphedema consultant. CLTs have more specific training than most medical professionals and can network parents to the best resources in the field.
- Initiate and adapt a treatment plan to commence CDT.

Be Patient and Cautious as Caregiver

Very young patients cannot communicate specifically what is bothering them. Without clear feedback, caregivers must adopt a relaxed and careful approach to compression therapy and always adopt a less aggressive mindset. Overly aggressive care is never productive for lymphedema patients regardless of age. But especially in pediatrics where all tissues are delicate, great care must be taken to avoid discomfort and most importantly injury. One must remember that a comfortable and happy patient will be a compliant patient. Moreover, this special child with a lifelong physical challenge who lacks the ability to control this imposed regimen must not be mistreated with untrained and dangerous compression procedures.

Parents can be consumed with worry and approach compression bandaging overzealously with the mistaken impression that "more pressure is better." This is typically due to the immediate reduction response to compression seen following bandage removal. However, as with anyone receiving compression therapy, aggression is far more likely to produce discomfort, pain, or skin infections, which can worsen lymphedema. As already stated earlier, the pediatric patient must be afforded more caution to avoid serious injury that may not be communicated to parents clearly and immediately by the child.

Similarly, MLD treatments delivered by the parent may be counterproductive if heavy-handed or rough. Lymphatic vessels are delicate, threadlike structures, which may spasm or become otherwise injured by inappropriate treatment. In the clinic, parents must invest time learning the appropriate skills. The importance of this investment cannot be overstated nor can the time spent in question-and-answer sessions with the therapist. The better educated the parent, the more likely they are to provide high-quality care for their child.

Therapist's objectives include the following:
- Discussing the comparative properties of short-stretch versus elastic bandages and garments.
  - Make sense of working and resting pressure, tension, and layering.
  - Describe the need for foam paddings (multiple reasons).
  - Explain LaPlace's law in simplified terms so that parents understand the shapes and placements of key padding materials, and the rationale.
  - Outline the signs and symptoms of intolerance, pain, or adverse effect.
- Discussing the principles of MLD and the techniques of the hands-on manipulation (strokes).
  - Impress the importance of light touch and working at the plane of the skin.
    - Practice it on the parent's skin. Reciprocate until it is correctly demonstrated.
    - Each stroke has a working and resting phase.
  - Convey a clear logic for the decongestive sequence to be followed.

- The involved limb is the last area to be treated (counterintuitive).
- The goal is a systemic improvement in drainage to the benefit of the involved limb/s.
  ○ MLD is NOT massage! It is a soft tissue manipulation that does not seek to improve or enhance blood circulation. There is no gliding, friction, or rubbing.
  - This can be very difficult for caregivers to comprehend.
  ○ Simplify strokes.
  - Single-handed techniques, no combination strokes are necessary.
  - One hand covers large body regions, so less hand placements are required.
  - Pump and stationary circles only. These are easy to learn and provide all of the benefits of MLD.

Play Sessions

Depending on age, most children will need to adjust to this "strange new routine," as well as to the intervening therapist. Time must be planned and budgeted for this necessary warm-up process using "play sessions" to create a feeling of comfort and safety, and orienting the child to the therapist's style.

Suggestions include the following:

- Set up a television or digital device in the treatment room as a welcome visual distraction.
- Bring favorite toys, music, and foods.
- Place a soft clean quilt on the floor and attempt treatment and bandaging from this vantage point.
- If it seems to benefit the session, allow a parent to hold the child on his or her lap while working.

During all sessions, continual verbal cueing is conducted with the parent, which is usually of great value. At first, this unstructured or playful format may seem less productive and become a source of further anxiety for the parent seeking immediate results; however, should this step be omitted, sensitive young children will not comply with any of the components of the program, ultimately creating an even less productive outcome.

Start with a Semi-Intensive Phase

Generally younger children (< 5 years) respond best to a "semi-intensive" approach, in that the total treatment duration is reduced to 2 weeks, versus 4 + weeks, as in adult programs. One benefit

to this adapted CDT model is that it allows for unused treatment sessions to be allocated over coming months. These sessions involve frequent follow-up visits where parent and therapist can review home care techniques and remain up-to-date concerning the overall condition of the child.

Therapist's objectives include the following:

- Build rapport with parent and child.
- Manage parent anxiety through education and by providing clinical perspective.
- Realize that adult approach is too intense and will be counterproductive.
- Learn the child's tolerance too and the effect of MLD and compression (if indicated).
  ○ Take charge before transferring tasks to the caregiver.
  ○ Learn what works.
  - Modify or discard anything that seems poorly tolerated or which appears a premature intervention or is too intensive.
  ○ Transfer caregiver tasks to the parent.
  - Require that caregivers demonstrate proper manual therapy.
  - Repeat during every session until safely performed.
- Schedule follow-up visits.
  ○ Frequency depends on therapists' confidence in caregivers' skills.
  ○ Initial follow-up within weeks, successive visits every 2 to 3 months.

Start with MLD and Self-Care Suggestions

For very young children of less than one year of age, therapists may be quite productive in administering MLD. This "massage-like" treatment, involving gentle, soothing skin manipulation, is usually well received by the infant. Parents can observe and repeat the agreed-upon treatment sequences at home, and may find that the best time to administer treatment is during nap times, or at night while the child is sound asleep. Older children of age 18 months to 3 years who are considerably more active and less agreeable to this routine may also benefit from similar timing.

The quality of touch required for proper MLD treatment is so gentle that children will become positively conditioned, and in time will view it as another form of loving touch from the parent and therapist. In time, children will also develop skills for self-care and can be engaged in self-MLD practice as they mature.

The goals of MLD are to create more efficient drainage within the affected area and systemically while offsetting the chronic skin changes associated with lymphedema. In children, the early intervention of MLD is extremely valuable in slowing or reversing these effects, especially on the dorsum of the hand and fingers and on the dorsum of the foot and toes. In some cases, the genital area is involved, making MLD application an essential home care component toward offsetting chronic skin changes.

Objectives of MLD for young patients:

- To establish a new routine so that this quality of touch is not foreign.
  - Expect that all children will respond to MLD favorably if experienced as gentle and loving.
- To productively intervene with safe therapy.
  - MLD may be the only form of therapy initially but offers many benefits.
- To provide a tool.
  - MLD can be done whenever a parent is holding the very young child.
  - May be best timed during naps or at night for very active children.
- To address difficult areas.
  - MLD is the only possible manual therapy for fingers, toes, and the genital region.
  - Bandaging is impossible or unsafe.
  - These regions tend to become chronic quickly in children making MLD a key tool.

5.7.5 Limitations of CDT

It is quite common for parents and CLTs alike to feel frustrated and limited while working with lymphedema children. Compared to adult patients, therapy often proceeds with full intensity and offers very predictable improvement in many different outcome areas that can be measured. These successes are partly due to the clear commitment and open communication that patients can make to the program. Adult patients have a tolerance to round-the-clock compression, are able to receive full body MLD, and can demonstrate self-care tasks to the CLT's satisfaction. The relationship is between therapist and each patient directly.

In pediatric patients, virtually all of this very skilled care falls upon the deeply invested caregivers who attempt to learn every required task. But in some instances, caregivers lack the aptitude, dexterity, temperament, or other resources to convey adapted CDT appropriately. In such cases, the CLT must decide how to modify, add, or subtract therapy elements or tools to maintain a safe and

effective home care plan. The chief limitations of CDT in very young patients are the lack of intensity of therapy and therefore less tangible treatment results initially. Compression is a very powerful tool that produces immediate measurable and visually apparent results. Although parents may be asked to refrain from compression until the child can tolerate this modality safely, they should know that more tools will become available by 1 year old in most cases. It is therefore important for therapists to convey the plan of care as continually unfolding to involve more opportunity to achieve effective results.

Compression Therapy

As mentioned earlier, compression therapy can be counterproductive if lacking great care and skill. Exercising this extreme caution becomes an additional expectation of parents, and must only be taught to responsible and cautious caregivers, with careful therapist assessment. In all cases, physician supervision is prudent even if unfamiliar with lymphedema to allow an open dialogue about the proposed modalities of therapy and to facilitate access if antibiotics, pharmaceuticals, or nutritional support are required (gastrointestinal absorption).

Some patients are simply too young to intervene with compression therapy. In other instances, a CLT exercising caution may consider applying a modified bandage in the clinic to gain a clearer picture of the potential for improvement based on the compression response. This customized pediatric bandage may not be practical for parental application until a later date, but may yield some important clues about the child's responsiveness to therapeutic compression.

With standing and walking (9+ months of age), lymphedema of the legs and feet may begin to worsen. This is the point in time where some compression strategies should be explored and employed. The only situation where intensive compression bandaging might be sanctioned earlier is with elephantiasis, a situation rarely encountered in infants. Therapist and parent must consider the benefits and tradeoffs carefully, as bulky multilayered bandaging impact the child's ability to safely "toddle." Bending the knees to crawl is made more difficult, and in the case of arm lymphedema, a bandage may largely compromise tactile skills and simple grasping tasks. For these reasons—which also include the child's compression tolerance level—an intensive phase of 2 weeks (10+ treatments) is usually adequate to deliver quality care, including home care education to astute parents.

Within this 10-day timeframe, the therapist's goals include the following:

- Achieving measureable softening and volume reduction without force.
- Learning the limbs' unique compression gradient for optimal long-term improvement.
- Effectively educating one or more caregivers in basic and tailored MLD techniques.
- Effectively educating one or more caregivers on the safe application of compression bandages.
- Measuring for any necessary compression garments, if appropriate.
- Educating parents on the signs, symptoms, and treatment of infections.

Compression considerations:

- Distracting the child is key.
  - Use videos, books, or toys to help settle the child so that a bandage can be applied. Be organized and work quickly yet safely.
- Therapist must take lead.
  - Never teach a technique before doing the technique.
  - Study the outcome of your own work and memorize your precise technique.
  - Replicate what is working, modify what is not working.
  - Learn the unique attributes of the limb and its response.
- Teach the caregivers, but:
  - Expect the technique may be too complex to master.
  - Distill the procedure to its essence so that it is achievable.
    - Add or subtract materials.
    - Package foam in sleeves.
    - Use ample tape to secure layers.
- Carefully assess parental mastery
  - Session-by-session improvement is the goal.
  - Unsafe bandaging must be discontinued.
- Assess the encumbrance for the child.
  - If worn while sleeping is less of a concern.
  - If worn while awake may be a concern for movement and general safety.

5.7.6 Age-Related Adaptations of CDT: From Birth to First Steps

Manual Lymph Drainage

MLD is always appropriate. Convey the following core principles to caregivers:

- Provide a rigorous stretch to the skin only.
  - No friction, squeezing, gliding, kneading, or rubbing.
  - It is not "massage." Refrain from using the word.
- Direction of stretch is always proximal on the involved limb.
- Each stroke has a working (stretch) and resting (relax) phase.
- Quality of touch is gentle, slow, and soothing.
- Demonstrate Dr. Vodder's pump and stationary circle techniques only.
  - Omit rotary and scoop techniques.
- Never neglect the toes and fingers to avoid chronic changes from occurring.
- Remember that "baby fat" overlays the edema and so defies palpable softening or pitting as indicators of the positive effect of MLD.
- Halting progression of swelling with subtle improvement are the current goals.
- Frequent treatment is beneficial, as it is the only modality suitable at this time.
  - 20 minutes per session, two to three times per day.
  - Nap times, night time, bonding times.

See Section 5.7 CDT Treatment Protocol Variations: **Primary and Secondary Lymphedema** for specific pediatric treatment sequences.

Compression

Avoid compression in infancy except in rare cases of severe lymphedema. Always seek physician's supervision to rule out other causes of such extreme pediatric swelling.

5.7.7 Age-Related Adaptions of CDT: From Standing Age to Toddler and Older

Manual Lymph Drainage

- Frequent daily treatments.
- Reinforce all core principles at all times.
- Practice with caregivers each follow-up visit.
- Observe and analyze the sequence for its effect and to modify.

Compression

In order to counteract gravity, compression therapy is warranted; however, all of the following precautions still apply (▶ Fig. 5.71):

5

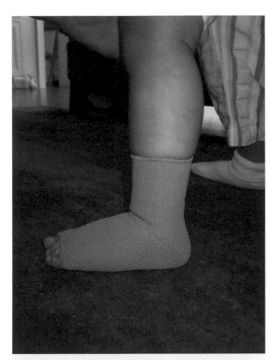

Fig. 5.71 Flat-knit pediatric anklet. Compression Class 1.

- Any sign of discomfort, pain, or intolerance must be mitigated.
- Signs of tourniquet effect must be rectified.
- Signs of retrograde lymph flow indicate poor technique, ill-fitted garment, or lack of gradient.
- Evidence of skin rash, abrasion, blistering, allergy, or excess erythema must be addressed and remedied.
- Misshapen limb contours indicate high pressures and/or poor garment fit. They also indicate a less than optimal gradient.

Both compression garments and bandages are possible options once a child is standing and walking. Each type of compression offers a different quality of pressure, which is beneficial as a long-term strategy for all ages and lymphedema presentations. However, with very young children and in the absence of chronic skin changes, elastic garments have several benefits.

Benefits of Garments

- Garments have a medically correct gradient pressure woven into the fabric.

- Bandages require the gradient to be created by the caregiver.
- Compression class (strength of support) can be controlled by the chosen class of fabric (always CCL 1).
- Compression garments can be measured to fit lightly and with a focus on the limb areas of concern.
- Garments are a single layer of fabric as compared to a bulky bandage; so they are
  - Less disruptive to gait.
  - Cooler to wear especially in warm climates or seasons.
  - Lighter in overall weight.
- Garments can be donned/doffed with less technical training.
  - Are less fallible to be being improperly placed.

Tradeoffs

- Garments are custom made and expensive.
- Replacement is more frequent due to rapid growth.
- Garments should be professionally measured for precise fit.
- Garments can be dangerous if precautions are not observed.
  - Never wear at night (round the clock).
  - Never allow rolling or bunching for prolonged periods.

5.7.8 Special Considerations for Compression Materials

Most bandaging materials are sized for the adult frame, and are too large for most young children or the infant patient. The following suggestions are important modifications in the materials' usage and are geared toward enhancing positive effects while mitigating the negative impact of pressure.

- Downsize materials.
  - Select 4-cm short-stretch rolls, replacing the standard 6 cm widths on hands and feet. Graduate to 6-cm short-stretch bandages or 8-cm materials as the maximum widths for limb segments.
- Protect the skin.
  - Velfoam is a special product gentle to pediatric skin. This fleece-lined foam padding material is well suited to delicate tissues and should be incorporated or substituted for other forms of padding (▶ Fig. 5.72).

5

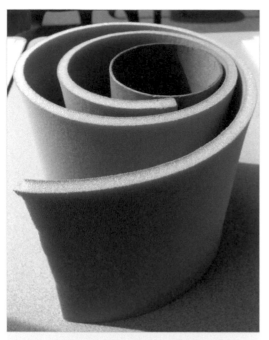

Fig. 5.72 Soft foam rolls for pediatric skin. Velfoam.

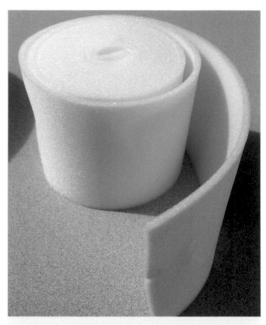

Fig. 5.73 Soft foam rolls for pediatric skin. Rosidal Soft.

- Synthetic cotton, foam rolls.
  - Artiflex, Cellona, and Rosidal Soft synthetic cotton or foam padding can also be used generously in combination with foam as an anti-shearing layer. Remember with rolls of material, shifting will occur, so flat foam should accompany these pads (▶ Fig. 5.73).
- Consider girth.
  - Omit the toes. Toes are usually too tiny to effectively wrap. A tourniquet effect is more likely on small circumferences, and great caution should be used if an attempt is made. Treat toes with gentle MLD, and firmer manual manipulation.
  - Select 4-cm materials for fingers which are best wrapped with traditional materials, such as Transelast or Elastomull. Take care to double the bandage into two-ply, as this will concentrate the bandage on a smaller skin area.
- Consider the order of materials.
  - Following lotion application, stockinette (TG, Tricofix) typically follows; however, even stockinette can be too harsh for pediatric skin. Apply synthetic cotton first followed by stockinette and foam or omit it altogether (▶ Fig. 5.74).
- The role of garments.

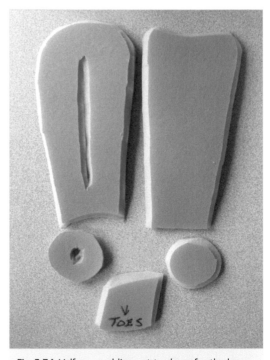

Fig. 5.74 Velfoam padding cut-to-shape for the lower leg.

- Elastic sleeves provide medically correct gradient pressure, which may be more precise than a caregiver's bandage.
  - Parents can rest assured that their "less-than-expert bandaging technique" can be corrected by daytime gradient compression.
- The child is liberated from cumbersome bandages during the daytime.
- Normal developmental milestones, such as coordinated crawling and walking, can be reached without delay.

5.7.9 Summary

Although early-onset primary lymphedema is troubling and challenging for the lymphedema specialist, it is devastating for the parents and others close to the child. Once the initial shock passes, most parents aggressively seek solutions only to find a dearth of clinical knowledge, insight, and competence. The well-trained lymphedema specialist becomes the most relied upon resource and fills the void with tangible, safe, and effective tools to be employed sensibly as the child matures.

This section strives to address the necessary modifications that must be made for young patients so that CDT can commence at low intensity, yet provide valuable therapeutic benefits. The single most important aspect of effective CDT with children is the realization that the parent or caregivers must be the focus and that they become a direct extension of the therapist for the majority of the child's daily life. Although CDT is the international gold-standard therapy for lymphedema, it is modalities are powerful and potentially dangerous if special pediatric precautions are not observed. This must be conveyed to the caregiver and reinforced frequently.

Primary lymphedema is only a disability if a person is told so. Most adult primary patients having lived as children or teens with the diagnosis do not live disabled lives, and having never known differently approach life with energy, zeal, and optimism. It is imperative that lymphedema specialists reinforce and reflect a healthy emotional and psychological perspective when treating these patients and interacting with parents.

Parents of these children are well served to consider allowing normal activities even those that involve physical contact or roughness and only retract if a true adverse consequence occurs. Infections are frequent in some but quite rare in many others, so should not be the reason to restrict a child from such activities without a prior history.

Immune deficiency although possible is highly variable and has little to do with severity of the lymphedema, so requires individual study in each patient's case. In all cases, as the child reaches 5 years of age or older, a more intensive approach to therapy is possible, yielding all of the benefits that are expected in adults. If the child can comply with therapy by remaining idle and helpful, lymphedema specialists have an opportunity to explore MLD and compression in far greater depth.

5.8 CDT Treatment Protocol Variations: Primary and Secondary Lymphedema

5.8.1 Adaptations for the Primary Lymphedema Patient

As known lymphatic dysplasia (hypoplasia/hyperplasia) is the underlying cause of lymphedema in primary lymphedema patients, the lymphatic system can be viewed as largely intact yet insufficient. But without imaging studies, it is always questionable whether or not a standard protocol involving the recruitment of intact neighboring territories (as in unilateral secondary patients) will yield the same predictable results as transport capacity may be reduced either regionally or systemically. While developing a plan of care, the therapist should ask himself or herself the following questions:

Regarding MLD

- Should MLD include the regional nodes to the swollen body part?
  - Are they still intact?
  - Have they ever been surgically sampled or excised?
- If treating the regional nodes, should treatment cross the watersheds to neighboring territories?
  - Is this thorough enough to ensure a good treatment outcome?
- What is the risk of triggering swelling in other body areas?
- Should treatment be aggressive or more cautious?

Regarding Compression

- Should the entire limb be wrapped when only a distal area is involved?
- Are there reasons to be concerned about triggering uninvolved areas with volumes of fluid movement?

- What modifications apply if multiple limbs are involved?
- Can the existing vessel pathways tolerate compression without adverse effects?

The following five primary patient treatment scenarios represent distinct challenges that are commonly encountered and serve to answer the above questions and concerns.

Scenario 1: Primary Lymphedema with Distal Limb Involvement Only

MLD Modifications (▶ Fig. 5.75)

In cases of primary lymphedema, the regional lymph nodes should ALWAYS be included in the MLD treatment sequencing. Although swelling exists in the same quadrant, the clinician cannot conclude with certainty that the regional lymph nodes are nonviable or noncontributory to therapy. In most primary lymphedemas, hypoplasia of nodes and vessels is the predominant genetic dysplasia.[77,78] Interestingly, in some cases, decades may pass without the full limb becoming involved, which reinforces the unique, unknown anatomical variations that have caused the insufficiency.

In these cases, if imaging studies could be performed without harm, a picture of distal, local lymphatic abnormality may be identified in the absence of any inguinal or proximal limb malformations. Indeed, in most cases of lymphedema, a clear underlying anatomical picture cannot be rendered. As such, clinician specialists are commonly challenged to adapt CDT to various patient types without clear guidance from diagnostic studies.

In this example, as the swelling is mild, it would stand to reason that the inguinal lymph nodes are themselves remote and are not yet secondarily congested by the proximal quadrant. The margins of the swelling show a normal girth (as compared with the other leg) at the proximal calf when measured. Adapting MLD to include the inguinal lymph nodes is a simple addition; however, as the distal aspect of the leg is the only area yet involved, the question should arise as to the relevance of treating the ipsilateral inguino-axillary anastomoses (IAAs).

In these particular cases, a productive treatment result is reached when the leg is treated as if it were intact and healthy (toward the regional nodes). The goal of MLD is therefore to stimulate lymphangio-activity locally and to guide the lymph toward the intact regional lymph nodes. To

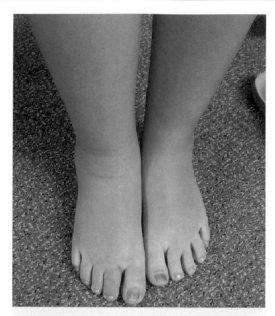

Fig. 5.75 Primary lymphedema: Distal limb involvement exclusively.

bypass the inguinal lymph nodes in an attempt to carry this distal accumulation of lymph remotely toward the axillary lymph nodes is difficult to rationalize given the full lower quadrant is not congested up to the transverse watershed. As such, function of these vessels is assumed to be intact due to lack of congestion rendering the direction of flow of hip, buttock, and lower abdomen and thigh still toward the inguinal lymph nodes (away from the watershed).

It is important to consider, however, that in cases of moderate or severe distal limb swelling without proximal involvement (large calf, normal thigh), due to the sheer volume of fluid moving through the proximal tissues under compression, that probable congestion will occur here during CDT. If this occurs, recruit the IAA. As this proximal area was formerly spared from edema, it is typical for these tissues to return to normal following the intensive phase.

Summary of MLD Modifications: Primary Lymphedema (Distal Limb Only)

- Always include lymph nodes even when the full quadrant is involved. We never know to what extent they may contribute to improvement.
- Treat to regional nodes in cases of distal limb involvement without crossing watersheds.

- Establish anastomosis in cases where involvement includes the proximal limb.
- Treat to neighboring regional lymph node groups with caution (see Compression Considerations below).
- Always involve the deep lymphatic system (venous angles, thoracic duct, abdomen).

Compression Considerations

Empirical proof supports the observation that compression on uninvolved proximal tissues causes an adverse effect on distal limb areas. This counterproductive result is most likely caused by impedance of normal drainage efficiency under high pressure. Edematous tissues soften and decongest under working pressure decreasing local pressure levels as a bandage is worn. Conversely, limb areas that are not swollen lack capacity to respond in this way because there is no decongestion from the pressure applied. Furthermore, since vessels are not "cushioned" by fluid, they may be effectively collapsed by compression, making them labor to work.

Clinical Implications

Compression bandaging is a highly efficient and powerful fluid mobilization modality. In primary lymphedema, the unknown transport capacity of the system (systemically and locally), coupled with variations in vessel and lymph node anatomy, cause compression effects to be less predictable. In general:

Avoid Compression on Uninvolved Tissues

- Wrap to below knee when edema margins end below knee and thigh is spared.
- Wrap to the proximal forearm if hand and forearm are involved, upper arm spared.

Include the Muscle and Joint Pumps of the Involved Tissue (the Natural Venous and Lymphatic Pumps).

Examples:
- If only the foot is involved, wrap to include ankle joint only (low boot height).
- If the toes up to the distal or mid-calf are involved, wrap to include ankle joint and calf muscle pump. Stop below the knee.
- If toes up to the knee are involved, wrap to include the ankle joint, calf pump, and knee

joints. (Stopping just above the knee can be technically difficult to achieve.)
- If the full leg is involved, wrap to the hip.

Examine Areas for New Congestion

If congestion occurs above the bandage and is caused by the bandage, adapt to the newly swollen tissues. Example:
- If a calf bandage stopping below the knee (knee high) produces knee and distal thigh congestion, bandage to the top of the leg.
- Consider alternating bandage coverage: half leg Monday, full leg Tuesday, and repeat, to alternately "congest" then "flush" proximal tissues.

Scenario 2: Primary Lymphedema (Unilateral Full Lower Extremity)

It is important to remember that primary lymphedema most often involves hypoplasia of the inguinal and pelvic lymph nodes (▶ Fig. 5.76). Kinmonth's studies revealed that hypoplasias are generally bilateral even when a single limb is clinically affected.[92] This fact must govern our thinking with regard to assessing the status of clinically intact, uninvolved tissues in treatment planning.

When the "margins" of the edema involve up-to-and-including proximal limb segments (upper arm or thigh), treatment to the regional lymph nodes only (as in Scenario 1 above) may prove insufficient to absorb the lymphatic loads during decongestive therapy. Upon closer inspection, it may be apparent that the swelling indeed encompasses the truncal aspect of the limb quadrant. Therefore in general whenever limb edema approaches a truncal watershed, establish anastomoses toward neighboring lymph node groups. However, the following considerations must be satisfactorily addressed before a safe plan of care can be established.

Considerations and Precautions in Unilateral Lower Extremity Primary Lymphedema

A thorough patient history should always be documented to determine or clarify the extent of involvement and assist in the treatment planning process. Key questions include the following:
- Is the contralateral leg patent or stable?
- Has the contralateral leg ever become edematous (stage 1), even intermittently?

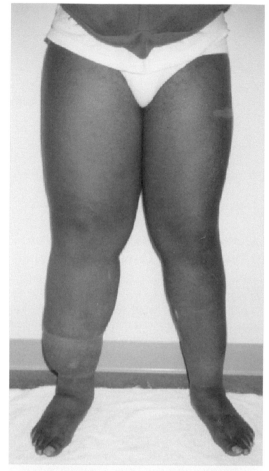

Fig. 5.76 Primary lymphedema: Full limb involvement unilaterally.

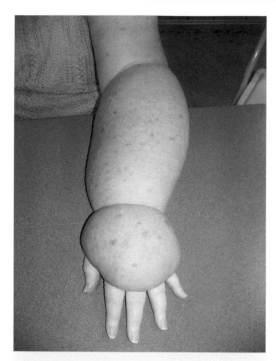

Fig. 5.77 Primary lymphedema: Unilateral upper extremity.

- Has the contralateral leg ever experienced cellulitis?
- Is the contralateral leg Stemmer's sign positive? (If so it is involved.)
- Are there any subclinical (stage 0) subjective complaints associated with this leg?
- Is there any current palpable/visible swelling that escapes patient's notice or is denied?

Should any of these questions be positively verified, it is extremely important that the clinician **avoid** the interinguinal anastomosis (IIA), so that the contralateral leg is spared additional lymphatic loads from the involved limb quadrant.

It is important to note that many patients with so-called single limb involvement actually do have bilateral limb symptoms; however, the subjective focus is on the more involved leg discounting or overlooking mild contralateral involvement.

If the contralateral limb is **clearly uninvolved** and is supported by a thorough patient history, it is the clinician's decision to utilize or avoid the IIA. As a rule:

- Always favor the ipsilateral IAA. (Spend more time here.)
- Inspect the contralateral leg closely prior to every treatment to assess any changes.
- Should contralateral leg edema appear, immediately halt treatment via interinguinal anastomoses.
- Compression therapy may be necessary to reestablish equilibrium in the contralateral leg.

Scenario 3: Primary Lymphedema (Unilateral Upper Extremity), Adult Age (▶ Fig. 5.77)

Primary upper extremity involvement is uncommon except in pediatric presentations (Milroy's disease), so rarely occurs spontaneously later in life. In nearly all cases of unilateral upper limb lymphedema, the contralateral arm is spared and remains so for life. Clinical experience reveals that treatment from the involved arm via the interaxillary anastomoses carries a very low risk of destabilizing the uninvolved arm. It should be noted that dysplasia (hypoplasia) dominates the lower extremity when compared with the upper limbs for unknown reasons. This observation has also been verified in experimental animal models.

As it relates to late diagnosis of adult Milroy's disease (as depicted here), expect the following challenges and benefits:

- Adults are more compliant with therapy, so allow for highly intensive therapy if necessary.
- Adults with primary lymphedema are generally exceptionally motivated to gain even modest improvements. Lymphedema has been a lifelong challenge. Finding well-trained therapists and a comprehensive system of therapy is most welcome.
- Expect highly fibrotic tissue, and a history of cellulitis. Frequent cellulitis hastens fibrotic skin changes.
- Explore variations in compression gradient to gain the most efficient long-term benefits from compression in home care. Remember that the anatomy is abnormal, so drainage may respond to these modifications. See the discussion in Scenario 1 for rationale and suggestions. Regarding MLD treatment, see section below, MLD Considerations: Milroy's Disease (Pediatric Age).

Scenario 4: Primary Lymphedema, Pediatric Ages (Upper Extremity and Lower Extremity Combined)

Most upper extremity primary lymphedema will be associated with Milroy's disease. Some patients find appropriate medical intervention at a very early age, others not until some decades later. Based on the points raised above in Scenarios 2 and 3, a treatment plan should be developed that minimizes risk to other uninvolved body areas. This plan should be governed by observation, palpation, medical history, and current stage of severity and further based on the most current understanding of this particular disease type (Milroy's).

In ▶ Fig. 5.70, the child has unilateral right arm and leg involvement with no evidence of left upper or lower extremity signs or symptoms. As previously noted, treatment from right to left arm crossing the midsagittal watershed via the interaxillary anastomoses (anterior and posterior) is considered low risk. Conversely, treatment of an involved lower extremity toward the contralateral inguinal nodes does carry the same high risk observed in all primary lower extremity lymphedema cases. Additionally in pediatric cases, examine for abdominal bloating (retroperitoneal ascites caused by intestinal dysplasia) and genital lymphedema during the course of treatment as the patient grows (see treatment section under "Pediatric Lymphedema"). It would be imprudent to assume that only the early expression of limb swelling will remain. As early onset proves a greater insufficiency than one that develops later in life, we must adapt to the full expression over time, which may change modestly or extensively.

The following suggestions mirror a current, conservative approach to delivering MLD to pediatric Milroy's patients. As the child ages, lymphatic territories continue to exhibit inherent functional strengths and weaknesses that influence therapeutic decisions with regard to further MLD protocol revisions. The sequences listed provide an overview without the precise incremental steps.

MLD Considerations: Milroy's Disease (Pediatric Age)

Involving Unilateral Leg

- Treat neck, abdomen.
- Treat the ipsilateral arm.
- Treat involved leg to ipsilateral inguinal nodes.
- No treatment to contralateral leg.

Involving Unilateral Arm

- Treat neck, abdomen.
- Treat arm to ipsilateral axilla.
- Treat arm to contralateral axilla (monitor signs of overload in arm).
- Treat arm to ipsilateral leg (monitor signs of overload in leg).

Involving Bilateral Legs

- Treat neck, abdomen.
- Treat to ipsilateral arms bilaterally.
- Treat each leg to include inguinal nodes.
- No treatment across inter-inguinal anastomosis.

Unilateral Arm, Unilateral Leg

- Treat neck, abdomen.
- Treat arm toward ipsilateral nodes and contralateral axilla.
- Treat leg to ipsilateral nodes and axilla if the ipsilateral arm is not involved.

- Treat leg to ipsilateral inguinal nodes only if the same side as involved arm.
- No treatment across IIA (unless closely monitored).

Unilateral Arm, Bilateral Leg

- Treat neck, abdomen.
- Treat arm toward ipsilateral nodes and contralateral axilla.
- Treat involved leg 1 to ipsilateral uninvolved axilla.
- Treat involved leg 2 toward inguinal nodes only (same side as involved arm).
- No treatment across IIA.

Bilateral Arms, Bilateral Legs

- Treat neck, abdomen.
- Treat each limb to ipsilateral regional nodes only.
- Do not establish anastomoses regardless of severity.

Compression Considerations: Milroy's Disease (Pediatric)

Multiple limb presentations in pediatric primary lymphedema patients must be carefully considered before compression therapy is administered.
  Concerns include the following:
- Skin tolerance to materials of a multilayered short-stretch complex bandage.
- Child's lack of clear communication or feedback if uncomfortable.
- Therapeutic pressure versus excessive pressure level on very small radii (Law of LaPlace).
- Disrupted gait, movement, balance, function, and impact on development.
- Parental oversight, ability, inclination to manage limb(s) with compression safely.

For the cited reasons, compression should be administered with great caution in all cases of pediatric lymphedema. Children younger than 12 months are generally considered too young to receive compression unless it is performed with great skill and experience. At 16 + months, compression garments can be administered as can skilled lymphedema bandaging with great caution. Although skilled bandaging can be performed by the therapist at an earlier point in time, parents will be rewrapping daily and have a strong tendency to use excessive pressure. Garments must always be custom-made and skillfully measured and should not exceed compression class 1 (CCL1).

Compression gradient and fit must be closely monitored because limb girths are small and relative pressure is higher than on adult limbs.

Summary of Compression Modifications

- Children younger than 12 months should (in general) not receive compression. (This is not an absolute contraindication but a strong precaution.)
- Children older than 12 months should receive only expert lymphedema care. (Seek mentorship if the therapist is inexperienced with pediatrics.)
- Garments do not disrupt gait, as does compression bandaging. Favor garments early on.
- Garments distribute pressure more evenly than bandages and may provide a better result.
- Bandaging regimen must consider the effect on developmental milestones.
- Tissue intolerance must be minimal. Sensitivity and tenderness are high.
- Pressure must not cause pain. Remember patient feedback is limited.
- As with adults, assess the edema margins and compress to include the joint and muscle pump only. Avoid excessive coverage to gain better drainage.

Scenario 5: Primary Lymphedema (Bilateral Lower Extremity), Adult Age

Since neither inguinal lymph node groups can accept fluid from the contralateral involved limb, the midsagittal watershed must be observed as a true "boundary" dividing both territories from shared workloads. As discussed, the ipsilateral regional inguinal lymph nodes should be utilized and are viewed as contributory to the reabsorption of edema. However, if a moderate or severe distal presentation exists, exclusive treatment to the inguinal nodes will most likely not yield good results.

  Treatment to the ipsilateral axillary lymph nodes bilaterally and preparation of the deep lymphatic system (neck, abdomen MLD sequences) create the substance of the protocol. In all cases of bilateral lymphedema, whether mild or severe, the midsagittal watershed must remain a boundary limiting work between territories. Regarding bandaging, each limb is treated with customized compression coverage depending on the margins of the edema and status of the tissues involved.

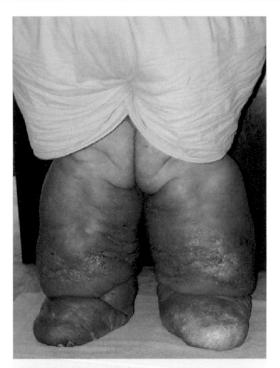

Fig. 5.78 Primary lymphedema: Bilateral lower extremity.

Mild Bilateral Primary Lymphedema

In cases of mild bilateral primary lymphedema (▶ Fig. 5.78), the therapist should
- Never cross the midsagittal watershed.
- Treat the inguinal lymph nodes of each limb.
- Establish both IAAs if the full limb is involved (see Scenario 1 above).
- Watch for genital involvement as the intensive phase progresses.
- Monitor arms for swelling, although a very rare complication.

Elephantiasis

In cases of elephantiasis, the key concerns are as follows:
- Renal function (ability to diurese).
  - Expect large volumes of fluid to shift to the central circulation.
  - Ascertain urine output, monitor closely.
  - Some patients require medical support.
- Congestion or retention in proximal tissues (thighs, trunk, genitals). Remember the anatomy is abnormal, drainage may be sluggish.

- Limb reduction is too rapid and overwhelms the proximal tissues.
  - Decrease intensity of compression, increase intensity of MLD.
- Rapid decongestion causes bandages to shift, losing grip and pressure.
- Tissue fragility and laxity (transformation may be too rapid), leading to pain, increased rates of cellulitis, small wounds.

5.8.2 Adaptations for the Secondary Lymphedema Patient

Secondary lymphedema by definition implies a variety of etiologies including trauma, untreated chronic venous disease, obesity, surgical compromise, and others. Depending on the severity of lymphatic injury, time line, and other exacerbating factors, secondary lymphedema can be deceptive regarding response to treatment. The intensity of treatment must be monitored based on actual response and further adapted to each patient accordingly. The following guidelines will assist in decision making to avoid overtreating very mild cases and undertreating more extensive presentations.

Scenario 6: Secondary Lower Extremity Lymphedema (Mild, Distal)

When secondary lymphedema is caused by inguinal lymph node trauma (surgery, radiation therapy, or other cause) simply stated, the only area of concern for the lymphedema therapist is the compromised territory (e.g., ipsilateral leg, lower trunk, buttock and hip, genital tissues). This more straightforward case presentation is typically treated with deep lymphatic preparation (neck, abdomen sequences) and recruitment of the ipsilateral axillary lymph nodes and contralateral inguinal lymph nodes via both anastomotic collateral pathways (interinguinal and inguino-axillary).

When these straightforward cases are seen soon after the clinical appearance of lymphedema, the margins of the edema may only involve the toes, dorsum of the foot, or ankle. To provide the most thoughtful and appropriate care, it is helpful to avoid aggressive CDT interventions, which may be viewed as excessive, cumbersome, and wasteful of patient and clinic resources.

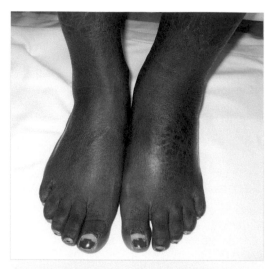

Fig. 5.79 Secondary lymphedema: Mild, distal involvement unilaterally.

Compression Suggestions

- As with mild distal primary lymphedema (▶ Fig. 5.79, Scenario 1), apply bandages or garments that cover only the involved area and access the local joint and muscle pump. This step helps avoid entrapment of fluid. As such:
  - For distal foot involvement: bandage to shoe height (low boot) and fit for an anklet (ankle-height) garment.
  - For foot and ankle involvement: bandage to a low-boot height or higher to below the knee. Alternate between the two versions and fit for calf garment (knee high).
  - For foot, ankle, or distal calf involvement, bandage to below the knee and fit for a calf garment (knee high).

Assess the Outcome, Then Modify

In modified bandages involving partial limb coverage, edema may saturate the tissues proximal to the bandage and remain visible and/or palpable following MLD. Since this is not an unexpected finding, more extensive coverage must follow to decongest. It is sometimes helpful to alternate between two different bandages to increase the steepness of the compression gradient. Such a protocol could involve the following:

- Monday—bandaging to ankle (result: more aggressive foot decongestion, but saturates calf),

- Tuesday—bandaging to knee (result: less aggressive foot decongestion, but decongests calf).
- Wednesday—bandaging to ankle (repeat).
- Thursday—bandaging to knee if necessary (repeat if findings continue).

The result of this modification is the ability to efficiently decongest a distal area while avoiding fluid deposition in proximal areas. Selection of the proper compression garment is indicated by the findings of these exercises. If the calf requires more support than was expected provide a knee-high garment. Conversely, if the calf regains stability, provide an ankle-high garment.

Note that distal arm and hand presentations can be approached in a similar fashion to improve decongestion of stubborn extremities.

MLD Suggestions

Some mild, distal swellings remain so for many months or even years without significant progression to proximal tissues. As such, it is reasonable to assume that the mechanical insufficiency does not yet represent a total failure in the quadrant. Simple compression support may be adequate to address the swelling sufficiently for some time. However, if MLD is employed, clinicians should likewise consider the extent and thoroughness of the protocol to avoid wasting time and resources. Modifications include the following:

- MLD should always include the deep anatomy (neck, abdomen, breathing).
  - The deep system is intact and will continue to drain the remaining intact inguinal lymph vessels and nodes and deep limb structures. MLD may increase the efficiency and collateral drainage through viable pathways.
- MLD includes proximal thigh, knee, and calf treatment.
  - If these tissues are currently edema-free, they are functioning. If not, fluid will begin to accumulate.
  - Remember that perforators exist between superficial and deep systems.

Clinical Observation

The typical treatment protocol for secondary unilateral lymphedema, which involves the ipsilateral axillary lymph nodes and IAA, may not be productive, so this can be omitted.

This conclusion is derived from clinical experience and the rationale for less intensive therapy is a supportive hypothesis. More extensive therapy remains an option. The therapist should consider the following:

- The lymphatic trauma may not be absolute; therefore, the anatomy may be partially intact.
- It is early in the timeline. More extensive effects of trauma may appear in time.
- In a mild or distal presentation, proximal lymphatic tissues within the involved quadrant are still functioning (tissue is not currently swollen).
- A superficial trauma may spare the deep anatomy, and vice versa.
- The deep lymphatic system is functioning, and perforators assist superficial collectors to empty, bypassing the trauma site.
- Functional reserve is higher in some individuals.
- Lympho-lymphatic anastomosis and healing occur at trauma sites.
- Functioning proximal lymphatic tissues (calf, thigh, truncal regions) counter fluid movement to the upper quadrant, draining toward remaining intact inguinal nodes. As such, fluid from a foot cannot cross the transverse watershed into an upper quadrant.

Scenario 7: Secondary Lymphedema —Unilateral Presentation, Bilateral Predisposition

Similar to unilateral primary lymphedema whereby the contralateral limb is "spared but predisposed," some secondary presentations elicit similar concerns and influence the plan of care prior to intensive CDT treatment.

Commonly mechanical failure of lymphatic vessels and nodes occurs asymmetrically (following a different timeline) even when both lower quadrants are subjected to proximal shared trauma or disruption. To avoid complications, clinicians must familiarize themselves with the type of trauma and assess the effects on the lymphatic anatomy to develop a sensible plan of care.

5.8.3 Underlying Diagnosis and Surgical Treatment Leading to the Development of Lymphedema

The therapist must understand and be aware of the following:

- Intrapelvic cancers generally involve sampling of lymph nodes from the pelvis bilaterally.
  - Although one leg is currently involved, the other is highly predisposed.

- "Radical" procedures by definition imply lymph node dissection.
  - Routine hysterectomy indicates only organ removal. The patient is not predisposed to develop lymphedema. "Radical" hysterectomy highly predisposes the patient to lymphedema.
- Radiation therapy for intrapelvic cancers may be either internally or externally administered.
  - External beam radiation (passing through the skin) may cause visual and palpable tissue changes. There will be tattoo markers indicating the field location. Damage may start at the skin but extensively affect deep tissues.
  - Internal radiation (brachytherapy) may be delivered via rods or seeds implanted vaginally or rectally. Tissue damage is not visible or palpable. The field is not clinically apparent, but long-term radiation effects must be expected. CDT contraindications still apply.
- The lymphatic drainage of intrapelvic and abdominal organs.
  - Surgeons sample the nodes draining the involved organs to stage cancer progression.
  - Surgeons will often sample nodes from both left and right nodal chains predisposing both limb territories to swell.
  - Disruption of deep nodes creates reflux toward intact distal nodes and vessels (pelvic nodes reflux into inguinal nodes and territories, etc.).

MLD Suggestions for Patients with Deep Lymph Node Removal

Pelvic or abdominal node sampling, whether dissection or irradiated, disturbs all distal nodes and territories to mechanical insufficiency. As such, MLD treatment directed from an involved leg to a currently uninvolved (yet predisposed) leg disregards the common drainage off both limbs to the deep system. This practice is considered high risk and is strictly contraindicated, as it will most likely trigger a contralateral swelling. Alternatively:

- Treat the deep system (neck, abdomen. and/or substitute diaphragmatic breathing if manual pressure is contraindicated).
- Treat the ipsilateral axillary lymph nodes.
- Treat the ipsilateral IAA.
- Treat the involved lower limb bypassing the inguinal nodes.
- Avoid the IIA.
- Always monitor the uninvolved contralateral leg for changes.

Compression Suggestions

If the entire unilateral quadrant is involved (ipsilateral: hip, lower abdomen, external genital, buttock), compression around the trunk may be helpful. However, since the contralateral lower quadrant is at high risk for lymphedema, the choices of compression must be carefully considered to avoid taxation of the as yet uninvolved limb.

Compression garment configurations include the following:

- Thigh-high coverage only, but neglect of proximal/truncal areas during the daytime.
- Pantyhose coverage, to offer additional compression support for the predisposed (uninvolved) leg.
  - This "preventative" coverage must be CCL1 and lightly measured to avoid taxation of local vessel structures.
  - Compressive panty portion may contribute necessary support to proximal tissues.
  - Never use pantyhose on one leg while only partially covering the other because it creates an effective tourniquet for the predisposed limb. This applies to primary lymphedema patients as well those with as yet unexpressed contralateral limb swelling.

5.9 Adapting CDT to the Palliative Patient

5.9.1 Set Realistic Goals

The application of CDT in the palliative context requires redefining the aims of therapy to reflect reality. A standard approach for the well patient will in many cases cause discomfort or intense pain and further draws upon diminishing energy. Without seeing quantifiable volume reductions, therapists may wrongly conclude that treatment is inappropriate or futile. In this situation, therapists should change gears and find other goals to pursue, creating a modified treatment plan that will be much appreciated by the patient, family, and the rest of the health care team. Providing comfort, relief from pain or other swelling-related symptoms, and maintaining or restoring function are outcomes of tremendous benefit. Early referral and intervention may help prevent or postpone the development of lymphorrhea, markedly swollen and painful limbs, and disability (▶ Fig. 5.80; ▶ Fig. 5.81).

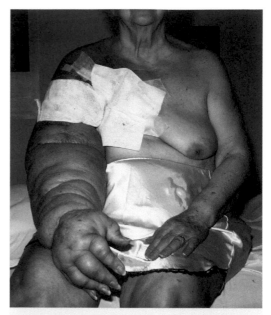

Fig. 5.80 Malignant lymphedema: Upper right quadrant, anterior view.

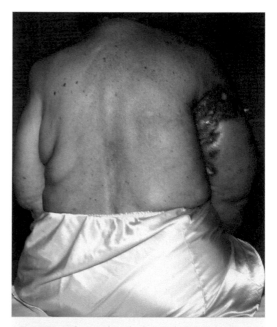

Fig. 5.81 Malignant lymphedema: Posterior view.

When cancer is in remission, outpatient rehabilitation settings strive for consecutive daily visits. However, the palliative patient typically requires flexibility to prioritize a multitude of other commitments and concerns, including medical oncology, accommodation for travel, and coordination of family support. When the lymphedema specialist initiates a course of therapy, interruptions must be expected and accommodated.[80]

With failing health, a true distinction between the two phases of CDT may be absent.[81] The patient graduating from clinic to home care may require continued intensive therapy, while clinic-based care may be less than the ideal intensity level due to a multitude of cited limitations. Intensive compression is generally warranted, as is regular MLD for the rich benefits each provides.[82] In both phases, family participation or community team involvement is crucial to safely carry out the therapist's recommendations and to accelerate learning from the very first visit. In situations of lymphorrhea, there is an absolute requirement for regular bandage removal, dressing change, and reapplication. This demands competent, attentive caregiver administration.[83]

Semi-intensive CDT continues to address the most important concerns, such as skin integrity, early identification and management of cellulitis, daily observation for adaptation to swelling margins, and ongoing pain management. Failing health may at some point result in an absolute contraindication to one or more modalities of palliative CDT, so careful and regular reassessment is paramount. Nevertheless, when patients and family members realize that the lymphedema specialist remains unconditionally committed regardless of these complications, an air of support, gratitude, and hope is maintained.

5.9.2 Strengths and Limitations of Each CDT Modality

Palliative Compression

Obstructive lymphedema is often resistant to attempts at volume reduction, refilling in minutes following removal of compression. Short-stretch bandaging provides containment, effectively arresting the progression of swelling that relentlessly stretches the skin. With synthetic cotton or foam padding layers, which gently embed in tissues, fluid displacement is maintained and successfully counters the sensation of "bursting" (▶ Fig. 5.81). Addressing this single swelling symptom significantly reduces pain and increases comfort. Exudative skin lesions require careful coordination with wound care specialists prior to redressing with compression. Range of motion is commonly limited or impossible when edema effectively splints the joints. Even modest edema reduction can free joints and improve function and mobility.

Elastic compression garments (medically correct gradient support stocking, sleeve, etc.) often fail to achieve comfort due to inherently high resting pressures, which constrict, roll, or cord if they are ill fitting. Sensations of throbbing are common as is immediate intolerance and exacerbation of pain. Low compression classes of elastic garments may be tolerated, but obstructive lymphedema overwhelms elastic threads regardless of compression class, and so cannot provide the required containment. Because of these concerns, many patients remain in short-stretch compression bandages and welcome the relief until the end of life.

Compression: General Modifications

- Low resting pressure is better tolerated.
- Decrease bandage tension overall.
- Use open cell foam to hold bandages secure. (Gently embeds in edema, is well tolerated.)
- Provide edema containment rather than aggressive reduction, to halt progression of swelling.
- Inspect frequently, care for skin then keep bandaged intensively.
- Wound management may require frequent change of absorptive layers.
- Avoid elastic materials: either too weak or cause of pain.

Palliative Manual Lymph Drainage

The terminally ill patient seeks MLD for swelling management, but an additional benefit lies in MLD's analgesic effect. Even as energy levels wane with disease progression, MLD remains productive for pain management, so it is always indicated even if abbreviated or modified according to other medical concerns. Since obstructive masses interrupt entire lymphatic quadrants, MLD primarily focuses on creating collateral flow in truncal territories, and secondarily in the limb.[84] Working closely with physicians, optimal pathways can be attended while avoiding superficial and deep tumor lesions. Although volume outcome measures may be difficult to quantify, treatment is essential to address skin tension–related pain, concomitant pain sources, lymphorrhea, range-of-motion limitations, and degraded skin integrity. MLD sessions are a rare and welcome extension of compassion, kindness, and human contact. The

5

extension of this service is the most prized aspect of CDT, as the tactile exchange that occurs during MLD forges close bonds between patient and caregiver.[85]

MLD: General Modifications

- Avoid contact with lesions, favor intact skin.
- Identify patent anatomical drainage (consult imaging studies).
- Limit unnecessary repositioning to conserve patient energy.
- Optimize comfort, bolster generously and with care.
- Emphasize analgesic benefit.
- Physician-directed plan of care: identify relative and absolute contraindications.

Palliative Skin Care: Management of Lymphorrhea

Excessive edema-related skin tension may generate fragile lymph cysts leading to rupture with copious leakage from the mechanical stresses of compression. Minor abrasion or injury combined with atrophic changes and dehydration set the stage for further erosion.[86] In some, dermal infiltrating tumors form nonhealing ulcers that progress until the end of life. Areas of skin-to-skin contact harbor moisture, fungal, and bacterial colonies. Multilayered compression can incorporate absorptive wound dressings, which are changed frequently to avoid maceration.[83] Frequent inspection identifies infections early and allows for assessment with each bandage reapplication. Odor control of necrotic lesions is important: lymphorrhea and anaerobic bacteria cause patient distress, self-consciousness, and loss of dignity. Topical preparations must be incorporated in wound dressings and skinfolds to mitigate this concern and allow patients to engage in social activities. Highly absorptive, nonadhesive materials including infant diapers can be incorporated successfully into a skilled bandage complex. Plastic backings or diapers can contain fluid, lessening saturation of multilayered bandage materials and minimizing maceration.

Skin Care: General Modifications

- Lymph cysts, blisters, and lymphorrhea are common.
- Control exudate to avoid maceration.

- Highlight hygiene and instruct caregiver from first day.
- Provide odor relief and manage fungal and bacterial colonies.
- Apply lotion generously and inspect for cracks.
- Protect fragile skin from mechanical stresses of compression.

Remedial Exercises and the Palliative Patient

Normal movement and activity should be encouraged whenever possible. In general, provided that pain control measures are optimized, remedial exercises are gentle enough to be acceptable to patients with advanced illness. However, standard lymphedema deep-breathing exercises may be a challenge, particularly if dyspnea is present. Metastatic disease in the bones may lead to a fracture risk even with minimal exercise: the therapist will need to be aware if such a risk exists. Muscle weakness or paralysis is a challenge that will require the prescription of more passive rather than active exercises.

Exercise: General Modifications

- Assess patient's capabilities, pain, ROM, strength.
- Assess general health with physician-directed plan; identify contraindications.
- Develop strategy with quality of life as goal.

Family Support and Education

The early involvement of family or a professional caregiver is of greatest importance in palliative CDT. The nature of palliative CDT requires manual therapy with each modality delivered with precision, understanding, and compassion. MLD can be learned quickly when simplified to its essence (e.g., single-hand vs. two-handed technique), and with careful mapping can be sequenced for frequent reapplication between clinic visits, maximizing analgesic and fluid reabsorption benefits. Compression management should never become the responsibility of the patient. Self-removal of a painful bandage or garment may be impossible and attempts at reapplication may cause dislocation, fracture, skin tears, and tourniquets. Constant monitoring of comfort, sensation, capillary perfusion, and skin integrity should occur every few hours if the patient is unresponsive.

5.9.3 CDT Management of Generalized Edema

Treatment strategies adapted to the terminally ill patient may closely resemble those constructed for typical primary and secondary lymphedema if disease progression is slow or if cancer therapy provides periods of disease control. Care plans vary widely depending on the extent and location of tumor involvement relative to lymphatic tissues (deep or superficial). Furthermore, renal insufficiency, liver failure, reduced cardiac output, and hypoproteinemia (monitored through serum albumin levels) may constitute relative or absolute contraindications.[80] Tolerance to compression is directly impacted by diabetic, neuropathic, or central nervous system disturbances and peripheral vascular complications that may cause therapy options to be significantly limited.[85]

Relative and absolute contraindications require particularly close physician-directed modifications based on assessment of drug interactions, severity of any organ failure, and potential interactions or exacerbations created by CDT modalities.[87] Acute CHF, acute DVT, thrombocytopenia, severe neuropathic or bone pain, advanced peripheral vascular disease (low ABPI), and complications of diabetes may constitute irresolvable challenges.[80,88]

Intermittent pneumatic compression (IPC) devices are particularly ill suited in the palliative context because almost invariably issues persist with edema at the root of the limb or limbs that may be exacerbated with IPC. A medical subcutaneous drainage technique as an alternative to, or in combination with CDT, has been reported in the literature for the treatment of edema in palliative care and merits further study.[89,90] This technique uses "butterfly"-type needles inserted into the subcutaneous space and attached via tubing to a drainage bag. It should be emphasized that this physical drainage has only been applied in the terminal phase and should not be a consideration before this time, as it invariably presents risk of infection and/or lymphorrhea (▶ Fig. 5.82).

Practical Adaptations for Lower Quadrant Edema

Unilateral lower quadrant edema commonly advances to both lower limbs, as disease progresses to the retroperitoneal nodes. Hypoalbuminemia (dynamic insufficiency) or physical obstruction (mechanical insufficiency) individually overwhelms lymphatic transport capacity or may

combine to create mixed edema. In general, the therapist's strategy involves axillo-inguinal collateral pathways (anastomoses) during MLD, as upper quadrant swelling is rarely triggered during fluid shifting. Attention to diaphragmatic-centered breathing drains deep lymphatics including the thoracic duct while neck treatment (supraclavicular fossa, venous angle) supports the central decongestive premise, benefitting the whole lymphatic system (▶ Fig. 5.83).

Compression bandaging may be so productive when applied to these mixed or low protein edemas as to overwhelm proximal territories. Genital involvement is common and may occur regardless of pressure level. As such, a focus on proximal

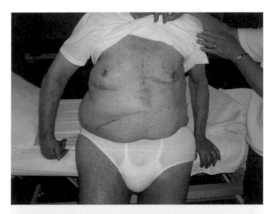

Fig. 5.82 Malignant lymphedema: legs, with trunk involvement.

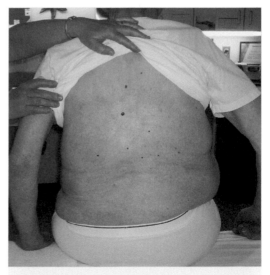

Fig. 5.83 Malignant lymphedema: Posterior trunk view.

congestion with sustained MLD aimed at emptying the trunk is the most sensible and productive strategy. Compression may be modified to address only one limb segment at a time to control the volume of fluid mobilized and allow for MLD to assist with absorption. In such cases, a bandage is applied from the toes to the knees and may be alternated to cover the full limb when it can be tolerated.

Dependency

Non–cancer-related disease processes may cause absolute or sustained periods of immobility generating low protein-dependent edema. In such cases, since the lymphatic system is largely intact, MLD treatment of regional nodes with attention to deep lymphatic anatomy (neck and abdomen) can help distal limb edema. If coupled with limb positioning against gravity (horizontal or elevated), swellings may not require compression. Bolstering of the genitals can be adequate to avoid tedious compression solutions while providing significant relief.[83]

Modified Approach (Lower Quadrants)
Specific MLD

- Incorporate all "general modifications."
- Establish bilateral IAA in most cases.
- Abdominal and or pelvic metastasis predisposes both lower quadrants to edema, no IIA.
- If unilateral limb is involved, IIA drainage may trigger contralateral lower quadrant; exercise caution.
- Quadrant is usually full to watersheds; compression exacerbates this status.
- Expect genital involvement and modify accordingly.
- Focus on quality of touch for soothing analgesic benefit.
- Limit positioning to accommodate comfort.
- Deep MLD techniques contraindicated in all involved areas.
- Breathing coaching without manipulation of abdomen if contraindicated.

Specific Compression

- Incorporate all "general modifications."
- Full leg bandage may overwhelm genitals, trunk. Adapt.
- Bandage to protect skin and absorb exudate and perspiration from skin-to-skin contact areas.

- Proximal limb segment may function temporarily as a reservoir for distal edema. Alternate full-leg, then half-leg bandage on alternate days.
- Distal limb (foot, ankle, toes) may be spared. Light compression may be adequate to maintain.
- If neuropathy exists, remain vigilant with visual inspection. Moderate intensity of compression or abandon compression strategy altogether if necessary.

Practical Adaptations for Upper Quadrant Edema

As with lower quadrant involvement, upper quadrant modifications are directed by the physician's assessment of disease progression. In general, superficial lymphatic territories (upper or lower) provide current, visual, and palpable feedback regarding obstruction of deep structures. In advanced disease, nonedematous quadrants are always at risk because there may be little capacity for receiving surplus fluid following collateral drainage with MLD. When the upper quadrant is drained to an ipsilateral lower quadrant, the Stemmer's sign is checked daily to gauge capacity to accept more fluid. A treatment plan may be severely limited if there is, for example, severe lymphatic obstruction from skin lesions, subcutaneous tumor, regions of radiation fibrosis, or mixed edema (venous thrombosis, hypoproteinemia). In these cases, therapists must rely largely on one predominant treatment modality (i.e., either MLD or compression).

Modified Approach (Upper Quadrants)
Specific MLD

- Incorporate all "general modifications."
- Establish axillo-inguinal drainage if no pelvic and abdominal metastasis (abdominal and/or pelvic metastasis predispose both lower quadrants to edema).
- Neck may be the only deep treatment option (with abdomen contraindicated).
- Breathing coaching without manipulation of abdomen if known metastasis.
- Assess: neck may have local involvement, so it is also contraindicated.
- Establish interaxillary drainage (if unilateral predisposition).
- Modify MLD to primary focus on the trunk (avoid lesions, be thorough).

- Limb may not be treated each session (emphasis on the trunk).
- No deep pressure in ipsilateral involved quadrant (intercostal, parasternal, paravertebral techniques).
- Bolster limb for comfort and protection if insensate.

Specific Compression

- Incorporate all "general modifications."
- Full-arm bandage may overwhelm breast, trunk, or ipsilateral neck: alternate with half limb, full limb strategy (fingers to elbow, then to axilla).
- Bandage to protect skin, absorb wound exudate, and perspiration from skin-to-skin contact (axilla).
- Hand may be spared; light compression may be adequate to prevent reflux.

5.9.4 Conclusion

Adaptations of standard decongestive therapies in palliative care are possible provided there is close collaboration with the palliative team in understanding the etiology of the edema and a clear impression of disease location and its impact on standard clearance pathways. The lymphedema therapist can be an invaluable member of the team, impacting quality of life by markedly improving physical and psychological comfort.

5.10 Lipedema Treatment: Understanding the Diagnosis and Patient Profile

As stated in Chapter 3 (Lipedema), there is considerable debate as to the precise pathophysiology and etiology of lipedema. Without a clear understanding of lipedema as a distinct disease process, patients routinely fall victim to inaccurate assessments and incomplete or even harmful guidance from the medical community.

5.10.1 Misguidance and Misdiagnosis

The characteristics of lipedema are distinctly different from lymphedema or general obesity, yet most patients are grouped with the obesity camp and follow general guidelines suggested for weight loss. Unfortunately, the body region most affected by lipedema (hips, legs) responds poorly to weight loss and as such further distinguishes it as a unique disease process. As with typical obesity, weight can be shed from the upper body, face, and neck with reduced caloric intake and increasing fitness. However, the characteristically thickened subcutaneous tissue of the hips and legs laden with adipose tissue will at most become softer. Since lipedema includes a tendency toward very loose connective tissue, it does not exhibit elasticity and restorative qualities, which allow the skin to recover as with typical weight loss. With this very low level of skin support, interstitial pressure is low, encouraging fluid to accumulate from poorly supported superficial veins and initial lymphatics.

Lipedema has been examined more in the literature in Europe, but the texts have not been widely translated. Poor access to this literature and inadequate domestic research has historically supported the rationale for ongoing disease mischaracterization. Regardless, as far as the patient is concerned, improper labeling of lipedema represents a callousness that is never productive and may create serious emotional conflict in this patient group.

5.10.2 Psychological Perspective and Personality Attributes

Although lipedema appears to be a variant of obesity, there are distinct differences in the personality profile of the two groups. In general, the causes of obesity are well documented and relate to low motivation toward physical activity coupled with a high intake of food with emotional distress. On the contrary, in the vast majority of lipedema cases, patients exhibit very high levels of motivation to lose weight with abundant emotional and physical energy to complete the tasks. In fact, this weight has been gained against their will or tendencies. Most comply with therapists' suggestions, including arduous tasks like self-bandaging, without complaint, and hold high hopes for a solution to their physical problem. With this high level of motivation, it is not uncommon to see an overcompensation in some patients toward the pursuit of weight loss through eating and activity disorders. Unfortunately, with repeated failure to achieve reduction in the leg and hips, more negative emotions may follow leading to desperation, disillusionment, depression, self-loathing, apathy, and secondary obesity.

5.10.3 Identifying Lipedema and Adapting Treatment

Through easy internet research, lipedema patients become familiarized with the various treatments available for swollen or enlarged limbs. However, without an accurate medical assessment, they commonly arrive at an incomplete self-diagnosis. In pursuit of solutions, patients often seek conventional treatments with the expectation that CDT, for instance, will yield the same results that are common in pure lymphedema. Once at the clinic, the CLT may be the first medical professional to identify lipedema accurately and, as such, it may come as a surprise and even a relief to receive a proper diagnosis for the first time.

Since the CLT maintains a responsibility to provide the most current overview of lipedema pathology, characteristics, and treatment options, it follows that the patient's considerable relief may be followed by shattered expectations. Many lipedema patients have been trialed with CDT to see what benefits may also be available for lipedematous limbs. But with well-documented failure, it is important to avoid employing modalities, methods, and treatment resources where no measurable benefit is appreciated. Unfortunately, many lipedema patients are welcomed into lymphedema programs without an edema component (venous or lymphatic), so are overtreated. In contrast, others are excluded due to poor comprehension of the diagnosis when a combined presentation (lipolymphedema) could be productively addressed. Evidently, there is much confusion about treatment options for lipedema in its variety of combined forms.

Various Forms

Pure Lipedema

This presentation appears early in the disease progression. Lipedema alone exists without secondary lymphatic or venous complications, so are characterized by the following attributes (▶ Fig. 5.84):
- Soft adipose from the ankles to knees, thighs, or pelvic crests.
- Bruises easily, hyperalgesia.
- No history of cellulitis.
- Foot sparing, Stemmer's sign negative.
- Non pitting (even in distal calf).
- No skin changes.

Lipolymphedema

This presentation represents the typical progression where lymphedema coexists with lipedema if no intervention (namely compression) is offered to halt the process (▶ Fig. 5.85). Lymphedema progresses through the stages of severity as it would with pure lymphedema. Lymphedema is considered a secondary consequence of the underlying untreated lipedema. It can be characterized by the following attributes:
- Soft adipose tissue from ankles to knees, thighs, or pelvic crests.
- Bruises easily, hyperalgesia.
- History of cellulitis possible (more likely with severity).
- Foot sparing still possible or mild, moderate, severe foot involvement; Stemmer's sign negative or positive.
- Mild, moderate, severe calf involvement, pitting edema; progresses proximal to groin with severity.
- Skin changes and pitting (typical for lymphedema).

Lipo-Phlebo-Lymphedema

This presentation represents a progression of the disease that involves the venous and lymphatic systems (▶ Fig. 5.86). It is important to note that the mixture of the three components can be any combination of severity (e.g., primarily lipedema with mild, moderate, severe venous disease, plus mild, moderate or severe lymphedema. It can be characterized by the following attributes:
- Soft adipose tissue from ankles to knees, thighs, or pelvic crests.
- Bruises easily, hyperalgesia.
- History of cellulitis possible (more likely with severity).
- Foot sparing still possible or mild, moderate, severe foot involvement; Stemmer's sign negative or positive.
- Hemosiderin staining, ulcers, lipodermatosclerosis.
- Prominent superficial veins and/or history of PTS.
- Mild, moderate, severe calf involvement, pitting edema; progresses proximal to groin with severity.
- Skin changes and pitting (typical for lymphedema).

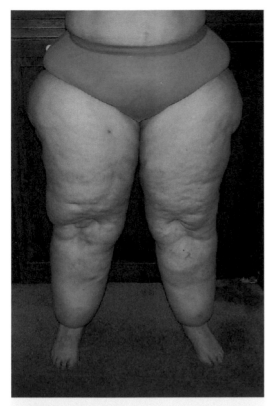

Fig. 5.84 Pure lipedema.

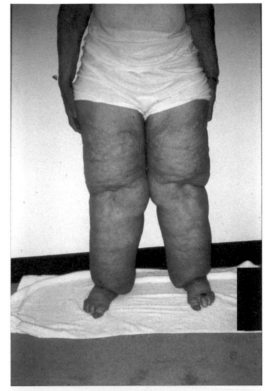

Fig. 5.85 Lipolymphedema.

Lympho-Lipedema

This presentation is where the lymphedema component coexists with lipedema and follows a parallel progression (▶ Fig. 5.87). As such, it is less accurate to say that lymphedema is secondary since a primary tendency may have existed from the onset. In some, it may appear that the lymphedema is a far greater proportion of the swelling, whereby a mild lipedema shows itself only with lymphedema reduction. It may also be the case that primary lymphedema in a person with a tendency toward obesity can be confused with lipedema. Regardless, a significant adipose component occupies the lymphedema-involved tissues and treatment will be most effective on the edema component. It can be characterized by the following attributes:

- Soft adipose from ankles to knees, thighs, or pelvic crests.
- History of cellulitis possible (more likely with severity).
- Foot sparing less likely; Stemmer's sign negative or positive.

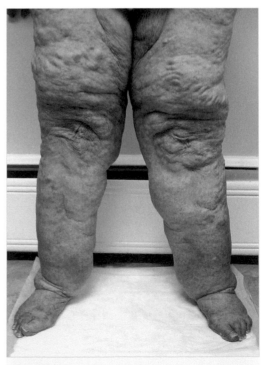

Fig. 5.86 Lipo-phlebo-lymphedema.

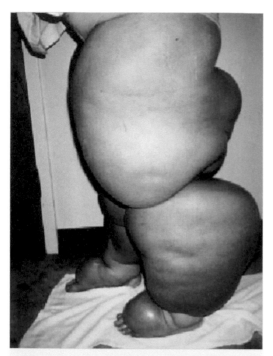

Fig. 5.87 Lympho-lipedema.

- Skin changes and pitting (typical for lymphedema).
- Less of a venous component.
- Lymphedema may mask underlying adipose tissue. Skin is not as soft.

5.10.4 Practical Guidelines for Therapy

Pure lipedema involves both a mechanical and dynamic insufficiency of the lymphatic system. Adipose congestion and increased skin compliance (less elasticity) comprise a physical challenge to the efficient production, collection, and linear transport of lymph by superficial lymph capillaries and vessels. With additional passive hyperemia from engorged superficial veins and increased capillary permeability, significant protein and water volume demands collection to retain interstitial fluid balance. Depending on the unique combination of adipose, venous, and lymphatic involvement with consideration for underlying inherited tendencies, treatment may be very simple or quite comprehensive.

Pure Lipedema Treatment

Compression of adipose tissue will not reduce adipose cells but favorably affects pericellular fluid stasis, which typically accounts for mild volume reductions. Although elastic garments may be all that are required in early onset, pure lipedema tissue hypersensitivity interferes with most attempts at compression. The high resting pressure of elastic garments coupled with the task of donning them, which allows for coiling, bunching, and cutting of the fabric, creates a difficult and painful first experience. Compression bandaging, in contrast, can be attempted successfully if generous synthetic cotton and foam padding are employed with the light resting pressure of short-stretch bandage layers. As a safeguard against intolerance to compression, MLD can be initiated with or without compression bandaging for the first few treatments to provide an analgesic benefit. Following a short intensive phase, compression bandaging can be discontinued, providing the best volume reduction for accurate measurement of garments. Suggested treatments are as follows:

- Apply MLD for analgesic effect with or without compression bandage.
- Sustain a short intensive phase for modest volume reduction and to improve tolerance to compression and garment fit.
- Discontinue bandaging, make a transition to garments for the long term (daytime only).
- Self-bandaging is not productive in most cases.
- Instruct patient on long-range expectations and supportive lifestyle.

Lipolymphedema Treatment

Whenever there is coexisting lymphedema, treatment should proceed as it would for a pure primary or secondary lymphedema. In the lymphedematous regions from ankles to knee and depending on duration, possibly involving the entire leg, tolerance to pressure is much higher. Volume reductions in these regions will be more significant and support a more productive therapist–patient relationship and long-range plan of care. Where lymphedema margins make the transition to lipedema, compression will again cause discomfort and yield only modest improvement. Since lymphedema requires constant attention, compression bandaging and garments will require time and attention during the self-care education process. Additional considerations for healthy living generally include weight management and exercise always performed in the compression garment. As adipose tissues receive the support they lack, exercise is more comfortable and productive leading to higher motivation to further improve the long-term outcome. With lipedema, however, it is important to set realistic expectations for further improvement in the regions of adipose congestion which may be very modest. Suggested treatments are as follows:

- Commence an intensive phase of CDT of sufficient duration to address the lymphedema stage of severity.
- Apply MLD and bandaging. Expect lymphedematous regions to be highly tolerant to compression.
- Conduct self-care education on compression bandaging and garments. Patients should continue this for the long term.
- Instruct patient on long-range expectations and supportive lifestyle.

Lipo-Phlebo-Lymphedema Treatment

Owing to the high skin compliance, many lipedema patients commonly exhibit visibly prominent superficial veins. If left untreated, secondary CVI will cause edema that characteristically improves with elevation and muscle pump activity. Since both vessel systems (venous and lymphatic) require support in compliant tissue to counteract a loss of interstitial pressure, compression alone is of benefit. When the venous system becomes involved, edema will improve significantly and reach a baseline quickly. This reduction is best achieved with compression bandaging so that the process is both comfortable and avoids fitting for garments that will become obsolete with reduction. It may appear that there is no lymphatic involvement due to the absence of typical signs. In many cases of lipedema when the lymphatic system fails, the foot continues to be spared and the Stemmer's sign remains negative. One sign that indicates lymphatic involvement is the tendency for compression bandaging to promote proximal movement above the bandage. For example, a knee-high bandage will not create a local reabsorption of water alone but will pump fluid proximally to be absorbed by lymphatic tissues. In this regard, MLD must be employed to improve uptake and transport of lymphatic loads unaffected by compression alone. Suggested treatments are as follows:

- Assess the involvement of venous and lymphatic systems.
- If venous edema, apply compression bandage only. Make the transition into long-term compression garments. Expect to reach a normal volume baseline.
- If combined venous edema and lymphedema, initiate an intensive phase of CDT. Proceed with self-care education for lymphedema management. Patients will continue this for the long term.
- Instruct patient on long-range expectations and supportive lifestyle.

Lympho-Lipedema Treatment

As described, there is an equal or greater lymphedema component in this combined form and, as such, a standard approach to treatment is required. The additional element of lipedema creates a lower expectation for achieving the appearance of near normalcy following a productive reduction. The patient should again understand that adipose tissue will not respond to compression except to halt any progression of the disease. Skin may be smoother from the tension of fluid and become soft with reduction, showing low elasticity and the underlying lipedema. Bruising and sensitivity may be less, allowing for a more comfortable and aggressive approach to therapy if required. Suggested treatments are as follows:

- Employ an intensive phase of CDT as with pure lymphedema.
- Expect a higher tolerance to compression.
- Long-term management is the same as for pure lymphedema.
- Do not expect a normal outcome, considering lipedema component.
- Instruct patient on long-range expectations and supportive lifestyle.

5.10.5 Alternative Treatments

Since lipedema commonly falls into the same category as obesity for most patients and clinicians, it is quite reasonable to seek or suggest more invasive and radical treatments that may have proven successful for purely obese patients. When diet and exercise fail, without current sound advice, liposuction, lipectomy, gastric bypass, skin reduction, or other surgical treatments may be sought. Considering the tendency for lipedema to secondarily affect lymphatic tissues, the likelihood of triggering lymphedema must be seen as a major risk.

5

Additionally, since the adipose distribution is not localized to one region (such as the lateral thigh or hips), surgical reduction must involve the entire limb to promise a cosmetic improvement. For these reasons and those associated with substantial invasive procedures, it is inadvisable to treat lipedema surgically. As the CLT, this position should be shared with the patient when embarking on a course of CDT to align patient expectations with reality, avoiding further damage into the future. Remind these patients that lipedema alone is far better than lipedema and lymphedema combined.

5.10.6 Compression Garments

Compression garments are a mainstay of long-term management for pure and combined forms of lipedema. When considering the optimal garment environment, material type, compression class, extent of coverage, and specific measuring techniques must be carefully considered. What most distinguishes lipedema as unique is the loose connective tissue that allows for increased skin compliance. In some, the texture allows for palpation of individual adipose lobules. In all cases, there is a remarkably soft texture that must be carefully considered for tenderness, injury, and counterproductive constriction within highly elastic fabrics. The slightest gathering of fabric can cause bruising and intense pain making the task of donning and removing garments an important one to master. In general, thicker flat-knit fabrics work best as they have less two-way stretch. Because they are measured to the true limb length with little additional longitudinal stretch, the opportunity for gathering is greatly minimized. Also, because of the coarse weave of these fabrics, loose tissues receive the structure and support that they lack. An important consideration for extent of coverage is the transition from compressed tissues to non-compressed tissues. Generally, whenever the lipedema extends to above the knee, a pantyhose is chosen even if the hips are spared. Although the lipedema diminishes at the thighs, a full leg stocking will end too abruptly without a sufficiently firm limb anchor. In these cases, the top edge rolls, cuts, and gathers creating great discomfort or pain. By continuing coverage to the waist fabric can smoothly make the transition from the proximal leg to the body part avoiding this tendency. Compression class (strength) must also be carefully considered to increase donning ease and long-term patient compliance. Empirical observation of many patient cases universally indicates that compression class 2, flat-knit garments are the preferred choice. These class 2 garments provide the right balance of structure, strength, and elasticity to accommodate donning and removal without undue struggle. Since a smooth and expeditious donning process avoids long periods of fabric accumulations with practice, the process can be completely comfortable and pain-free. In some patients where lymphedema is also present, a class 3 garment may be beneficial as a second step evolving from a period in class 2 fabrics.

A final unique attribute of many lipedema and lipolymphedema presentations is the transition from calf to foot. This so-called bell-bottom appearance presents a challenge for measuring and fitting due to the dramatic decrease in circumference that occurs over a short distance. When measuring, please consider the following suggestions for flat-knit class 2 pantyhose:

- Due to low elasticity of skin, consider measuring over the stocking to be replaced. This sublayer will provide firmness and lift tissues that otherwise fall due to gravity.
- If measuring for the first time, use moderate tension where the tissues are softest. To avoid cutting, be quick at each point and adjust the numbers by estimation tighter if necessary rather than by applying firm tension with the tape.
- In general, firm tension as compared with recording "true" circumferences provides the best fit. Adipose tissue can be "gathered up" by a snug-fitting garment without discomfort and provides better therapeutic control.
- Use light pressure at the proximal thigh (point "G"). This allows the fabric to evenly make the transition to the body part.
- When measuring the knee (point "E"), avoid the popliteal crease. Bend the knee to 45 degrees and measure from the apex of the patella to include tissues of the thigh just above the crease. This will create a better fit traversing a very prominent fold.
- At the ankle (point "Y") dorsiflex to 90 degrees and measure from the heel to include tissue of the distal calf. This avoids falling below the fold and getting an artificially small measurement.
- At the ankle (point "B"), measure the most distal circumference of the calf at the "bell-bottom."

For illustrations of the measuring points and comprehensive instructions on how to take measurements, see Section "5.16 later in this chapter.

5.11 Application of Compression Bandages

Successful treatment of lymphedema requires the use of a vast assortment of compression materials, which are applied using specialized bandage techniques. Only trained individuals with a thorough knowledge of lymphedema and its implications should apply compression bandages to patients with lymphedema.

General goals in compression bandaging are the following:
- To create a palpable compression gradient from the distal to the proximal end of the extremity.
- To create a functional, effective, comfortable, and durable compression environment.

Functional: Joint and muscle movements should be only minimally restricted; joints are bandaged in a functional position.

Effective: The pressure values should be high enough to achieve the goals outlined in Chapter 4, Effects of Compression Therapy, but not limit arterial blood supply or cause tourniquet effects, discomfort, or pain.

Comfortable: The skin and other structures (tendons, bony prominences, areas of small circumference) are protected with specialized padding.

Durable: Bandage materials should be applied to minimize slippage. This is important because the patient wears the compression bandages while decongestive exercises are performed.
- To create a structure for the external short-stretch bandages to adhere to.

Lymphedematous extremities are often abnormally shaped, and deepened skinfolds are present in the vicinity of joints. These uneven circumferences and lobuli are padded to create a more physiological structure for the compression bandages.

5.11.1 Required Materials

The use of various compression materials is essential to reduce limb volume safely and effectively. The following is a list of materials that are commonly used in skin care and compression bandaging for lymphedema and related conditions. To avoid allergic reactions, all materials used should be free of latex. The leading manufacturers for compression materials in the United States are Lohmann & Rauscher and BSN-Jobst. The materials listed can be obtained from specialty distributors (▶ Fig. 5.88).

Lotions

Patients are instructed for proper cleansing and moisturizing techniques to maintain the health and integrity of the skin. Suitable neutral or low-pH ointments and lotions commonly used in lymphedema are Lymphoderm and Eucerin.

Stockinettes

These tubular bandages are made from cotton and are used as an underlay to protect the skin from the padding materials and the bandages from lotions and perspiration. An assortment of different sizes to accommodate smaller extremities (children) as well as extremely large lymphedematous extremities are available from both manufacturers. Brand names are TG or K (Lohmann & Rauscher) and Tricofix (BSN-Jobst).

Stockinettes are packed in rolls of approximately 22 yards (~ 20 m), which is generally sufficient for

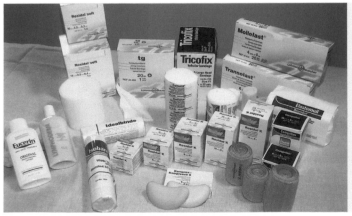

Fig. 5.88 Materials used in lymphedema management.

the duration of the decongestive phase of the treatment. A portion of this roll is cut before each bandage application to fit the length of the patient's extremity and should be replaced with every treatment.

Gauze Bandages

Made from elastic cotton material, gauze bandages are applied on fingers and toes and also are used to bandage male genitalia. Gauze is available as cohesive bandages, which are often used with male genitalia. Gauze bandages may be applied to keep foam pieces (padding) in place. They are available in different widths and colors (white and beige). Brand names are Mollelast or Transelast (Lohmann & Rauscher) and Elastomull (BSN-Jobst). Gauze bandages should be used for one application only and replaced with every treatment.

Padding Materials

Padding ensures an even distribution of pressure supplied by the short-stretch bandages and avoids tourniquet effects around the circumference of the extremity. These materials are applied on top of the stockinette and under the short-stretch bandages. Different materials can be used for the purpose of padding, such as nonwoven synthetic bandages, soft foam, compression pads, and ready-made bandage liners.

Synthetic Padding Bandages

These can be used over the entire length of the limb (except phalanges) and to pad deep skinfolds and creases. Synthetic padding is available in different widths; brand names are Cellona (Lohmann & Rauscher) and Artiflex (BSN-Jobst). Nonwoven synthetic padding should not be washed and should be replaced when dirty (usually once a week).

Soft Foam

Foam materials provide sufficient padding and prevent bandages from sliding. Soft foam is available as foam rolls or sheets. Foam rolls (Rosidal Soft from Lohmann & Rauscher) provide extra-soft padding and are more durable than synthetic padding bandages and soft foam sheets. The interlocking surface area of foam rolls makes the compression bandages slip-resistant. Foam rolls can be used in place of, or in addition to, nonwoven

synthetic padding bandages and 6-mm-thick foam sheets. Foam rolls are washable and available in different widths and thicknesses.

Sheets of soft foam (generally 3 feet × 6 feet [91 cm × 183 cm], with a recommended density of ~ 1.6 lb per cubic foot [~25.6 kilos per cubic meter]) may be cut by the clinician into individual sizes and patterns to provide extra-soft and uniform pressure distribution. Custom-cut foam pieces may be used in abnormally shaped extremities and lobuli to provide a more even surface area for the compression bandages to adhere to. They are held in the proper position with gauze bandages. Foam materials with 6 to 12 mm thickness are typically used. A 6-mm-thick foam is less bulky, has minimal rebound effect, and spreads the pressure more evenly than nonwoven synthetic padding bandages. A 12-mm-thick foam is more bulky, more durable, has a moderate rebound effect, and distributes the pressure very evenly. Foam sheets cannot be washed and are typically used throughout the decongestive phase.

Bandage Liners

In suitable cases, conventional padding options, such as synthetic padding bandages and soft foam materials, may be replaced by ready-made bandage liners, which should be made of comfortable, durable, and machine-washable materials. Well-crafted bandage liners contain specially designed channels, which enhance directional flow of lymphatic fluid. The addition of chipped soft foam particles used for padding creates localized pressure and helps reduce fibrotic tissue. Bandage liners are available in a variety of sizes for the upper and lower extremities.

High-Density Foam

This material is used to increase the radius of an extremity in certain areas, such as the palmar surface of the hand and the area between the malleoli and the Achilles tendon. As discussed in Chapter 4, La-Place's law, the surface pressure of a bandage increases if the radius decreases. It is therefore necessary to pad areas of concavity to achieve an increase in radius, thus preventing extremes. High-density foam has fibrinolytic qualities and is applied in areas of lymphostatic fibrosis, with the goal of softening fibrotic sections in the tissue. Foam rubber pieces are available as rolls, sheets, and precut pieces (oval and kidney shapes). The edges of foam rubber pieces used in compression bandaging should be beveled to avoid pressure marks on the skin; the edges of precut pieces are beveled by the manufacturer. To protect the patient's skin as well as the foam rubber pieces from lotions and perspiration, the pieces should be covered in stockinette. High-density foam rubber is available under the brand name Komprex (Lohmann & Rauscher). Komprex rubber foam is typically used throughout the decongestive phase.

Chip Bags and Swell Spots

Chip bags are used to soften "stubborn" areas of lymphostatic fibrosis in appropriate cases. Bags may be fabricated by the clinician using small foam cubes (~ 6–18 mm) that are placed in a stockinette. The open ends of the stockinette are sealed with tape. Contents of the chip bags may be composed of cubes made from soft foam (mildest effects), high-density foam (most aggressive effects), or a mixture of both (not too aggressive). The fibrinolytic qualities of the foam are enhanced by a "micromassaging" effect to the tissues produced by the foam cubes. It is important to understand that chip bags work well, but more aggressively than foam pieces by themselves. Upon removal of the chip bags following a period of wearing the compression bandages, deep indentations on the tissue surface may be observed. Chip bags should not be incorporated in the compression bandage on a daily basis. The use of chip bags is up to the clinician's discretion, but they cannot be used with patients on anticoagulant medication, hemophilic patients, or over varicose veins, and if they cause discomfort or pain.

Readily available swell spots (see ▶ Fig. 5.19) containing soft foam particles are a convenient alternative to therapist-manufactured soft foam cube chip bags. They are available in different shapes and can also be used to provide contoured padding and compression in difficult regions, such as the genital area and face.

Short-Stretch Bandages

Compression therapy, such as MLD, exercise, and skin care, is a major element of CDT. In most cases of lymphedema, the elastic fibers in skin tissues affected by lymphedema are damaged and unable to provide adequate resistance against the musculature working underneath, and the blood and lymph vessels within these tissues. External compression compensates for the elastic insufficiency of the affected tissue, providing the resistance

necessary to maintain the reduction of the swelling and to prevent reaccumulation of lymphedematous fluid.

Compression bandages are used during the decongestive (intensive) phase of CDT. In this sequence of the treatment, the volume of the affected limb changes almost on a daily basis, and it is necessary that external compression adapts to these changes. Bandages are much better suited for this task than compression garments (sleeves, stockings), which would have to be refitted constantly. Garments are used in the second phase of CDT, when the limb is decongested and volume changes are minimal.

Several layers of these textile-elastic bandages have to be applied to achieve the desired pressure values and effects on the swollen extremity. Short-stretch bandages are available in different widths (4, 6, 8, 10, and 12 cm). The length of short-stretch bandages is ~ 5.5 yards (~ 5 m); 10- and 12-cm-wide bandages are also available in lengths of ~ 11 yards (~ 10 m). These double-length bandages simplify the application of compression bandages on the thigh, as well as the application of self-bandages by the patient. Short-stretch bandages should be cleaned when dirty (usually once a week), and when there is a noticeable decrease in elasticity. Washing guidelines for compression bandages are outlined in the following.

Why Short-Stretch Bandages Are Used for the Treatment of Lymphedema

Crucial in lymphedema management is to provide the skin tissues with a solid counterforce against the muscles working underneath, particularly while standing, sitting, walking, or performing therapeutic exercises. The subsequent increase in the tissue pressure during muscle activity promotes lymphatic and venous return, and prevents fluid from accumulating in the skin. It is equally important to prevent the bandages from exerting too much pressure on the tissues during rest, which could cause a tourniquet effect and effectively prevent adequate return of these fluids.

There are two distinct types of compression bandages—short-stretch and long-stretch bandages. The difference refers to the extent the bandages can be stretched from their original length. Short-stretch bandages are made from cotton fibers, which are interwoven in a way that allows for ~ 60% extensibility of their original length, whereas long-stretch bandages, commonly known as "Ace" bandages, contain polyurethane, which allows for an extensibility of more than 140% of the original length.

The extent to which a bandage can be stretched specifies the two main qualities of pressure in compression therapy—the working pressure and the resting pressure. The working pressure is determined by the resistance the bandage provides against the working musculature underneath, and is active only during muscle activity, and therefore temporary. The pressure the bandage exerts on the tissues at rest (i.e., without muscle contraction) is known as the resting pressure, which is permanent. Relevant to these pressure qualities are the number of bandage layers, the tension with which these layers are applied, and, most importantly, the type of bandage used.

The high working pressure of short-stretch cotton bandages provides the necessary solid counterforce and makes them the preferred compression bandage in the management of lymphedema. Owing to the low resting pressure of short-stretch bandages, tourniquet effects are prevented, provided these bandages are applied correctly.

Long-stretch ("Ace") bandages have the exact opposite effect and are not suitable for lymphedema management. The low working pressure these bandages provide does not offer adequate resistance, and fluid would inevitably accumulate. In addition, the high resting pressure of long-stretch bandages could constrict veins and lymph vessels during rest.

During the evaluation, the clinician determines the quantity of materials needed for the application of the compression bandages during the decongestive phase of the therapy. To ensure successful intervention, adequate supplies have to be on hand before treatment starts. Either the treatment center keeps a sufficient quantity of compression materials in stock or the patients themselves are responsible for ordering the materials needed from a distributor before the initial treatment. Approximate stock quantities for lymphedema treatment centers are listed in Chapter 6, Suggested Materials to Start Up a Lymphedema Program.

> The life of short- and medium-stretch bandages can be considerably extended by using two sets, one to wear and one to wash. Manufacturers recommend replacing the bandages every 3 months if used daily.

Wide-Width Short-Stretch Bandages

These bandages are available in widths of 15 and 20 cm and are applied primarily on the thorax and abdominal areas. Wider bandages are also applied over the narrower short-stretch bandages on the thigh to increase stability or to hold larger foam pieces in place. Brand names are Idealbinde (Lohmann & Rauscher) and Isoband (BSN-Jobst).

Tape (~ 1 inch or 2.5 cm wide) should be used to affix the bandage material and not clips or pins. Sharp bandaging clips or pins may cut into the patient's skin and provide an avenue for infection.

Washing Guidelines for Compression Bandages

Machine Wash versus Hand Wash

As with compression garments, if compression bandages are not washed on a daily or regular basis, skin cells and oils will become trapped in the fibers and damage the integrity of the textile. Compression bandages may be machine or hand washed, depending on the preference of the user. A machine wash is preferred because it will get the bandages cleaner. Once they go through the spin cycle, they are easy to hang and will dry much faster. Daily washing is recommended, especially if lotions or creams are being used. When washing garments in a machine, it is recommended to place the unrolled bandages in a mesh laundry bag to protect the fabric during the washing cycle. A gentle cycle should be utilized.

Bandages should be washed in warm water (40–60 °C/104–140 °F); if the bandages are extremely dirty, they may be boil washed (95 °C/203 °F).

It is best to have more than one set of bandages (one to wear and one to wash). These should be applied alternately to allow the elasticity to recover and to prolong their effectiveness.

Tips for hand washing procedures:

1. Start by filling a bowl, bucket, sink, or small tub with water.
2. The compression bandages should be dipped gently into the water to dampen.
3. Add a small amount of washing solution (see below).
4. Let the compression bandages soak for a few minutes.
5. For better cleaning, gently rub the fibers of the compression bandages together without stretching them excessively.

6. Then, empty the tub and refill with water; dip or rinse the clean compression bandages thoroughly to rid the bandages of residual salts and oils from perspiration.
7. Gently squeeze the compression bandages to remove excess water.
8. Refer to the following drying options.

Washing Solutions

Harsh cleaning agents, solvents, petroleum-based cleaners, etc., can destroy the thin fibers of compression bandages. Mild soaps or detergents should be used, free of bleach, chlorine, fabric softeners, or other laundry additives. Some compression garment manufacturers offer garment washing solutions, which are formulated to remove oil, body acids, and skin salts quickly and easily without damage to the fabric; using these specially formulated solutions is also recommended for compression bandages and will help extend their lifespan and keep them firm.

Bandages may be washed up to 50 times without losing their elasticity. While proper care will increase the lifespan of short-stretch bandages, they will need to be replaced about every 6 months, or when the bandages lose their "stiffness" and recoil.

Drying Guidelines

Compression bandages should be air dried. If using a dryer, the dial should be set on a no-heat (maximum low-heat) drying cycle because excessive heat exposure may weaken or even damage the textile of the bandages. When bandages are air dried, it is important not to pull, squeeze, or wring out the residual water from the material excessively. Rolling up the compression bandages in a towel and gently squeezing the towel before laying them out to dry speeds up the drying process; bandages should never be left rolled up in a towel.

Whether bandages are line dried, or laid flat to dry, exposure to direct sunlight should be avoided. It is recommended to place a towel on a drying rack and lay the bandages on top to dry. It is not advisable to hang the bandages directly on a rack or pole to drip dry because the weight of the water could stretch the material.

Ironing of short-stretch bandages is not necessary or recommended. When the bandages are removed from the wash, they should be hung so that they are flat and not twisted. Once they are

dry, they should be tightly rolled for storage and future application.

Care of Other Materials Used for the Application of a Padded Short-Stretch Compression Bandage

Padding bandages, foam rolls, and gauze bandages have a much shorter lifespan. Padding bandages lay much closer to the skin and tend to collect oils, body acids, and skin salts. The "fresher" the padding bandages, the softer they are and the more cushioning they provide. The same principles apply to gauze bandages (for finger and toe wrapping). Once gauze begins to lose its shape and becomes soiled, it is time to discard it and open a fresh roll.

Stockinettes or tubular bandages (used directly on the skin as an underlay between the skin and bandage materials) can be washed. They will fray after a couple of washes and lose their shape. Tubular bandages can be purchased in rolls and it is a good idea to replace them with a new layer after a couple of uses.

5.11.2 Lymphedema Bandaging: Selecting Foam Padding

The following list can assist the lymphedema therapist while constructing a thoughtful and sophisticated compression bandage. It should be expected that daily round-the-clock compression of several weeks' duration is likely to create comfort concerns at key anatomical points, and in the worst case scenario, soft-tissue damage and circulatory disturbance. The patient's experience of wearing compression, be it positive or negative, is directly linked to the long-term success of the program and of the patient's compliance as regards home care.

Objectives and Considerations for the Use of Foam Rubber Pads

The objectives (goals) for each multilayered bandage complex are to
- Create a palpable, even, compression gradient in the affected limb.
- Create padding and protection around bony prominences and tender areas.
- Protect skin and soft-tissue structures from undue irritation or harm.

- Create a structure for the external short-stretch bandages to adhere to.
- Create a durable compression environment that endures and allows for daily activity.
- Create a dynamic environment for the muscle pump ("rebound effect").
- Create a teaching strategy for home care replication and optimization.
- Breakdown deposits of scar tissue (lymphostatic fibrosis).
- Create a comfortable environment to improve long-term compliance.

Long-Term Compliance in Home Care

It must be emphasized that sustainable treatment success is largely dependent on daily, uninterrupted compression therapy involving compression garments of the medically correct gradient and multilayered short-stretch bandaging. Remember that the experience of wearing compression in the intensive clinical phase, be it positive or negative, is directly linked to patient' home care compliance and is a further reflection on the success of the program and the skill level of the therapists involved. The chief concerns related to poor compliance include the following:

- Discomfort caused by ill-fitting garments or poorly applied bandaging.
- Lack of appropriate education and guidance regarding the bandaging technique and regimen.
- Poor motivation, inspiration, and belief of the patient and/or therapist.
- Multiple diagnoses, which further complicate the long-term strategy.
- Lack of support in the family and health care community.

Materials and Considerations

The use of various compression padding materials is essential to the process of safely and effectively reducing limb circumference. The compressive outer layer is always the same: a short-stretch, nonelastic, pure cotton bandage (Rosidal/Comprilan). In CDT, it is important to realize the superior qualities of foam technology as compared with synthetic cotton padding materials. Once these materials are implemented on a regular basis, therapists notice many dramatic differences, effects, and productive qualities.

The following points can be used to evaluate the qualities of a variety of foams as compared with synthetic cotton. By becoming familiar with the various foams available. choices can be made to tailor the padding strategy precisely as desired for maximum therapeutic effect. Please note that even the negative attributes are far more beneficial than using cotton padding or no padding.

- Take time to customize the fit of foam padding applications; anatomically correct fit will ensure even coverage and enhanced comfort.
- The templates provided in CDT training manuals can be followed when selecting shapes for different anatomical areas.
- If used, be aware of allergic reactions or contact dermatitis and aggressive, harsh response on the skin where foam overlaps or embeds itself.

Gray Foam Sheets Open Cell

¼ inch thickness, 3 feet × 6 feet (6 mm × 0.91 m × 1.82 m).

Positive Attributes

- Good starting point for most patients (less threatening on first treatment day).
- Spreads pressure more evenly than synthetic cotton (no spiral pressure marks or bunching).
- Limbs can be wrapped in one continuous layer (no need to bevel edges).
- Effectively protects against abrasions of short-stretch layers (Comprilan and Rosidal contain "coarse" weaves).
- Least bulky (as compared with other sheet foams).
- Easy to cut, less complicated to fit to limbs, requires less precision.
- Can act as a sublayer under more aggressive foams.
- Economical.

Negative Attributes

- Generates very direct pressure due to less thickness and structure. May not be comfortable for all patients.
- Least durable (as compared with other foams); wears out quickly.
- Least structural integrity (as compared with other foams); may buckle or sag.
- Minimal "rebound effect" (muscle pump dynamic); less productive at fluid mobilization.

Gray Foam Sheets Open Cell

½ inch thickness, 3 feet × 6 feet/12 mm × 0.91 m × 1.82 m.

Positive Attributes

- Patients often graduate to ½ inch (12 mm) foam following ¼ inch (6 mm) foam (as the need for comfort increases and edema decreases).
- Generates pressure more comfortably and less directly (as compared with ¼ inch [6 mm] foam).
- Spreads pressure very evenly (allows for a uniform compression gradient).
- Limb should be "pressed" not encircled (allows for reduction between two pieces).
- Moderate durability (as compared with other foams).
- Moderate structural integrity (as compared with other foams).
- Moderately bulky (as compared with other foams).
- Has moderate to high "rebound effect" (muscle pump dynamic).
- Economical.

Negative Attributes

- Edges must always be beveled (allowing pressure marks to be minimized). Requires time.
- May be too bulky (objectionable to some patients).
- Takes more skill to cut and fit.
- Edges must be beveled or pressure marks may injure skin.

Gray Foam Sheets Open Cell

1 inch thickness, 3 feet × 6 feet (2.5 cm × 0.91 m × 1.82 m).

Positive Attributes

- Very durable (as compared with other foams).
- Very high structural integrity (excellent for splinting, bridging folds, and defects).
- Most protective if the objective is to avoid injury or a trauma site; most bulky (not appropriate for covering entire limb).
- Best application: paralysis (dorsum, palm splint), elephantiasis (bridging deep creases, offsetting very high pressures).

Negative Attributes

- Too bulky if used in large pieces. Never encase an entire limb.
- Must be carefully beveled at all times.
- Difficult to maneuver.
- May be too aggressive on tissues if used in a high pressure bandage.

Komprex Closed Cell

1 cm thickness, 50 cm × 1 m.

This orange foam is specially blended for close contact with the skin. It is one of the only closed cell foam rubber products used in lymphedema bandaging.

Positive Attributes

- Highest durability, structural integrity, and density (ideal for long-term home care).
- Highest intensity: Use Komprex only after working with 6- and 12-mm gray foams. Graduate into Komprex if more intensity is required.
- Very high "rebound effect" (muscle pump dynamic).
- Limb should always be "pressed" not encircled (allows for reduction between two opposing pieces).
- Can be used in combination with other foams (layered, laminated with gray foams).
- Hypoallergenic (but should not be chosen on this factor alone).
- Most effective for softening lymphostatic fibrosis.

Negative Attributes

- Less comfortable, very aggressive pressure (best for patients with advanced fibrosis).
- Most difficult to cut and shape.
- *Time consuming*: Edges are always beveled (allowing pressure marks to be minimized).
- Pressure marks can be severe if edges are not beveled professionally.
- Most expensive foam.

Komprex-Binde Closed Cell

0.5 or 1 cm thickness, 8-cm-wide rolls.

This white foam is another version of medical grade closed cell foam rubber.

Positive Attributes

- Softer than orange Komprex.
- Offers more comfort and does not collapse like open cell foam.
- May be laminated with other foams.
- Highly durable.
- Very structural.

Negative Attributes

- Edges must be beveled.

- Never spiral to cover the limb; pressure marks will be harsh and counterproductive to drainage.
- Is only available in narrow rolls; therefore, use for smaller crafted pieces only.
- More expensive than gray open cell foams.

Komprex II Open Cell

65 cm × 65 cm.

This white foam is made up of parallel foam cylinders sewn between fabric. It has an uneven surface created by the cylinders, which are aligned in rows.

Positive Attributes

- Provides high and low pressure areas to soften fibrotic tissue (3D effect).
- Gentle effect as compared with Schneider pack applications.
- Washable, reusable, and durable.

Negative Attributes

- May not be advisable for every patient type (lipedema, fragile skin, soft edema).
- More costly.

Velfoam Open Cell

8-mm thickness, 50- or 150-mm-wide rolls.

Because of the fleece lining on each side, this padding material can be used directly against the skin.

Positive Attributes

- Excellent inside stockings and sleeves and gloves (protects popliteal and cubital creases).
- Excellent as padding for very sensitive areas such as the face, breast, and genital areas.
- Good starting point for padding in pediatric lymphedema.
- Accepts Velcro hook applications.

Negative Attributes

- Will not create the structure and comfort of the sheet foams (too thin).
- Comes in rolls, so it is best in small pieces; not to be used for full limb coverage.
- Relatively expensive.
- Requires washing or frequent disposal and replacement.

Rosidal Soft White Foam Roll

3 or 4 mm thickness, 10 or 12 cm width.

Used as a substitute for cast padding (synthetic cotton).

Positive Attributes

- Washable and reusable, economical.
- Grips better than synthetic cottons.
- Conforming quality and low elasticity create grip.
- Can be cut without tearing. Good for customized applications.

Negative Attributes

- Structure is not sufficient to hold bandage securely if used as the sole padding.
- Elasticity can cause high "resting pressure" if applied aggressively.

5.11.3 Lymphedema Bandaging: Practical Guidelines

Guidelines for application of compression bandages to both mildly affected limbs and advanced presentations involving abnormal body contours and massive edema.

Principles and Goals of Compression Bandaging

Principle: Rationale for Short-Stretch Bandage Materials

Generate Low Resting Pressures

A low constriction force is applied which increases patient comfort when at rest and ensures against blood circulatory disturbances. This is achieved by eliminating elastic threading from the individual compression bandage resulting in a cast-like "sheath," which does not shorten around the limb at work or at rest.

Generate High Working Pressures

The bandage creates a high resistance to refilling because, due to its nonelastic composition, it will not stretch or accommodate under the pressures of gravity, new fluid formation, or accumulation of mobilized fluids. This preserves the decongestive results between each treatment.

Construct a Compression Gradient

The area most distal to the trunk on an affected limb is compressed with greater force than an area more proximal. This seminal bandaging principle is achieved for each patient through the application of short-stretch bandaging materials in multiple layers. A compression gradient can be accomplished with the following techniques.

Technique: Methods of Application Will Create Predictable Results (Basic or Advanced)
Vary the Widths of Bandages

By selecting bandage rolls of increasing width, pressure is distributed over a greater surface area with each layer and on proximal limb areas.

Apply More Bandage Turns Distally Than Proximally

By starting each roll on the distal aspect of the limb, a thicker sheath is developed distally, and a thinner sheath is developed more proximally.

Standard Bandage Spacing

By overlapping each preceding bandage turn a standard amount (+~ 50%), the bandage will be more concentrated at the distal aspect of the limb where bandages are narrower.

Standard Bandage Tension

To generate even tension around the limb, each bandage should be applied uniformly around the full circumference. This is achieved by a standard "pull/tension" on the bandage, as it is passed from one hand to the other, each hand addressing 180 degrees of the full circumferential pressure.

The Goal of Each Bandage Is Always the Same (Basic or Advanced)

It is important to realize the complementary relationship between MLD and bandaging in the achievement of this treatment objective. Bandaging alone is not sufficient to guarantee reduction and alone may create significant complications. Therefore, to prevent complications, the following steps should be considered:

Prevent the Return of Evacuated Lymph

The high working pressures generated by multilayered short-stretch bandaging resist the forces responsible for refilling, such as gravity and active and passive hyperemia. Exercise, heat, friction, and low-grade inflammation or dependent positions are usually the cause.

The Influence of Starling's Law (Microcirculation)

By increasing interstitial tissue pressure via application of external compression, ultrafiltration of tissue fluid is decreased (less lymph formation). Likewise, reabsorption of interstitial fluids through the venous circulatory system is improved (less water in tissues). In combination with MLD, protein-rich fluid (lymph) enters the lymph capillary (increasing lymph formation/volume).

Reduce Limb Volume (Progressive Confinement)

All compression bandaging mobilizes fluid by "squeezing" the edematous subcutaneous tissue spaces. However, it is more therapeutically sound and technically safe to approach lymphedema bandaging with a less aggressive mindset, which could be characterized as "progressively confining the limb to size." It is important to understand that MLD alone will measurably decrease limb volume with each treatment; however, fluid will return spontaneously. Therefore, the goal of each bandage is to preserve the results of the MLD treatment with an immediate bandage application. The result is continual linear reduction without aggressive squeezing, thus preventing the swollen compartment from refilling. Without undue application of force, through the use of multiple low tension layers, skin integrity is preserved, guaranteeing comfort and short- and long-term compliance.

Break Down Depositions of Scar Tissue

Lymphedema is a disease process involving accumulation of fluid and connective tissue in the form of chronic tissue inflammation followed by lymphostatic fibrosis (metaplasia). More productive

5

and intensive than MLD, skilled bandaging alone creates remarkable softening and scar tissue reversal in the majority of patient presentations regardless of severity or duration.

- Incorporate the appropriate materials into each bandage: the mechanical breakdown of fibrous tissue is often achieved with localized placement of denser grades of foam padding (Komprex) and increased pressure. Foam cube packs (Schneider packs) and other specialized padding materials employ a similar strategy involving "deeply embedding" padding materials to leave pressure marks or "pits" in the target areas of fibrosis. These careful and thoughtful strategies create a softening effect, which can be maintained and further improved upon.
- Require patient activity within the bandage: A powerful component of CDT involves creating an exercise program that is tailored to the unique capabilities of the patient. When all exercises are performed wearing the bandage, complex mechanical forces combined with a customized padding strategy manipulate the fibrotic tissues and facilitate the softening of hardened tissues.

Improve the Muscle and Joint "Pump"

Lymph drainage is enhanced by performing exercises and even simple daily activities within a high working pressure bandage complex. Without bandage support, the insufficient lymph collector valves (as those of veins) allow a continuous column of fluid to develop, which results in stasis, reflux, and further accumulation during exercise.

- Bandaging supports the insufficient valves. Continuous external support allows for valvular patency and the intrinsic contractility of each lymphangion to resume normal function, thus restoring fluid propulsion and promoting further decongestion.
- Bandaging harnesses the forces of muscle contraction. The edematous compartment between the muscle fascia and the bandage sheath is squeezed by the action of the engorged muscle as it contracts and relaxes. Coupled with the high working pressures of the unyielding bandage, a natural pumping action is created which enhances proximal fluid movement.

Create Comfort for Patient Compliance

The goal of comfort cannot be overstated. Each therapist should strive to experience the bandage vicariously to draw upon the sense of empathy and better understand the demands of intensive therapy. With comfort come patient satisfaction, trust, loyalty, teamwork, and a much higher likelihood of continued home care participation. (See also Section 5.11.2)

Advanced Bandaging: Practical Guidelines

The basic principles of lymphedema compression bandaging also govern the approach to advanced patient presentations. However, to achieve success in complex patients with elephantiasis, thoughtful deviation is necessary from standard approaches. As lymphedema therapists, we must apply many more tools and techniques than are required in more moderate cases.

Use More Compression Bandages

There is no standard number of bandages for advanced cases. Use as many layers as it takes to create the necessary gradient, support, and structure. Remember that very large limb girths consume bandages with less coverage and generating higher pressures on a large radius (La-Place's law) will require more force and structure. Consider double-length (10 m), short-stretch bandages to minimize waste from starting and ending multiple bandages.

Use Generous Amounts of Foam Padding

Bandage pressures may be considerably higher in advanced cases. To offset discomfort, choose thicker bulkier types of foam. This bulk can also be achieved through lamination (layering) of different types and densities of foam. Take time to create a padding strategy that addresses fibrosis, creases, and fragile skin and allows for movement. There is no limit to the amount of padding that can be utilized to achieve these goals.

Create Additional Structure

Expect advanced cases such as elephantiasis to respond to CDT with dramatic daily volume reductions. These reductions do, however, cause bandages to shift, slacken, or fall and create loss of tissue support, bunching and injury, potential areas of tourniquet, and refilling of fluid. The selection of more structural foams such as

Komprex or 1-inch (2.5-cm) gray foam will "splint" the bandage in place and offset this tendency. The application of more bandage layers will assist this process adding more structure.

Use Higher Pressures

Moderate cases of lymphedema respond to moderate pressures. The benefits of lighter wrapping are numerous, such as preservation of skin integrity, enhanced comfort, lighter overall bandage weight, improved patient compliance, and easier home care education. In advanced cases, we may not be able to reach a satisfactory reduction without increasing the overall compression to levels which are considerably higher. This is generally attributed to the extent of fibrosis. It is sometimes predictable that large volumes of fluid will be shifted between treatments. Starting with firm pressure may be necessary in an effort to offset shifting as the bandage softens from fluid that is rapidly mobilized.

Use the Edema as a Padding

An empirical observation to consider is one that initially offsets discomfort in very edematous limbs. Patients report higher levels of comfort and tolerance to aggressive bandaging initially, when there is the most fluid and fibrosis, which serves as an inherent (intrinsic) padding. As volume decreases, however, so does the benefit of this cushion. Most patients will become progressively less tolerant as edema reduction occurs. At this phase of treatment, overall pressure is reduced and padding may be increased.

Adjust the Compression Gradient Daily

Elephantiasis patients typically require deviation from the standard gradient. Abnormal folds, lobular outgrowths, and severely fibrotic skin may be resistant to standard gradients of pressure. Therefore, the therapist may be required to temporarily increase pressures in a proximal area such that they are equal to or greater than that of the distal limb. This deviation can be done temporarily with no adverse effect, provided that it is not performed at each treatment. Typically stubborn areas will yield when pressure is focused and the attention can then be shifted to the next more distal area. In this fashion, proximal decongestion will eventually lead to distal limb improvement, where distal areas are characteristically more advanced. Likewise in some cases of severe distal involvement of

the hand, foot, calf, or forearm, the gradient may again require careful study to achieve a benefit. It is not uncommon for proximal pressure to worsen a distal region even when a correct standard gradient is created. In these limbs, a steep decrease in pressure may proximally be the only method to achieve a distal improvement.

Protect Skinfolds and Creases

In advanced cases where limb contour is extremely abnormal, avoid allowing bandages to cut into creases and skinfolds, otherwise a tourniquet may develop and skin breakdown is likely. First, pack the fold areas with generous amounts of synthetic cotton or gentle foam scraps. This step not only fills in the void but assists in opening these areas to air circulation, mechanical stimulation, and daily cleansing. Next, create an enclosure for the area using structural foam, (thick gray or Komprex) so that the external compression layers traverse (span) the creased areas and avoid following these defects.

Temporarily Omit Difficult-to-Reach Skin Areas

In an example involving calf tissues draping over the foot, contacting the floor, it may be impossible to adequately cover the most distal areas in the first few sessions. As a strategy, first work to achieve a generalized softening throughout the calf, which will create the necessary skin slackening to gradually reposition the tissues in the bandage. The exposed area should always be covered for protection from direct contact with the ground using tubular gauze, and in most cases this challenge is only a temporary problem.

Incorporate Elastic Materials with Caution

The safety and control afforded by the use of nonconstricting (nonelastic) bandaging materials cannot be overstated. However, in advanced elephantiasis, it may be nearly impossible to secure the bandage sheath securely between daily treatments due to the rate of reduction. The solution may be to include elastic "Ace" bandages causing the bandage to cling to the limb and shrink down with each subsequent reduction. It must be emphasized that elastic bandages can be contraindicated in certain patient profiles and that the application must never be directly against the skin.

5

These wraps must always be applied external to a padding layer (Komprex, thick foam) and not traverse the joints.

Additional Guidelines for Applying "Elastic" Bandages

- Never extend elastic bandages to more than 50% of the stretch.
- Ensure that each bandage layer is perfectly flat.
- Never let the bandage exploit creased skin areas.
- Never let the bandage cut in at joint areas.
- Use only one or two layers in a multilayered bandage.

Incorporate Elastic Garments into Bandage

Many patients with advanced lymphedema have worn (used) elastic garments that can be of service to the therapist's compression strategy. Pantyhose may be cut into shorts at any point above the knee, then applied either as the last layer to assist in keeping bandages in place or as the first layer to create sufficient grip for additional layers to adhere to.

Address Lymphostatic Fibrosis More Aggressively

Severely thickened skin areas will not generally respond to mild bandaging methods. However, it is imperative to correctly identify fibrosis and differentiate it from tight, saturated tissue areas, which are often misinterpreted as fibrosis. Commonly, hyperkeratosis that is evident on the skin correlates to chronic underlying scar tissue. In general, these areas can take more aggressive pressure and padding (Komprex) early in treatment. In other cases, epidermal skin integrity is good, but the underlying dermal tissues are dramatically thickened and scarred. In any scenario, the initial goal of treatment is to first decongest the fluid component of the swelling. This can be easily evaluated with weekly measurements, which will reveal a reduction plateau. Yet, if the limb size is still far from a normal baseline, it is safe to assume that much of the remaining swelling can be attributed to thickened skin, fibrosis, and/ or adipose tissue.

Guidelines for Application of "Schneider Packs"

- Chose a density of foam that is appropriate for each skin type.

- Hyperkeratosis as in advanced elephantiasis can take larger cubes of gray foam or very small cubes of Komprex.
- Normal epidermal skin external to more advanced dermal thickening should only be addressed with small gray foam cubes.
- Avoid using "Schneider packs" on a daily basis.
- Alternate with flat sheets of foam that assist in establishing a consistent gradient.
- Gradient pressure is difficult to achieve through bulky cube packs; therefore, proximal flow can be difficult to achieve.
- Do not send the patient home with Schneider packs unless they have been well trained to use them.

5.11.4 Upper Extremity Bandaging

Recommended materials for applying a compression bandage on the upper extremity during the decongestive phase of CDT (phase 1) are listed below. The following quantities represent two sets of compression bandages:
- One bottle of skin lotion.
- One box of stockinette (tubular bandage) in the appropriate size.
- One to two boxes (20 individual rolls in a box) of gauze bandages (4 or 6 cm width).
- Four to six synthetic nonwoven padding bandages (10 cm) or two Rosidal Soft foam bandages (10 cm).
- Two short-stretch bandages (6 cm), or two short-stretch bandages (4 cm, for smaller hands).
- Two short-stretch bandages (8 cm).
- Four to six short-stretch bandages (10 cm).
- Two short-stretch bandages (12 cm).
- Tape to secure the bandages.
- If necessary, one sheet of soft foam (~ 6 mm: 23 cm thickness).
- If necessary, one sheet of Komprex or one roll of soft foam rubber.

Application

Generally, bandages are applied with an even pre-stretch of ~ 30 to 40% and an overlap of ~ 50 to 70%. The patient should be in the sitting position.

Skin Care

Wash and bathe the skin, then apply the appropriate lotion thoroughly.

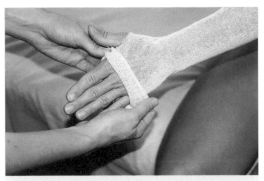

Fig. 5.89 Application of stockinette.

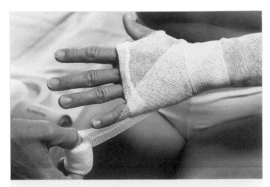

Fig. 5.90 Application of gauze bandages on the fingers.

5

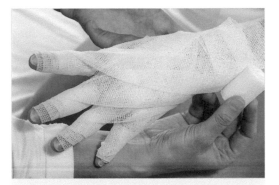

Fig. 5.91 Application of gauze bandages on the fingers; fingertips remain unbandaged.

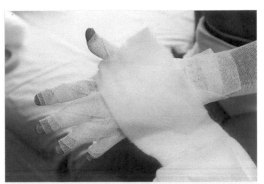

Fig. 5.92 Application of padding materials on the hand.

Stockinette

The tubular bandage should be cut to a length that allows for an overlap of ~ 12 cm on the proximal end of the extremity. This overlap is used to extend over and cover the complete compression bandage on the proximal border to protect it from axillar perspiration. A hole is cut for the thumb on the distal end (▶ Fig. 5.89).

Finger Bandages

The patient's fingers are spread slightly, and the hand is in pronation. A bolster should be placed under the elbow to support the patient's arm.

Start the first gauze bandage with a loose anchor turn around the wrist (▶ Fig. 5.90), then proceed over the dorsum of the hand to the little finger (or the thumb). The fingers should be bandaged with light pressure from the distal to the proximal ends with ~ 50% overlap. The fingertips are not covered. Leave the finger over the dorsum of the hand toward the wrist, apply a half turn (complete anchoring turns should always be avoided) around

the wrist, and proceed to bandage the remaining fingers in the same fashion (▶ Fig. 5.91). The borders of the gauze bandage should not slide or roll in on the distal and proximal ends of the fingers. One-and-a-half to two gauze bandages are typically necessary to bandage all fingers. Any unused part of the second gauze bandage should be wrapped spirally (not circularly) around the forearm.

Upon completion, the fingertips should be checked for proper circulation. The bandages should not slide over the knuckles when the patient makes a fist, and no skin area over the fingers should be visible.

Padding Materials

Nonwoven synthetic padding (Artiflex, Rosidal) or soft foam rolls (Rosidal Soft) are used to pad the hand and arm. A hole is cut for the thumb (▶ Fig. 5.92); the padding bandage is secured around the wrist with a circular turn. The hand is then padded down to the knuckles using two to

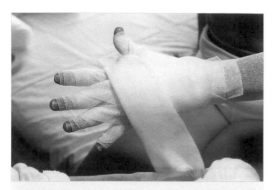

Fig. 5.93 Application of padding materials on the hand.

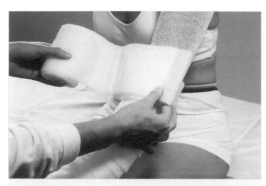

Fig. 5.94 Application of extra padding materials on the antecubital fossa.

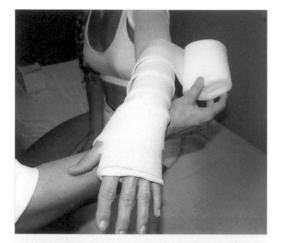

Fig. 5.95 Application of padding materials (soft foam roll) on the arm.

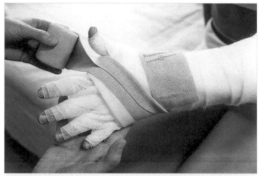

Fig. 5.96 Application of 6-cm bandage on the hand.

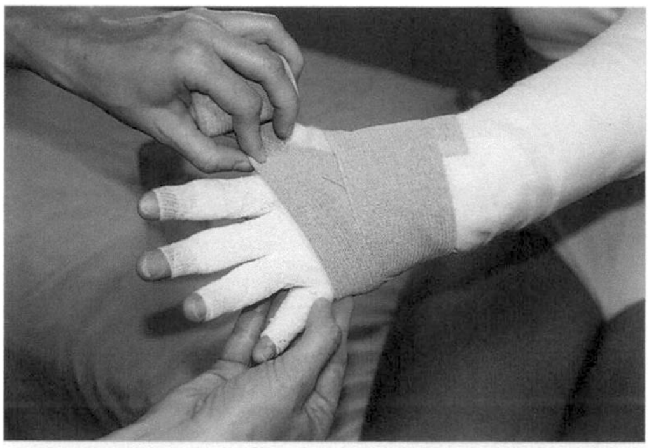

the forearm and upper arm. The cubital fossa is protected with extra layers of padding (▶ Fig. 5.94). Two rolls of padding bandages typically are used for an upper extremity (▶ Fig. 5.95).

Short-Stretch Bandages

Starting a 6-cm-wide bandage with a loose anchor turn around the wrist, the hand is bandaged to include the knuckles, with the patient spreading the fingers slightly (▶ Fig. 5.96). To avoid irritation in the web space between the thumb and the index finger, the bandage should be folded over about one-third of its width (depending on the size of the hand), without twisting the bandage (▶ Fig. 5.97). The bandage is anchored between each turn around the hand with half turns on the wrist (thenar area). To avoid bulking, the fold on the hand should alternate between the proximal and distal border of the bandage with each turn (▶ Fig. 5.98). The double bandage layer resulting from folding the bandage provides increased pressure on the distal portion of the hand, where the swelling is usually more pronounced. Any

Fig. 5.97 Folding of the 6-cm bandage on the dorsum of the hand.

four circular turns, with the padding bandage folded in half (▶ Fig. 5.93). The padding bandage then proceeds in the proximal direction to cover

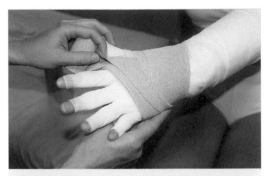

Fig. 5.98 Alternating folds to avoid excessive pressure.

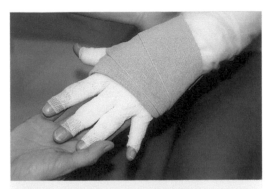

Fig. 5.99 Finished bandage on the hand.

5

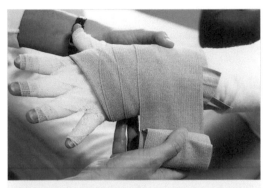

Fig. 5.100 Application of the 8-cm bandage on the hand and forearm.

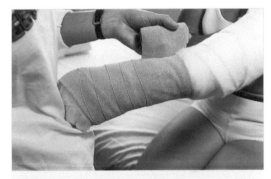

Fig. 5.101 Application of the 8-cm bandage on the forearm.

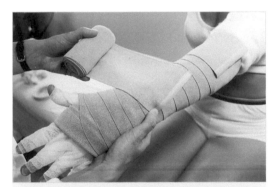

Fig. 5.102 The 10-cm bandage starts on the area of lowest pressure.

remaining bandage material is used on the forearm (▶ Fig. 5.99).

The successive bandages are applied in opposite directions to each other. This provides for a more functional and durable bandage. The next bandage (8 cm) starts on the wrist, with a loose anchor (▶ Fig. 5.100) in the opposite direction of the first bandage, and proceeds to cover the forearm and

the elbow area (depending on the size of the extremity). Typically, the bandages are applied with ~ 30 to 40% stretch and 50 to 70% overlap in a circular manner. While bandaging the forearm, the patient should make a fist and push the arm against the therapist's abdominal area (▶ Fig. 5.101). This technique provides for a functional bandage on the forearm and prevents tourniquet effects during the use of the forearm musculature while wearing the bandage. The next two bandages (either two 10 cm or one 10 cm and one 12 cm) are applied in opposite directions to each other. To provide a smooth gradient from distal to proximal, the individual bandages are started in areas of soft pressure (▶ Fig. 5.102). The therapist continues to check the gradient of the compression bandage during the entire process of application. Feedback from the patient is necessary and helpful. It is important that the bandage ends in the axillary fold to prevent accumulation of fluid between the armpit and the proximal end of the bandage (▶ Fig. 5.103). Compression bandages are secured with tape, and the proximal overlap of the stockinette is folded over the external bandage.

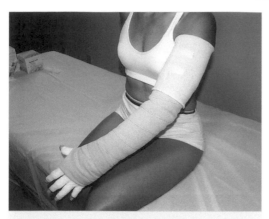

Fig. 5.103 Complete bandage on the upper extremity.

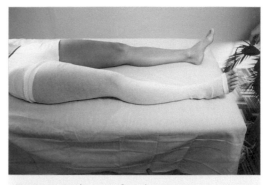

Fig. 5.104 Application of stockinette.

5.11.5 Lower Extremity Bandaging

The following is a list of recommended materials for applying a compression bandage on the lower extremity during the decongestive phase of CDT (phase 1). The quantities listed represent two sets of compression bandages:

- One bottle of skin lotion.
- One box of stockinette (tubular bandage) in the appropriate size.
- One to two boxes of gauze bandages (4 cm width).
- Two high-density foam pieces (kidney shape).
- Six synthetic nonwoven padding bandages (10 cm) or two to three Rosidal Soft foam bandages (10 cm).
- Four to six synthetic nonwoven padding bandages (15 cm) or two to three Rosidal Soft foam bandages (15 cm).
- Two short-stretch bandages (6 cm).
- Two short-stretch bandages (8 cm).
- Six to eight short-stretch bandages (10 cm).
- Eight to 12 short-stretch bandages (12 cm).
- Four wide-width short-stretch bandages (15 or 20 cm, depending on the patient's size).
- Tape to secure the bandages.
- If necessary, one sheet of soft foam ~3 feet × 6 feet (~12 mm thickness).
- If necessary, two sheets of Komprex or two rolls of soft foam rubber.

Application

Generally, bandages are applied with an even pre-stretch of ~ 30 to 40% and an overlap of ~ 50 to 70%. To bandage the foot and the lower leg, the patient should be in the supine position and should stand on the floor during the application of the compression bandages from the knee up to the groin.

Skin Care

Wash and bathe the skin, then apply the appropriate lotion thoroughly.

Stockinette

The tubular bandage should be cut to a length that allows for an overlap of ~ 12 cm on the proximal end of the extremity. This overlap is used to extend over and cover the complete compression bandage on the proximal border (▶ Fig. 5.104).

Toe Bandages

Start the first gauze bandage with a loose anchor turn around the dorsum of the foot (in the MTP joint area), then proceed to bandage the big toe (▶ Fig. 5.105). Enter the toe over the dorsum, apply two or three circular turns, and leave the toe again over the dorsum; avoid sliding or rolling of the bandages in the web space area. The tips of the toes remain unbandaged. Proceed to bandage the remaining toes (except the fifth toe, which generally is not involved in the swelling) in the same manner (▶ Fig. 5.106). One 4-cm gauze bandage (usually folded to half width) is generally sufficient to cover the toes. Any unused part of the gauze bandage should be wrapped spirally (not circularly) around the foot. Upon completion, the tips of the toes should be checked for proper circulation.

Padding Materials

Nonwoven synthetic padding (three rolls) or soft foam rolls (two rolls of Rosidal Soft) are applied on

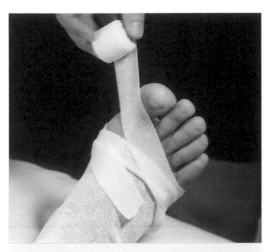

Fig. 5.105 Gauze bandages start with a loose anchoring turn around the dorsum of the foot.

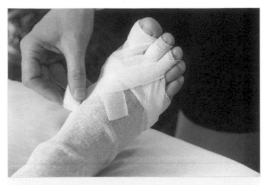

Fig. 5.106 Application of gauze bandages on the toes.

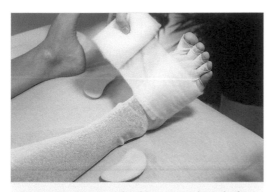

Fig. 5.107 Application of padding materials on the foot.

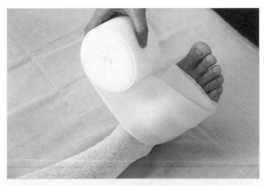

Fig. 5.108 Application of padding materials (soft foam roll) on the foot.

the foot and lower leg (▶ Fig. 5.107; ▶ Fig. 5.108). Komprex foam kidneys are secured between the medial and lateral malleolus and the Achilles tendon with the padding bandages (▶ Fig. 5.109). Synthetic padding bandages may be doubled over the shin area to provide additional protection.

Short-Stretch Bandages

Using a 6- or 8-cm-wide bandage (depending on the size of the foot), do a loose anchor turn around the metatarsus (▶ Fig. 5.110). The foot is bandaged down to the web spaces with three or four circular turns in the MTP joint area. The bandage should roll from lateral to medial (toward the big toe) and is applied without tension on the foot. The same bandage proceeds to cover the heel, using the "heel lock" technique, which provides additional support for the ankle and keeps the bandage from sliding (▶ Fig. 5.111; ▶ Fig. 5.112). During the application of compression bandages on the heel, the ankle is in ~ 70 to 90 degrees of dorsiflexion.

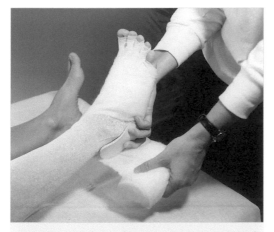

Fig. 5.109 High-density foam (Komprex) pieces behind the ankles are held in place by padding bandages.

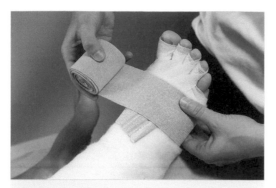

Fig. 5.110 Loose anchor turn around the metatarsus with the first short-stretch bandage.

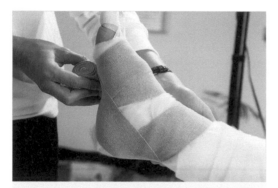

Fig. 5.112 "Heel lock" technique around the medial ankle.

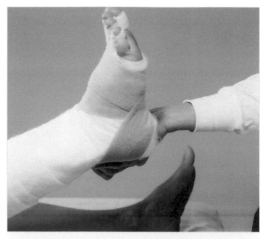

Fig. 5.111 "Heel lock" technique around the lateral ankle.

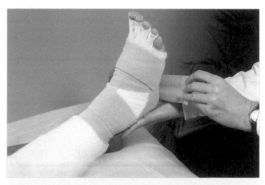

Fig. 5.113 Complete application of the first short-stretch bandage on the foot.

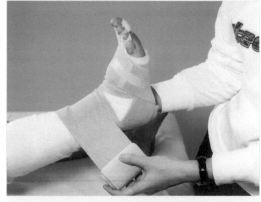

Fig. 5.114 Start of the second short-stretch bandage with a loose anchor around the ankle.

The bandage is guided from the plantar surface toward the Achilles tendon, covering the area between the heel and the lateral malleolus, from here around the ankle to the area between the medial malleolus and the heel, and again down to the plantar surface of the foot (▶ Fig. 5.113). Proceed with a circular turn without tension around the foot, and repeat the heel lock technique until the bandage is used up; secure with tape. The next bandage (8 or 10 cm) starts above the ankle with a loose anchor in the opposite direction to the previous bandage (applying compression bandages in the opposite direction to each other prevents bandaging the foot in eversion or inversion; i.e., it provides for a functional bandage and adds durability). The goal is to cover the heel and the foot with the second bandage in a circular technique (▶ Fig. 5.114; ▶ Fig. 5.115). The lower leg is bandaged with 10- or 12-cm-wide bandages (typically two to four rolls). To provide a smooth gradient from distal to proximal, the individual bandages are started in areas of soft pressure

5

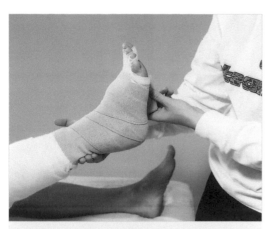

Fig. 5.115 The heel and foot are covered with the second short-stretch bandage.

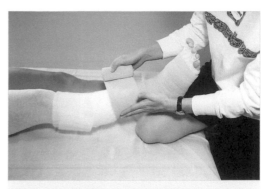

Fig. 5.116 Bandaging of the lower leg.

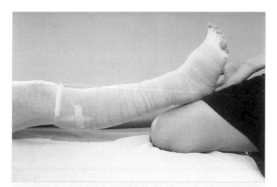

Fig. 5.117 Finished bandage on the lower leg and foot.

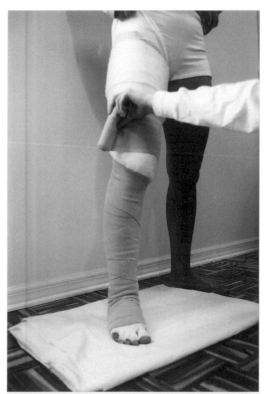

Fig. 5.118 Application of short-stretch bandages on the knee using the figure-eight technique.

(▶ Fig. 5.116). The therapist continues to check the gradient of the compression bandage during the entire process of application. Feedback from the patient is necessary and helpful. Secure the last bandage on the lower leg with tape (▶ Fig. 5.117).

The remaining compression bandage is applied with the patient in a standing position. The patient should shift the body weight to the extremity being bandaged, with the knee slightly bent. Padding materials using nonwoven synthetic padding or soft foam rolls are applied on the knee and thigh. When using synthetic padding bandages, the layers may be doubled in the popliteal fossa to provide additional protection. The knee and thigh should be bandaged using 12-cm-wide short-stretch bandages (typically four to six rolls). The first bandage starts with a loose anchor turn below the knee, proceeding to cover the knee using the figure-eight technique (▶ Fig. 5.118; ▶ Fig. 5.119).

The remaining thigh is bandaged in a circular manner up to the groin area; the last bandage (or each individual bandage) is secured with tape (▶ Fig. 5.120). An additional 15- or 20-cm-wide medium-stretch bandage may be applied on the thigh to add stability.

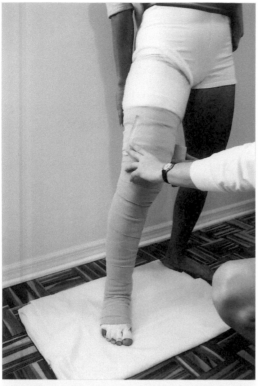

Fig. 5.119 Application of short-stretch bandages on the thigh starting with a loose anchor turn.

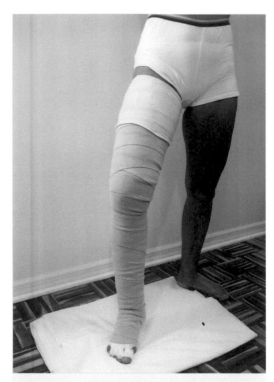

Fig. 5.120 Finished bandage on the lower extremity.

Hip Attachments

If the lower truncal quadrants are involved in the swelling, or to prevent the compression bandages on the leg from sliding, the hip may be bandaged using one or two rolls (depending on the size of the patient) of 20-cm-wide short-stretch bandages. (*Note:* hip attachments are applied directly on the skin; the patient wears the underwear on top of the bandages.) Start the first bandage with a loose turn around the proximal thigh to secure (▶ Fig. 5.121), then proceed to cover the trunk, guiding the bandage from the lateral thigh to the opposite iliac crest (to prevent sliding, at least one-third of the width of the bandage should be cranial to the iliac crest). From here, apply a complete circular turn around the trunk, and proceed with the bandage over the buttocks back down to the thigh (▶ Fig. 5.122). Proceed with the same technique until the lower trunk is thoroughly covered. Circular turns on the proximal thigh should be avoided to prevent tourniquet effects. Upon completion, the bandage is checked again for correct pressure gradient. If two rolls of bandages are needed for

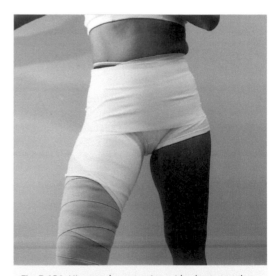

Fig. 5.121 Hip attachment using wide short-stretch bandages (15–20 cm).

the hip attachment, the ends may be sewn together to simplify the application.

5

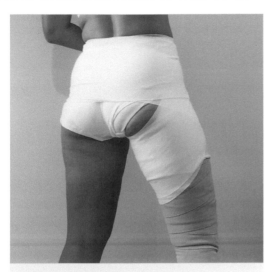

Fig. 5.122 Hip attachment, posterior view.

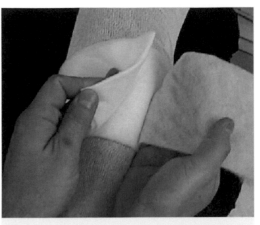

Fig. 5.123 Application of synthetic cotton to the elbow.

5

5.12 Bandaging Procedures Using Foam Padding

5.12.1 Arm Bandaging Procedure Using Foam Padding (in Detail)

In this bandage procedure, synthetic cotton (Artiflex or Cellona) will be used at the elbow and wrist/hand areas only. Foam padding will be used as a general replacement for synthetic cotton on all other limb areas. See ▶ Table 5.2 for a summary of steps and materials for arm bandaging using foam padding.

Stockinette and Synthetic Cotton

Following application of the stockinette, select the appropriate size of synthetic cotton padding and apply a generous layer at the elbow folding it into extra layers (▶ Fig. 5.123).

To increase the level of protection at the cubital crease, double the Artiflex or Cellona into multiple-ply coverage.

Tip: 10 cm width is usually the most appropriate size for most arms.

Fix Foam Padding into Position

Next affix the foam padding templates using a 15-cm Isoband or Idealbinde fixing bandage. In these

Table 5.2 Steps and materials for arm bandaging using foam padding

Step	Material
Lotion	Eucerin or other low-pH lotion
Stockinette	TG or Tricofix
Cotton (elbow, hand, or wrist)	Artiflex, Cellona, or other
Bandage for affixing foam (forearm or upper arm)	Isoband, Idealbinde, or other
Finger bandage	Transelast or Elastomull
Foam (dorsal hand)	Gray ¼ inch or 12-mm foam or Komprex
Bandage for affixing foam (dorsal hand)	6-cm bandage
Short stretch (hand wrap)	6-cm Comprilan or Rosidal K
Short stretch (forearm or elbow wrap)	8-cm Comprilan or Rosidal K
Short stretch (wrist to top of arm no. 1 and no. 2)	10-cm Comprilan or Rosidal K
Short stretch (as necessary)	10- or 12-cm Comprilan or Rosidal K

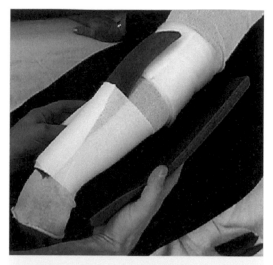

Fig. 5.124 Application of foam padding with a short-stretch fixing bandage.

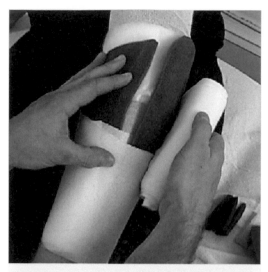

Fig. 5.125 Securing the forearm.

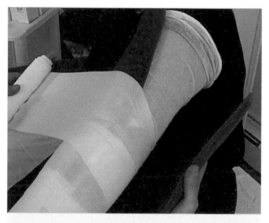

Fig. 5.126 Securing the first upper arm.

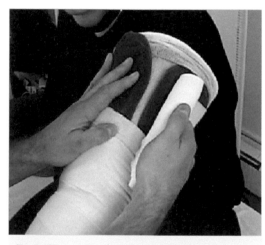

Fig. 5.127 Securing the second upper arm.

pictures, a thicker foam pad (12-mm gray foam) is being applied in two separate pieces (▶ Fig. 5.124; ▶ Fig. 5.125).

Tip: This fixing bandage is a structural and compressive layer. Apply moderate tension and attempt to cover all areas of foam with wide spacing and even distribution. Smooth and mold the foam to create a firmly anchored padding layer. Once the Isoband or Idealbinde is in place, apply tape to fasten.

Keep the patient's arm in a straight and outstretched position so that the foam padding will remain undisturbed. This will result in a firm

elbow joint, which is prone to loosen prematurely (▶ Fig. 5.126; ▶ Fig. 5.127).

Apply Compressive Finger Bandage

Apply a pre-folded finger bandage (Elastomull or Transelast Classic) by lightly anchoring at the crease of the wrist proximal hand area. This anchor may be over the foam or just distal to the foam at the base of the hand.

Tip: Stand facing the seated patient. Have his or her arm outstretched and supported by a bolster at the elbow. Position the hand with the palm

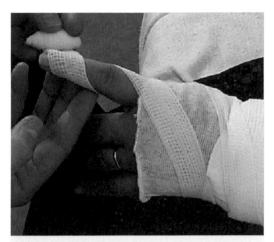

Fig. 5.128 Application of a compressive finger bandage.

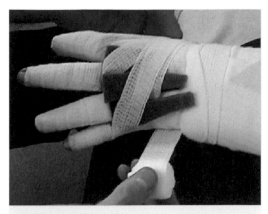

Fig. 5.129 Application of foam on fingers and intercarpal spaces.

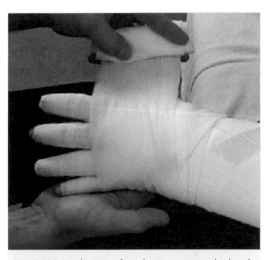

Fig. 5.130 Application of synthetic cotton to the hand.

facing downward; fingers should be straight and spread.

Choose a Direction and First Finger

Continue by selecting a direction. If proceeding in an ulnar-to-radial arm direction, wrap the thumb first followed by the index finger. Guide the bandage toward the lateral margins of each finger, spiral toward the nail bed then back to the base with even overlaps and tension (▶ Fig. 5.128).

Tip: There is no correct direction when starting; however, if choosing the opposite direction (radial to ulnar), begin by wrapping the little finger followed by the ring finger. This will create a consistent geometric pattern for learning the procedure and memorizing the final look and coverage of the bandage.

Lock Finger Foam Padding in Place

In this example, pieces of foam have been incorporated into the finger turns and are also placed in the dorsal intercarpal spaces (▶ Fig. 5.129). These foam additions do not change the pattern that is followed and add to the therapeutic effect by displacing fluid and reshaping swollen tissues.

Apply Synthetic Cotton to the Hand or Wrist

This layer is not a compression bandage and thus should be applied lightly and with even overall distribution. At the knuckle area do not cover the extended fingers. Use the knuckles as a distal most landmark (▶ Fig. 5.130).

Tip: The knuckles represent the starting point for the dorsum pad and compression layers. If the fingers are covered with synthetic cotton, foam padding and compression layers will also be started too low and create interdigital pressure areas. Open the hand wide, spreading the fingers to clearly visualize the knuckles.

Anchor 6-cm Short-Stretch Bandage to the Wrist

Lightly anchor the first short-stretch compression bandage to the wrist and immediately fix foam padding against the palm and dorsum.

5

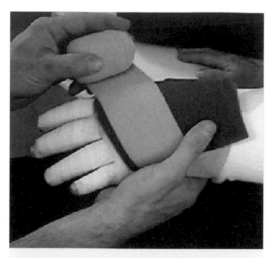

Fig. 5.131 Application of a foam pad to the dorsum with a 6-cm short-stretch bandage.

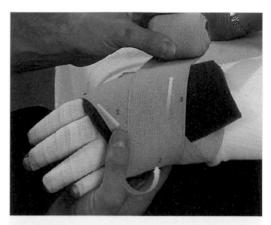

Fig. 5.132 Covering the dorsal hand. 1. Follow metacarpophalangeal joints; 2. Cross palm; 3. Cross dorsum behind thumb.

Position and Anchor the Pads

Secure the pads by positioning both at the edge of the metacarpophalangeal (MP) joints, which are aligned with the synthetic cotton. Continue to pack and mold this pad while proceeding through the pattern of turns (▶ Fig. 5.131).

Tip: This will be a bulky application. It therefore requires continual, gentle molding and packing to draw the air out of the foam and position the pads firmly in place.

Cover the Dorsal Hand with a Standard Pattern

The first compressive turn (after the anchor) involves another turn directly over the MPs, in front of the thumb. Next, proceed under the palm to the lateral hand then cross the dorsum on an angle toward the area behind the thumb near the wrist (▶ Fig. 5.132).

Continue Over the MP Joints

Next proceed under the palm to the lateral hand, then traverse the dorsum again toward the MP joints twice (▶ Fig. 5.133).

The Triangle

After the first of these two turns, notice a small, narrow triangle over the MP joints that is not covered. Cover the triangle each time it appears staying in front of the thumb, allocating structure and

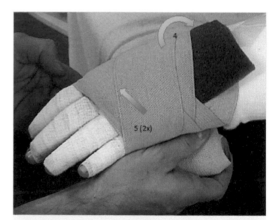

Fig. 5.133 Covering the dorsal hand. 4. Cross palm to lateral hand; 5. Cross metacarpophalangeal joints creating triangle pattern.

working pressure where it is most needed (▶ Fig. 5.134). Secure the tape at the bandage ends (▶ Fig. 5.135).

This alternating pattern "in front of and behind the thumb" creates the triangle and then covers it up. In doing so, extra structure and pressure is localized over the MP joints.

Palpate the Resulting Bandage

Once the hand bandaging is nearly completed and the firmness and layering are sufficient, proceed to run the remaining bandage out onto the forearm.

Tip: Palpation is the key to creating a correct result. Bandage turns alone do not make a firm

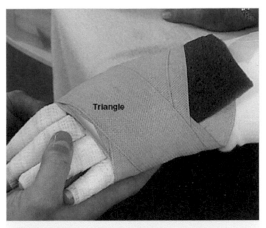

Fig. 5.134 Second pass covering the triangle.

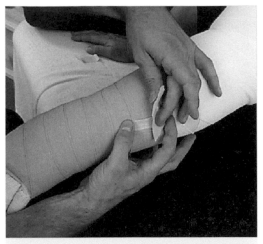

Fig. 5.135 Application of tape at the bandage ends.

5

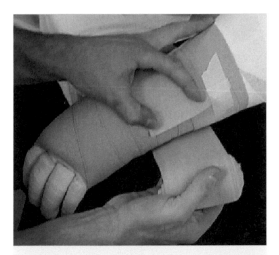

Fig. 5.136 Securing an 8-cm short-stretch bandage at the wrist.

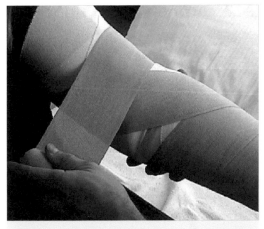

Fig. 5.137 Spiraling a bandage to the elbow, crossing at an angle to the cubital crease.

bandage. Always educate your hands by assessing the result before moving forward. The hand is now completed. There is rarely a reason to apply more than one 6-cm bandage on the hand. We have selected a narrow bandage (6 cm) to accommodate the size of the hand and localize the bandage pressure. Use the entire bandage if necessary.

Anchor an 8-cm Short-Stretch Bandage at the Wrist

Start an 8-cm bandage near to the flexion crease of the wrist. Avoid covering the thenar aspect of the hand. Reinforce the wrist twice before continuing upward. Spiral with even spacing (~ 50% overlap) and even tension toward the elbow (▶ Fig. 5.136).

Crisscross at the Cubital Fossa

To avoid having the bandage fall into the cubital crease (parallel to the crease) the first time, it is covered, traverse at a steep angle (▶ Fig. 5.137). Maintain tension and encircle the upper arm completely (▶ Fig. 5.138). Direct the bandage downward on an opposing angle toward the forearm and traverse the cubital crease creating an X

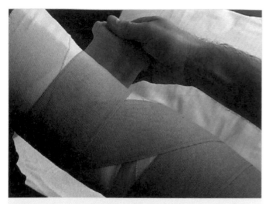

Fig. 5.138 Anchoring around the upper arm.

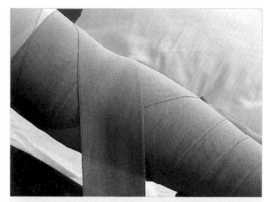

Fig. 5.139 Creating an X over the cubital crease.

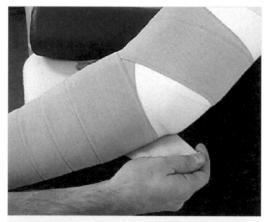

Fig. 5.140 Finishing a 8-cm short-stretch bandage covering the elbow.

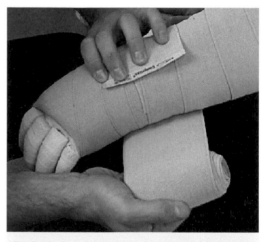

Fig. 5.141 Securing a 10-cm short-stretch bandage at the wrist, spiraling to the top of the arm.

(▶ Fig. 5.139). Proceed to cover the olecranon with the remainder of the bandage evenly spaced upward, turns perpendicular to the axis (▶ Fig. 5.140). Do not repeat the X a second time.

Anchor a 10-cm Short-Stretch Bandage at the Wrist

At the wrist and above the thenar aspect of the hand, encircle more than once to establish compression before migrating upward (▶ Fig. 5.141).

Tip: If the anchor is not firm, the result will be bandage coverage but without compression resulting in a loose wrist.

Proceed proximally with even spacing (50%) and even tension toward the axilla. Finish the bandage at the top of the arm and proceed to apply a second 10-cm bandage.

Anchor a Second 10-cm Bandage

Apply a second 10-cm bandage at the area of the wrist as with the first. Encircle more than once if necessary to establish compression. The second or even third 10-cm bandage may be applied in a herringbone pattern.

Tip: If the wrist feels finished, start the bandage a short distance proximal to avoid excessive compression.

Herringbone Technique

If another 10-cm bandage is necessary, anchor at the wrist but begin to alternate the angle at a tangent to the limb axis. This will result in a pattern with intersecting points occurring in a line toward the axilla. The herringbone technique avoids "bands" of pressure and "accordion" type slippage

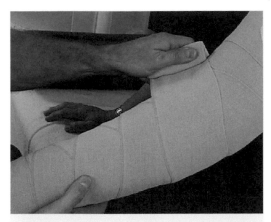

Fig. 5.142 Application of a second 10-cm bandage at the wrist with herringbone pattern to the top of the arm.

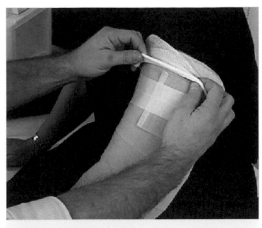

Fig. 5.143 Application of tape to secure roll-down tubular gauze stockinette.

5

as the limb decongests and the bandage relaxes (► Fig. 5.142).

Tip: By including the herringbone technique, a more structural result is possible creating adherence and stiffness. This technique consumes the bandage more quickly and thus covers less distance.

Fold Stockinette

Fasten the bandage at the top of the arm. Gently pull the extra tubular gauze stockinette out of the top of the bandage and fold over to create a finished bandage. This step avoids losing the stockinette end, which may create irritation or be rolled like a cord within (► Fig. 5.143).

Compression Bandaging for the Paralyzed Limb

Limb paralysis and lymphedema sometimes coexist. Prior to the development of modern radiotherapy techniques, breast cancer treatment risked significant brachial plexus injury as well as regional lymphatic disruption. Fortunately, the incidence of limb paralysis has dropped precipitously with the advancement in technique. However, survivors of antiquated methods still populate lymphedema clinics.

Regardless of cause, limb paralysis independent of lymphadenectomy and/or radiation therapy is subject to dependency, venous hypertension (dependent edema), and infection, which secondarily erodes the healthy function of lymph vessels and results in venous and lymphatic (combined)

insufficiency. In time, combined insufficiency (high water and protein loads) will result in characteristic tissue changes and immune dysfunction associated with pure lymphedema.

Lymphedema with limb paralysis is considered appropriate for CDT, but as it relates to administration of compression modalities (both elastic and nonelastic) all precautions should be taken.

Precautions and Contraindications

Areas of caution and special consideration include the following:

- The inability to integrate feedback from the patient's experience of compression (lack of sensation).
- Extreme fragility of thinning, atrophic skin with loss of hydration.
- Increased prominence of bony and tendinous landmarks.
- Atypical swelling patterns. Atrophic skin may permit swelling in the palm, plantar surfaces, and digital pads. The web spaces may migrate forward, and degloving is possible.
- Joint laxity and atrophy of the ligaments allows bones to reposition when compressed (especially in the feet), and gravity-induced subluxation of proximal joints such as the shoulder and hip can occur.
- Effect of diminished muscle and joint pump mechanism for return of venous blood and to facilitate lymph drainage.
- Heightened injury risk for bones and nerve structures during the intensive phase of CDT.

Absolute contraindications include the following:
- Forced compliance with rigorous exercise programs.
- Forced range of motion in areas of contracture, subluxation, or radiation damage.
- Application of high pressure bandages or strong elastic garments.
- Self-donning and removal of compression bandaging and garments.
- Strong manipulations during MLD (edema techniques or fibrous tissue techniques).
- Manipulation of radiation fibrosis.
- Improper bolstering during therapy (limbs must be secure in position).
- Excessive added weight from large, bulky bandage materials.

Principles

As many concerns are centered around the application of compression, to mitigate adverse consequences therapists must consider the impact of physical forces, such as by LaPlace's law and the dynamics of working pressure and resting pressure.

Less Is More

The goal of each bandage is to decongest the limb without further injury to the involved tissues, nerves, underlying skeletal structures, and joints. Therefore, as a rule observe the principle of "less is more." Even with functional limbs, therapists are well served by erring on the side of less aggressive pressure; however, in cases of flaccid paralysis, this guiding principle is an imperative. Assess the result of a light, thoughtfully padded compression bandage, and then adapt accordingly. If light compression achieves a controlled gradient flow and a reduction in volume, there is no need to increase pressure or intensity.

Use High Working Pressure, Low Resting Pressure

Based on empirical observation, combined insufficiencies (high water and high protein loads) are very responsive to compression. Without the muscle pump function, these deeply pitting edemas (indicating less lymphostatic fibrosis in the early stages) require the structural containment of a high working pressure multilayered bandage to offset gravity and the force of these high water loads. Structure halts swelling progression; slowly

returns water to the venous limb for reabsorption; and, with a well-crafted gradient, progressively confines the limb to a decongested state promoting lymph flow to the trunk.

Conversely, high resting pressures constrict and localize pressures on prominent tendons and bones. Depending on the degree of soft-tissue atrophy, prominent areas become even more pronounced with surrounding edema reduction, and without sensory feedback directing modifications in the bandage procedure, slight constriction or locally elevated pressure can cause significant tissue damage and ulceration.

LaPlace's Law

Atrophic hands are highly susceptible to injury from compression and thus require careful analysis of the cross-sectional shape (oval). Even the severely swollen hand remains oval and thus has smaller radii on the radial and ulnar aspect while maintaining larger radii on the dorsal and palmar surfaces. Functional hands, although also oval in cross-section, will elicit pain or discomfort signals to redirect compression for modification from excessive intercarpal pressure. The insensate limb has no such feedback mechanism.

The partial solution is to use bulky dorsal and palmar pads sized to the full width of the hand to allow the short-stretch bandage to generate a "downward press effect" while minimizing contact with the sides (intercarpal pressure).

The following procedure has been developed for lymphedema with flaccid paralysis of the arm, but the principles and elements may prove helpful to any patient not tolerating intensive compression bandaging. The components can be easily applied to the lower limb with slight modifications based on the same core principles.

Careful Surveillance

As a final consideration and safeguard against avoidable injury, plan to see this patient type on the first day (or consecutive days) of the intensive phase both in the morning and afternoon. This careful surveillance allows for inspection and assessment of the compression strategy and makes preemptive modifications possible early on. It should be noted that slight erythema over prominent landmarks (hot spots) may develop into open lesions without an immediate bandage modification.

5

5

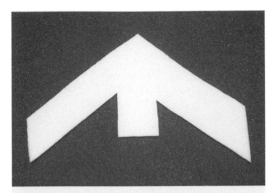

Fig. 5.144 "Arrow"-shaped synthetic finger padding.

Bandaging Procedure

1. *Apply lotion:* Generously apply lotion to the entire limb avoiding unnecessary accumulation of moisture. Allow a moment for evaporation if necessary. Maceration should not be permitted on any bandaged limb.
2. *Create finger protection:* Using synthetic cotton or foam (Rosidal Soft as shown), fabricate finger protection. These pieces are shaped like an arrowhead and effectively wrap around each finger with an extension for the crease. This piece serves to protect the interdigital spaces and flexion crease on the palmar aspect of each finger (▶ Fig. 5.144; ▶ Fig. 5.145; ▶ Fig. 5.146).
3. *Reverse steps; apply cotton to the hand first:* Typically, the stockinette application follows the application of lotion; however, in keeping with concerns related to skin injury, these steps are reversed. Using synthetic cotton, wrap the hand and wrist lightly from the MTP joints to the distal flexion crease of the wrist omitting the thumb hole. By applying synthetic cotton first, the web space of the thumb is protected from the edge of the stockinette, which has a hole cut for the thumb. Even in functional limbs, this hole can be either too small or get drawn back into the web space with high force. In addition, any rolling of extra stockinette at the MTP joints (causing pressure marks) is offset by cotton protection.
4. *Apply cotton/foam to the fingers and fix into place:* With the arm completely supported by the treatment plinth, position each fabricated finger piece into place and fix with one turn of a standard finger bandage. This finger bandage lightly holds these pieces and prevents them from shifting following the standard finger

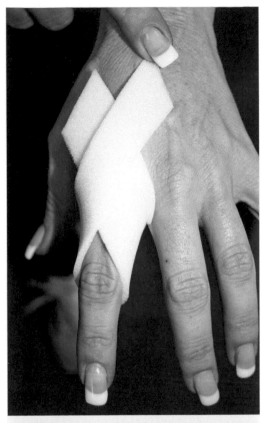

Fig. 5.145 "Arrow" applied to the finger; dorsal view.

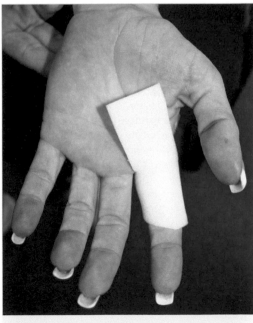

Fig. 5.146 "Arrow" applied to the finger; palmar view with "tab extension."

425

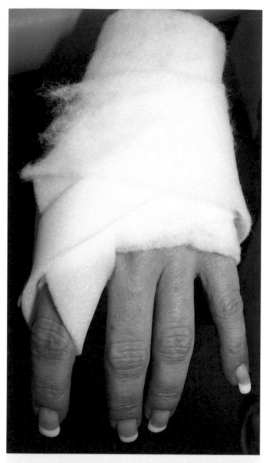

Fig. 5.147 Padding procedure 1. Apply cotton to the dorsum, then fix "arrow" to the index finger.

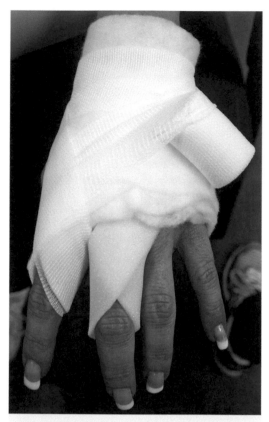

Fig. 5.148 Padding procedure 2. Fix the index finger with a finger bandage, one turn only.

wrapping pattern across the hand (▶ Fig. 5.147; ▶ Fig. 5.148; ▶ Fig. 5.149).

5. *Create compression on each finger:* Apply a standard finger bandage (two-ply, folded gauze) to each finger to create compression (▶ Fig. 5.150). If the fingers are very swollen, this bandage can be applied with moderate tension and close spacing, creating a thick uniform covering. Take a moment to inspect the base of the finger assessing that the tab of cotton protects each flexion crease (▶ Fig. 5.151). No rolling of the bandage edge can be tolerated here to ensure ongoing skin integrity. As the hand has full cotton coverage, the finger bandage, if meticulously applied, lays flat and is not able to cut at any aspect of the wrist where it anchors.

6. *Apply cotton at the elbow:* Stockinette is a simple open cotton weave and, with moisture, can be abrasive. To avoid direct contact with the cubital crease and prominent olecranon, first apply a layer of synthetic cotton. This may be as generous as required (or cover the entire arm) to provide adequate protection. Keep the cotton flat and smooth and use low tension.

7. *Apply the stockinette:* Select the appropriate size tubular gauze stockinette and cut a hole for the thumb. Pull the stockinette into place and notice that the thumb hole is buffered from direct contact with the web space by synthetic cotton (▶ Fig. 5.152). Take a moment to smooth the underlying cotton so that compression creates the least pressure marks.

8. *Position the arm foam:* Using a fixing bandage, secure the forearm and upper arm foam into position (▶ Fig. 5.153). As pressure will be very low, thin gray open cell foam (¼ inch/6 mm thickness) is a suitable starting point for providing necessary protection. Take care when handling the arm to support the elbow (from hyperextension) and the shoulder, which may already suffer subluxation.

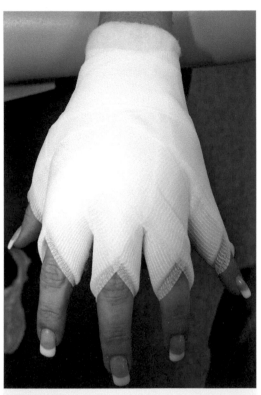

Fig. 5.149 Padding procedure 3. Repeat on all fingers.

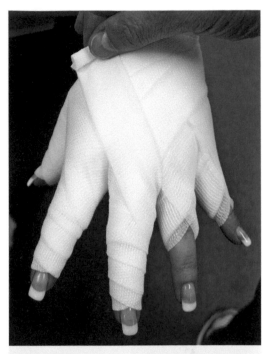

Fig. 5.150 Padding procedure 4. Apply a compressive finger bandage on top of padding.

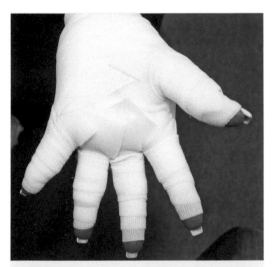

Fig. 5.151 Tabs protect flexion creases at the palm.

9. *Wrap the hand:* The standard pattern for wrapping a hand should be followed precisely (see Anchor 6-cm Short-Stretch Bandage to the Wrist). However, additional care should be taken at every step to avoid injury.

   a) Replace the typical foam padding with double-thickness padding on both the dorsal and palmar aspects. This may require two-ply ½-inch (12 mm) thick open cell gray foam or one piece of 1-inch (2.5 cm) thick open cell gray foam (▶ Fig. 5.154).

   b) Cut the foam to a dimension that is slightly wider than the hand with cotton padding in place. Bevel the edges, making certain they face away from the hand.

   c) While wrapping, gently press the hand flat against the plinth to broaden the hand with each turn. Tension the bandage across the palm and dorsum rather than downward on the sides to avoid pulling the hand into a cupped position. This molding step will draw the foam down and flatten and splint the hand wide.

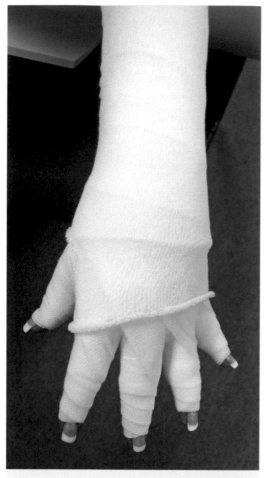

Fig. 5.152 Application of cotton to the arm length, then stockinette to the arm with a hole at the thumb.

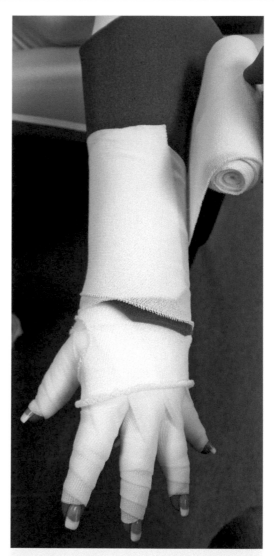

Fig. 5.153 Securing foam to the arm length with a short-stretch fixing bandage.

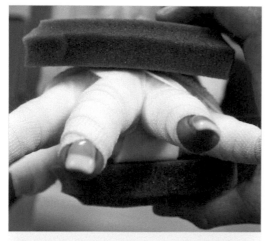

Fig. 5.154 Application of foam pads to the hand. The dimensions are wide and thick to protect radial and ulnar aspects of the hand.

These steps observe LaPlace's law, by shaping the hand from an oval to round (cross-section) while creating a steep "drop-off" at the lateral hand, which avoids contact with prominent bones and enhances the downward press effect.

1. Wrap the arm:
   a) Apply an 8-cm short-stretch bandage starting from the wrist (distal flexion crease) and proceed to the elbow with low tension and

even spacing. If the arm is to be positioned into a sling (recommended), stop this bandage before the cubital crease. If the arm will remain straight (although not generally recommended), proceed with the X pattern at the elbow. This step further protects the cubital crease regardless of position.

b) Apply a 10-cm short-stretch bandage from the wrist to the top of the arm with even spacing and low tension. If the arm is to be bent to accept a sling, bend it now to a 90-degree angle before crossing the elbow. Consider the apex of the olecranon to be a typical pressure point and assess whether additional padding is necessary such as a foam "donut"-shaped piece. Cross the cubital crease with light tension only.

c) If more pressure is desired, apply a second 10-cm short-stretch bandage in a similar fashion. Remember that low tension with multiple layers will not rest with high pressure but will create a high structural integrity. Observe the effect of each day's bandage to assess the need for further modifications.

5.12.2 Leg Bandaging Procedure Using Foam Padding (in Detail)

Before Applying Foam

Apply lotion to the limb and select a stockinette that is of a size appropriate for the calf. Allow a few centimeters of extra length so that it can be folded over the top of the calf bandage when finished. Next bandage the toes (a review of toe bandaging can be found in this section). Finally, apply synthetic cotton at the foot, ankle, and around the knee but not covering the calf because foam replaces cotton in most areas.

See ▶ Table 5.3 for a summary of steps and materials for leg bandaging using foam padding.

Dorsiflex the foot from the beginning of this procedure to simulate a functional position. This step will help with foam positioning, comfort, and function. Consider applying the bandage with the patient in the supine position to offset the effects of gravity on the swelling.

Table 5.3 Steps and materials for leg bandaging using foam padding

Step	Material
Lotion	Eucerin or other low-pH lotion
Stockinette (calf or thigh)	TG or Tricofix
Toe wraps	Transelast or Elastomull
Cotton (knee, ankle, or foot)	Artiflex, Cellona, or other
Bandage for affixing foam (calf or thigh)	Isoband, Idealbinde, or other
Foam (for dorsum)	Precut piece of gray Vi inch (12 mm) Komprex
Bandage for affixing foam (dorsum)	6-cm Comprilan or Rosidal K
Short stretch (Roman sandal)	6-cm Comprilan or Rosidal K
Short stretch (HAS)	8-cm Comprilan or Rosidal K
Short stretch (ankle to knee two times)	10-cm Comprilan or Rosidal K
Short stretch (knee to mid-thigh: no. 1, knee to top: no. 2, distal thigh to top: no. 3, ankle to top: no. 4, and additional short stretch (as necessary)	12-cm Comprilan or Rosidal K

Abbreviation: HAS, heel–ankle–sole.

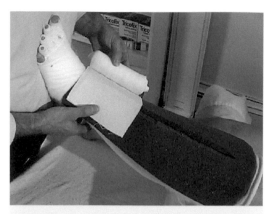

Fig. 5.155 Securing foam to the lower calf with a short-stretch fixing bandage.

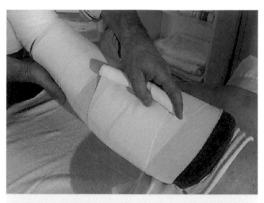

Fig. 5.156 Securing foam to the upper calf with a short-stretch fixing bandage.

Fix Foam in Place

Using a 15-cm-wide, white, short-stretch bandage, affix the anatomically crafted foam pieces into place with the beveled edges facing away from the skin (▶ Fig. 5.155). Anchor the anterior piece first with tension and then fix the posterior piece. Keep the bandage smooth and neat to avoid cutting into unprotected areas and cover all of the exposed foam.

Correct the Fit

The fixing bandage should act as a prewrap, drawing the foam pieces firmly against the limb, adding mild compression and a base of structure (▶ Fig. 5.156).

> The tibial relief is designed to relieve pressure on the prominent tibial bone; therefore, the "slot" must be centered, beveled, and positioned carefully to alleviate discomfort.

The Foot Portion

First Compression Bandage: The "Roman Sandal" Pattern

When working with foam padding, make sure that the calf pieces are already in place before beginning the foot bandage. This will ensure the ankle is already protected from the first two bandages. Next, anchor the 6-cm bandage to the edge of the MTP area without covering the toes, proceed twice to secure the gray foam in place (▶ Fig. 5.157).

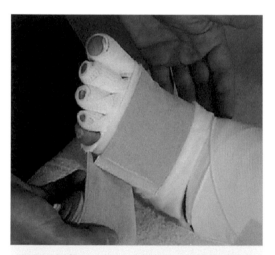

Fig. 5.157 The Roman sandal pattern. Anchor a 6-cm short-stretch bandage to the metatarsophalangeal region.

Continue to Anchor Additional Pads

If using a second dorsal pad (in this case, Komprex), place it into the bandage with the next turn so that it is adjacent to the first piece and is secured beneath the maximum number of layers (▶ Fig. 5.158). Notice that the padding is beveled and these edges face outward to minimize harsh impressions in the swollen tissues.

Place Ankle Pads Into "Roman Sandal"

Proceed directly from the base of the toes toward the heel crossing the malleolus either medially or laterally fixing one ankle pad in place (▶ Fig. 5.159). Keep the bandage low along the floor plane but above the curvature of the heel.

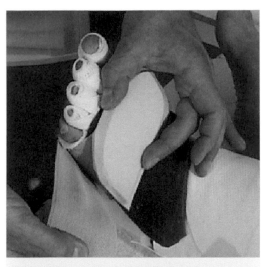

Fig. 5.158 The Roman sandal pattern continued. Secure the dorsal foam pads with the next turn.

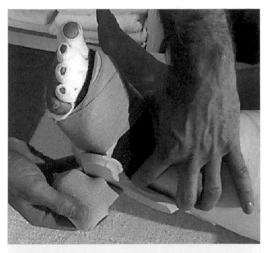

Fig. 5.159 The Roman sandal pattern continued. Secure the ankle pads.

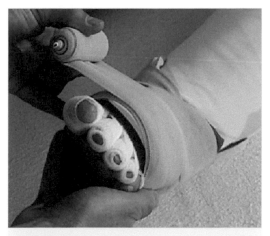

Fig. 5.160 The Roman sandal pattern continued. Cross the dorsum at the metatarsophalangeal joints.

Cross the Achilles tendon and immediately fix the second ankle pad in place. Again keep the bandage low to the floor, maintain tension, and mold the pads firmly against the bony structures.

The direction chosen toward medial or lateral ankle first is sometimes subject to the anatomy of the foot. Consider either direction to get the best finished bandage placement.

Repeat Crossing the MTP Joints

From the malleolar area, proceed directly to the MTPs and cover them at the edge of the foam padding. As with the hand bandage, you will see a triangular area of fabric. Proceed fully around the forefoot twice remembering to mold and pack the foam padding into position covering this triangle (▶ Fig. 5.160). Adjust the foam manually toward the edge of the MTPs, as it is likely to shift backward.

Repeat the Heel Anchor

Proceed from the toes toward the heel again, migrating slightly further away from the floor plane. Pack and mold the padding against the malleolus and continue out to the toes again. In most cases, the entire bandage can be used ending anywhere in the pattern (▶ Fig. 5.161).

Second Compression Bandage: The Heel–Ankle–Sole (HAS or ASH) Pattern

Start at the Ankle

The second bandage is used in a repeating pattern which may begin anywhere in the cycle. It is demonstrated here as starting at the ankle and leading to the sole, then heel (ASH). Anchor the 8-cm short-stretch bandage at the distal calf slightly above the ankle. This anchor can be wrapped twice around to give a firm base for this repeating pattern (▶ Fig. 5.162).

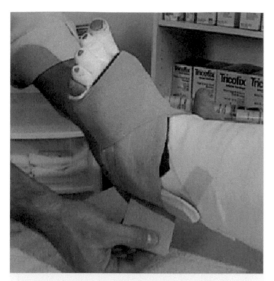

Fig. 5.161 The Roman sandal pattern continued. Graduate higher around the ankles with each pass.

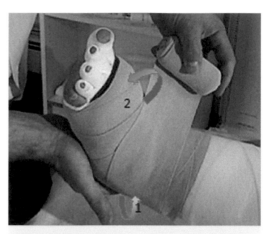

Fig. 5.162 Heel–ankle–sole pattern. Anchor an 8-cm short-stretch bandage at the ankle (1). Proceed to the sole crossing the dorsum (2).

Remember to dorsiflex the foot to simulate a functional standing position. This creates room for the tibialis anterior tendon to tense and relax. Maintain this position until the calf bandage is complete.

Locate the Underlying Bone Prominence

Use a finger to feel for the bony structures so as to locate the pad in the soft areas surrounding them. Remember these pads are meant to sculpt the limb to normalcy and avoid increased pressure on prominent structures.

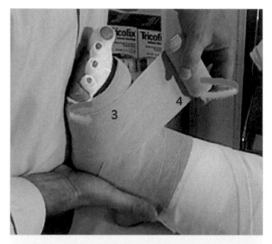

Fig. 5.163 Heel–ankle–sole pattern continued. Proceed from sole to heel crossing the dorsum (3, 4).

The dorsal foot also harbors the cuneiform bone, which in many cases is prominent in high-arched feet. Careful tensioning, foam crafting, and molding create a more tolerable, comfortable bandage.

Cover the Sole

Direct the bandage at a steep angle toward the sole to cover the arch. Apply tension to the sole and lateral foot, then lay the bandage with moderate tension across the tender tibialis anterior tendon (▶ Fig. 5.163).

Pressure quickly builds at the tender area of the tibialis anterior tendon. Take care to avoid applying tension until under the arch. This will lock the bandage materials together and avoid them shifting backward into the dorsal foot and tendon area.

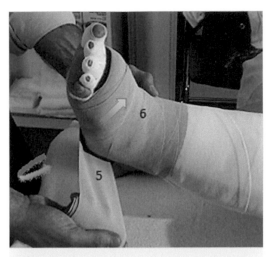

Fig. 5.164 Heel–ankle–sole pattern continued. Hook the bandage on the heel securely (5). Proceed around the ankle (6). Continue pattern as required.

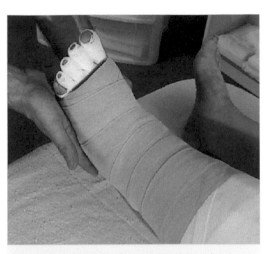

Fig. 5.165 Application of an additional 8-cm bandage to the distal calf.

5

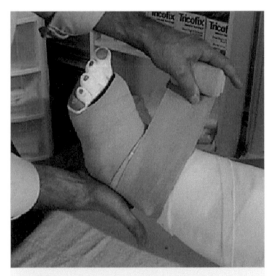

Fig. 5.166 Securing the first 10-cm short-stretch bandage to the distal flexion crease of the calf.

Cover the Heel

From the dorsum proceed directly to the heel. Cover the heel with centered distribution so that the bandage is well anchored and cannot slip off the apex of the heel (▶ Fig. 5.164). Proceed directly to the ankle again and repeat the sole, heel, ankle, and sole pattern until sufficient pressure and structure is achieved.

Finish the HAS Bandage

When the bandage looks and feels finished, run any excess bandage material out onto the calf with even spacing (50%) and apply tape.

> If the foot is small, do not apply the entire bandage or excessive pressure will develop. If the foot is quite large, a second 8-cm bandage, partially applied, may be necessary (▶ Fig. 5.165).

Calf Portion

Third Compression Bandage

Using a 10-cm short-stretch bandage, anchor at the distal calf twice to secure firmly (▶ Fig. 5.166).

> This bandage should not cover the foot because the Roman sandal (6 cm) and HAS pattern (8 cm) are properly sized to localize the pressure and make up sufficient layering. Keep this bandage oriented to the distal calf, but try to avoid excessive buildup over the tibialis anterior tendon. Maintain the foot in a dorsiflexed position.

433

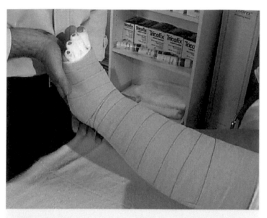

Fig. 5.167 Spiraling to the top of the calf. Application of the tape.

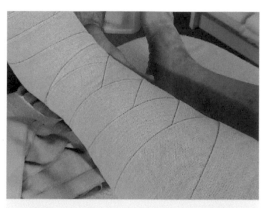

Fig. 5.168 Application of the second 10-cm short-stretch bandage with herringbone pattern to the full calf.

Complete the First Layer

Using even spacing (~ 50%) and moderate tension, spiral to the top of the calf and apply tape (▶ Fig. 5.167).

Use the popliteal crease as a landmark and avoid cutting into the area. The posterior foam piece ends here, protecting against direct contact with the skin. Although synthetic cotton is in place, it does not sufficiently protect the area from multiple layers.

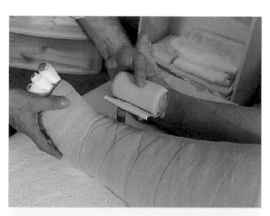

Fig. 5.169 Application, if required, of the third 10-cm short-stretch bandage in a spiral pattern.

Fourth Compression Bandage: The Second Layer

Starting again at the distal flexion crease between foot and calf, anchor a second 10-cm short-stretch bandage twice to firmly reinforce the compression before advancing upward (▶ Fig. 5.168). Produce a herringbone pattern with equal spacing and tension, noting an intersect point on the tibial aspect of the calf.

Herringbone Pattern

This pattern creates structure, decreases "banding" from multiple circumferential turns, and weaves the bandage producing noticeably increased structure.

Do not use the herringbone pattern exclusively because it results in a different allocation of bandage, which may be too dense. Notice how the herringbone pattern consumes the bandage in a shorter area of coverage; this method can be a challenge for spacing of turns.

Fifth Compression Bandage: Start the Third Layer

As with the first and second layers, anchor the third 10-cm bandage at the distal calf (▶ Fig. 5.169). Be mindful of excessive pressure buildup here and spiral with even spacing and tension to the top of the calf.

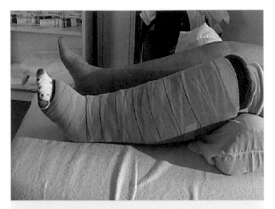

Fig. 5.170 A finished calf bandage.

In this example, we have blended spiral and herringbone patterns together to create turns that are perpendicular to the limb axis, and also at an angle to the axis.

Final Result

The finished calf bandage should look neat and smooth with even bandage allocation (▶ Fig. 5.170). Take a moment to palpate the end result feeling for gradient and structure.

This bandage may be adjoined to the thigh for a full leg application. If so, it will receive additional layering that extends from ankle to thigh. If this is the case, the current bandage should be at 75% of finished pressure, leaving room for finished pressure levels. It is most important to keep the foot dorsiflexed at all times, and palpate the result of each bandage applied.

Knee and Thigh Portion

It is generally helpful to position the patient in a standing position for the completion of the full leg bandage procedure. With weight in the leg and the knee either straight or slightly bent, apply the remaining layers. Having maintained proper positioning during foot and calf wrapping (dorsiflexion), the patient should now report being comfortable in the standing position.

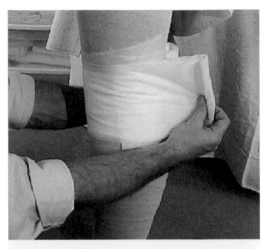

Fig. 5.171 A thigh bandage: Application of synthetic cotton to the knee.

Apply Stockinette to Thigh

With the patient in a standing position, cut a tubular gauze stockinette of appropriate size to fit the full length of the thigh. Allocate extra length to allow for coverage of the knee, overlapping the proximal calf, and for folding over the finished bandage at the top.

The fit of the stockinette should be snug to add grip for foam and external bandages to stay securely in place.

Apply Synthetic Cotton at Knee

Encircle the knee with 15-cm synthetic cotton, increasing the coverage behind the knee by folding the material into double-ply (▶ Fig. 5.171).

The popliteal crease is a common tender spot due to joint articulation, bent knee positioning, and prominent tendons. For this reason, extra care must be given to offset friction and cutting forces.

Affix the Foam Padding into Position

Position the anterior foam pad and encircle the knee with a 15-cm fixing bandage locking it into

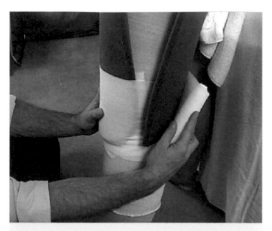

Fig. 5.172 Securing foam to the thigh with a short-stretch fixing bandage.

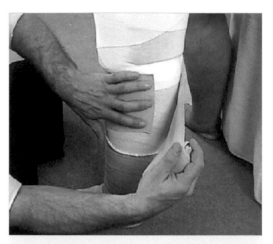

Fig. 5.173 Application of the first 12-cm short-stretch bandage below the knee.

place (▶ Fig. 5.172). Use moderate tension and mold the foam, keeping the bandage smooth, especially behind the knee. Immediately position the posterior thigh pad and encircle the thigh again, locking it in place.

Cover all of the Padding

The 15-cm fixing bandage is wide enough to cover the entire visible surface of padding. The goal is to create a basement layer of compression and structure while firmly fixing the padding into position. Once this is accomplished, the following layers will be better able to exert compression rather than continue to fix the padding. Additionally, where overlap exists (knee), this fixing layer molds and shapes away the excessive bulk.

The pads have been crafted of thicker foam and therefore require beveled edges to minimize pressure marks. Beveled edges must always face away from the skin for the safest result.

Maintain Proper Positioning

To accomplish a firm knee joint, keep the patient in a straight-legged position. Avoid "testing out" the bandage prior to finishing all layers.

For patients who are nonambulatory, a semibent or fully bent (90-degree) position is recommended. For the ambulatory patient, joint articulation will generally soften a firm bandage; therefore, a firm start is recommended.

First Compression Bandage: Apply the First Layer

Using a 12-cm short-stretch bandage, anchor below the knee on the proximal calf (▶ Fig. 5.173).

Angle Upward Behind the Knee

Immediately traverse the posterior knee at a steep angle toward the mid-thigh.

To illustrate, the picture shows a posterior view. This steep angle crossing the popliteal crease produces less "cutting force" increasing comfort. Anchoring at the mid-thigh versus the distal thigh ensures this angle, which is only necessary to complete once. All subsequent layers can traverse the crease at various angles.

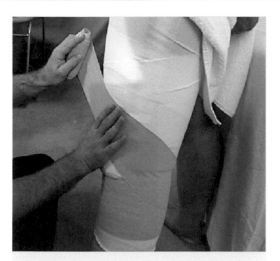

Fig. 5.174 Encircling the thigh. Anchor securely, proceed upward creating an angle across the popliteal crease (posterior view).

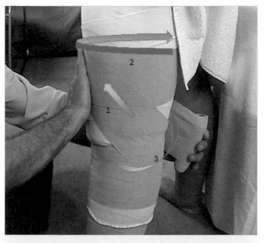

Fig. 5.175 Knee wrapping procedure: 1. Angle upward, 2. Secure around the thigh one full turn, 3. Angle downward completing the X over the popliteal crease.

Encircle the Thigh, Complete an X Behind the Knee

Maintaining moderate to firm tension and a straight, weight-bearing leg, encircle the mid-thigh (▶ Fig. 5.174).

The thigh must be fully encircled to "lock" the bandage anchor to the thigh. Immediately angle the bandage steeply downward toward the calf at an opposing angle, creating an X over the popliteal crease (▶ Fig. 5.175).

This X created two layers of insulation and lays at a tangent to the popliteal crease. This projects against the additional bandage layers that are oriented parallel to the crease by pushing outward.

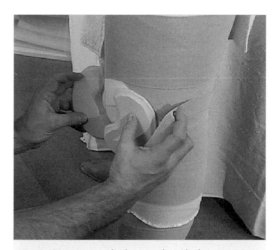

Fig. 5.176 Securing the knee pads with the remaining bandage (if required).

Incorporate Additional Knee Pads and Lock Pads Firmly into Position

Using the remainder of the 12-cm bandage, position additional pads into place and apply tape to hold the bandage end (▶ Fig. 5.176).

Knee pads are optional. The pads shown here are dense and may not be appropriate for all patients. Customization of padding is a major key to exceptional treatment outcomes.

Feel for the underlying bony structures while carefully positioning the pads as they are meant to distribute higher pressure, resculpting the limb to a natural contour.

Second Compression Bandage

Anchor the second 12-cm short-stretch bandage directly over the knee, taking time to pack and mold the bulky knee padding inward (▶ Fig. 5.177). Be careful to pull evenly and with care behind the knee. Keep the bandage smooth, laying neatly at all times. With even spacing (~50%) spiral to the top of

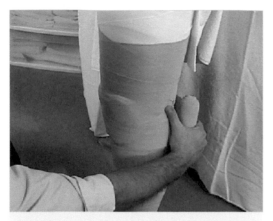

Fig. 5.177 Application of the second 12-cm short-stretch bandage starting over the knee.

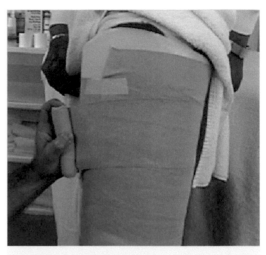

Fig. 5.178 Spiraling to the top.

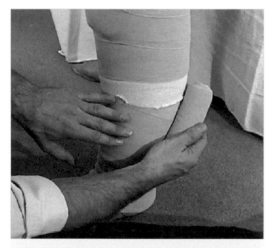

Fig. 5.179 Application of a third 12-cm short-stretch bandage starting at the ankle, spiraling to the top.

the thigh using the remaining bandage length. Apply tape to hold (▶ Fig. 5.178).

Third Compression Bandage

Anchor a third 12-cm bandage just above the knee and create a herringbone pattern toward the top of the thigh (▶ Fig. 5.179). The herringbone pattern consumes the bandage in a shorter area resulting in less coverage and denser buildup. Space the bandage more generously (25% overlap = 75% spacing) to avoid problems and do not use herringbone in two layers consecutively without practice.

Note: Large limb girth will consume the bandage very quickly; therefore, consider a double-length bandage on the largest limbs. Do not feel limited to three to four layers when bandaging. Mild to moderate tension with multiple layers creates a soft castlike bandage resulting in high "working pressure" and low "resting pressure."

Fourth Compression Bandage

Anchor a fourth 12-cm bandage at the distal calf reinforcing the calf bandage pressure if more is desired, integrating the lower and upper leg segments into a continuous gradient.

Remember that the calf segment did not receive finished pressure and can accept additional coverage. If the calf is too firmly wrapped, this coverage may be excessive and result in discomfort. Plan the bandage spacing so that it reaches the top of the thigh with a wide spiral.

This may necessitate very wide spacing without overlap. Remember, the outermost layers of a lymphedema bandage are meant to distribute pressure over wider surface areas; therefore, wider spacing is beneficial toward creating a gradient effect.

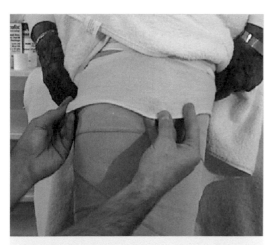

Fig. 5.180 Addition of a fourth (if required) 12-cm short-stretch bandage to the thigh with herringbone pattern. Fold over the stockinette.

Apply More Layers if Necessary

Palpate the bandage to decide if additional layering is required to achieve the desired level of pressure and structure. More layers are optional and can be incorporated if needed.

Check for Gradient

It is imperative that each finished bandage be thoroughly palpated to ensure that a therapeutic environment has been achieved. Palpate the full limb thoroughly and in its full dimensions to ascertain, structure, tension, smoothness, and completeness. These subtle factors can only be mastered with instructor evaluation and feedback followed by further practice.

Fold Over Extra Stockinette When Finished

When the bandage is complete and passes final inspection, pull the remaining stockinette upward to reduce slack. Fold the extra length over the top edge creating a finished product (▶ Fig. 5.180).

> It is important to budget extra stockinette length to avoid exposing the skin to the foam and to secure it from rolling down inside the bandage.

5.13 Genital Lymphedema Treatment

No complete and thoughtful discussion of lymphedema therapy should omit detailed guidelines for the treatment of genital swelling. Unfortunately, there are vast gaps in knowledge among the ranks of most certified therapists due to the personal and intimate nature of these necessary discussions. It has been the author's experience that although direct discussion may be unpleasant, patients are forever grateful that someone cared to open a dialogue and if necessary provide direct therapeutic adaptations of CDT to the involved regions.

5.13.1 Secondary Genital Lymphedema

Genital involvement often accompanies lower extremity lymphedema, although the rate of occurrence has not been well documented. This may be due to the fact that patients were 91% more likely to be identified with lymphedema when enrolled in studies using objective measurement methods rather than those comparing subjective assessments.[89] Understandably, due to the deeply personal nature of any revelations, genital lymphedema as a subset of the lower quadrant is not openly reported or offered up for discussion in most clinical evaluations unless pointedly addressed.

Following review of this detailed section, it may become apparent how important a thorough evaluation, inclusive of genital assessment, is (either via inspection or questioning) to the comprehensive treatment of the lower quadrants.

Considering the fact that lower quadrant melanoma, urogenital, and gynecological cancers are treated with inguino-femoral and/or iliac lymphadenectomy often followed by radiation therapy, drainage of the legs and external genitals are equally disrupted. It has been observed that lymphedema risk increases considerably for patients undergoing pelvic dissections (as compared with other procedures) and further increases with radiation therapy in all cancer groups. Observations regarding the effect of adjuvant radiation therapy have been thoroughly documented in multiple breast cancer–related lymphedema studies.[91]

Genital lymphedema is common in filariasis and is caused by parasitic obstruction and secondary injury of the inguinal lymphatics. As such, patient evaluation must always include considerations of geographic residence and/or travel destinations where filarial parasites remain rampant.

Recent onset (newly detected) genital lymphedema where historically the swelling has been limited to the legs must receive immediate physician referral to rule out lymphatic obstruction due to undiagnosed or recurrent disease. In all cases, genital lymphedema indicates a proximal lymphatic impairment of draining regional lymphatics and thus must elicit suspicion and investigation of underlying causes. Until an obstruction has been ruled out, the diagnosis of primary genital lymphedema would be premature.

5.13.2 Primary Genital Lymphedema

As with secondary genital lymphedema, primary incidence is difficult to assess. Estimates published by Kinmonth[92] in the 1980s and supported by others[91] fall within the range of 10% congenital, 37% praecox, and 33% tarda occurrences. Etiologies are cited to be any of three possible abnormalities: genetically determined aplasia or valvular incompetence, lymphatic obstruction of unknown cause, or lymph node fibrosis also without a determined cause. Primary genital lymphedema is uncommon in Milroy's disease (5%) and is more likely to appear in the teens and early 20s with a tendency toward affecting males. Considering that females are far more likely to develop primary lymphedema, it is suspected in cases of genital lymphedema that male anatomy with its dependent, highly extensible external tissues and narrowing toward the scrotal root creates an unfavorable challenge to drainage. In the majority of cases, primary genital involvement is accompanied by one or both legs, which precedes the development of genital lymphedema by several years.[93]

5.13.3 Predisposition to Develop Lymphedema

As the vast majority of genital lymphedema is due to a known cause typically related to cancer treatment, it is helpful for CLTs to analyze the cancer treatment history. Pathological reports and/or direct consultation with the surgeon and radiologist can expedite the formation of a clear plan of care devoted to constructing the most effective and efficient MLD procedure and compression strategy.

Superficial Lymphatic Disruption

Based on the training received in basic and advanced level lymphatic anatomy and physiology, lymphedema therapists can devise a thoughtful, logical, and defensible plan of care aimed at achieving more productive treatment outcomes. For example, disruption of the superficial inguinal nodes has no adverse effect on the deeper situated iliac and lumbar nodes or trunks. Furthermore, if the treatment procedure remains unilateral, the contralateral inguinal nodes will not become impaired. This overview lends itself to the realization that both the deep abdominal drainage pathways and superficial anastomotic collateral pathways to the contralateral inguinal nodes, and also the ipsilateral axilla, are viable treatment objectives and may prove to support a more favorable and predictable outcome.

Deep Lymphatic Disruption

Whenever surgery and/or radiation therapy involves the intrapelvic (iliac) or abdominal (lumbar) lymph nodes, all tributary regions drained by these structures (superficial nodes and lymph collectors) must be considered secondarily disrupted. In this scenario, it is common to mistake the otherwise "intact" inguinal nodes as viable limb and genital drainage pathways. However, with proximal disruption, these still "intact nodes" and vessels cannot drain efficiently to the deep system. Similarly, in cases where unilateral leg lymphedema had been caused by deep lymphatic disruption, the (as yet) spared contralateral limb remains at high risk of future involvement. Treatment should therefore always omit the nodes distal to a disruption to avoid reflux and potential strain on uninvolved at-risk territories.

Understanding the basics of surgical procedure, the diseased organ or structure removed, and its lymphatic drainage is essential to developing a safe and highly efficient plan of care. There are many instances of harmful or ineffective therapy causing unintended contralateral leg or genital swelling due to treatment plans that have neglected to conduct a thorough analysis of viable collateral drainage. In this regard, pneumatic compression devices disregard scientifically sound rationale, which is why they have been predictable triggers for the development of genital lymphedema in a multitude of leg patients.[1]

5.13.4 Complications

The most frequent unforeseen complications of genital involvement include changes to the skin. Although the formation of hyperkeratosis and papillomatosis is expected in advanced stage extremity lymphedema, genital skin is particularly susceptible to hypertrophic change. Depending on the extent of lymphatic disruption or structural malformation, reflux exploits the skin's extensibility and inherent thinness. Visible clear fluid-filled vessels (cysts) may be abundant and in some cases a white color may indicate chylous reflux. These blisterlike cysts (dilated lymphangions) rupture easily, leaking copious amounts of lymph. Owing to the mechanical challenge of ambulation, sitting and standing, clothing, moisture, and size of the edematous genitals, scrotal cysts are extremely vulnerable to injury.

With vast amounts of resident skin bacteria, the genital region lends itself to recurrent infections especially attributable to ruptured cysts. The presence of fragile cysts is the most common aggravating factor for recurrent erysipelas and cellulitis with lymphorrhea in the genital region. In one study, 85% of patients with genital lymphedema experienced one or more infections annually.[93] For this reason, the issues of hygiene, self-care compression, antibiotic administration, and even the patient's suitability for surgical intervention must be considered carefully. In cases of cutaneous fistula with chylous reflux, introduction of bacteria to the gastrointestinal region is a life-threatening concern, which may necessitate surgical intervention. Recurrent leakage creates malodorous and macerated skin which can be embarrassing, disabling for sexual function, and devastating to quality of life. In many patients, a quiet desperation for answers in the absence of responsible guidance leads to vulnerability to submit to radical and regrettable treatment interventions.

5.13.5 Surgical Treatment

The rationale for surgical excision procedures (including amputation) on limbs has been to remove nonhealing lesions, infection prone tissues, gross enlargement, or to address the threat of mortality in patients who have already experienced sepsis. In most instances, CDT replaces these radical procedures, which involve considerable comorbidity, sparing limbs from disfigurement or even subsequent amputation caused by poor wound closure.

In contrast, with regard to genital lymphedema, surgical procedures have proven of great benefit when there is a history of recurrent infection associated with leakage impacting quality of life. In cases where the external genitalia are markedly disfigured, rendering sexual interaction painful or impossible to perform, surgery may also warrant consideration. Recurrent infections are known to worsen the stage and severity of the involved regions and when accompanied by malodorous leakage interferes significantly with socialization and enjoyment of others. In young adults, these complications may prove a disastrous emotional challenge, significantly altering normal development.

In one cohort, nearly half of patients undergoing reduction surgery reported being "cured," while others indicated that significant improvement occurred only following a second operation 5 to 7 years later. In women receiving excision surgery, two-thirds reported no need for a second procedure at the 10-year mark.[93] In another study, nearly 40% experienced a complete elimination of further infection with a significant number of others achieving dramatic reductions in antibiotic use.[94] Unfortunately, it is suspected that only with total removal of all diseased skin, can recurrence of cysts be prevented.

Hydrocele

It is suspected that as many as 30% of male genital lymphedema is associated with hydrocele, a fluid-filled space (tunica vaginalis testis and/or spermatic cord) that accumulates serous fluid. Upon palpation, this accumulation, which causes a noticeable enlargement, should not be mistaken for genital lymphedema. The involved testicle will feel enlarged, yet the scrotal skin will remain thin and pliable. Since hydrocele may occur in isolation, the course of treatment would not involve CDT, but with consultation it is likely to require surgical intervention. If hydrocele is combined with scrotal lymphedema, there may be a noticeable asymmetry where one testicle is involved; however, true scrotal lymphedema generally masks the testicle with thick edematous skin, making evaluation of hydrocele more difficult. As such, genital lymphedema is NOT lymphedema of the testicles but involves the scrotal sac and penile skin. It is advisable to seek physician's guidance if there is a suspicion of hydrocele providing a coordinated effort to address one or both diagnoses appropriately.

5.13.6 Conservative Therapy

Prior to any potential surgical intervention, an intensive course of CDT should be employed to assess its effectiveness. For some patients, genital treatment with CDT is a remarkably productive strategy, rendering invasive procedures unnecessary. In those electing to have surgery, CDT serves a productive preoperative function by decongesting involved tissues sufficiently to aid in postoperative healing and improve regional lymph drainage.

Setting the Stage for CDT

Gender Pairing

From the viewpoint of delivering optimal care, it is productive to consider pairing genders. Unfortunately, with the predominance of female therapists and abundance of male genital lymphedema patients, this ideal plan will likely prove impossible to achieve. Regardless of pairing considerations, requiring a significant other's direct participation in the clinical session satisfies the goal of assisting with optimal home care management while addressing the unusual but possible liability related to perceptions of unprofessional conduct. In general, whenever a pediatric patient is treated with or without genital involvement, a second adult must be present. Considering the multidisciplinary backgrounds of CLTs, each clinician should observe relevant practice guidelines, which outline limitations that may exclude direct genital contact.

Gloves

To create a thoughtful emotional and physical boundary, CLTs should don surgical gloves prior to establishing contact with genital tissues. In all other skin areas, skin-to-skin contact during treatment provides a second strong message that conveys empathy and a willingness to provide caring human contact. Additional benefits of wearing gloves include hygienic protection from lymphorrhea and lower risk of introducing pathogens to highly susceptible tissues.

Develop a Plan of Care

Genital lymphedema is accompanied by leg lymphedema in the majority of patients. From the perspective of CDT, decongestion of the entire lower quadrant is the only productive approach that warrants consideration. That said, many patients are solely focused on a genital treatment plan because of the numerous, undeniable, and troubling challenges it alone presents. To close this gap in the objectives of both parties, therapists must have a dialogue with the patient in order to reach an understanding that represents the most productive course of treatment and long-term efficacy. Treatment of the genitals without decongestion of the lower quadrant(s) ignores the fact that the entire territory shares the same regional lymph nodes and deeper pathways. Although genital reduction can be achieved, it will be short-lived (artificial) if concomitant treatment of the leg or legs is not conducted. Discussion of these logical realities is generally convincing and gains the approval of most patients.

Pertaining to the therapist's initial, inherent discomfort with treatment of genital lymphedema, which is almost universal, it should be noted that opting out of genital treatment, yet choosing to treat an involved leg, is neither possible nor responsible and will effectively worsen the genitals, which will accommodate fluid evacuated from the treated leg. As such, therapists who object to direct genital contact must refer these patients to someone open to and capable of treating without hesitation.

Even though some lymphedema patients receiving CDT are candidates for semi-intensive therapy (less than 5 days per week, one treatment per day), genital lymphedema requires daily intensive therapy. Since decongestion involves diuresis, for male patients urination requires repeated removal and reapplication of penile and scrotal compression bandages. This skill can only be acquired by immediate daily education and training sessions, which develop proficiency while further protecting against cumulative erosion of fragile skin due to bandage misapplication.

Document and Assess the Edema Margins

Following physician consultation and evaluation for CDT candidacy, record volumetric and circumferential measurements and further document with pictures. Owing to the fact that the labia, scrotum, and penis are difficult and awkward to measure, illustrative documentation can prove highly valuable and informative for assessing progress. To improve the validity of these pictures, photograph from a standard position, distance, view, and background. This consideration will allow for unambiguous comparisons that verify and support the progress achieved.

Continue by taking full bilateral leg measurements assessing subtle or gross involvement to be addressed in the treatment protocol. In some instances, benign secondary genital lymphedema presents with swelling that encompasses the proximal thigh, hip, and buttock while temporarily sparing the distal thigh and legs. It should be noted that malignant lymphedema is also generally described as a proximally pronounced swelling. As such, these clinical signs should elicit physician instructions to identify any current disease process responsible for this atypical clinical presentation.

Palpate the skin of the suprapubis, lower abdomen, hips, and buttocks recording your assessment with descriptions, measurements, and/or pictures for future reference. It is not uncommon to note swelling that encompasses all tissues up to the transverse watershed. Decongestion of the genitals relies upon ipsilateral trunk decongestion; therefore, these clear proximal margins will dictate the thoroughness required for the MLD sequence.

Draping

To facilitate a less stressful or anxious course of therapy, most patients appreciate thoughtful draping of the genital region. Once an MLD treatment sequence has been established, complete all the steps required prior to MLD before exposing the genital region. Undrape only at the time of direct contact and redrape immediately following completion of MLD and bandage application.

Start with Compression

Although each treatment session always includes MLD followed by compression bandaging, it is prudent to prioritize the compression procedure. The foremost consideration involves the necessity for frequent urination, which will require skilled patient reapplication of the bandage. Since each therapy session encompasses only a fraction of the day, this task will fall upon the patient or caregiver from the very first session. The second consideration is the practical and technical challenge of wrapping, which in genital treatment is always a highly customized procedure. Furthermore, by bandaging the genitals, first the therapist can inspect for results but also preserve the benefits of the previous bandage. Loose scrotal skin refills

rapidly without constant compression. Prioritizing this procedure will allow ample time to study, solve, and adapt to problems that may present early on.

Train the Patient or Caregiver

Prioritizing bandaging also builds necessary confidence in the therapist and defines the procedure as a stepwise and teachable task. It is recommended that a first bandage be applied, removed, and reapplied repeatedly by the therapist until the most thoughtful approach to compression is defined. Once a system is defined, taking into account special considerations such as shape, size, tenderness, skin fragility, folds, or bandage adherence, proceed to the task of patient and/or caregiver instruction. In general, most patients feel that self-care autonomy is a valuable goal here and support a teaching strategy that eliminates the need for reliance on the therapist. Once this procedure is defined, the maximum amount of remaining time can be allocated to a thorough MLD sequence, which sets the stage for improved genital drainage and will contribute to less rapid refilling.

The Manual Lymph Drainage Sequence: Step by Step

The following MLD sequence can be applied for both primary and secondary genital lymphedema. In general, the patient position that provides the highest degree of comfort is supine unless the genital swelling is mild. To avoid prone positioning, lying on the side may be preferred to gain access to the lumbar and gluteal regions in patients requiring this pretreatment step. In others where no hip or buttock involvement is detected, the entire treatment may be performed in the supine-only position.

Treatment position: The patient lies supine; the therapist stands on the right side of the patient.

1. *"Short" neck treatment (supraclavicular fossa or SCF):* Place fingers on either side of the neck and resting flatly to cover the area bordered by the acromion, clavicle, and lateral neck (SCF). If a depression exists, gently apply pressure on the trapezius muscle so that full skin contact is achieved. Avoid resting with pressure on the clavicle or upper chest. Use stationary circles by initiating stretch toward posterior and medial, both hands working in unison.

Treatment of the SCF is adequate for its therapeutic contribution to the genital lymphatic drainage sequence in that it prepares the venous angles (lymphovenous anastomosis), which empty the thoracic duct and all tributaries. Electively if the sequences involving the shoulder and cervical regions are included, they will not provide therapeutic value (to the genital region) but may succeed in developing contact and trust with the patient.

2. *Abdominal treatment (two part: visceral, deep)*: The orientation of this sequence involves addressing five distinct regions, which follow the colon drainage.
    a) Effleurage:
       1. Soft strokes with the fingers in the direction of the colon using firm contact to avoid hypersensitivity.
       2. Soft strokes with the fingers alternating from hip to hip across the midline in a paint-brush–like motion.
       3. Soft strokes with the fingers from the pubic symphysis superiorly along the midline, under the ribcage, and toward lateral, then returning to the point of origin.
    b) Treatment of the colon (visceral):
       1. *Left lower quadrant:* Rest the first hand (i.e., the hand nearer the feet) on the lower quadrant above the left pelvic crest and rest the other hand on top. Apply a stationary circle in a gentle supinating motion in several sets before repositioning.
       2. *Right lower quadrant:* Avoiding the area of the bladder and using the same manual orientation, apply stationary circles to the lower right quadrant of the abdomen. If necessary, repeat the same technique in a more lateral position within the same quadrant for larger abdomens.
       3. *Right upper quadrant:* Switch hands so that the hand nearer the head is placed gently against the abdomen while the other hand rests on top. Locate the hands under the last rib (hepatic flexure) region of the quadrant. Apply a stationary circle in a gentle supinating motion in several sets before repositioning.

4. *Transverse colon:* Using the same manual orientation, move the hand position toward the midline and between the ribs. Be careful to stay beneath the xiphoid process, and gently apply stationary circles in a supinating motion.
5. *Left upper quadrant:* Maintaining the same manual orientation, reposition the hands under the left ribcage (splenic flexure) and apply stationary circles in a gentle supinating motion.
6. *Return to left lower quadrant:* Finish the sequence as it was started (step a) completing a sixth step to the sequence.

c) *Treatment of the thoracic duct, cisterna chyli (deep)*: Treatment position—legs are elevated (wedged) or bent at a 45-degree angle, and head is slightly elevated (pillow).
   1. *Breathing coaching and awareness:* Diaphragmatic breathing is the key to effective treatment. Spend the first moments of the treatment ascertaining the strength and fullness of the patient's deep-breathing technique.
   2. Coordinate hand position with breathing cycle:
      • As the patient exhales, place the hand over the area of treatment. Follow the exhalation with gentle pressure in a downward spiral.
      • During inhalation, create a resistance ("a heavy hand") and instruct the patient to lift the hand with a strong, deep diaphragmatic breath.
      • Once the inhalation is complete, quickly reposition the hand to another aspect of the abdomen (hand placement) and follow the exhalation with gentle pressure in a downward spiral.
      • Repeat the above three-step breathing sequence on five distinct points visiting nine hand placements. Coordination must involve resistance on the inhalation and repositioning on the exhalation in an unbroken and natural breathing rhythm. The five points or regions illustrate the five distinct regions of hand placement. However, the order varies from that which was outlined in step b, treatment of the colon (visceral).

As illustrated, the five regions are visited in the following order rendering nine hand placements (▶ Fig. 5.181).

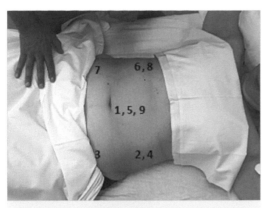

Fig. 5.181 The nine hand placements.

1. Center.
2. Left upper quadrant.
3. Left lower quadrant.
4. Left upper quadrant.
5. Center.
6. Right upper quadrant.
7. Right lower quadrant.
8. Right upper quadrant.
9. Center.

Since the order of hand placements starts in the center, revisits the center, and ends there, we could conclude that a special emphasis has been placed on applying pressure directly over the cisterna chyli. Likewise, the upper left and right quadrants receive two hand placements each, lateral to the thoracic duct and cisterna chyli. The two points distal to this region, the left and right lower quadrants, receive only one hand placement and may be considered more remote to the thoracic duct and therefore are less of a focus during this treatment.

1. *Treatment of the RIGHT axillary lymph nodes*: Treatment position—the therapist stands at the side of the patient.
   a) Support the patient's arm at the elbow with the hand at lower end of the patient's body and apply stationary circles with the other hand. The arm is abducted to 90 degrees and the therapist faces toward the feet.
   b) During the first set, the direction of the stationary circle is inward (toward trunk) from distal to proximal on the medial (brachial) aspect of the arm. Do not advance the working hand.
   c) The second hand placement (second set) is centered on the axillary fossa. Adduct the arm enough to soften the pectoralis and latissimus muscles allowing for full skin contact in the fossa. Apply a stationary circle without advancing the hand in the same inward moving direction.

2. *Establish the RIGHT IAA*: The therapist stands on patient's left side (reaching across).
   a) Standing on the LEFT side, establish the RIGHT IAA anastomosis using a "traffic jam" approach. The "traffic jam" approach implies that the neighboring quadrant (ipsilateral upper quadrant) is progressively decongested as if cars were moved 1, 2, 3 from a traffic jam. This allows congested tissues to drain into noncongested tissues more efficiently.
   b) For the "first pass," start above the transverse watershed and apply the alternating stationary circle technique dynamically (advancing) to the axillary nodes. For the "second pass," start one hand width into the involved lower quadrant (below the transverse watershed) and treat toward the axillary nodes. For the "third pass," start a width of two hands below the watershed (at the right hip) and continue to the axillary nodes. Use consecutive passes from hip to axilla repetitively.

3. *Decongest the RIGHT ipsilateral lower abdomen and suprapubis*: Therapist stands on the patient's LEFT side (reaching across).
   a) Following establishment of the IAA, treat the lower abdomen and suprapubic region with rotary techniques toward the IAA. Observe the midsagittal watershed as a boundary (do not cross) and direct fluid toward the right IAA. Follow up with stationary circles crossing the transverse watershed toward the axillary nodes.

4. *Treatment of the LEFT axillary lymph nodes*: Therapist stands on the patient's LEFT side.
   a) Follow steps as outlined for the right axillary lymph node treatment (step 3).

5. *Establish the LEFT IAA*: Therapist stands on the patient's RIGHT side (reaching across).
   a) Follow steps as outlined for right IAA treatment above (step 4).

6. *Decongest the LEFT ipsilateral lower abdomen and suprapubis*: Therapist stands on the patient's RIGHT side (reaching across). Follow steps as outlined above (step 5).

7. *Treatment of the external genitals*: This is described for the male patient. However, all steps can be followed as written for the female patient up to step f. The therapist will stand on both sides treating symmetrically and duplicate

the steps. Gloves should be donned for the following steps.

a) Standing at the side of the patient, expose the genital region. Separate the legs to allow space to perform the techniques. Using the hand that is toward the lower end of the patient, pull the scrotum to the side and apply stationary circles with the headward hand to the entire surface (left or right aspect). Envision the working phase of the stroke directing fluid toward the suprapubic region. After several strokes, follow up with rotary techniques in the suprapubic region directed toward the IAA. Repeat again for several minutes or as time permits.

Suprapubic strokes may be passing close to or over the inguinal nodes; however, these nodes (although intact) must be viewed as congested and are not viable collateral drainage pathways.

b) For the posterior aspect of the scrotum (perineum), perform stationary circles envisioning the drainage crossing the "chaps/gluteal" watershed. Direct strokes posteriorly.

c) Switch sides and repeat steps a and b focusing on the side opposite to where you are standing.

d) Bend the knee on your side and apply alternating stationary circles to the proximal posterior thigh reaching close to the perineum/posterior scrotum and directing fluid across the "chaps/gluteal" watershed. Perform again for several repetitions.

e) Switch sides and repeat step d.

These steps (d and e) allow the patient to remain in the supine position for the entire session. The supine-only position is suitable only when the hips, buttocks, and legs are spared swelling. When leg and/or lower trunk involvement exists, it is helpful to turn the patient on each side to allow for a "modified lumbar and gluteal" treatment. This additional step will help ensure adequate truncal preparation for efficient genital drainage.

Treatment of female genital lymphedema: All steps can be performed as outlined earlier. The natural separation between the left and right labia creates a clear change in drainage direction. Modify the hand placement to encompass the entire labia (as described for the scrotum) so that the full length of one, two, or three fingers (instead of the whole hand) can apply stationary circles.

f) *Treatment of the penis*: If the penis is spared involvement or is retracted (enveloped) into the scrotum, this step is neither possible nor necessary. Using one hand as a firm support, rest the penis and apply stationary circles to the entire shaft of the penis focusing on a light circular motion directed toward the suprapubis. Depending on the size and level of involvement, the penis can be approached by first focusing on the proximal aspect then on the distal aspect.

g) *Treatment of the foreskin*: Lymphedema can be the most pronounced and severe in the foreskin. For patients with a foreskin, perform focused stationary circles with the fingertips exploring the texture, pliability, and fibrotic involvement. This step will also provide valuable information upon which to base custom-compression considerations.

h) Apply compression bandaging to the genitals (male patients) to preserve the benefits of therapy. If there is no leg involvement, the session can conclude. Otherwise follow step i either before or after applying the compression bandages.

i) *Treatment of the leg(s)*: If one or both legs are also involved, perform a standard secondary unilateral or bilateral leg treatment. Each leg is treated toward the hip with a great emphasis on avoiding the genitals and midsagittal watershed. In primary genital lymphedema patients, the inguinal nodes can be treated but are not the target of collateral drainage.

Compression Bandaging for Male Genital Lymphedema

Genital lymphedema may involve the scrotum and penis combined or only one region. In the following description of practical bandaging steps, the penis and scrotum are approached as singular compression challenges. When the penis and scrotum are simultaneously involved, address the penis first to avoid a more difficult wrapping procedure. The second benefit to this order is that the adherence of the scrotal bandage is improved. If the penis is spared involvement and is not engulfed by the scrotal swelling (which is common), there is no indication to wrap unless there is a migration of fluid into the penis.

One of the most challenging aspects of genital bandaging in male patients is the tendency to erode the skin, which creates pain, open skin lesions, and increased risk of infection. For this reason, special consideration must be given to any compression procedure and in particular the materials applied. Foam padding has proven indispensable on limb lymphedema; two of its benefits include the ability to displace fluid (then occupy the space) and add structure to stiffen the bandage, which creates a safe container for the compressed tissues. Since most varieties of foam cannot be applied directly to the skin without risk of allergy, a special type (Velfoam) is used to address this concern. Velfoam is a fleece-backed, open cell foam made for direct skin contact. It is thin enough to avoid bulk, is washable, reusable, and, importantly, accepts Velcro hook tabs.

The following sequence outlines the scrotal wrap followed by the penile wrap and shows a finished bandage where each is separately completed. The order (scrotum first) is shown for clarity and illustrative purposes only.

Materials required: Velfoam, scissors, Velcro hook tabs, gauze, Lenkelast, or Ace.

Wrapping the Scrotum Separately

The following procedure can be performed with or without penile involvement. As stated earlier, the scrotal bandage always follows the penis wrap if one is required. The rationale for using Velfoam straps in the scrotal bandage complex is to create better adherence but more importantly to give skin protection against the abrasive qualities of the gauze or coarse woven wraps.

Rationale

The root of the scrotum passes into the perineum posteriorly and pubis anteriorly which creates a flaring of the skin. When wrapped, this flaring (widening) causes the compressive materials to roll into a cord and with movement and moisture create abrasion, injury, and pain. Additionally, for a patient without the necessary dexterity and flexibility or help of a therapist or caregiver, reaching these areas blindly can set the stage for an inadequate and unsafe bandage. The following foam application will create a safe, comfortable barrier to offset the rolling of fabric while acting as a harness to assist with overall adherence.

Position

Standing, legs slightly spread and leaning against an elevated massage table, plinth, or conventional bed.

1. Using a strip of Velfoam (5 cm wide), estimate the length by placing it behind the scrotum and as high as possible toward the perineum. Allow the end to overlap and fix closed with Velcro (▶ Fig. 5.182).
2. Take a second Velfoam strip and attach it with Velcro from left to right following the contour of the scrotum (▶ Fig. 5.183).
3. Add an additional narrower strip (2.5 cm wide) from left to right under the penis if more protection is desired. This understrap may prove

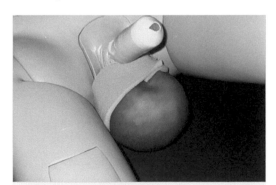

Fig. 5.182 Securing a Velfoam strip to the base of the scrotum.

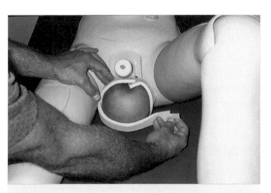

Fig. 5.183 Securing a second Velfoam strip from left to right.

5

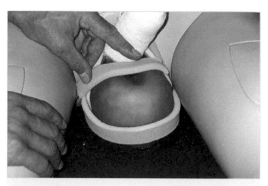

Fig. 5.184 Securing a narrow Velfoam strap under the penis at the base.

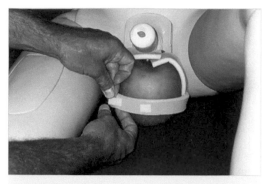

Fig. 5.185 Application of an adhesive-backed Velcro hook along the straps.

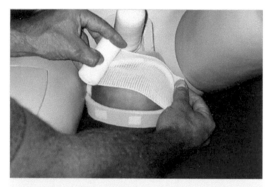

Fig. 5.186 Application of gauze to the scrotum allowing the hooks to embed in the fabric.

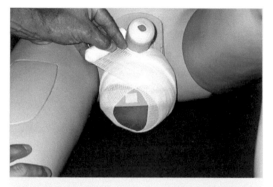

Fig. 5.187 Continued thorough coverage of the entire scrotal region.

helpful at protecting the underside of the penis (▶ Fig. 5.184).

4. Apply adhesive-backed Velcro hook tabs every 5 cm or as needed along the entire apparatus. With the hooks facing outward, these tabs help ensnare the gauze as it passes over, effectively holding the gauze layers in place (▶ Fig. 5.185).

5. Apply gauze of any width (4, 6, 8, or 10 cm) that seems proportional to the mass of tissue being wrapped. Since the areas most likely to receive abrasion are protected, chiefly the penile root and perineum, posteriorly firm tension and molding can be used to create a strong external compression. If necessary, finish with an elastic bandage to additional resting pressure (▶ Fig. 5.186; ▶ Fig. 5.187; ▶ Fig. 5.188).

Wrapping the Penis Separately

1. Begin by cutting a piece of Velfoam to the approximate length and girth of the edematous penis. Take time to trim the foam edges with a bevel so that the pressure diminishes at the edges

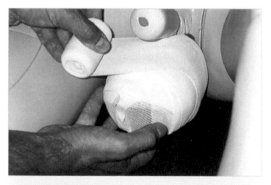

Fig. 5.188 Application (in desired) of a medium-stretch bandage to increase pressure.

minimizing pressure marks. To encompass the entire length, cut a gentle arc to accommodate the underside of the penile root. Trim the edges to avoid overlap and fix closed with small rectangular Velcro tabs. If there is an edematous foreskin, place a second foam "cap" over the end to increase the pressure (▶ Fig. 5.189; ▶ Fig. 5.190).

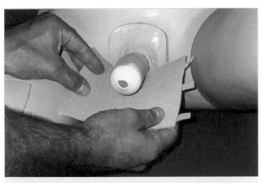

Fig. 5.189 Fitting and application of Velfoam to the penis.

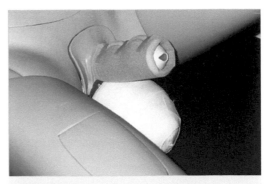

Fig. 5.190 Securing the closing with Velcro.

5

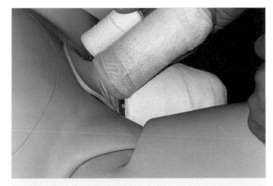

Fig. 5.191 Application of gauze emphasizing gradient pressure.

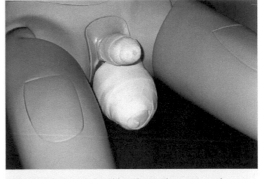

Fig. 5.192 A completed bandage: The penis and scrotum are separately wrapped.

2. Select a standard gauze finger or toe wrap of ~ 6 cm width and apply an even, smooth distribution to the entire enclosure. Avoid touching the skin at the root area and keep all material within the margins of foam as this is the prime rationale for using Velfoam. Be careful to allocate more gauze material to the distal aspects, generating a compression gradient that would otherwise be absent. As with limb lymphedema, inspect the result after every bandage removal to assess the effectiveness of the gradient and make further adjustments in materials allocation to the next wrap (▶ Fig. 5.191; ▶ Fig. 5.192).

The Foreskin

When the foreskin becomes edematous, it will extend far out from the shaft and glans of the penis creating a closed slit, which makes urination and hygiene an added challenge. Decongesting this area may occur satisfactorily without special measures beyond the general wrapping procedure described earlier. In others, the foreskin proves very difficult to decongest and as the most distal region is most prone to developing fibrotic skin changes. In such instances, special pieces of foam may be applied to aggressively "press" the skin. This may be done with the introduction of small pieces of closed cell foam (Komprex) applied during the general wrapping procedure.

Another approach involves creating a foam plug that is inserted into the foreskin, opening the cavity to create a firm core to wrap against. Unlike limbs, which have a skeletal core, the flaccid foreskin in particular and even the shaft of the penis respond less productively to pressure without the resistance of solid core. For this application, cut the finger off a surgical glove, insert open cell foam, and lubricate the outside before inserting. Follow this procedure with a complete wrap of the penis or a separate wrapping segment for the foreskin.

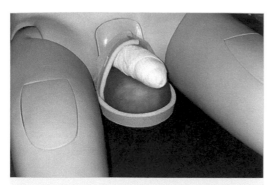

Fig. 5.193 An integrated bandage: Application of the harness from the scrotum to above the wrapped penis.

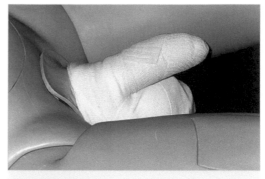

Fig. 5.194 Application of a scrotal wrap, securing turns above the penis.

Integrating the Penile and Scrotal Wraps

The benefit of applying separate wraps is to allow only one area to be removed and reapplied as necessary. This allows for far greater flexibility with urination, which may be frequent while also accommodating spontaneous scrotal volume reduction. Unfortunately, the most difficult variable to control is the tendency for these fluctuations to result in poor bandage adherence. To address this technical challenge, it is helpful to integrate both the penile and scrotal wraps into one procedure.

1. Wrap the penis as outlined in the above steps.
2. Apply the scrotal harness so that it grips the base of the penis (▶ Fig. 5.193).
3. Consider applying an understrap (illustrated above in ▶ Fig. 5.184).
4. Complete the scrotal wraps including bandage turns that follow the straps that cross over the base of the penis (▶ Fig. 5.194).

Since reductions of the scrotum can be dramatic and occur within hours, the entire complex may require immediate downsizing. Although this is exciting progress, it is recommended that therapists and caregivers study the wrapping procedure carefully to apply the safest bandage with consistency. Without an emotional attachment to an immediate and total remission of swelling, a comfortable, tolerable, and controlled reduction can be achieved. Unfortunately, in most instances, a total reversal cannot be accomplished and thus a compression strategy will be required in the long term. As such, proficiency and safety are the chief aims of any compression strategy involving the genital

region. With practice and confidence, the reduced swelling volume will allow for a reduction in padding and pressure, which sets the stage for achieving the goal of a highly simplified, low-intensity maintenance program. In the best cases, a compression garment with a scrotal pouch may prove productive during the day followed by circumferential wrapping nightly or as required.

Alternative Materials

To provide additional pressure, semielastic or strong elastic bandages can be applied over the gauze layers. These high resting-pressure bandages shorten with swelling reduction, which may be helpful to adherence, but require great care and control during application. It is recommended that light tension be used and that the materials lay flat to avoid rolling and increased local pressure. These materials include Lenkelast or ACE bandages.

Compression Garments for Genital Lymphedema

General Considerations

There are several pros and cons to elastic compression garment applications for genital lymphedema management. Perhaps the most important requirement for the selection of a compression garment is a comprehensive understanding of the edematous areas to be compressed. One of the most common mistakes made in the selection of a garment is to configure the coverage to accommodate only the involved area, disregarding the propensity for neighboring high-risk areas to swell. In fact, to exclude coverage of high-risk areas often acts as the precipitating factor for onset of swelling. The same observation applies to misjudging and neglecting the hand's compression requirements, where swelling currently involves only the same arm.

As discussed earlier, most external genital lymphedema occurs when pelvic or lumbar lymph nodes are disrupted by surgery and/or radiation therapy. Since lymph node sampling generally involves the left and right pelvic lymph nodes, both lower quadrants are subjected to a decrease in transport capacity.

Male or female genital lymphedema benefits from elastic garment coverage in the pelvic region. For example, the hips, abdomen, and external genitals require the so-called body part or panty portion which is always fabricated with extensions into the legs for comfort (bike shorts). Even if the target area is only the external genital area, the entire lower quadrant is at risk if not involved. As such, it is the therapist's responsibility to apply compression to both full lower limbs. Appropriate configurations include the following:

- Pantyhose (compression class can vary for left leg, right leg, and panty portion).
- Bike shorts to be worn with two full-leg stockings.
- Capri pants with two knee-high stockings.

Improper configurations include the following:
- Bike shorts (only).
- Pantyhose one full leg, one short leg.
- Capri pants, no knee-high stockings.
- Bike shorts, plus two knee-high stockings.
- Panty portion, no leg extensions.

Male Considerations

Compression garments alone are never appropriate or adequate to address genital lymphedema. Although they may lift the tissues and slow down the increasing volume, they lead to fungal infections by decreasing airflow and harboring moisture. If upward support is all that is offered, the penile and scrotal tissues will mold to that shape and begin to thicken permanently. Circumferential compression bandaging gently supports the skin and allows for improved uptake and transport of lymph, reduces the formation of new lymph, dries the skin, and maintains the natural shape. For this reason initially, compression garments are worn over the genital wraps to improve adherence and offset the effects of gravity.

Another successful strategy for compression garment application in male patients is to place a bulky pad into the area of the pubis where fluid is

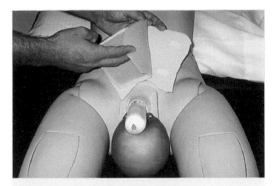

Fig. 5.195 Suprapubic padding (for the male patient).

often harbored. The panty portion of the garment must accommodate this bulky pad but responds by gently pulling it inward against the swollen tissues. Although this pad creates undesirable bulk, it can be very effective therapy for a challenging body region and may be removed following decongestion and stabilization (▶ Fig. 5.195).

Scrotal pouches: Most garment manufacturers will accommodate requests for special pouches. Extra fabric here allows spaces for bandages and bulk without excessive lifting forces. In general, a compression class 1 fabric provides ample structure and support. In the "cut-and-sew" fabric types used in burn garment applications, a uniform-strength, light-fabric pouch can be attached to shorts and be wrapped over the top. With reduction, the pouch can be inexpensively tailored to a smaller size. This type of approach works best for patients with no penile involvement because there is no hole for the penis in this pouch.

In summary, as a long-term management strategy, a scrotal pouch may be helpful during the daytime by liberating the patient from excessive, noticeable bulk. It may also create the lift and allow for the room required to cover the bulky bandage. However, the standard, extensible crotch panel of pantyhose may suffice. To offset the shape distortion, loss of air circulation, and the tendency for fungal infections, and to achieve a controlled reduction, bandaging should be performed for a portion of each day with or without an external scrotal pouch.

Female Considerations

To exert compression comfortably and safely in females, an elastic garment is the only solution capable of accommodating the labia. In all cases, the standard, highly extensible crotch panels

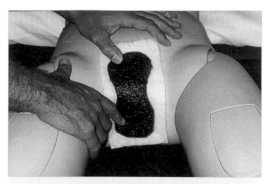

Fig. 5.196 Labial padding (foam and synthetic cotton).

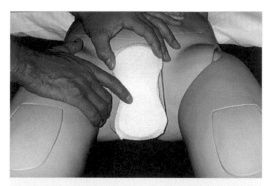

Fig. 5.197 Labial padding (foam within stockinette).

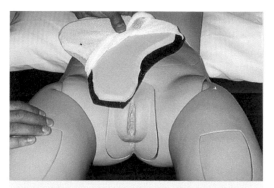

Fig. 5.198 Combined labial and suprapubic padding configuration.

typically made to increase air circulation and decrease pressure must be replaced with compressive, structural fabric to generate higher pressure. With this added fabric integrity, specially shaped padding pieces can be created to exert pressure on one or both labia as well as the suprapubic region. As discussed, the bulkier the foam, the more inward pressure can be achieved as the pad is pulled back against the body. Similar to the male patient, it is important to consider tolerance to the materials, avoiding contact dermatitis, abrasion, or pressure sores.

Since the female patient requires an upward and inward pressure at all times, there may not be sufficient rest from constant compression which may lead to intolerance and poor compliance. It may be advisable to sleep without compression or take breaks for a few hours daily to allow the skin to breathe and recover from the aggressive feeling of genital compression (▶ Fig. 5.196; ▶ Fig. 5.197; ▶ Fig. 5.198).

In all cases, fluid stasis creates subtle but progressive tissue thickening (lymphostatic fibrosis), which responds favorably to pressure and mechanical stimulation. To retain skin pliability, thinness, and softness, special pads with uneven surfaces (chip bags) can be used to alternate with flat foam pads as part of a long-term strategy. These pads should encompass all involved areas to include the suprapubic region.

Another consideration for augmenting pressure may involve analyzing daily function and occupational positioning. In this regard, straddling positions (bike seats or modified chairs) may provide added compression benefit. For female pediatric genital lymphedema, consider toys that require straddling (bikes, rocking horses, etc.) because they may be sensible adjunct tools.

Self-MLD

There are important situations where self-MLD proves beneficial to long-term success. However, in some instances it can be counterproductive due to improper or aggressive technique. In genital lymphedema, careful self-administered MLD is essential and serves to liberate the patient from therapist's treatment of the genitals, which allows the clinical session time to be allocated to truncal decongestion and compression strategies. Although lymphedema therapists should always inspect and provide quality checks of these tasks, self-administered MLD allows the patient to take control and engage in ongoing, frequent self-care of a highly personal problem.

In all cases, regular deep breathing sessions set the stage for improved whole body lymphatic drainage efficiency. Spontaneous reductions have been observed with deep breathing alone and thus should not be underestimated for effectiveness.

5.14 Truncal Lymphedema

5.14.1 Lymphedema of the Thorax

Breast or chest wall lymphedema is often over-looked and remains underdiagnosed.[95] Frequently, the patient's interpretation of his or her symptoms may not be accurate due to postoperative deficits in sensation following axillary dissection because of injury to the intercostobrachial nerve.[96] Sensations of "fullness" or excess tissue may be attributed to altered anatomy related to surgery. Since this symptom often predates any congestion in the region, patients are unlikely to notice when actual edema appears. Furthermore, some patients may be hesitant to inspect the area due to body image issues. While it is understandable why many patients fail to identify edema in the thorax, it remains imperative for clinicians to adequately diagnose the presence of truncal lymphedema, as the risk for developing complications is the same as for limb edema.[96] This requires complete examination of the thorax in all patients with ipsilateral cancer treatment or limb edema. While limited research on risks associated with untreated truncal congestion exists, our physiological approach to the treatment of lymphedema necessitates attention to this region.[97,98,99] Failure to recognize early stages of truncal edema can indeed adversely affect patient outcomes. Lack of treatment of truncal edema may result in pain or discomfort in the upper quadrant of the trunk and/or the extremity while also contributing to higher levels of patient anxiety or distress. Furthermore, higher pressures in the truncal region can reduce already limited lymphatic return from the adjacent limb.[97]

Symptoms and Presentation of Breast Lymphedema

The symptoms of breast lymphedema are different from limb edema in many ways. Lymphedema of the breast may begin quickly and is commonly non-pitting in its early stages. It should be distinguished from inflammation that is related to radiation, particularly in women with large breasts, where detection of edema may be masked by underlying breast tissue. As with limb edema, truncal edema is commonly characterized by sensations of "heaviness," presence of redness or erythema, discomfort, or pain. Patients can be distressed due to fears about recurrence or inflammatory breast cancer. In a prospective study by Degnim et al, erythema was present in 79% of study participants with breast lymphedema. Following surgery, participants with breast lymphedema were also 65% more likely to report symptoms of "heaviness" ($p < 0.0001$) than patients without breast lymphedema.[100]

Patients with breast edema report higher pain levels and more sensitivity to pressure. While this may be due to a neurosensory response to the edema in the thorax, this characteristic is generally considered unique to truncal lymphedema. Differential diagnoses such as cellulitis, mastitis, Mondor's disease (thrombophlebitis of the superficial veins of the chest wall), and costochondritis should also be considered. Seroma formation should be ruled out. Some patients may even undergo skin biopsy to rule out recurrence, inflammatory breast cancer, or angiosarcoma—any of which can occur in cases of chronic breast edema.[101] Hematoma formation following breast surgery is rare, but when it occurs it may cause significant discomfort and edema in the breast.

When evaluating breast lymphedema, an exact description of the location of the edema should refer to quadrants of the breast or reference its position with relation to the top or bottom of incisions. In some cases, a patient may have changed bra sizes to accommodate the edema, and this allows for easier quantification of the edema. In other circumstances, a wound assessment template can be used to quantify the size of an area of localized fibrosis. Incisional scars should be mapped and described in terms of mobility and adherence. Photos are extremely useful because measurements are difficult to reproduce. Custom compression garment measurement forms or relevant references can provide templates, but these can be time consuming and lack validity studies.[99] As with all measurement strategies, however, using a consistent technique is paramount to identifying progression or improvement.

Lateral Breast Edema

In a relatively recent prospective analysis, 124 patients were followed up for signs and symptoms of breast edema over the course of 1 year. Initial postoperative edema was ruled out by scheduling the first study visit at 3 months.[100] Breast edema was identified by clinical examination in 31% (38 of 124) of patients. The investigators then localized breast edema by quadrant, noting that lateral breast edema was present in 78% of the 38 patients with newly diagnosed lymphedema, with the lateral inferior and medial inferior quadrants most commonly involved (74 and 50% of patients, respectively). The study also described incidence of symptoms among women with and without breast edema including breast heaviness (65 vs. 22%, $p < 0.0001$), redness (62 vs. 29%, $p = 0.0006$), and swelling (59 vs. 22%, $p < 0.0001$). Despite these symptoms, the authors found relatively low levels of distress among patients with lateral breast edema compared to higher levels of distress with more severe edema.

The impetus to treat breast edema, however, extends beyond quality of life, given the known increase in health-related concerns and complications related to lymphedema. Minimizing the risk of infection (cellulitis) and preventing progression of lymphedema are two key reasons to identify and treat breast lymphedema. Larger patients may have redundant skin along the lateral aspect of mastectomy incisions, known as "dog-ears."[96] These flaps can be irritating to the ipsilateral limb, and the skin folds may become sites of localized fungal infection. Additionally, patients find that when edema accumulates in this region, the added friction can worsen the edema as well. In cases where the inframammary fold is maintained, edema usually collects in the dependent portion of the breast.[100] Inferior bra bands may also contribute to breast edema by trapping it and hastening fibrosis through chronic fluid stasis. ▶ Fig. 5.199 shows significant lateral breast pitting edema with contribution from a poorly fitting bra.

Chest Congestion with Limb Edema

This is perhaps the most intuitive type of truncal lymphedema, as it often may occur in the anterior or posterior truncal quadrants in the setting of upper limb lymphedema. Surgical removal of axillary lymph nodes impairs drainage of the corresponding truncal quadrant, thus contributing to lymphedema of both the limb and the remaining portion of the associated root area. Diagnosis of the limb edema may occur more readily than identification of nearby truncal edema. This is likely due to decreased awareness of truncal lymphedema as well as the need for patients to undress for proper diagnosis.

While truncal congestion or lymphedema adjacent to an affected limb seems intuitive, many therapists do not adequately inspect and quantify this edema. This is imperative. As mentioned previously, some of this underdiagnosis may be due to excessive reliance on patient report. Owing to the common sensation loss in this area, women are much less likely to describe these symptoms. As such, taking the time to fully inspect the truncal quadrants in their entirety is an essential part of the evaluation of breast cancer patients. Patients may be reluctant to undress as well due to body image issues after mastectomy, and clinicians often sense this reluctance and are hesitant to request patients to undress fully. This, however, can greatly compromise the evaluation and treatment of the individual. The clinician must carefully look for changes in tissue folds, as edema can "fill" natural tissue folds and even increase space between folds. See ▶ Fig. 5.200 for an illustration of truncal lymphedema identified by alterations in the lateral tissue folds. A side-by-side comparison illustrates this best, although this may not be possible for patients with bilateral involvement. In

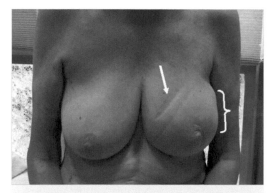

Fig. 5.199 Lateral breast edema (bracket) with a contribution from a poorly fitting bra (arrow) in a patient 4 months after left lumpectomy with axillary dissection.

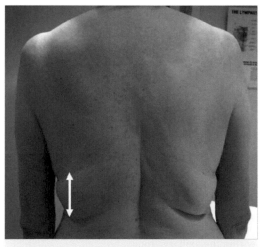

Fig. 5.200 Truncal edema illustrated by increased space between lateral tissue folds (arrow).

cases of bilateral truncal congestion, impressions left by undergarments may help identify congestion. Characteristic of most forms of lymphedema, there should be asymmetry in the amount of congestion even in situations of bilateral involvement.

Regarding treatment for this variant of truncal edema, thorough decongestion of adjacent unaffected quadrants is vital. Identifying target lymph nodes and establishing anastomoses are not sufficient. Rather, extensive truncal decongestion, including deep techniques when possible, is critical to alleviating edema before it becomes chronic. Scar management will likely be a necessary component of treatment due to fluid trapping above or below incisions. Surgical drain scars are often thickened in edematous areas. Scar management in parallel with lymphedema treatment can improve drain scars and assist with lymphatic drainage (see discussion on scars and lymphatic flow).

Surgical Considerations

Modified radical mastectomy, when done in conjunction with axillary dissection, typically includes the removal of level I and II axillary nodes, located lateral to the pectoralis minor muscle and below the axillary vein.[96] Level III axillary nodes (those medial to the pectoralis minor muscle) are not typically removed due to an unfavorable added risk of lymphedema which is not offset by lower morbidity or risk of cancer recurrence. Lymphatic drainage of the breast occurs predominantly through these lateral axillary lymph nodes, but several other pathways exist as well. Thorough utilization of these alternate drainage pathways is essential during MLD therapy to help maximize native pathways to drain breast tissue after axillary dissection.

The pectoral nodes, located at the medial wall of the axilla between the second and seventh ribs, are believed to be the predominant drainage routes for the breast, as evidenced by the relevance of tumor location in the risk of breast edema.[102] As a result, pectoral nodes should be included in all upper truncal quadrant sequences for MLD therapy. The parasternal and internal thoracic nodes assist with drainage toward the medial aspect of the breast near the interaxillary anastomosis. Epigastric and intercostal nodes also help provide deeper drainage pathways. A final and important pathway, the apical nodes are classified as level III within the axillary group, and these nodes are also likely to be preserved during surgery but may be included in radiation treatment.

In recent years, many surgeons have used sentinel node biopsy (SNB) techniques to help minimize lymph node removal during breast cancer resection.[102] The incidence of lymphedema is reduced overall by approximately one-third using SNB, and breast edema may potentially be less likely to occur following SNB.[103,104] However, other studies have not shown a relationship between SNB and lower rates of breast edema, likely reflecting the lack of standardized criteria for the diagnosis of chest wall or breast edema.[100,102] A prospective study of 144 women, conducted by Boughey et al, found no association between breast edema and the type of axillary surgery (SNB vs. axillary node dissection, $p = 0.38$), or number of axillary nodes removed ($p = 0.52$). Instead factors most strongly associated with breast edema included body mass index (BMI; $p = 0.004$), incision location ($p = 0.009$), and whether a prior surgical biopsy had been performed ($p = 0.01$).[105] In another prospective analysis, by Rönkä et al, breast edema was identified in 48% of 160 women who underwent axillary clearance (AC) surgery with positive nodes, 35% of women with axillary clearance and negative nodes, and 23% of those undergoing SNB alone ($p = 0.001–0.0001$ between SNB and AC groups).[106] In the prospective study conducted by Degnim et al, roughly 50% of 124 women developed breast lymphedema following axillary node dissection.[100] Goffman et al performed a retrospective analysis of 240 patients undergoing radiation and reported a 9.6% incidence of breast edema.[107] This study also identified predictors of breast edema among patients undergoing SNB including tumor location (upper outer quadrant of the breast) and greater BMI. Although patients with tumors in the upper outer quadrant of the breast had a higher incidence of breast edema ($p = 0.0042$ when compared with other locations), the tumor quadrant was not a significant predictor of lymphedema of the limb.

One challenging variant of lymphedema involves the management of patients with autologous transverse rectus abdominis myocutaneous (TRAM-flap) breast reconstruction as these individuals may have as many as three incisions in each upper truncal quadrant in addition to the large transverse incision in each of the lower truncal quadrants.[108] Often pedicled TRAM-flap recipients are advised to avoid wearing bras due to possible compromise of blood flow in the inframammary region. Patients should be encouraged to discuss this with the surgeon while therapists should become knowledgeable about local surgeons' techniques and preferences. Breast edema in these patients may be difficult to diagnose because areas of fat necrosis or flap loss may obscure edema or contribute to fluid stasis. Consultation with a reconstructive surgeon is advised to better understand the breast anatomy in a patient with lymphedema, or if you are unsure what processes are occurring in the reconstructed breast. Abdominal lymphatics may be compromised as a result of harvesting the donor flap for breast reconstruction. Research on microlymphatic transfer during TRAM procedures is ongoing as this approach could assist in reducing truncal lymphedema in this population.[109] Recipients of the latissimus-flap reconstruction technique are also at risk for lymphedema. Chang and Kim reviewed 444 consecutive breast reconstructions (394 free flaps and 50 latissimus dorsi flaps) at one institution and found no difference in the incidence of lymphedema based on type of breast reconstruction.[110] Moreover, of 38 patients with pre-existing lymphedema, breast reconstruction proved not to worsen lymphedema, and 23.7% of patients actually demonstrated a significant improvement in lymphedema.[110]

Radiation and Lymphedema of the Thorax

Radiation is a major contributor to the development of breast lymphedema. The inflammation and other tissue effects caused by radiation also adversely affects lymphatic vessels and lymph

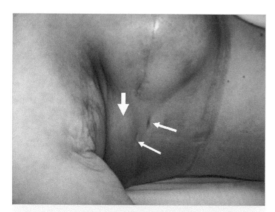

Fig. 5.201 Radiation-related breast edema. Note the sharply demarcated skin changes representing the edges of the radiation field, with thoracic edema located within the region of tissue damage (thick arrow). The scars from prior surgical drains (thin arrows) also appear "deep" and provide further evidence of edema in the lateral thorax.

nodes within the radiation field (see ▶ Fig. 5.201). Clarke et al found that radiation-related (late onset) breast edema, noted in 41% of 74 patients in this study, was less reversible than early-onset thoracic edema.[104] A retrospective review by Back and colleagues documented a 21% incidence of breast edema immediately after breast irradiation in 234 patients. Tumor location is highly relevant because many patients undergo boost doses of radiation to the tumor site, which may also impact the risk of developing breast lymphedema.[107] Other predictors of lymphedema related to radiation factors included hypofractionation (large doses given less than once a day) and full axillary irradiation after nodal dissection. As with the surgical techniques described earlier, the lymphedema therapist must understand the exact regions that have been irradiated so that the most effective MLD sequence may be provided for each individual patient.

Although the effects of radiation to lymphatic tissue have been well described, postoperative breast tissue that has been irradiated has also been shown to have higher levels of lymphatic drainage than the contralateral untreated breast.[111] While this may seem counterintuitive, ongoing inflammation following radiation likely contributes to persistent lymphatic flow. Perbeck et al found a fourfold increase in the lymph flow of the operated irradiated breast (and a 2.5 increase in the operated nonirradiated breast) at 2 to 5 years after treatment.[111] These findings suggest that there is a change in subcutaneous lymph circulation both after surgery and radiation. The authors speculated that radiated fibrocytes lead to increased collagen production and incomplete resorption of deposited collagen. The increased burden on the lymphatic system due to surgery and radiation, accompanied by decreased transport of fluid due to mechanical insufficiency, makes clinically relevant lymphedema likely to develop within the radiation field.

Of clinical importance to the therapist treating postradiation edema in the thorax are the other effects of radiation. In addition to the effects on the lymphatic system, bone demineralization can occur as a result of the destruction of osteoblasts. Use of deep techniques during MLD within the radiation field is unwise for at least 3 months after treatment.[112] In addition, careful inspection of the skin is mandatory before each MLD session to assess for skin burns or breakdown prior to massage or garment application.

Other Factors Contributing to Thoracic Lymphedema

While the etiology of seroma formation following surgical treatment is not well established, it is considered to be one of the most common postoperative complications, and may be a significant predictor in the development of truncal lymphedema. Fu et al found that patients with symptomatic seroma (seroma requiring needle aspiration) were 7.78 to 10.64 times more likely to develop lymphedema of the trunk or upper extremity ($p < 0.001$).[113] Patients with seroma also demonstrated an increase in lymphedema symptoms, such as heaviness, tightness, firmness, pain, or impaired mobility. It is thought that the accumulation of serous fluid which comprises a seroma contributes to local tissue inflammation, resulting in soft-tissue fibrosis, and thus increasing the risk of developing lymphedema.[113] The elevated infection risk in patients requiring repeated needle aspirations of a seroma will increase the risk of lymphedema as well.

Another factor important to consider when evaluating for thoracic lymphedema is the presence of axillary web syndrome (AWS) or cording. The formation of cording following axillary surgery can result in discomfort, pain, and a loss in mobility for patients. The exact etiology of axillary cording remains not well understood. It is thought that cording could be a variation of Mondor's disease, as resected cords may demonstrate thrombosed and dilated lymphatics, and at times, thrombosed superficial veins.[114] Studies have found the incidence of cording to be as high as 72% in patients following axillary lymph node dissection (ALND), versus 20% in patients following sentinel lymph node biopsy.[114] Relatively few studies examine the possible correlation between AWS and onset of lymphedema. In a randomized, single blind, clinical trial conducted by Torres Lacomba et al, it was suggested that the damage that occurs to the lymphatics in an ALND can produce an overload to the lymphatic system, resulting in the onset of lymphedema.[115] Thus, the rationale is that it is beneficial to the patient to address axillary cording early in the treatment plan, thereby reducing the risk of developing lymphedema.

Clinically, we know that surgery permanently lowers lymph transport capacity, but obstructive undergarments can temporarily impair transport as well. The most likely culprit is a poorly fitting bra. Trapped fluid, combined with inflammatory changes and altered lymphatic circulation, can set the stage for chronic chest wall or breast lymphedema. As fluid becomes trapped above the lower border of the bra, the resulting reactive fibrosis alters the tissue texture and may trap additional fluid. While clinicians agree that breast edema is progressive in nature, as with lymphedema of the limb, treatment is therapeutic.

It is important to note, however, that undergarments alone are not always the cause of new thoracic lymphedema. Sometimes fluid can become trapped between incisions and the border of the bra, or between two incisions alone. The ideal therapeutic interventions at this point include finding alternative (and perhaps lightly compressive) undergarments as well as scar management. It is imperative to eliminate fluid accumulation in the area long enough to lower the amount of interstitial protein, so that reaccumulation of lymphedema may be minimized or prevented. Of note, fat necrosis (a process that occurs following reconstructive therapy) should not be mistaken for areas of soft-tissue fibrosis. These naturally occurring necrotic regions following breast reconstructions are much more firm to the touch and can be bumpy as well.[116] Do not attempt to treat these areas because MLD is ineffective for areas of fat necrosis. Similarly, chronic seroma formation can be further irritated by manual techniques. Patients can often hinder adequate healing of a chronic seroma by aggressive self-care and manipulation. As such, differential diagnosis of truncal lymphedema is imperative to ensure patient safety and treatment efficacy.

As always, the patient who presents with an acute onset of truncal and/or upper extremity edema requires a cautious approach. Patients with indwelling central venous catheters can have an increased risk of developing subclavian vein thrombosis. Individuals with subclavian DVT also may present with discomfort in the ipsilateral shoulder or neck, edema in the ipsilateral upper extremity or supraclavicular region, dilated cutaneous veins, jugular venous distinction, or upper extremity cyanosis.[117]

Treatment of Breast Lymphedema

The most important modality in the treatment of truncal lymphedema is MLD.[100,107] MLD sequences must include sufficient truncal pretreatment of deep pathways, adjacent anterior and posterior thorax sequences, as well as peripheral deep techniques (intercostal, parasternal, and paravertebral techniques). Treatment of the involved breast tissue itself should be included while keeping in mind nonaxillary drainage pathways and relevant anastomoses. In cases of acute breast edema, MLD alone may resolve the edema. Multiple sources on breast lymphedema suggest early-onset breast edema to be self-limiting—resolving in 3 to 18 months with minor intervention (MLD alone).[100, 106,107] Of the 38 cases of breast edema followed up in the prospective analysis by Degnim et al, however, only 23 of 33 patients compliant with treatment (combination of MLD with or without compression) had improved symptoms, while others had no change (4) and/or worsening of symptoms (3).[100] Worsening of breast edema despite treatment did occur in three cases despite the application of MLD, compression bra (two), and compressive wrapping (one). Lack of improvement or compliance in some cases may be, in part, due to the lower levels of distress regarding mild breast edema, when compared with limb edema.

Although MLD may be sufficient for some patients with breast lymphedema, more challenging clinical presentations or patients with a higher level of distress about lymphedema may need additional modalities such as compression, Kinesio tape, or low level laser therapy. In addition, many patients with posterior thoracic lymphedema may require compression of the thorax with bandages or compressive garments. Circumferential wrapping with Isoband or Idealbinde can be a great way to determine whether or not a patient can tolerate compression in this region for longer periods of time with compression garments (see section on bandaging materials). The SuperWrap product line by Fabrifoam provides a thin, foam inner layer, which helps the product to stay in place. This product also has a Velcro attachment on one end. Mildly compressive "shapewear" camisoles may provide sufficient increase in interstitial pressure to offset truncal edema as well. These are available at many local department stores. The incorporation of foam "pads" made with closed cell foam or a combination of foams can assist with applying concentrated pressure on a problem area (see ▶ Fig. 5.202). For more diffuse truncal edema, a compression vest may be necessary (see 5.16.5). These can be made to overlap with a compression sleeve for a seamless transition in patients with concomitant limb edema.

Kinesio taping has shown promise in the treatment of lymphedema.[54] Developed by Dr. Kenzo Kase, this unique tape was designed to mimic the skin's own elasticity. The wave-like glue pattern on the back of the tape acts as a neurosensory stimulus which helps decrease pain and edema. Relatively few studies exist on the use of Kinesio tape in the treatment of lymphedema. A prospective study by Finnerty et al examined the effects of Kinesio tape on breast lymphedema, and while a change in circumferential measurements was difficult to establish, the study did find that Kinesio tape contributed to an overall improvement in tissue texture. Kinesio taping may also be beneficial in reducing scar tissue contractures, which will facilitate an improvement in lymph flow.[118] Kinesio taping strategies for the treatment of breast edema include the "fan" application, which works to remove trapped fluid by facilitating movement of lymph fluid into regions of the trunk without impaired lymphatic drainage. This is best utilized along the lateral trunk to direct fluid toward any intact ipsilateral inguinal lymph nodes.

Low level laser therapy (LLLT) (see 3.11.6) can be therapeutic in this region due to its ability to soften tissue fibrosis and surgical scars. For example, Dirican et al found that 76.4% of breast cancer-related lymphedema patients had improved scar mobility after LLLT was incorporated into a traditional CDT program.[119] In addition, patients noted improved shoulder range of motion and decreased edema and pain following two rounds of LLLT. In another study randomizing 50 women with post-mastectomy lymphedema to LLLT versus placebo, shoulder mobility and hand strength were increased, while limb volume was decreased among the patients treated with LLLT three times a week for 12 weeks.[120] The authors hypothesized that LLLT may work to increase lymph vessel diameter and contractility, improve wound healing, reduce scar adhesion to underlying tissues, and

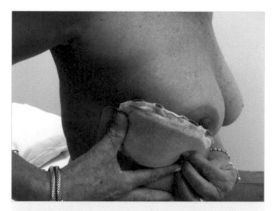

Fig. 5.202 Treatment of lateral breast edema with elastic tape and lateral breast pad insert (foam chips on the skin side, ¼ inch (6-mm) gray foam facing out).

reduce the risk of skin infection. Demir et al performed a randomized control trial using LLLT on the oral mucosa of rats postoperatively, finding the LLLT group had accelerated wound healing and improved epithelialization.[121]

It is relevant to note that treatment of the trunk with pneumatic compression has not demonstrated a significant improvement over pneumatic treatment of the arm alone.[98] It must be stated, however, that patients in this study (42) did not have clinically diagnosed truncal lymphedema (only clinically significant arm lymphedema). A follow-up study on the efficacy of pneumatic treatment on 10 patients with clinically apparent truncal lymphedema was performed to evaluate this potential treatment approach for this population.[33] Though the authors demonstrated a significant reduction in truncal edema symptoms, no significant reduction in truncal girth was reported.[99] Further studies are needed to determine the efficacy of pneumatic compression devices in this population.

5.14.2 Lymphedema of the Abdomen

In general, edema is easier to identify in smaller regions of the body, and thus diffuse abdominal edema can easily go undetected. As with thoracic fluid, lymphedema in the abdomen can exist with or without limb edema. Since lymphedema typically begins distally, abdominal congestion is most commonly a secondary phenomenon which occurs as a result of proximal backup during the development and treatment of limb lymphedema. Obstructive lymphedema due to malignancy is associated with proximal congestion, peau d'orange skin changes, and associated pain. While palliative treatment can improve patient comfort, it should only be performed under close physician supervision due to other ongoing medical processes. Lymphedema in the abdomen related to obesity can take on a "cobblestone" appearance of the skin, secondary skin lesions including localized cellulitis or discolorations and regional pain. One of the differential diagnoses for truncal lymphedema is abdominal edema-related chylous reflux, most often caused by direct damage to the thoracic duct.

Causes of Abdominal Lymphedema

The contributions of surgery and radiation to the development of lymphedema in the abdomen are similar to those in the thorax. Surgical removal of inguinal lymph nodes and/or pelvic lymph nodes can result in secondary lymphedema of the abdomen and lower extremities. Radiation of these areas, such as in the treatment of urologic cancer, contributes to the incidence of lymphedema as well.[122] The use of sentinel lymph node biopsy in the treatment of vulvar cancer has reduced incidence of lymphedema in the legs and, presumably, the abdomen.[123] Surgical techniques such as vertical rectus abdominus (VRAM) flap transfer show promise in improving lymphatic drainage of the lower limb and groin region as well as reducing occurrence of cellulitis.[109]

In addition to these primary causes, abdominal lymphedema can result from progressive lower limb lymphedema, or as a secondary phenomenon from leg compression or MLD therapy. Patients with lymphedema of the lower extremities are at risk of developing abdominal lymphedema since lymphatic fluid from distal regions must drain via the abdominal lymphatic network. As such, significant leg and genital congestion can result in backup in the abdomen. The borders of compression garments as well as other undergarments (as shown in ▶ Fig. 5.203) can trap edema in the abdomen, thus expanding the affected areas. The rationale for treatment of abdominal lymphedema extends beyond patient comfort. For starters, chronic lower limb lymphedema will not improve unless abdominal lymphedema is addressed. Furthermore, the risk of secondary genital lymphedema is worrisome, as its development brings a significant increased risk of cellulitis as well as functional mobility restrictions.[98] Treatment of lower limb lymphedema without pretreatment of the abdomen, such as with repetitive use of pneumatic compression devices, can result in adjacent truncal congestion. In one retrospective analysis, 23 of 53 patients who used pneumatic compression developed truncal congestion ($p < 0.001$).[1]

Massive localized lymphedema (MLL) describes obesity-related lymphedema in the proximal lower limbs or abdomen and is also associated with higher cellulitis rates.[124] Characteristics of MLL include peau d'orange appearance of the tissues, and one case series of five patients with chronic MLL demonstrated a concern for secondary angiosarcoma potentially related to the chronic edema, inflammation, and fibrosis.[124] While obesity-related MLL is difficult to treat, reduction in weight in parallel with reduction in lymphedema provides a combined approach to therapy which helps reduce the risk of secondary

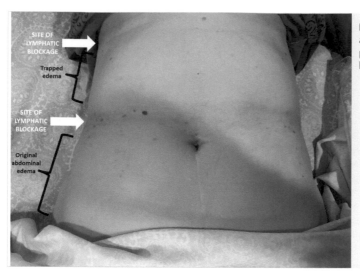

Fig. 5.203 Abdominal edema trapped above top band of waist-high compression garments and below inferior bra band.

complications of lymphedema and the underlying disease etiology.

Treatment of Abdominal Lymphedema

Treatment of abdominal lymphedema begins with MLD. Visceral and deep techniques (see 5.2) should be employed if no contraindications exist. Expansion of truncal sequences to include medial to lateral techniques on the abdomen itself may be necessary if the patient's abdomen is large or edematous. Deep techniques on the posterior lower quadrants including quadratus lumborum technique and lumbar paravertebral techniques should be utilized. Diaphragmatic breathing can be repeated several times during and after treatment to enhance deep lymphatic drainage.

The application of compression to the abdomen can be challenging. Compressive bandaging with the "hip spica" technique bilaterally using Isoband or Idealbinde bandages is a good start. This leaves the groin open to allow the patient to use the bathroom without removing bandages. Shapewear garments such as Spanx or compressive biker shorts can supply longer term compression or can be applied over bandages. For larger patients, abdominal binders such as those used for lumbar support can provide adjustable compression. When ordering compression garments, custom flat-knit garments with truncal compression extending up to or beyond the navel are best. Chronic compression with open crotch garments are discouraged as they can allow fluid to pool in the genital region. Foam pads using a combination of open and closed cell foam allow for increased compression in problem areas. Owing to the need for these items to be washed regularly, commercially available Swell Spots or other washable quilted garments are recommended. Patients with abdominal lymphedema who exhibit recurrent cellulitis must be closely assessed for genital involvement. It may be necessary to consult with infectious disease specialists to assist with the management of these infections.

5.15 Bandaging in the Presence of Wounds

Specialists in lymphedema treatment are likely to see wounds in their practice. This is not because lymphedema as a disease process causes wounds but rather because lymphedema is often associated with pathologies of other organ systems that lead to wounds, most often circulatory pathology (which can cause venous, arterial, or diabetic ulcers) and/or injury to the skin (maceration of skinfolds or mechanical disruption of edematous tissue). Previous sections of this chapter have examined the close connection between venous pathology and lymphatic impairment, as well as treatment of wounds.

In this section, we will discuss the application of compression in the presence of open wounds and will focus on the lower extremities, as that is the most common region of the body in which CLTs will see open wounds. In the lymphedema literature, there is little discussion of compression over wounds other than to say some version of: "apply the short-stretch lymphedema bandage after treating and dressing the wound."[125,126] Wound care literature on the other hand discusses compression for edema extensively, focusing primarily on the debate between single-layer compression versus multilayer compression and the differences between elastic compression bandages and inelastic compression bandages.[127] In recent years, wound care literature is coming to accept a skilled short-stretch bandaging approach as a truly valuable skill set in the larger arsenal of wound care.[128] In many cases, management of edema is the primary factor in healing a wound. With our understanding of wound healing and the innate connection of the lymph system to all edemas, we come to realize that the lymphedema bandage is the best tool to use with wound-associated edemas. We will discuss factors that should be taken into account and modifications that could be made by the therapist when applying a short-stretch compression bandage if a wound is present.

5.15.1 Precautions and Contraindications

The clinician must first assess for potential contraindications and/or precautions that might lead to adverse outcomes if compression is applied inappropriately. Contraindications include DVT and arterial occlusive disease.

Arterial status must be assessed and adequate for application of compression. This assessment may be done clinically (e.g., palpation of arterial pulses, capillary refill test, presence of intermittent claudication)[128] and, if indicated, thorough noninvasive diagnostic studies such as ankle brachial index (ABI) and TcPO$_2$. These tests are discussed in depth in section "Wounds and Skin Lesions" in Chapter 3. ABI values less than 0.5 indicate severe arterial occlusive disease and compression is contraindicated. We will discuss later how a clinician can address edema in the presence of mildly reduced arterial inflow. DVT must be ruled out before application of compression. The primary test to rule out DVT is a duplex Doppler ultrasound. In the presence of a positive DVT test, compression is contraindicated until there is documented clearance for compression by the referring physician and the patient is on a therapeutic level of anticoagulation.

Additional precautions to consider include reduced sensation in diabetic patients, patients with peripheral neuropathy (not related to diabetes), or patients with sensation impairments due to other possible neurological pathologies. Also, a common contraindication/precaution that may be seen in edema/wound patients is heart failure.

Treatment of wounds with compression is best approached in two distinct phases. The first phase is direct wound care. The second phase is skilled application of a short-stretch compression bandage.

5.15.2 Treat the Wound

As noted earlier, a detailed look at the proper management of wounds is addressed in Chapter 3. In many cases in which a patient with significant edema in conjunction with a wound is referred to the lymphedema specialist, the wound care plan has already been determined by the referring clinician. Therefore, in the first phase of a treatment session, fully complete the wound care as per the plan determined by the referring clinician. Otherwise, it is recommended the treating therapist to refer to Section 3.13 Wounds and Skin Lesions in Chapter 3 for guidance on wound bed treatment and dressing application.

Managing Excess Drainage

Often the most important consideration for the lymphedema specialist when treating patients with highly draining wounds is managing copious amounts of exudate. The range of wound care products includes many that are designed specifically to absorb high volumes of exudate. Even in a case in which the referring provider has directed the specifics of the primary wound dressing, it may fall to the CLT to choose an adequate, absorbent secondary dressing for exudate management.

There are two reasons to adequately manage wound exudate. The first is to prevent the accumulation of exudate in the wound bed or on the surrounding intact tissue. This can lead to delayed wound healing or additional skin breakdown through uncontrolled maceration of tissue. The second reason is to prevent the exudate from collecting external to the wound dressing and therefore on the compression bandage materials. Lymphedema bandage materials are meant to be reused, but soiled bandage materials should not be reapplied to a patient.

Occasionally, the therapist will come across a clinical case in which the drainage from the wound, or even weeping from the surrounding edematous tissue (termed "lymphorrhea"), is not adequately contained by even the most absorbent wound care products. In these cases, the therapist may need to look beyond the typical wound products to find more conventional products for absorption of fluid. These include feminine pads and diapers. As the purpose is to absorb excessive drainage, they can be safely and strategically placed in addition to the primary wound dressing but prior to application of the compression bandage to absorb excess exudate (see Section 5.15.4).

Frequency of Visits

An additional consideration when factoring exudate management into the treatment plan is frequency of treatment visits. In the CDT model of lymphedema treatment, the default treatment frequency is five times a week. Yet in many typical outpatient wound treatment clinics, the usual frequency is once a week. If the clinician is working in a clinic in which the default frequency is once a week, it may be necessary to temporarily increase the frequency of patient visits until the exudate is brought under control. This may mean daily treatments at the initiation of treatment, which can be reduced incrementally as the lymphorrhea and wound drainage are brought under control. This higher frequency of visits not only keeps exudate from soiling compression bandage materials but also promotes a shorter length of treatment by limiting the adverse effects of exudate on intact tissue and in the wound bed.

5.15.3 Apply Compression

Once the wound is properly dressed and exudate management has been addressed, the second phase is application of the lymphedema bandage directly over the completed wound dressing. It may be appropriate in many cases to refer to 5.11.3 earlier in this chapter for guidance on the application of a standard short-stretch compression bandage with foam, addressing edema from the toes to the knee. (Due to the combination nature of the edema in many wound patients, in most cases, the combination edema can be effectively addressed with short-stretch bandages to the knee only.) As with all lymphedema bandages, the CLT pays close attention when using the standard bandage approach to create an effective compression gradient. Following LaPlace's law, the CLT uses foams of different densities and proper spacing and layering of bandages with consistent, even tension to achieve effective but also safe compression.

Modify the Standard Lymphedema Bandage

However, the challenge that occurs with many wound patients, due to the frequent presence of pathologies in addition to lymphedema, is that the shape of the limb may not allow for an effective and safe compression gradient when using the basic lymphedema bandage. Several of the more common variants in the shape of the limb are outlined below. These include the inverted champagne bottle, the columnar-shaped leg, and the reverse cone shape.

Inverted Champagne Bottle Shape

Many patients with severe venous pathology will present with an inverted champagne bottle shape to the leg: a very narrow and tightly bound lipodermatosclerotic fibrosis at the ankle and distal leg, with the proximal leg demonstrating more typical lymphedematous fibrosis with pitting and expanded circumference of the limb. This might also be termed a severe (rather than gradual) cone shape to the limb. The goal of any lymphedema bandage is to create a compression gradient over a more gradual cone shape. The therapist can address this issue by increasing the circumference of the limb distally, artificially creating the more gradual cone shape needed for safe compression. Increasing the circumference of the limb distally can be achieved by building up the limb with additional or thicker gray foam, by using additional layers of cotton padding or a combination of the two.

A second strategy to consider for the inverted champagne bottle-shaped leg is to modify the allocation of layers of bandage to the limb. As we know that, given the same radius of the limb under the bandage, the number of bandage layers is directly proportional to the level of compression (i.e., more layers over a certain part of the limb equal more compression, fewer layers equal less compression), and that equal layers of bandage over a cone shape (progressively increasing radius) leads to an effective compression gradient, the basic lymphedema bandage makes use of the gradual cone shape to create a safe and effective

5

compression gradient. In the case of an inverted champagne bottle shape, it makes sense to space the layers of bandage wider (fewer bandage layers over skin) at the narrow, distal portion of the leg, and then space the layers of bandage closer at the wider, proximal portion of the limb. This will create a safe, effective, and gradual compression gradient. As the lymphedema bandage uses more than one bandage from the ankle to the knee, this modification of layers of bandage can be done with just one bandage to make a more gradual modification to the basic lymphedema bandage, or may be done with a second or even third short-stretch bandage to have a greater impact on the gradient. The number of bandages applied with modified spacing is a matter of clinical judgment for the therapist in each individual case and can be modified visit to visit as the shape of the limb is brought steadily to a more normal, gradual cone shape.

Columnar Shape

The absence of a cone shape (also called "a columnar shape") also requires a modification to the basic lymphedema bandage to create an effective compression gradient. A columnar-shaped limb is not an uncommon presentation in a patient with a wound. In this case, as the radius is essentially unchanging from the ankle to the knee, taking the standard approach of evenly spaced layers of bandage applied over even layers of foam would result in an absence of compression gradient. Again, there are two possible modifications to the bandage that can generate the gradient compression needed to reduce the edema.

The first is to artificially change the shape of the limb by building up padding layers in the proximal portion of the limb, making the proximal limb wider than the distal limb and therefore approaching a cone shape. The second is to modify the allocation of layers of bandage so that there are more layers distally than proximally, thus creating greater pressure distally. As with the inverted cone shape modifications, this closer spacing can be done with just one bandage or more than one bandage, depending on each patient's unique presentation and the level of modification indicated. As the shape of the limb is changed over the course of treatment by appropriately applied short-stretch compression, it is likely that the limb will become gradually more cone-shaped and the clinician will need to change the bandage approach

so that it is more in line with the standard lymphedema bandage.

Reverse Cone Shape

Occasionally, a clinician may encounter a wound and edema patient in which the shape of the calf is more of a reverse cone shape, with a wider radius at the distal leg and ankle, and a smaller radius on the proximal calf. Clearly, a standard lymphedema bandage would not result in an effective compression gradient if applied to this limb. As we have seen earlier, the goal is to approximate a gradual cone shape by using extra padding layers to modify the shape of the limb and/or modifying the allocation of bandage layers to create more pressure distally and less proximally. In the case of a reverse cone shape, it may make sense to use both strategies: build up the radius proximally with foam and cotton padding layers and also to increase the bandage layers distally while applying fewer bandage layers proximally. Therefore, the clinician may add extra turns of cotton padding and 12-mm (or thicker if indicated) gray foam to the proximal limb. This should result in an approximation of a column shape. Then, as with the strategy to address a columnar-shaped limb as noted earlier, the compression bandages can be applied with greater overlap distally and less overlap proximally. As additional layers of bandage are applied, it will be up to the clinician to continue applying bandages with extra bandage layers distally, or to return to the standard approach of even spacing of the bandage layers throughout the limb.

If comorbidities include diabetes or neurological impairment that hinder protective sensation, these must be taken into account when devising a safe as well as effective compression bandage. Compression always carries the risk of impairment of arterial flow and potential ischemia with tissue necrosis; therefore, take precautions to, first, pad the bandage adequately with foam to guard against the occurrence of ischemia (typically, this can occur at bony prominences such as the navicular, the tibial crest, the malleoli, and the lateral borders of the first and fifth metatarsal heads); and second, to allow for adequate visualization of the toes to allow for neurovascular checks. Often, in patients with neurologic impairment, the level of pressure due to the bandage can be less than would be seen with the standard lymphedema bandage. Therefore, fewer total bandages may be applied to lessen the overall compression level.

5

5

Suggestions for patients with arterial compression are outlined as follows.

Arterial Insufficiency

In patients with decreased arterial perfusion, diagnostic studies quantifying the lack of arterial perfusion should be obtained. Literature now supports light short-stretch compression to address edema in patients with an ABI of 0.5 or above. Even so, it makes sense to apply lower levels of compression by applying fewer layers of bandages. Also, patients with lower levels of arterial perfusion will be more susceptible to ischemia at bony prominences. Therefore, in this case, the goal when applying short-stretch compression bandages is to guard against ischemia while also providing edema reduction with an adequate compression gradient. To guard against ischemia, extra open cell, gray foam padding with appropriate relief cut into the foam at sites of bony prominences should be incorporated into the bandage. It may be helpful to think of the application of foam under the bandages as a fully encompassing cushion or pillow to the limb, which, when the short-stretch compression is applied over the top of it, helps evenly transmit the compression forces to the limb while at the same time softening the pressures at points of concern such as bony prominences. Then the light compression force is achieved by modifying the standard lymphedema bandage—primarily by using fewer bandages so that there are fewer layers over any point of the limb. This can be done by using just two bandages: one bandage to cover the foot and ankle using the Roman sandal combined with the HAS pattern, and one bandage to cover the leg from malleoli to proximal calf. It is also possible to apply just one short-stretch bandage: start with one cycle of the Roman sandal pattern, one cycle of HAS and finish with a spiral to the calf.

5.15.4 Negative Pressure Wound Therapy and Compression

CLTs who encounter wounds in their practice may also encounter negative pressure wound therapy (NPWT), also known as "vacuum-assisted-closure," or generically "wound-vac." Lymphedema may be a concomitant disease in addition to the primary wound diagnosis that indicates the need for NPWT, or a direct factor in a wound that is the indication for NPWT. In either case, compression may be indicated directly over the NPWT.

NPWT application and management requires proper training. Untrained clinicians should not attempt to apply, fix, or manage the dressing or the settings of a NPWT pump. Given the properly trained clinician has established the need for NPWT, and if compression therapy is indicated for this situation, compression may be applied over the NPWT. Therefore, it is best if the wound specialist and the lymphedema specialist collaborate in order to ensure safe and optimal outcomes. Per guidelines of one manufacturer of NPWT devices,[129] compression is not contraindicated when using NPWT as long as

- Compression is indicated for the pathology underlying the ulcer presentation.
- Caution is exercised against pressure points that may result in tissue damage or discomfort to the patient.
- A trac pad is not placed under any form of compression.
- Care is taken to prevent further trauma and/or pressure when placing NPWT tubing particularly over bony prominences.

It is commonly thought the goal of NPWT is to remove fluid from a wound, but it is much more than that. The purpose of NPWT can be listed as follows:

- Apply controlled, localized negative pressure to help draw wound edges.
- Provide a closed, moist wound healing environment.
- Promote perfusion and granulation tissue formation.
- Remove exudate and infectious materials as well as edema.
- Stimulation of cell proliferation.
- Reduction in wound volume.
- Removal of free radicals from the wound.
- Decrease wound bioburden.
- Prepare the wound bed for closure.

Compression therapy is shown to decrease excess proteins seen in chronic ulcers[130]; therefore, the goals of compression/CDT are in line with the goals of NPWT, that is, to promote healing of the integument through removal of excess fluid and wastes.

There is a paucity of literature speaking specifically to the use of compression with NPWT. When literature addresses compression used in conjunction with NPWT, it mentions multilayer compression, but does not offer specifics on the technique of compression application. This author is aware from personal interaction with clinicians from around the country that many clinics are applying compression over NPWT.[131]

In applying compression to a limb with NPWT, the primary concern is to avoid disruption of the trac pad and the vacuum tubing. The trac pad is the firm plastic disc applied over the foam of the NPWT that then connects to the tubing that adjoins the wound site to the vacuum pump. Applying compression directly over the trac pad, the tubing may press these firm objects into the wound bed or against intact skin, potentially leading to skin injury, or may cause impingement of the trac pad or tubing, interfering with the function of the NPWT. As trained lymphedema specialists take into account varying tissue types and boney prominences when customizing compression to individual patients, modification of bandage application falls within the CLT skill set when taking the trac pad and tubing into account.

The NPWT application and setup should be complete before initiating the compression bandage. Collaboratively, the wound specialist may be sure to orient the vacuum tubing in a direction that works best with the compression bandage, which is typically directed laterally and/or superiorly. The following are suggested modifications when applying lymphedema short-stretch compression with foam over a limb that also has NPWT. The creative clinician may devise other modifications that supply effective compression without adverse outcomes.

Suggested Compression Modifications

The compression bandage should be a typical lymphedema bandage based on the lymphedema presentation and shape of the limb, regardless of the wound or presence of NPWT. Once the basic bandage strategy is determined, minor modifications due to the presence of NPWT are considered. Simply stated, the goal is to place foam relief around the trac pad, then to apply the compression bandage material such that the trac pad and tubing are completely or mostly *outside* of the short-stretch bandages. If these goals are met, there can be effective compression without disruption of the NPWT or adverse tissue responses due to pressure over the tubing or trac pad.

Lower Extremity Modifications

The following suggestions are based on lower extremity compression bandaging and presume the use of ½-inch gray foam in the standard fashion, which is fully encompassing the calf as well as dorsal foot and incorporating malleolar foam pieces. *As a note, the use of closed cell orange foam around the trac pad is not recommended.*

A small hole is cut into the stockinette at the position of the trac pad, and the tubing of the NPWT is threaded through this hole when the stockinette is applied. If the wound/trac pad is on the calf, either anteriorly or posteriorly, a limited cut is placed in the gray foam from the medial or lateral edge to the location of the trac pad. The external surface of that cut is beveled slightly. This cut from the side of the large piece of foam allows the foam to be placed over the limb (and over the wound dressing of the NPWT) in the normal position while allowing the vacuum tubing to extend external to the foam. The cut in the foam also then becomes the relief for the trac pad, as the gray foam will surround the trac pad but allow it to protrude through the foam. The bandage to secure the foam can then be applied, with emphasis on light tension. The light tension is to account for an uneven overlapping of the bandage layers as the foam-securing bandage is applied around the trac pad and tubing, where it protrudes through the gray foam padding. Because there is light tension in the foam-securing bandage, it is then permissible to fold the securing bandage in order to allow it to pass closely by, but not over the trac pad. The vacuum tubing should also remain outside of the bandage.

The remaining layers of the compression bandage are the typical short-stretch bandages applied with the typical approximately 50% tension. These bandages are applied in a spiral or herringbone pattern. Depending on the number of bandages used, as the spiral pattern is altered slightly in order to avoid covering the trac pad and tubing, it is important that a spiral in the opposite direction is used in a succeeding bandage in order to help ameliorate the alteration of bandage layers around the trac pad. It is also advisable to incorporate one or two herringbone patterns, if the number of bandages allows, with the "X" of the herringbone occurring in the plane of the trac pad. This will allow for the upward and downward portions of the "X" to skirt around the protruding trac pad.

According to the authors, the final short-stretch bandage, when applied, may be allowed to cover the trac pad as so many preceding bandages have accounted for protecting the trac pad and tubing from unwanted pressure. In addition, all the layers of foam and bandage provide an appreciable level

5

of relief for the small amount of pressure the final bandage places directly over the trac pad and tubing. The tubing will then extend from under the final bandage laterally and/or superiorly and can then be secured to the outside of the compression bandage with tape. The experienced CLT will recognize that the decreased layers of bandage directly over the wound and trac pad means the level of compression in that area is less than the other areas of the compression bandage. The fluid-removing effects of the NPWT largely compensate for disruption of gradient pressure within the bandage. This illustrates the supportive nature of these two modalities when used together.

5.15.5 Summary

Wound patients with lymphedema or mixed etiology edemas can be challenging for the lymphedema specialist, but also very rewarding. The specialized knowledge and skills of the lymphedema specialist are uniquely suited to healing wounds in the presence of edema. The CLT is often that final puzzle piece required to heal wounds that have otherwise been non-healing for months or even years.

5.16 Measurements for Compression Garments

To ensure preservation and improvement of the therapeutic success achieved in phase 1 of the treatment, it is imperative that a compression garment is chosen that meets the patient's individual needs. To select the correct style (ready-made or custom-made), compression level, length, and, if necessary, fastening systems, the patient's age, physical abilities (and limitations), lifestyle, type of lymphedema, and any other conditions must be taken into consideration.

Most manufacturers provide compression garments in a variety of sizes. Custom garments should be ordered if the extremity is either too large or too small for standard-size garments or if a single compression garment with a compression level of more than 50 mm Hg is necessary. The length of a compression garment is indicated by a system of letters used by the manufacturers. These letters represent the measuring points on both ends of the garment; an arm sleeve that covers the extremity from the wrist (measuring point C) to

the axilla (measuring point G), for example, is called a C-G sleeve. An open-toe stocking covering the lower extremity from the foot (point A) to the groin (point G) would be referred to as an A-G stocking.

Only trained individuals with a thorough understanding of lymphedema and its implications should take measurements. Ill-fitting and ineffective compression garments not only produce poor results but also can be dangerous to the patient.

To increase effectiveness, it would be beneficial to have an assistant present at the time of measurements to complete the data on the measuring forms.

Measurements should be taken at the end of the intensive phase of CDT (phase 1), when the extremity is at its most reduced state. Ideally, the measurements should be taken early in the morning, at the end of a treatment, or after the compression bandages have been removed.

Materials needed to take measurements include a measuring board obtained from the manufacturer. These boards simplify the measuring process and increase accuracy. Other materials needed are a metric system measuring tape (measurements should be taken in centimeters), a nontoxic skin marker, a pen, and a measuring form (order form).

5.16.1 Measuring for Stockings and Pantyhose

Circumferential as well as length measurements are required. The skin of the patient should be marked with a nontoxic, nonpermanent marker on each circumferential measuring point (these markings also determine the length measurements). The length measurements are taken on the inside of the leg from each circumferential point to the sole of the foot (▶ Fig. 5.204).

If the lymphedematous leg is unusually shaped, the positions of the circumferential measurement points, as well as the length measurements, should be taken first on the unaffected extremity. This technique helps identify the position of the measuring points on the affected extremity.

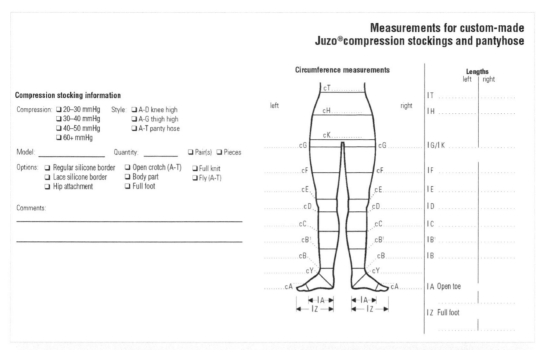

Measurements for custom-made Juzo®compression stockings and pantyhose

Compression stocking information

Compression: ❏ 20–30 mmHg   Style: ❏ A-D knee high
           ❏ 30–40 mmHg   ❏ A-G thigh high
           ❏ 40–50 mmHg   ❏ A-T panty hose
           ❏ 60+ mmHg

Model: _____   Quantity: _____   ❏ Pair(s) ❏ Pieces

Options: ❏ Regular silicone border   ❏ Open crotch (A-T)   ❏ Full knit
        ❏ Lace silicone border   ❏ Body part   ❏ Fly (A-T)
        ❏ Hip attachment   ❏ Full foot

Comments:

Fig. 5.204 Measurement form for compression stockings and pantyhose (with permission from Juzo USA, Inc.)

Required Measurements for Custom-Made Knee-High Stockings (A-D)

Circumferential measuring points (indicate the position of all measuring points with nontoxic, nonpermanent marker):

- *Point cA*: Around the metatarsal heads, horizontally around the base of the fifth metatarsal base. This measurement should be taken loosely and also be checked with the patient standing as the foot may splay in weight bearing with an increase in circumference. If this measurement is taken too tight, garment pressure in the areas of the first and fifth metatarsal heads may be too uncomfortable.
- *Point cY*: Around the instep and the heel at a 45-degree angle, taken with the ankle in maximum active dorsiflexion. For compression higher than level III, it is generally recommended that at least 1 cm be added to the measurement for additional comfort during wear.
- *Point cB*: Around the smallest circumference above the malleoli. This is the point of greatest compression of the garment when worn. Several measurements are recommended to ensure the location of this point, and then marked. This measurement should not be taken tightly.

- *Point cB1*: Around the lower leg at the transition between the Achilles tendon and the calf musculature (plantar flexion in the ankle helps find this measuring point).
- *Point cC*: Around the largest circumference of the calf.
- *Point cD*: Smallest circumference of the knee, in the area of the fibular head. It is recommended to have the patient flex the knee with the tape measure in place to ensure the garment will not cut into, or roll at the back of, the knee while the patient sits. However, the garment should be long enough to include the entire calf musculature. In patients with a columnar calf, the addition of a silicone band may be necessary to keep the garment in place.

Length measurements: For open-toe stockings, take the length measurement from point cA to the heel (I–A); if a closed toe stocking is required, the length measurement from the longest toe to the heel is taken (I–Z). The length measurements from the sole of the foot (even with the floor or the measuring board) to the circumferential measurement points cB to cD are taken with the ankle in 90 degrees of dorsiflexion.

Required Measurements for Standard-Size Knee-High Stockings (A–D)

- Circumferential measuring points: points cB and cC.
- Length measurements: from the floor to circumferential measuring point cD (determines the length of the stocking).

Required Measurements for Custom-Made Thigh-High Stockings (A–G)

Circumferential measuring points in addition to the ones taken for A–D stockings (indicate the position of all measuring points with nontoxic, nonpermanent marker):

- *Point cE*: Around the popliteal fossa and the patella with the leg slightly bent.
- *Point cF*: Around the middle of the thigh. Because the thigh often has a larger circumference at this point and may have very soft tissue, the circumferential measurement may be taken more firmly to address the need to contain this tissue effectively.
- *Point cG*: Horizontally around the proximal end of the thigh with the patient standing.

Length measurements: Taken on the inside of the leg between the floor and each circumferential measuring point.

Required Measurements for Standard-Size Thigh-High Stockings (A–G)

- Circumferential measuring points: Points cB, cC, and cG.
- Length measurements: From the floor to circumferential measuring point cG, on the inside of the leg.

Required Measurements for Custom-Made Pantyhose (A–T)

Circumferential measuring points in addition to the ones taken for A–G stockings (indicate the position of all measuring points with nontoxic, nonpermanent marker):

All measurements are taken with the patient standing.

- *Point cK*: Taken at the same height as measuring point cG, but includes the circumference of both thighs and buttocks.
- *Point cH*: Around the greatest circumference of the hips. In patients with a pendulous abdomen, the application of a wide bandage (20 cm), or having the patient wear lightweight spandex shorts to support the tissue, is recommended to assist in taking accurate measurements.
- *Point cT*: Around the waist, just above the iliac crest. It is recommended that this measurement should be taken above the apex of the abdomen to ensure that the garment will have adequate purchase to avoid slipping down during wear. It is rare that a garment measured to end below the umbilicus will stay in place. In practice, this measurement point may not be at the true waist in an individual with a large abdomen.

Depending on the condition, the abdominal part of the compression pantyhose may be ordered with full, partial, or neutral compression. Adjustable and highly elastic abdominal parts are available (pregnancy, postsurgical conditions). Front openings may be ordered for male patients.

Length measurements between the floor and up to circumferential point cG are taken on the inside of the leg. Length measurements between the floor to points cH and cT are taken on the outside.

Required Measurements for Standard-Size Pantyhose (A–T)

- Circumferential measuring points: Points cB, cC, cG, and cH.
- Length measurements: From the floor to circumferential measuring point cG.

Depending on the condition, the abdominal part of the compression pantyhose may be ordered with full, partial, or neutral compression. Adjustable and highly elastic abdominal parts are available (pregnancy, postsurgical conditions). Front openings may be ordered for male patients.

5.16.2 Measuring for Arm Sleeves

Circumferential as well as length measurements are required. The skin of the patient should be marked with a nontoxic, nonpermanent marker on each circumferential measuring point. The length measurements are taken on the anterior arm from the wrist (point c) to each circumferential measuring point (▶ Fig. 5.205).

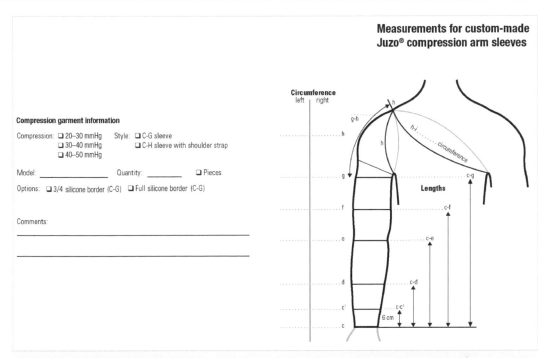

Measurements for custom-made Juzo® compression arm sleeves

Compression garment information

Compression: ☐ 20–30 mmHg Style: ☐ C-G sleeve
☐ 30–40 mmHg ☐ C-H sleeve with shoulder strap
☐ 40–50 mmHg

Model: _____ Quantity: _____ ☐ Pieces

Options: ☐ 3/4 silicone border (C-G) ☐ Full silicone border (C-G)

Comments:
_____
_____

Fig. 5.205 Measurement form for compression arm sleeves (with permission from Juzo USA, Inc.).

Required Measurements for Custom-Made Arm Sleeves (C–G)

Circumferential measuring points (indicate the position of all measuring points with nontoxic, nonpermanent marker):

- *Point c*: Around the smallest circumference of the wrist, on the transition from the hand to the forearm.
- *Point c1*: This measurement is necessary for arm sleeves worn in combination with compression gauntlets. The measurement is taken around the forearm, 6 cm (may vary; see Section 5.16.3 later in this chapter) proximal to circumferential measuring point c.
- *Point d*: Around the forearm, at the midpoint between point c and the elbow.
- *Point e*: Around the elbow, in the cubital fossa, with the arm slightly bent 30 to 40 degrees to allow for ease when the garment is worn as the elbow is always flexed during wear. A patient's occupation should be taken into account, as a person who sits at a computer all day has more acute flexion angle at the elbow for long periods of time and it may be correct to measure with a more acute elbow angle.

- *Point f*: Around the middle of the upper arm.
- *Point g*: Around the proximal end of the upper arm, in the axillary fold. This measurement point can be easily determined with a paper placed up into the axilla with the arm on the patient's side. The paper is folded forward over the arm and the spot is marked.

If a shoulder cover and strap is required:
- *Point h*: Vertically around the axilla and the shoulder.
- *Point h–i*: This measurement is necessary to acquire the length of the shoulder strap. It is taken circumferentially from measuring point h across the thorax to the opposite axilla.

Length measurements are taken from the circumferential measuring point c along the anterior arm (the arm is in supination) to each circumferential measuring point.

For arm sleeves with a shoulder cover and strap, an additional length measurement is required:
- *g–h*: This length is taken on the outside of the shoulder between circumferential measuring points g and h.

5

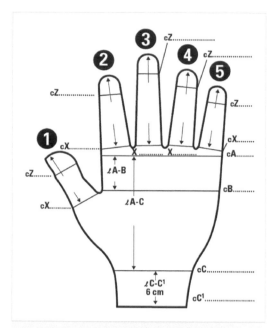

Fig. 5.206 Measurement form for hand and finger compression garments (with permission from Juzo USA, Inc.)

Required Measurements for Standard-Size Arm Sleeves (C–G)

- Circumferential measuring points: Points c, e, and g.
- Length measurements: From circumferential measuring point c to circumferential measuring point g along the anterior arm (forearm in supination).

5.16.3 Measuring for Hand and Finger Compression Garments

See ▶ Fig. 5.206 for an example of a measurement form for hand and finger compression garments.

Required Measurements for Compression Gauntlets with Finger Stubs or Closed Fingers

Circumferential measuring points (indicate the position of all measuring points with nontoxic, nonpermanent marker):

Though many patients find that they are able to control swelling with only a sleeve, for increased activities, strenuous exercise, or plane flights, additional compression for the hand is prudent.

With any history of hand swelling, a glove is preferred for appropriate compression. Compression gloves are ordered with open fingertips to accommodate better function. Gloves and gauntlets are ordered separately from an arm sleeve to allow the patient to remove the hand compression for functional activities. It is rare for a sleeve to be ordered with the gauntlet or glove attached unless deemed necessary for better edema control.

The fingers should be slightly spread for points cA and cB:

- *Point cA*: Around the metacarpus (bases of the second and fifth metacarpal bones).
- *Point cB*: Around the metacarpus, at the web space between the thumb and the index finger (parallel to point cA). In elderly patients with atrophy of the intrinsic muscles of the hand, this measurement may be smaller than point a. In this instance, the point b measurement must be adjusted so that it is not smaller than the one on point a, as otherwise fluid may be trapped in the distal hand during wear.
- *Point cC*: Around the smallest circumference of the wrist, on the transition from the hand to the forearm.
- *Point cC1*: Around the forearm, 6 cm (see also length measurement C–C1) proximal to the circumferential measuring point cC.
- *Point Cz*: Around the distal end of each finger and the thumb, at the point where the end of the finger portion is desired (finger stubs should not end in the joint/crease area of the finger).
- *Point Cx*: Around the proximal end of each finger and the thumb. Point Cx can be easily identified using the crease on the palmar surface of the finger bases. This measurement should be taken carefully without tension, as the circumference of fingers is small and too much compression is likely if measured with tension.

Length measurements for the hand are taken with reference to point Ca. Finger and thumb lengths are taken from the web space to just proximal to the nail bed. It is recommended that finger lengths do not end at the joint lines given this is a common reason for discomfort and a potential source of skin irritation. Length measurements can be taken either directly from the palmar surface of the hand or from a paper tracing of the hand, which should be done with the patient's hand pronated. Depending on the manufacturer, both methods may be acceptable and it is recommended that the therapist choose one method and use it consistently when measuring for better accuracy.

Due to LaPlace's law, gauntlets and gloves may not be completely effective in controlling hand swelling. Several suggestions may improve this control and should be considered in determining length measurements. If the a–b measurement is too long, for example, there will be excess fabric on the dorsum of the hand, which will lead to less compression than may be applied if this length was more precise. Patients will often request that the finger lengths be shorter than covering the full length of the finger to the nail bed. However, when the patient flexes the fingers during wear, this may cause a tensioning of the fabric covering the dorsum of the hand and contribute to better edema control. Shortened finger lengths in a glove eliminate this tensioning effect.

A–B: Distance between circumferential measuring points cA and cB. Take measurement with open palm.

C–C1: Distance between circumferential measurements cC and cC1. This measurement determines the length of the wrist extension. If an extension shorter than 6 cm is desired, circumferential measurement cC1 should be taken at the appropriate point.

Cz–Cx: The length of each finger is measured between the circumferential measuring points cZ and cX.

For a gauntlet with closed fingers, the lengths of the fingers between circumferential measuring points Cx and the fingertips are taken.

Required Measurements for Compression Gauntlets with Thumb Stub (No Finger Swelling)

Circumferential measuring points (indicate the position of all measuring points with nontoxic, nonpermanent marker):

- *Point cA*: Around the metacarpus (bases of the second and fifth metacarpal bones). The fingers should be slightly spread for this measurement.
- *Point cC*: Around the smallest circumference of the wrist, on the transition from the hand to the forearm.

No length measurements are necessary for standard-size compression gauntlets.

5.16.4 Compression Neck and Chin Straps and Face Masks

Pressure garments for the face are available as neck and chin straps and as partial or full-face masks. Full-face masks may be ordered with or without openings for the eyes, nose, or mouth.

Depending on the severity and chronicity of the swelling, compression garments for the face may be ordered in knitted materials or other synthetic fabric.

Custom-made face masks in knitted materials generally provide firmer and more durable compression, but they often have a long turnaround time and are costly to produce. Face masks made of other materials (often used in burn care and postfacial surgery) are manufactured using the more cost-effective "cut-and-sew" technique. These garments are available in standard sizes, but they tend to be less durable.

It is crucial that the patient's airway is not obstructed with the use of the garment and careful consideration must be given to the coverage chosen. Allowance can be made for a tracheotomy tube when ordering a garment; it is recommended that the manufacturer be consulted before ordering a garment with this requirement. Coverage of both eyes in a compression mask is also discouraged for safety reasons in the event of an emergency. If compression is necessary over the eyelids, a separate, easily removable form of compression is recommended to allow the patient to adjust the pressure over the eyes and to be able to see immediately when necessary.

Many patients can control swelling by using only a chin strap-style garment because their swelling is limited to the submandibular or neck area. Patients must be carefully instructed to remove this type of compression immediately if any facial swelling occurs. In this case, the patient will probably require a full face mask for adequate control of the swelling. Custom-made masks are sometimes necessary to begin CDT and the mask is adjusted with foam inserts to maintain compression as the swelling reduces. The patient is then measured for a better fitting mask for long-term use as the swelling plateaus. Garments manufactured for postoperative edema control following plastic surgery procedures can offer a more cost-effective solution if the edema is not severe.

5.16.5 Compression Garments for the Upper Thorax and Breast

Compression bras: These garments typically are used if swelling in the mammary gland is an issue (▶ Fig. 5.207).

Advantages: Velcro closure in the back allows for adjustments, fashionable, available in a variety of

5

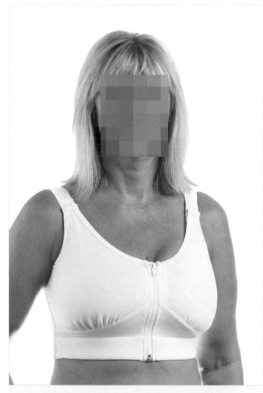

Fig. 5.207 Compression bra (with permission from Wear Ease, Inc.)

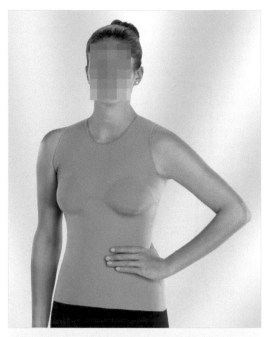

Fig. 5.208 Compression vest (with permission from Juzo USA, Inc.)

standard sizes, only one circumferential measurement on the chest (below the breast) required, relatively inexpensive.

Disadvantages: Closure in the back may be difficult to reach; does not provide sufficient support in truncal swelling; and the low cut in the axillary area may allow fluid to accumulate.

Compression vests: These custom-made garments are available in different compression levels (18–21 mm Hg and 23–32 mm Hg) and are appropriate for patients with a tendency to swell in the upper quadrant(s). Compression vests may be ordered as slip-ons or with optional closure systems (Velcro, zipper), which may be located in the front or back. Vests can be ordered with attached compression arm sleeves (▸ Fig. 5.208, ▸ Fig. 5.209).

Required Measurements for Compression Vests

Circumferential measuring points (indicate the position of all measuring points with nontoxic, nonpermanent marker):

- *Point h*: Vertically around the axilla and the shoulder. The arm should not be elevated during this measurement.
- *Point t*: Around the waist (just below the last rib).
- *Point n*: Around the chest, under the axilla.

Length measurements:
- *s–s*: This measurement determines the neck opening. It is taken on the front of the neck between the desired points of the neck opening on the shoulder height (point s represents the height of the shoulders).
- *qu–r*: This measurement determines the lower portion of the neck opening and is taken between the desired points of the opening.
- *r–s*: Determines the height of the opening between the shoulder height (point s) and the lower portion of the neck opening (point r).
- *m–s*: The length between the waist measurement (point m) and the shoulder height (point s).
- *m–n*: The distance between the circumferential measurements on the waist (point m) and the chest (point n).

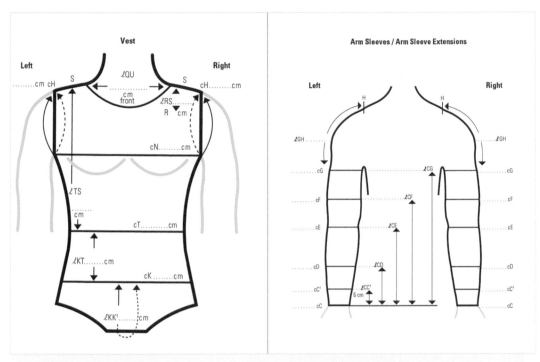

Fig. 5.209 Measurement form for compression vest (with permission from Juzo USA, Inc.).

5.16.6 Fitting Compression Garments upon Delivery

One of the most highly anticipated moments in the process of treating a patient for lymphedema is when their compression garments are delivered and the patient comes for the fitting.

Components of successful fitting

There are several components to successfully fitting garments and introducing the patient to the use of their garments.

Considerations

- Ensure the patient has maintained a stable limb volume while awaiting the delivery of the garments.
- Independence in self-bandaging or the patient must continue treatment until all garments arrive from the manufacturer.
- Timing for ordering garments should be as early as feasible upon the plateauing of limb volume, then continued treatment can focus on addressing tissue textural changes that persist until the garments are available.

- Limb volume should be remeasured first during a fitting session for two purposes:
  - To check stability of the volume since the garment was measured/ordered.
  - To provide a baseline at fitting for reassessment after the patient has independently used the garment for at least 1 week.
- A patient should not be discharged from care until the effect of garment use has been reassessed and stable limb volumes are assured.

Donning/Doffing

Correct donning/doffing techniques are extremely important because a well-fitted and effective garment that cannot be donned is useless. It is recommended that a clinic have at least several of the different styles of donning aides available for the patient to experiment with. The most important donning tool, however, remains EDUCATION and a pair of gloves that allow for a good grip of the garment so the garment can be massaged into place while protecting the garment from snags or other damage. There are several different styles of gloves that provide adequate "grip" on the glove surface for this purpose. All garment manufacturers sell donning gloves, but they are also widely available in garden centers as "work gloves." These are usually cotton-knit with the appearance of having been "dipped" in rubber for the fingers and palm. However, be aware of patients with a latex allergy. There are knit gloves available with a silicone "drizzle" to add grip for this patient population. Open toe lower extremity garments allow for the use of slippery limb covers that can be removed following garment donning exiting through the open toe. These are available for the upper extremity as well. One of the most important things to teach a patient is to don/doff the garment without gathering the garment up into a bunch, which negates the ability to stretch the garment to any degree to don/doff easily. Turning the garment inside out for half of its length or to the heel can facilitate this process. Manufacturers provide written instructions for appropriate donning in most cases. Evenly spreading the fabric over the entire limb is important. Please ensure that the patient can also doff the garment. It is recommended that the garments be turned over at the top and "peeled-off" to preserve the fabric and hence the compression in the most distal part of the garment. This avoids strongly pulling at that end and is particularly important for the removal of elastic compression gloves at the fingertips.

Additional Considerations

At the time of delivery, assess the garment before fitting for correctness of the garments' manufacture:

- Correct compression class.
- Whether all options are included as ordered.
- Correct color.

After the patient dons the garment for the first time, assess the fit:

- Correct length.
- Comfortable in garment.
- Adequate suspension of the garment in sitting/standing and with activity.
- No compromise of circulation or numbness.

Improving Comfort and Fit

Most manufacturers recommend that a garment be washed and worn every day for 3 to 4 days at a minimum to adequately assess the garment fit when new. Slight improvement in fit of a garment can be achieved by "easing" the garment especially in the most distal parts by washing and then allowing the garment to dry while slightly

stretched. For gloves and toecaps, inserting a chunky marker or cork into the too tight digit and allowing the garment to air dry repetitively can accomplish this. In an arm sleeve, stretching the washed garments' wrist portion over the shoulder of a wine bottle for the first 5 to 7 cm of length to air dry may provide sufficient "ease" over several days. Foam padding inserted into the glove may be necessary to achieve adequate control of dorsal wrist swelling. Velfoam pads inserted in the popliteal fossa or antecubital fossa may reduce skin irritation in those regions. It is strongly recommended that therapists apprise themselves of all options available for any garment line, as many comfort issues can be addressed by careful consideration before placing an order.

All manufacturers have policies regarding restocking or remaking of garments that do not fit well. These policies should be familiar to ordering therapists and patients should be educated about these policies at the time of original order. It is rare that a garment cannot be reordered to achieve appropriate fit and function. Manufacturers' regional sales representatives can be especially useful when garment-fit issues arise and should be contacted directly through the manufacturer or durable equipment provider.

5.17 Compression Bandaging Alternatives: Guidelines to Choosing the Right Home Care Systems

Multilayered short-stretch compression bandaging has few limitations and thus remains the most adaptable and readily customized compression application for lymphedema. As bandaging requires a high level of skill, it is best suited to the domain of the CLT. Unfortunately, there remains a long-term requirement for continued compression bandaging in home care to preserve the decongestion achieved during therapy and in many cases to ensure further improvement with diligent upkeep.

Prior to the appearance of compression bandaging alternatives, skills were developed through continual education of each patient or caregiver. This hands-on education process would usually start at the midpoint of intensive therapy. At this point in the continuum of care, patients have usually achieved remarkable improvement, establishing trust and faith that continued self-care will be a worthwhile investment. Importantly, having studied the limb's response to multiple bandage applications, the therapist conveys key instructional pointers to help the patient with unique modifications, which have proven to benefit the limb's specific needs.

5.17.1 Rationale for an Alternative

The impetus for developing alternatives is noble because every patient experiences an unwelcome adjustment in lifestyle when adapting to these new demands. In fact, the majority of patients with lymphedema report strong emotions related to continued self-bandaging, ranging from simple frustration to depression or rage. Simply stated, the single most likely reason for lack of adherence to the home care program is a self-bandaging regimen.

5.17.2 Important Considerations

Both the patient and therapist welcome alternative systems promising to address this major quality-of-life concern by simplifying the bandaging procedure. Compression systems offering abbreviated procedures imply less time, energy, and frustration, and thus are easy to discuss with the patient. The universal truth of chronic lymphedema management, however, is that it requires a thorough solution. To gain an appreciation for the therapeutic requirements of any alternative, therapists and patients must consider whether it
• Provides the essential qualities of high working, low resting pressures.
• Provides a compression gradient.
• Complies with LaPlace's law.
• Minimizes pressure marks, preserving skin integrity.
• Maintains or improves limb decongestion.
• Maintains or improves fibrosis.

Further practical requirements include the following:
• Ease of donning and removal.
• Ease of compression procedure, with precise daily replication.
• Protection against self-injury.
• Affordability.
• Durability.

5.17.3 Product Categories

The following categorical overview provides guidance as to the type of device and its benefits and trade-offs. It is most important to thoroughly consider the therapeutic and practical requirements listed before pairing device and patient.

Padding Sleeves

In most instances, these products are sized to "stretch into." As such, they have a low resting pressure and no working pressure. Some padding sleeves are meant to act as a basement layer to be wrapped over with typical short-stretch bandage materials. Although they do make the process of padding the arm easier, these sleeves will still require all of the standard outer bandage layers and the necessary time to be skillfully applied. It is important not to assume that the padding sleeve alone functions as an adequate substitute for bandaging.

Best patient profile

Very mild stage 2 (clinically apparent at all times), low volume, and without fibrosis.

Elastic Outer Sleeves

Lightweight elastic sleeves can be worn on top of the padding sleeve. These increase the resting pressure minimally but offer no working pressure. They are appealing alternatives but cannot perform well except in very early-stage lymphedema. As the outer compression layer is worn on top of the padding, a compression gradient can be difficult to achieve and does not address LaPlace's law regarding the hand.

Best patient profile

Very mild stage 2 (clinically apparent at all times), low volume, and without fibrosis.

Padding Sleeves with Foam Chips

These products are based on the original "Schneider Pack" idea incorporating small foam chips into the bandage complex for softening of fibrosis. As the foam chips are meant to embed into the swollen tissue, they are not indicated for many patient types. Outer elastic sleeves can be worn on top or short-stretch compression bandage layers. It is advisable to wear bandaging for the benefits of working pressure, but pressure marks are a concern for some diagnoses and tissue types.

Best Patient Profile

- Lymphedema with fibrosis.
- No history of cellulitis.
- No capillary fragility or lipedema component.
- No wounds.
- Not for pure venous edema.

Nonelastic Sleeves

Without foam padding as an underlayer, these products perform best when worn over a compression garment, which provides the gradient for limbs that are not conical in shape. This sublayer also provides even distribution of pressure to minimize pressure marks and alone they provide all working pressure (no resting pressure); therefore, they are, in principle, considered safe for around-the-clock wear. In fact, these alternatives are best for daytime wear because when sleeping they lack the structure to stay securely in place. Additionally, with the removal of the underlayer of the compression garment, intense pressure marks can develop if nonelastic sleeves are worn alone at night.

Best Patient Profile

- Pure venous edema (adds extra support during the daytime).
- Pure lymphedema requiring additional calf support (simulates high working pressure of bandage without bulk during the day).
- Lymphedema without foot or hand involvement.

Padding Sleeves with Nonelastic Outer Jackets

Solutions like these offering dedicated layers of padding and short-stretch jackets are the best simulations of a compression bandage. These materials are further tensioned against the limb with D-rings and long straps affixed with Velcro. These high working pressure, low resting pressure environments strive to achieve with one layer what bandaging achieves in multiple layers, reducing the workload and time investment considerably. Depending on fit and product type, pressure marks may result as fluid is molded and pushed into low-pressure areas. As there is a high degree of variability in these systems, foam padding liners and strapping need to be considered carefully. None of these products address the hand sufficiently; therefore, bandaging must still be applied unless the hand is spared involvement.

Best Patient Profile

- Upper or lower extremity lymphedema with spared involvement of the hand and foot. (Hands and feet may require modified bandaging.)
- Mild or moderate severity. (Stage 3 patients may require more tailored long-term strategies.)
- Where limb decongestion occurred in the clinic without high-intensity bandage pressures.

5.17.4 Maximizing the Benefits of Alternative Devices

Regardless of the stated strengths and shortcomings of compression alternatives, an almost unanimous need exists to support improved quality of life. Some patients experience these alternatives as true lifesavers, allowing them to get on with life and come to terms with the demands of living with lymphedema. Although, in theory, every patient should receive an alternative compression system at the time they enter the home care phase; in reality, there may be significant hurdles to overcome before improvements are found and these alternatives match the performance of standard compression bandaging.

Therapists must vigilantly seek the best solutions to long-term management. This includes the potential to further improve treatment outcomes achieved in the clinic. Lymphedema becomes more chronic if left partially treated (poorly decongested). When thorough decongestion is satisfactorily achieved, it must be maintained for true limb stabilization and the numerous associated benefits. It should be noted that some patients initially protest against continued self-bandaging but become less averse when they see the benefits it offers. As such, it may be best to champion continued self-bandaging for a time and make the transition to an alternative when suitable. Others may be completely capable but are unwilling to comply with the suggestion. This patient type may present challenges with any self-care requests and thus may require further interviewing to assess the level of commitment to a partnership in therapy. In some cases, this patient does not lack commitment but rightly understands that bandaging will either be too emotionally taxing or impossible to adhere to for practical reasons. Conducting this discussion is important to better understand where the perceived "finish line" is before the therapist begins consideration of the alternatives most suitable for the individual.

5

Critical Observations

- First ascertain if the patient is a candidate for an alternative system early in the clinical phase of therapy. For advanced-stage patients, no alternative provides the level of detail and tailored compression necessary to achieve stabilization and improvement. However, if home care support is absent and the patient would be unable to self-apply bandaging, the need is clear. In such cases, it becomes necessary to adapt and modify the alternative to tailor the compression strategy where possible.
- Decongest the limb as thoroughly as possible during the intensive phase. A decongested limb is easier to manage, is less massive, requires fewer tailored compression solutions, and utilizes fewer materials, resulting in less bulk.
- Study the unique character of the limb as it decongests. Every limb is different; therefore, by "learning the limb," the therapist can apply this knowledge to the overall strategy, measuring and selection of compression garments, and alternatives.
- Considerations:
  - What is the best pressure? Some limbs respond to light pressure, others to strong pressure.
  - Is there fibrosis? If lymphostatic fibrosis exists, aggressive pressure may be required regionally.
  - What is the pattern of decongestion? Some limbs decongest evenly, others in segments.
  - Is there extra skin, fold points, fragility, or adipose tissue to contend with?
  - What gradient works best? At times, proximal pressure causes a distal problem in the hand or foot, forearm, or calf. This should inform subsequent compression choices, materials, fit, and pressure levels.
  - Is the hand or foot involved? Is the condition mild, moderate, or severe?

Following this analysis and based on the product category and product attributes, select the alternative that provides the level of sophistication required to address the needs of the limb.

5.17.5 Patient Education and Long-Term Compression Therapy

At the transition point in therapy where patient education in self-bandaging is required, instead switch to self-application of the chosen alternative device. Let the patient leave with the product as if he or she were wearing a bandage in order to assess the benefits and shortcomings on the next treatment day. By taking control on the first day, the therapist should apply only the alternative device, incorporating astute observations about the limb's unique requirements. This simulation (experiment) will provide abundant feedback about the strengths and shortcomings of this alternative as compared with the bandage. From here, sensible modifications may be possible depending on the device category.

5.17.6 Suggested Modifications by Product Category

Padding Sleeves with Nonelastic Outer Jackets

As this category of product is the most sophisticated, it best approximates the attributes of a multilayered short-stretch bandage complex. Be careful not to alter the product unless you are not concerned about voiding the warranty. Weak pressure regions may be bolstered by inserting additional padding to the inside of the existing pads with Velcro. Areas such as the ankle, dorsum, knee, or elbow may benefit greatly from this step. If the limb has been benefitting from a particular foam type, such as closed cell orange foam, and a particular shape and pattern, these can be transferred. Observe the level of tension used for each Velcro strap to achieve the pressure required, then mark them with tape, Velcro tab, or other method so that this tension level can be easily duplicated by the patient at home. If fragile, tender, or vulnerable areas of the limb require protection, add synthetic cotton or an alternative protective dressing before applying the device.

Padding Sleeves with Foam Chips

If this product is being chosen, consider carefully the effect of the foam chips on the skin. If only a light elastic outer sleeve is being trialed, remember that this system is not true to the principles of the compression bandage because no working pressure is being applied. In most cases, additional layers of compression bandage will be applied to create containment, which will amplify the effects of the foam chips. Consider applying a protective underlayer of synthetic cotton, thin foam, or more basically a short-stretch fixing bandage on areas that receive harsh pressure marks. To improve performance on the hand or foot, consider adding dorsum pads on top of or underneath the device to amplify the pressure in keeping with LaPlace's law.

Nonelastic Sleeves

These very simple devices close with either interlocking or sequential overlapping strips of material. As stated earlier, they perform best with a sublayer of compression garment to equalize pressure and reduce marks. Because there is no foam, a thin layer can be added to improve the effect. However, this foam must not be too thick or bulky, as the device lacks the capacity for tension and may buckle or otherwise fail.

Final considerations should include the patient's ability to afford comparative devices and the durability of the spectrum of devices under consideration because they may be far less expensive when the manufacturer assures durability.

5.18 Treatment Considerations in Managing the Morbidly Obese Patient

5.18.1 The Problem

Between 2000 and 2005 in the United States, morbid obesity was reported to have increased by 50% for individuals with a BMI of 40 and by 75% in individuals with a BMI greater than 50.[132] These patients often have numerous comorbidities causing peripheral edema (cardiac, pulmonary, venous insufficiency, etc.) as well as diabetes, and are commonly seen in busy lymphedema clinics due to primary or secondary lymphedema or lipedema.[133] These patients are often not active, with a reduced musculoskeletal pump, and have sleep apnea symptoms.

If questioned, many morbidly obese patients report that they do not sleep in bed due to a need for elevation to breathe comfortably. In these cases, a recliner is preferred or sitting fully upright to sleep with the legs never elevated to the level of their heart during sleep. In such instances, these patients do not have the assistance of reduced gravity to aid constant congestion in leg veins. A heavy abdominal apron causes pressure against the groin while sitting and adds pressure against venous and lymphatic return.[134] All of these factors contribute to unrelenting venous hypertension in the lower extremities.

Progressive venous insufficiency is commonly caused by obesity, which can lead to the combined insufficiency characterized by phlebolymphedema.[135] One group of authors studied obesity-induced lymphedema patients with lymphoscintigraphy. All patients had a BMI > 30 (obese). BMI had a predictive value for lymphatic dysfunction. Patients with a BMI higher than 60 had abnormal lymphoscintigraphy and patients with a BMI less than 50 had normal lymphatic functioning. The authors recommended that patients be referred for bariatric surgery if they present with a BMI below 50 to avoid developing lymphatic dysfunction with weight gain that leads to crossing a threshold where lymphatic function diminishes.[136]

Will massive weight loss lead to improved lymphatic function? A case study and small case series suggest that once the weight threshold is crossed with development of lymphatic dysfunction, it is not reversible for most patients.[137] Studies of the physiology of the interstitium in obesity have demonstrated a reciprocal relationship between obesity and lymphedema—obesity can lead to impaired lymphatic function, but impaired lymphatic function also causes increased fat deposition through increased adipocyte activity and decreased clearance of macromolecules in adipose tissue.[138]

Treatment outcomes can be greatly improved by recognition of untreated conditions such as sleep apnea and morbid obesity, addressing these issues prior to initiating treatment for lymphedema. It requires sensitivity to discuss weight management. A good online resource is "Talking With Patients about Weight Loss: Tips for Primary Care Providers" from the National Institutes of Health.[139]

5.18.2 Equipment

It is essential that the safety of a patient and the treating therapist be considered during program planning for the morbidly obese patient commonly encountered in lymphedema clinics. Most therapy equipment is rated to support a patient of 350 pounds. For this population, a lymphedema clinic must have specialized equipment and facilities for treating patients who are heavier (at least 650 pounds), including treadmills, lobby furniture, treatment room equipment, restroom, and shower facilities. This patient population requires a wider treatment table with the ability to elevate the head of the bed to at least 45 degrees, as many patients are unable to breathe comfortably lying flat. Being able to safely lower and elevate the treatment surface is also critical to allow for safe patient

5

transfers and good therapist ergonomics during treatment to avoid injury to either person. In particular, the treating therapist must avoid attempting to support a limb with their own body for bandaging, as the limb may easily weigh in excess of 100 pounds, increasing the risk of injury to the therapist. A rolling stool or bolster is preferable for limb support.

A digital wide-based scale is also essential, as because a majority of patients who exceed 350 pounds often do not know what they actually weigh. Standard clinic's weight scales do not exceed a 350-pound capacity. Furthermore, the obese patient, in many cases, is unable to stand with feet together to fit on the scale for assessment.

5.18.3 Treatment Challenges

The literature describes this patient population as one that develops "massive localized lymphedema"[140] or localized lobules of soft tissue with advanced edema with signs of peau d'orange and fibrosis on the most dependent surfaces of the lobule. These lobules are commonly seen on the medial leg or arm, abdomen, or suprapubic region and are thought to develop as regional lymphatics become compressed and obstructed by heavy folds of dependent fat or chronic skinfold infections.

Lobules can be a difficult treatment challenge as they lead to a very irregular limb shape, which creates a challenge to the creation of a good gradient during compression bandaging. Some lobules may weigh up to 60 or 70 pounds and defy attempts to be suspended upward or to accept adequate compression bandaging applied in the conventional way. Addressing the lobule with bandaging encompassing it and then incorporating this into the full limb bandage can be effective. Surgical resection may be necessary to debulk; however, a compression strategy must still be employed postoperatively to avoid recurrence.

Deep skinfolds are common and offer numerous challenges. They can harbor anaerobic and/or fungal infections due to a common lack of appropriate hygiene coupled with dark, moist conditions in the depth of the fold. Meticulous cleansing and drying of the skin is essential during each treatment. Antifungal topical agents such as nystatin powder or spray-on metronidazole formulations are often beneficial in eliminating and/or preventing fungal and bacterial infections. The areas within deep skinfolds are usually extremely delicate due to the lack of stimulation. Stimulation is important to create a healthier skin surface.

Skinfolds may be packed open with soft padding to stimulate the skin and begin the process of eliminating the fold altogether as the surrounding tissue is further decongested. Compression within the skinfold can be achieved by inserting soft rolls constructed from strips of foam or rolled, thick wound dressing pads. As such, foam of 2.5 cm thickness offers good structure for this purpose. During this process, foam must be beveled for softened edges and covered with soft materials to avoid abrasion. Stockinette should be applied to the limb *after* skinfolds have been packed because the surface of knitted stockinette can itself be an irritant due to its coarse texture.

Skinfolds must often be "bridged" by foam sheeting to prevent exploitation by the overlying compression bandage layers. Thicker and stiffer foams are necessary in many cases to provide essential structure when bandaging over soft, frequently proximal tissues of the limb. This consideration provides a better "purchase/grip" of the bandage to the limb preventing slippage. Laminating layers of foam using a spray adhesive can assist in the creation of pieces applied to abnormal contours. In highly congested tissue, a very rapid early reduction in swelling often causes bandage slippage and, in fact, should be expected. It is helpful to educate the patient that bandaging applied early in treatment *will* be prone to slippage.

This avoids the patient losing confidence in the prescribed treatment in the early stages when a very large amount of decongestion in the tissues is expected and often very rapidly. To address this tendency, an intermediate layer of medium- or high-stretch bandage can provide the entire bandage with a better "grip," reducing slippage from one treatment to the next. The therapist should be prepared in any case to "rethink" the bandaging complex from day to day as the limb shape changes rapidly. Commercially available spandex bike shorts or old stretched-out garments can assist suspension of a lower extremity bandage when donned over the top of the compressive bandage.

In the outpatient setting, when bandaged to the groin bilaterally, it is often difficult for a patient to ambulate and function. In this instance, it may be feasible to bandage both lower extremities to the knee during daily clinical sessions while advancing the bandage to the groin for one leg at a time on alternate days. Alternately, another strategy may involve teaching the patient to advance the bandage to the groin in the evening while removing only the thigh bandage for better mobility the following day.

Custom flat-knit garments are generally necessary for long-term compression when treatment ends due to several factors: irregular limb contours, a need for strong containment and compression of the decongested tissue, and a persistence of skinfolds. Morbidly obese patients also have difficulty with donning garments due to a limited ability to reach. Custom garments allow for modular applications (i.e., knee-high AD or thigh-high AG garments layered with knee-length GT "bike shorts" or ankle-length "Capri pants"). Garments to "the waist" must often be measured to extend above the level of the umbilicus ending above the apex of the abdomen. If this step is not considered, the garment will not have sufficient grip to prevent slippage when worn.

Suspenders are often helpful to suspend the garment. Donning is greatly eased when an individual garment piece (AD, AG) is applied to each limb separately rather than as a one-piece configuration (i.e., pantyhose, AT). Patients often request an open crotch in a waist hi garment to make toileting easier. This is strongly discouraged because an open crotch, with no support for the delicate genital tissues, may be the precipitating factor for the development of genital swelling in a patient who previously was without this problem.

When measuring for custom flat-knit garments, wrapping the limb with saran wrap or a layer of fixing bandage can "lift" the tissue, as it would be lifted during donning of the garment to allow for more accurate measurement of how the tissue will be supported by the flat-knit garment. This is especially important if a massive reduction has been achieved with loose, hanging tissue.

Low-profile bandage alternatives are often the best choice for nighttime compression. They can also function well as daytime compression solutions, offering increased ease of donning with more effective compression than elastic garments can provide. Low-profile bandage alternatives can supplement the containment of lower leg tissue allowing for an overall lower compression class in the flat-knit garment and for greater ease in donning with application of the bandage alternative as a second layer, achieving adequate edema control.

During treatment, it is particularly important to include exercise in each day's clinical session. This patient population is often very sedentary. As such, activation of the musculoskeletal pump while wearing compressive bandaging greatly enhances the effect of compression. Weight loss is an important component contributing to a sustained long-term improvement in edema following intensive treatment (▶ Fig. 5.210; ▶ Fig. 5.211; ▶ Fig. 5.212; ▶ Fig. 5.213; ▶ Fig. 5.214).

There is a tendency for the patient to focus on their leg swelling symptoms to the exclusion of

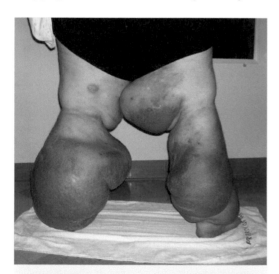

Fig. 5.210 This series of clinical photos (▶ Fig. 5.210; ▶ Fig. 5.211; ▶ Fig. 5.212; ▶ Fig. 5.213; ▶ Fig. 5.214) demonstrates the effect weight loss can have on achieving a good result with complete decongestive therapy. On evaluation, this patient had lost 70 lb (~32 kg). He weighed approximately 450 lb (205 kg) before weight loss began.

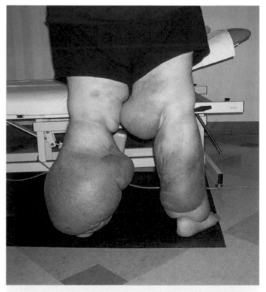

Fig. 5.211 Treatment began 6 months later when the patient was able to schedule transportation. He had lost an additional 70 lb (~32 kg). Note the improvement in the right lower extremity even before treatment commenced.

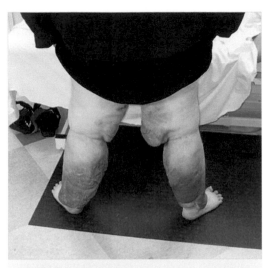

Fig. 5.212 The patient after seven complete decongestive therapy treatments.

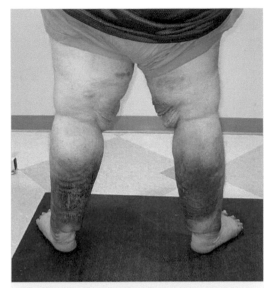

Fig. 5.213 At the end of the treatment course over 3 months, the patient was fitted with custom flat-knit thigh highs with a bike pant.

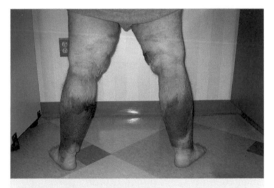

Fig. 5.214 At the 6-month follow-up, the total weight loss to date was approximately 250 lb (113.5 kg).

the causation of their symptoms, namely, their obesity. Exercise is part of a healthy lifestyle and has been shown to provide important benefits addressing many of the comorbidities experienced by this obese population. Exercise alone cannot lead to significant weight loss, but has proven important toward maintaining weight loss.

5.19 Lymphedema Therapy in the Home

Traditionally, treatment of lymphedema has been primarily conducted in the outpatient setting. However, with medical advancements, increasing life expectancy, changes in insurance benefits, and decreased hospital length of stay, there is an under-recognized population of patients living with lymphedema who are confined to the home. This community of patients is too medically fragile to leave home safely and independently to seek outpatient lymphedema therapy. Unfortunately, few home care agencies or independent practitioners currently provide lymphedema treatment, thus leaving homebound patients with a limited ability to access medically necessary services. Lymphedema practitioners must consider the needs of all individuals and advocate providing treatment across a full continuum of care.

Medicare has specific qualifications to delineate homebound status.

To be homebound means

*"You have trouble leaving your home without help 'like using a cane, wheelchair, walker, or crutches; special transportation; or help from another person.' Because of an illness or injury, or
Leaving your home isn't recommended because of your condition, and you're normally unable to leave your home because it's a major effort. You may leave home for medical treatment for short, infrequent absences for non-medical reasons, like attending religious services. You can still get home health care if you attend adult day care." Medicare and Home Health Care, medicare.gov, revised 2016.*

Many lymphedema patients fall within the Medicare homebound guidelines. Reduced functional mobility, limited activity tolerance, and the high risk of infection associated with chronic fluid stasis and open wounds may limit a person's ability to obtain appropriate treatment. At times, the edematous limb may be so large that it is the cause of mobility deficits, resulting in homebound status. This type of patient should not be discriminated against because of an inability to leave the home to seek outpatient services. There is an ever increasing need for home care agencies who deliver evidence-based lymphedema therapy. The home care team must include a CLT or nurse to ensure safe and effective treatment. Ongoing cross training for the home health team is essential for a successful program.

Lymphedema treatment in the home setting offers patients improved access to care. CDT can help prevent the progression of the lymphedema and decrease the risk of cellulitis and wounds often associated with protein-rich fluid stasis. This helps reduce the rate of complications, re-hospitalization, and reduce health care costs.

5.19.1 Complications in the Home Care Setting

A unique set of treatment challenges present themselves when CDT is provided in the home. Multiple comorbidities, impaired functional mobility, limited independence with activities of daily living, range of motion, and strength deficits all impact how the lymphedema clinician delivers treatment. These same obstacles are often what prevent patients from leaving their homes and complying with traditional lymphedema care. Other common complications include wounds, cardiovascular, circulatory, neurological, immune, endocrine, and pulmonary diseases. Because of the severity of comorbidities common in this patient population, the lymphedema therapist must understand the complexity of care. It is not recommended for the newly trained lymphedema therapist to begin their lymphedema career in this care environment.

5.19.2 The Home Environment— Opportunities and Challenges

From equipment to support to hygiene, the physical environment presents its own distinct opportunities and challenges. In a traditional outpatient setting, access to high-low tables, rehab equipment, and therapy aides within a sanitary and protected clinic are readily available. In contrast, home care settings vary drastically and the therapist may encounter living conditions that enhance or impede delivery of lymphedema treatment. When working with homebound patients, the therapist must modify the five components of CDT to accommodate environmental limitations for successful outcomes.

Proper body mechanics are essential to protect the therapist but are more challenging than in a clinical setting. The therapist may need to utilize pillows, gardening pads, and protective plastic barriers to promote safe body mechanics, as well infection control. Ideally, hospital beds replace high-low tables for treatment. If hospital beds are unavailable, MLD and compression application may be completed with the patient in a bed, sofa, recliner, or chair, depending on what is available and accessible.

Recliners commonly replace beds and present their own unique challenges. While a recliner aids in mobility and can provide a comfortable sleeping position, it can also hinder the flow of lymphatic fluid in the area of the abdominal and inguinal lymph nodes. When used in place of a bed, a recliner can further impede lymphatic circulation in the extremities and create pressure points or areas of lower resistance where fluid will accumulate such as the unsupported calf. Additional pillows or padding materials may be placed to provide support and relieve pressure for the affected limb(s). Whether utilizing a recliner or not, many patients are unable to transition into a prone position; therefore, adaptations must be considered to MLD sequences and positioning altered for beneficial decongestion.

Another potential obstacle that may hinder successful outcomes is the cleanliness of the home. Good hygiene is critical to lymphedema treatment. While many patients have the ability to care for themselves and their homes, others do not. In these situations, the therapist must educate and assist the patient and family in creating a clean and healing environment for optimal outcomes. This can include washing bandages, changing bed linens, or even vacuuming the floor to reduce the risk of infection. Assistance from family, friends, and outside community resources may be explored if the patient is unable to maintain a healthy living environment. Social work referrals may be warranted if resources are limited.

While pets provide emotional companionship, they can also provide a challenge to the home care therapist. Most commonly seen pets include dogs, cats, birds, and reptiles. Pet dander, scratches, saliva, bites, and excrement will affect skin hygiene and can contribute to infection, skin breakdown, and decreased wound healing. Ongoing observation may reveal unexpected interactions between patients and their pets. Examples of these interactions can include the following: Cats clawing the lymphedematous limb as if it were a scratching post and spraying bandages and wound supplies, dogs licking wounds and lymphorrhea off the skin, birds pecking at open wounds on insensate skin, and bed linens and bandages littered with animal hair or fur. In these cases, additional education regarding skin protection and meticulous hygiene should be provided. These suggestions may be met with resistance and must be presented tactfully because the pet may be a patient's sole source of companionship.

5.19.3 A New Care Setting— Administrative Guidelines and Considerations

Home care therapists must be creative and diligent when treating lymphedema patients to ensure the effectiveness of therapy within the constraints of the home setting. A strong clinical foundation is necessary for the therapist to effectively treat this population. Experience in an outpatient or inpatient setting is imperative to build a foundation on which to modify home techniques and achieve successful outcomes. Furthermore, a network of other CLTs is helpful to solve problem, develop creative solutions, share best practices, and consult on alternative methods to help patients progress.

Administration and therapists must agree upon and understand the duration of treatment and expense of supplies needed to support a lymphedema home care program. Because of travel distances, patients in the intensive phase are typically seen three times a week. The duration of these visits is often longer than the typical outpatient treatment due to the inherent complications and medical or mobility obstacles. Productivity standards will need to be adjusted and visits weighted to compensate for the increased time spent providing lymphedema treatment versus traditional occupational, physical, and speech therapy.

A retrospective study conducted at Florida Hospital Home Care Services, Inc., presented at the National Home Care Conference in 2004, found that lymphedema treatment in the home was cost-effective. Not only was there a reduction in agency visits, there was a decreased length of stay, decreased certification periods, and incidents of cellulitis. Additionally, hospital readmission rates were reduced and more than 89% of patients showed improvements in functional outcomes.

At times, traditional therapy may accompany lymphedema treatment due to ADL and mobility issues. Medicare and most insurance companies will not reimburse for two visits from the same discipline in 1 day, even if one of the visits is dedicated only to lymphedema. Therefore, communication between therapists of the same discipline is imperative to prevent nonbillable visits. In these cases, it is recommended for the lymphedema therapist to treat the patient on Monday, Wednesday, and Friday, while the traditional therapy from the same discipline is delivered on Tuesday and Thursday. If possible, it is helpful if a different clinician provides the traditional therapy to keep the focus of each visit dedicated to either lymphedema or functional OT/PT/ST.

A multidisciplinary approach also includes skilled nursing services. When working as a team with nursing and therapy, it is recommended that the agency provide a yearly competency for non-certified staff to better address the needs of the lymphedema patient. A basic understanding of multilayered compression bandaging, use of compression garments and bandage alternatives, meticulous skin care, side effects, and contraindications for therapy results in successful outcomes.

Because many lymphedema patients have wounds, the agency will need to have policies regarding which discipline provides wound care services. If both lymphedema and wound care are addressed by the same clinician, there is a risk that vital components of treatment will not be completed due to time constraints. If nursing is completing the wound care, it is important to coordinate nursing and lymphedema services for immediate reapplication of multilayer compression bandages. Having a nurse visit the home just prior to the lymphedema therapist allows both clinicians to focus on their areas of expertise and provide treatment more efficiently.

5

5.19.4 Appropriate Referral Protocols

Lymphedema protocols specific to home care need to be developed to identify patients who are physically and cognitively appropriate to receive lymphedema services in the home. If the patient is not physically able to actively participate in self-treatment or is cognitively not able to follow instructions, a caregiver must be involved in the daily treatment. A written protocol is necessary for the admission coordinator to identify candidates who will benefit from lymphedema in the home care setting. Not every referral will be appropriate and having a screening tool will help delineate those patients who can be safely treated at home versus those who would be better served in the inpatient or skilled nursing setting. The therapist must adhere to the parameters established by their agency to ensure successful outcomes.

Considerations for protocols include the following:

- Assess if the patient meets the criteria for home-bound status under insurance guidelines.
- Weight limit specific to men and women. This will help reduce the risk of injury to the therapist and the patient. If the weight exceeds the defined limit, the patient would be more safely cared for in a setting that would provide for additional skilled personnel and equipment to treat the edematous limb(s) and provide nutritional/weight management guidance.
- Cognition and the ability to follow simple verbal instructions. Owing to the complexity of self-management and safety with lymphedema care, patients must be able to direct and guide their care or have a dedicated caregiver to assist.
- Driving distance. The home care agency must identify the parameters or limits of travel time and mileage acceptable for their agency. This is also a factor to consider in the cost-effectiveness for the home care agency.
- Identified caregiver/support system. The most important protocol to establish is a consistent and dedicated caregiver so that once home care is discharged, ongoing management is continued to prevent multiple readmissions.
- Willingness of the patient to follow through with purchase of compression. Because most home care patients are insured by Medicare, they generally have to self-pay for compression garments. It is important they understand the cost of compression garments and bandaging alternatives.

- Contraindications. At times, hospitals may refer patients who were having lymphedema treatment prior to admission or who were being treated in acute care. These patients may not yet be stable for CDT in the home where they are not monitored 24 hours/day as they are in the hospital. Patients must have time to stabilize after acute events before treatment can safely be initiated in the home. Thus, a list of contraindications, especially active CHF and DVT, will help intake personnel screen potential clients before accepting them for care.

5.19.5 The Five Components of CDT in the Home Care Setting

Manual Lymph Drainage

- MLD protocols may need to be creatively adapted to the patient's abilities, physical space constraints, and the setup of the home. Home care lymphedema therapists work independently without support staff and, at times, in less-than-ideal conditions. Although all four Vodder's hand techniques are important, the stationary circle and the pump are the most utilized due to patient positioning and safety of the therapist's body mechanics.

Compression Bandaging

- As discussed in previous chapters, compression bandages are used primarily in the intensive phase for decongestion. It is helpful for a home care therapist to travel with a stock of bandaging and wound care supplies in their car. This allows the bandages to be distributed immediately to prevent a delay in care. In the United States, these supplies are currently considered in the bundled payment for treatment reimbursement. Because of the fragility and high risk for falls in this population, bandaging strategies may need to be modified. Due to comorbidities, the therapist must be cautious regarding the number of bandage layers utilized to prevent skin breakdown and fluid shifts. A foam layer is imperative to promote skin integrity and help keep the bandages from slipping between visits. For lower extremity home bound patients, rarely do bandages extend beyond the knee due to the risk of falls and difficulty with transfers. If the patient presents with swelling in the thigh, a bandaging alternative or modified bandaging techniques may be utilized. Non-skid footwear is essential to decrease the risk of falls.

Compression Garments and Alternatives

By definition, home-bound patients cannot easily leave the home. Thus, the home care clinician must be proficient measuring and fitting for compression garments and alternatives. Rarely can this population don, doff, or tolerate compression garments at the medically necessary compression classes. Layering or combining lower levels of compression garments or bandaging alternatives can assist with maintaining reduction during phase 2 of treatment versus utilizing one higher level compression garment. Functional mobility, hand dexterity, upper extremity strength, oxygen saturation levels with exertion, ability to bend forward to touch the toes, and skin integrity need to be assessed when making the recommendations and fitting garments or alternatives.

Local durable medical equipment (DME) suppliers and supportive vendor representatives are vital to obtaining products that will help with the self-management phase once home care services have been discontinued. It is helpful for the therapist to obtain samples of various forms of compression garments and alternatives as well as don/doffing devices to allow a patient to make an educated choice before purchasing a product. Several treatments may be required to assess use of various forms of compression, donning devices and to determine what is most appropriate for the patient. Some patients do not have the endurance to tolerate donning or doffing compression more than one or two times during a session as they transition between phase 1 and phase 2 of treatment. Thus, multiple visits may need to be dedicated to practice these techniques, allowing the patient to become independent with self-care.

Meticulous Skin Care

- The home care patient may be more prone to cellulitis. Depending on the support system, they may be less able to clean the home, bathe adequately, or properly care for their limbs/skin. Education to promote meticulous skin care is crucial to reduce the risk of recurrent infections. Assessment and recommendations for appropriate medical equipment to promote independence and safety with bathing can be an important part of the care plan. An occupational therapy or home health aide referral to instruct the patient on new skills for improved carryover of safe and consistent bathing techniques will help reinforce proper skin care. Social workers may provide patients with information on local or government programs available to assist with house cleaning and bathing after discharge from home care.
- Skin maceration is a common occurrence due to wound exudate and incontinence. Skin barrier creams, incontinence pads, maxi pads, and adult diapers incorporated and secured by tubular gauze, over wound dressings, help reduce soiling of bandages and protect skin. Skin hydration is critical even in this moist environment. Patient education must focus on use of low pH moisturizers and strategies on how to reach and apply the lotion to the affected areas avoiding wound beds. A long handled sponge or lotion applicator may be incorporated to increase patient compliance.

Education

Education must begin with the patient and family/caregiver on the first visit. Information regarding the course of treatment and each component of CDT should be emphasized. Written handouts with pictures or diagrams left in the patient's home will provide basic information regarding lymphedema treatment and become an important reference after discharge. These handouts should address lymphedema education, signs and symptoms of cellulitis, risk reduction practices, skin care, remedial exercises, and compression techniques. Additionally, a list of contraindications for treatment should be provided so that the patient understands when a call to the agency is warranted or if the bandages need to be removed. A patient must be able to remove his bandages or have a caregiver who can do this should it become necessary. It is expected that more time and visits will be needed for the patient to fully comprehend the lymphedema home program. For example, repetitious education may be necessary to review and simplify home programs, including remedial exercises and donning/doffing of bandages/alternatives and garments for successful carryover.

Remedial Exercises

Remedial home exercise programs must be simple and concise to promote compliance. Consideration for mobility deficits, limited activity tolerance, decreased ROM, and comorbidities will determine the extent of the exercises recommended.

5.19.6 Practical Applications and Useful Tips

Though the suggestions listed below are not the "ideal" methods that would be utilized in a clinical setting, they may help promote independence and provide practical solutions when functional and financial constraints limit options. DME coverage may differ when a patient receives home care services versus outpatient rehabilitation. Therefore, creative solutions and problem solving may include the following:

- The therapist should inform the patient that approximately 1 hour prior to the scheduled therapy visit, bandages must be removed and rerolled. If the patient is physically able, it is also helpful if skin is cleansed and hydrated.
- Educate the patient to remove the bandages if they become soiled due to weeping, wound exudate, or incontinence to promote skin hygiene.
- Use of one layer of tape with tabbed edges to secure bandages to the most proximal aspect of the limb will ease independence of doffing bandages. The less the use of tape during application, the easier it is for the patient to remove bandages.
- Skin barrier creams to proximal and sensitive skin areas will assist with the promotion of skin integrity of incontinent patients.
- Many home care patients have little disposable income to contribute toward expensive compression garments, alternatives, and DME. Therefore, patients who sew can fabricate their own compression alternative with items purchased at a craft or fabric store. Various types of foam that can be found in these stores, covered by bathing suit material or spandex, may facilitate compression therapy at night. Homemade alternatives can be secured with Velcro, D-rings, or short-stretch bandages.
- Patients who cannot afford to purchase and replace cotton or foam for use under bandages can substitute a fleece blanket cut into strips, a soft quilted mattress pad, or soft cotton T-shirts placed under short-stretch bandages to fill in concavities.
- Small paint-brush rollers with thick padding and sticky-paper lint rollers can be used by patients to extend their reach in order to complete self-MLD and to reduce fibrosis.

- Creative use of a thick plastic grocery bag can facilitate donning both upper extremity and open-toe lower extremity compression garments.
- Gloves are essential to ease donning and doffing compression garments. Donning gloves may be substituted with gardening gloves or automotive gloves found in grocery and big box stores. Medical rubber gloves or basic dishwashing gloves will not work well and cause frustration.
- A rubber shelf liner can help smooth out wrinkles in a compression garment used around the hand like a glove, especially with patients who have hand limitations with strength or range of motion.
- To facilitate donning or doffing closed-toe lower extremity garments, non-skid pads placed on the floor can be used. Examples include computer mouse pad, rubberized shelf liner, a cut yoga mat, or a gardening mat. A rubber backed bath mat placed upside down on carpet may also work. The rubber in these items will grip the garment and help slide it over the heel.

5.19.7 Conclusion: Building a Bridge

In conclusion, lymphedema therapy in the home is an important service filling a critical gap and offering treatment to a segment of the population that has been traditionally underserved. Patients may complete the entire course of CDT in the home or start in the home and then transfer to an outpatient setting when medically appropriate. When the home care company is part of a hospital system, inpatient, outpatient, skilled nursing, and home care therapists can collaborate to provide a smooth continuum of care. This network of lymphedema therapists should establish written protocols to help promote patient compliance improve functional outcomes and provide a cost savings to the hospital system. If a home care agency is not part of a hospital system, therapists are encouraged to incorporate an interdisciplinary approach to provide optimal outcomes for their patients.

Home care therapists have the unique opportunity to intervene within a patient's own environment, customizing treatment services within their home setting. Clinicians creatively assist patients to achieve their maximum potential with lymphedema management based on individual abilities and environmental limitations. By empowering patients to use what is readily available to them within a cost-effective means, lymphedema patients are apt to be more compliant as the treatment suits their lifestyle. Most of all, by providing care in the home, patients no longer have to go without treatment because they are unable to access an outpatient facility. Although delivering lymphedema therapy services in the home may require unique and customized delivery techniques, adherence to the basics of CDT will result in successful outcomes.

5.20 Patient Education

Successful lymphedema management requires a well-trained lymphedema therapist and a properly set up treatment environment conducive to special requirements in the care and management of lymphedema.

5.20.1 Lymphedema Therapists

Lymphedema therapists can be physical therapists and their assistants, occupational therapists and their assistants, physicians, nurses, chiropractors, or massage therapists who have undergone specialized training in CDT. Several schools in the United States educate and certify therapists in proper lymphedema management; these schools meet the training standards outlined by the Lymphology Association of North America (LANA) and the minimum requirements for lymphedema therapy training outlined in the position paper of the National Lymphedema Network (NLN). Unfortunately, currently there are no mandatory training standards for lymphedema therapists, and some health care professionals claim to be lymphedema therapists, but have not actually attended and successfully graduated from one of these recognized training programs. A newly formed association, the North American Lymphedema Education Association (NALEA), which is an alliance of major training programs in North America involved with lymphedema education, is encouraging the development of national standards in lymphedema education for therapists who perform combined (also known as complex or complete) decongestive therapy, or CDT. NALEA member schools are in agreement as to the minimum educational framework required to graduate specialized lymphedema therapists with refined manual skills based on medically sound, evidence-based knowledge.

To assist patients in finding properly trained lymphedema therapists, several organizations established "therapist locators" on their websites. These provide assistance in locating a qualified therapist, who meets recommended training standards. The National Lymphedema Networks resource can be located on their website (www. lymphnet.org; accessed March 4, 2016). The Lymphology Association of North America provides a link at their website as well (www.clt-lana.org; accessed March 4, 2016). The American Lymphedema Framework Project (ALFP) developed a mobile web application software labeled Look4LE, which provides a common directory of trained lymphedema specialists with an online registration and validation system. Patients are able to install this free web application to search for certified lymphedema specialists worldwide.

A high level of competency and skill is needed to master all components of CDT. Patients should make sure that the lymphedema therapists in the facility are specifically educated and trained in lymphedema management, and meet the training standards outlined by LANA, and the minimum requirements for lymphedema therapists as outlined in the position paper of the NLN.

Successful lymphedema management requires, in most cases, daily treatments in the intensive phase; it is therefore desirable that the treatment facility employs two lymphedema therapists to cover for absence and for professional exchange and support.

Providing patients with appropriate information and education facilitates long-term success of lymphedema management. A dialogue between the patient and the lymphedema therapist covering all relevant aspects of lymphedema management should be initiated early on in the intensive phase of the treatment. Sufficient knowledge of the patient regarding his or her condition is the key to compliance. Patients need to know what causes lymphedema to understand fully why self-management is a necessary component of CDT (easy-to-understand terms should be used; a sample patient information form is given in Chapter 6, Sample Forms). Patients should be informed about the possible consequences if self-care for lymphedema is neglected. Knowledge about the risks involved in certain activities (air travel, extremes in temperature, etc.) helps avoid the recurrence of symptoms.

At the end of the intensive phase, the patient should have the necessary skills to perform self-bandaging and self-MLD techniques safely and

5

effectively and to execute a customized program of decongestive exercises. A thorough understanding of preventive measures (see Do's and Don'ts for Upper Extremity Lymphedema and Do's and Don'ts for Lower Extremity Lymphedema later in this chapter) as well as of high- and medium-risk activities for lymphedema should be achieved at the time the patient makes the transition into phase 2 of the treatment.

5.20.2 Self-Bandaging

During the intensive phase of the therapy (phase 1), the compression bandages applied by the therapist may slide somewhat over the treatment-free weekend days. Sliding is usually limited to the upper arm or thigh. The patient should be able to reapply the bandages in these areas to avoid reaccumulation of fluid and/or tourniquet effects caused by bunching up of the compression bandages. It is therefore necessary to involve the patient in the bandaging process as soon and as much as possible. At the end of the first week of treatment, the patient should be able to apply padding and compression bandages on the proximal parts of the extremity without major difficulty.

To maintain and improve the success achieved in the first phase of treatment and to further reduce and soften areas of fibrotic tissue, most patients have to continue to wear bandages at night. Even patients who do not experience an increase in extremity volume during the nighttime and who do not have any areas of fibrotic tissue may experience fluctuation in limb volume at times (due to lifestyle, menstrual period, weight gain, climate, etc.). It is therefore imperative for long-term success that every patient learns appropriate self-bandaging techniques while under the care of an experienced and properly trained lymphedema therapist.

To support patient compliance, it is essential to keep the self-bandaging techniques as simple as possible. It cannot be expected that a patient will be able to use the same techniques as the lymphedema therapist. The use of high-density foam without the supervision of the clinician is not advisable. Bandages in the self-management phase are primarily worn at nighttime, when the patient sits or lies down. Much less bandage pressure is needed to achieve the beneficial effects of compression therapy. The quantity of materials is therefore much lower than during the intensive phase of therapy, during which the compression bandages are worn 22 to 23 hours a day.

Upper Extremity

The following is a list of the recommended materials for applying a compression bandage during the night on the upper extremity (self-management phase). The quantities represent two sets of compression bandages, which are recommended for hygienic reasons (one to wear and one to wash):
- One bottle of skin lotion.
- One box of stockinette (tubular bandage) in the appropriate size.
- One to two boxes (20 individual rolls in a box) of gauze bandages (4 or 6 cm width).
- Two to four synthetic nonwoven padding bandages (10 cm) or two Rosidal Soft foam bandages (10 cm).
- Two short-stretch bandages (4 or 6 cm).
- Two to four short-stretch bandages (10 or 12 cm).
- Tape to secure the bandages.

Application

Bandages generally are applied with an even prestretch of ~ 30 to 40% and an overlap of ~ 50 to 70%. The patient should apply the bandages while sitting on a table.

All materials should be arranged in the order in which they are applied; two or three strips of tape per compression bandage (~ 12 cm long) should be prepared. Padding bandages are not taped.

Skin Care

Appropriate skin care products are applied thoroughly, without causing redness of the skin.

Stockinette

The tubular bandage should be cut to a length that allows for an overlap of ~ 12 cm on the proximal end of the extremity. This overlap is used to extend over and cover the complete compression bandage on the proximal border to protect it from axillar perspiration. A hole is cut for the thumb on the distal end.

Finger Bandages

Fingers are slightly spread, and the palm of the hand faces down. A bolster should be placed under the elbow to support the weight of the arm.

Start the gauze bandage with a loose anchor turn around the wrist, then proceed over the back of the hand to the little finger (or the thumb). The fingers should be bandaged with light pressure

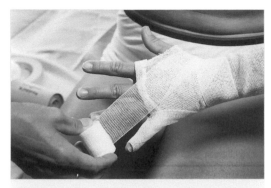

Fig. 5.215 Application of gauze bandages on the fingers.

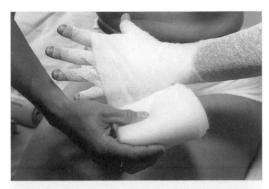

Fig. 5.216 Application of synthetic padding bandages on the hand, including the knuckles.

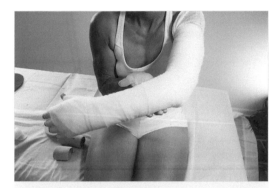

Fig. 5.217 Padding of the arm using synthetic padding bandages.

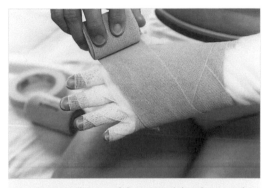

Fig. 5.218 Application of short-stretch bandages on the hand and wrist.

from the nail bed up with ~ 50% overlap (▶ Fig. 5.215). The fingertips are not covered. Leave the finger with the gauze bandage toward the back of the hand and proceed to the wrist; apply a half turn (complete anchoring turns should be avoided) around the wrist, and continue to bandage the remaining fingers in the same fashion. The borders of the gauze bandage should not slide or roll in on the distal and proximal ends of the fingers. One gauze bandage is generally used to bandage all fingers. Any unused part of the second gauze bandage should be wrapped spirally (not circularly) around the forearm. The finger bandage should never start or end at a finger. Upon completion, the fingertips should be checked for proper circulation.

Padding Materials

Nonwoven synthetic padding or soft foam rolls (Rosidal Soft) are used to pad the hand and arm. A hole is cut for the thumb; the padding bandage is secured around the wrist with a circular turn. The hand is then padded down to the knuckles using

two to four circular turns (▶ Fig. 5.216). The padding bandage proceeds to cover the forearm and upper arm. Two rolls of padding bandages are used to cover the hand and arm (▶ Fig. 5.217). Do not use tape to secure the padding materials.

Short-Stretch Bandages

Starting a 6-cm (or 4-cm)-wide bandage with a loose anchor turn around the wrist, the hand is bandaged to include the knuckles with slightly spread fingers (▶ Fig. 5.218). The bandage is anchored between each turn around the hand with half turns on the wrist. Any remaining bandage material is used on the forearm (▶ Fig. 5.219). The end of the bandage is secured with two strips of tape. The subsequent bandage (10 or 12 cm) is applied in the opposite direction from the first bandage. This provides for a more functional and durable bandage. The bandage starts on the wrist with a loose anchor and proceeds to cover the forearm, elbow area, and upper arm with circular turns and ~ 50% overlap (▶ Fig. 5.220). A third bandage may

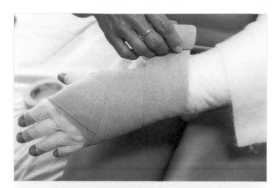

Fig. 5.219 The remaining short-stretch bandage is used to apply compression on the forearm.

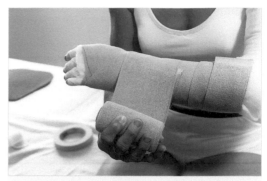

Fig. 5.220 Application of the second short-stretch bandage starting at the wrist.

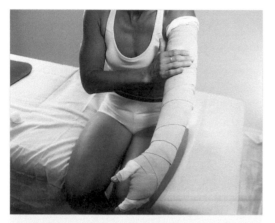

Fig. 5.221 Finished compression bandage on the upper extremity.

be used if necessary. It is important that the last bandage ends in the axillary fold to prevent accumulation of fluid between the armpit and the end of the bandage (▶ Fig. 5.221).

The end of the bandage is secured with two or three strips of tape, and the overlap of the stockinette is folded over the bandage.

Lower Extremity

The following is a list of the recommended materials for applying a compression bandage on the lower extremity during the self-management phase of CDT (phase 2). The quantities represent two sets of compression bandages, which are recommended for hygienic reasons (one to wear and one to wash):

- One bottle of skin lotion.
- One box of stockinette (tubular bandage) in the appropriate size.
- If toe bandages are necessary, one to two boxes of gauze bandages (4 cm width).
- Two high-density foam pieces (kidney shape).
- Three to five synthetic nonwoven padding bandages (10 cm) or two Rosidal Soft foam bandages (10 cm).
- Two to four synthetic nonwoven padding bandages (15 cm) or two Rosidal Soft foam bandages (15 cm).
- Four to six short-stretch bandages (10 cm) or two double-length (11 yards/10 m) 10-cm rolls.
- Four to six short-stretch bandages (12 cm) or two double-length (11 yards/10 m) 12-cm rolls.
- Tape to secure the bandages.
- If necessary, additional foam pieces provided by the therapist.

Application

Bandages generally are applied with an even pre-stretch of ~ 30 to 40% and an overlap of ~ 50 to 70%. All materials should be arranged in the order in which they are applied; two or three strips of tape per compression bandage (~ 12 cm long) should be prepared. Padding bandages are not taped.

To bandage the foot and the lower leg, the patient should be sitting, with the foot of the affected leg resting on another chair or on the knee of the other leg. Bandages from the knee up to the groin are applied while standing.

Skin Care

Appropriate skin care products are applied thoroughly, without causing redness on the skin.

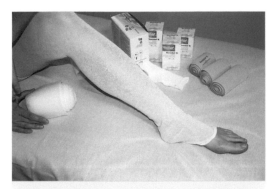
Fig. 5.222 Application of stockinette on the leg.

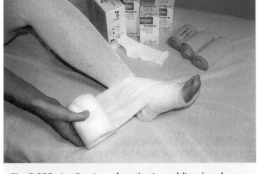
Fig. 5.223 Application of synthetic padding bandages on the foot, ankle, and lower leg.

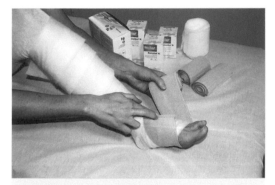
Fig. 5.224 Start of the first short-stretch bandage with a loose anchor around the foot.

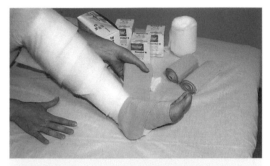
Fig. 5.225 The ankle is in 70–90 degrees of flexion while applying bandages around the heel.

Stockinette

The tubular bandage should be cut to a length that allows for an overlap of ~ 12 cm on the proximal end of the extremity. This overlap is used to extend over and cover the complete compression bandage on the proximal border (▶ Fig. 5.222).

Toe Bandages (If Necessary)

Start the first gauze bandage with a loose anchor turn around the foot, then proceed to bandage the big toe. Approach the toe from the dorsum of the foot, apply two or three circular turns, and leave the toe again over the dorsum of the foot. Avoid sliding or rolling of the bandages in the web space area. The tips of the toes remain unbandaged. Proceed to bandage the remaining toes (except the fifth toe, which generally is not involved in the swelling) in the same manner. One 4-cm bandage (usually folded to half width) is generally sufficient to cover the toes. Any unused part of the gauze bandage should be wrapped spirally (not circularly) around the foot. Upon completion, the tips of the toes should be checked for proper circulation.

Padding Materials

Two or three rolls of nonwoven synthetic padding, or one or two rolls of soft foam (Rosidal Soft), are applied on the foot and lower leg (▶ Fig. 5.223). Komprex foam kidneys are secured between the medial and lateral anklebone and the Achilles tendon with the padding bandages. Synthetic padding bandages may be doubled over the shin area to provide additional protection.

Short-Stretch Bandages

Starting a 10-cm-wide bandage with a loose anchor turn around the foot, the foot is bandaged down to the web spaces with three or four circular turns (▶ Fig. 5.224). The same bandage proceeds to cover the heel in a crisscross fashion. During the application of compression bandages on the heel, the ankle is in ~ 70 to 90 degrees of flexion (▶ Fig. 5.225; ▶ Fig. 5.226). Secure the bandage with tape. The next bandage (10 cm) starts above the ankle with a loose anchor in the opposite direction of the previous bandage (applying compression bandages in the opposite direction to

5

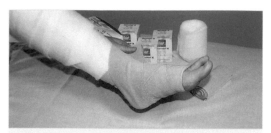

Fig. 5.226 Short-stretch bandages around the ankle are applied in a crisscross fashion.

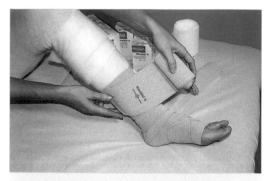

Fig. 5.227 The second short-stretch bandage starts with a loose anchor around the ankle.

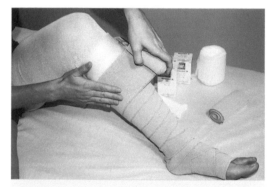

Fig. 5.228 Application of short-stretch bandages on the lower leg.

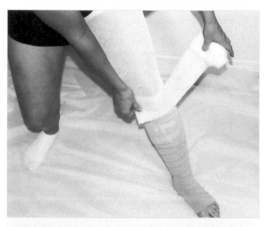

Fig. 5.229 Application of synthetic padding bandages on the knee and thigh.

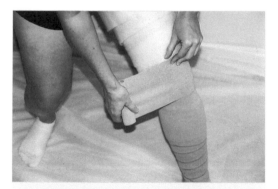

Fig. 5.230 Application of short-stretch bandages on the knee and thigh.

each other prevents bandaging the foot in a non-functional position; i.e., it provides for a functional bandage and adds durability). The goal is to cover the lower leg up to the knee using circular turns (▶ Fig. 5.227; ▶ Fig. 5.228). Secure the bandage on the lower leg with tape. If a double-length bandage is used, the foot as well as the lower leg may be bandaged using the same roll.

The remaining compression bandage is applied while standing up, and the body weight should be shifted to the extremity being bandaged, with the knee slightly bent. Padding materials using non-woven synthetic padding or soft foam rolls are applied on the knee and thigh (▶ Fig. 5.229). When using synthetic padding bandages, the layers may be doubled in the back of the knee to provide additional protection. The knee and thigh should be bandaged using two or three rolls of 12-cm-wide short-stretch bandages (or one double-length roll). The first bandage starts with a loose anchor turn below the knee, proceeding to cover the knee and parts of the thigh using circular techniques (▶ Fig. 5.230). The remaining thigh is bandaged with the next bandage roll. Secure the bandage with tape, and fold the overlap of the stockinette over the bandage (▶ Fig. 5.231).

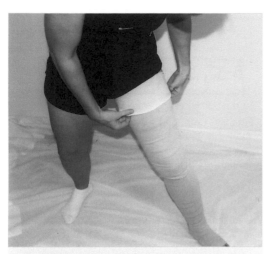

Fig. 5.231 Finished compression bandage on the leg.

5.20.3 Exercises

The positive impact a well-tailored regular exercise program can have on a healthy lifestyle, improvement of general well-being, increased energy level, and stress and weight management is well known. Additional benefits of exercises for those individuals at risk of, or have, lymphedema include improved limb flexibility, range of movement, and most importantly increased lymphatic drainage and venous return from the swollen areas, which can result in reduction of limb size and subjective limb symptoms.

Research indicates that the transport of lymph fluid and proteins from swollen areas increases during and after exercises. Studies show that lymph flow increased fivefold in the first 15 minutes and two- to threefold during the remaining time of a 2-hour exercise protocol.[141,142] In addition to the benefits to the lymphatic system, it is known that muscle activity and diaphragmatic breathing also have a considerable impact on venous blood returning from the extremities back to the heart, which in turn also positively affects fluid management within the interstitial spaces; increased venous return is of particular importance for those individuals affected by lower extremity lymphedema.

To better understand these effects, it is necessary to take a look at the anatomy and physiology of the lymphatic and venous systems (see also Chapter 1, Anatomy).

The lymphatic system is closely associated with the blood system and represents an accessory route by which lymph fluid flows from the body's tissues back into the blood stream. Contrary to the blood system, the lymphatic network and its vessels do not form a closed circulatory system. It begins with small lymphatic vessels (lymph capillaries) in the body tissues, and continues with successively larger lymphatic vessels (collectors and trunks), which ultimately connect to the venous part of the blood system via the venous angles, which are composed of the internal jugular and subclavian veins on either side of the neck. While the flow of blood through the arteries and veins is uninterrupted, the transport of lymph fluid through the lymph vessel system is interrupted by lymph nodes. The lymphatic system has no central pump; lymph vessels produce their own propulsion system with a network of smooth musculature located in the walls of lymph collectors and trunks.

The superficial lymphatic vessels are located between the muscle layers and the skin. With activity, the muscle contracts and relaxes against the skin, which increases lymphatic activity and return of lymph fluid. In many cases of lymphedema, the elastic fibers in skin tissues affected by lymphedema are damaged and unable to provide adequate resistance against the musculature working underneath, and the blood and lymph vessels within these tissues; therefore, it is advisable to wear compression bandages or garments during exercise. External compression compensates for the elastic insufficiency of the affected tissue, providing the resistance necessary to improve lymphatic return and to maintain the reduction of the swelling.

The blood circulatory system represents a closed system with the heart as its central motor, and blood and blood vessels as the other structural elements. The main purpose of the blood vessels is the uninterrupted supply of all body tissues with nutrients and oxygenated blood, and the removal of metabolic waste and carbon dioxide from the tissue cells. The blood pressure inside the venous part of the blood system is considerably lower than the pressure in the arterial side; pooling of venous blood, especially in the lower extremities, is prevented by a system of valves inside the larger veins, which helps ensure the efficient transport of venous blood back to the heart. A sufficient return of blood to the heart would not be possible without a functioning valvular system and the help of the muscle and joint pumps, diaphragmatic breathing, and the suction effect of the heart during its relaxation phase (diastole).

The positive impact on lymphatic and venous return of muscle and joint activity during exercise, especially while compression garments are worn, and abdominal (diaphragmatic) breathing exercises, explains the benefits of a well-rounded and tailored exercise regimen for those individuals affected by lymphedema of the extremities.

Which Exercises Can Be Incorporated into the Patient's Self-Management Regimen?

There is no real consensus on the type of exercise regimen for individuals affected by lymphedema. Research suggests that a program of progressive exercises, that is, starting with gentle exercises and increasing intensity moderately over time, tailored to each patient's needs and abilities, is not likely to increase the risk of lymphedema.[143]

Although research has shown that strenuous exercises can be undertaken by those individuals at risk of, or already having, lymphedema without negative effects,[141,142] it is advisable to start the exercise regimen slowly, which avoids the risk of increased swelling, strains and injury to muscles, and allows the individual to observe how the edematous extremity responds to exercise.

Flexibility and stretching exercises (Yoga), swimming, water aerobics, and walking can be beneficial additions to the decongestive exercise program. Higher impact activities may exacerbate the symptoms associated with lymphedema and should be avoided. However, in some cases, it is not an easy task to come up with a general statement of which exercises should be avoided for individuals with lymphedema. Many patients find it important to continue their pre-lymphedema activities, even if these activities are considered "high-risk" (see Do's and Don'ts for Upper Extremity Lymphedema and Do's and Don'ts for Lower Extremity Lymphedema) for lymphedema. Tennis or golf, for example, does not rank very high on the list of beneficial activities for individuals with upper extremity lymphedema. For patients with lymphedema of the leg, kick-boxing and step-aerobics are activities that bear a great risk of injury and are considered "high-risk activities." However, for many individuals engaging in these activities, exercise plays such a vital role in their daily routine that giving up these "high-risk activities" could have a serious impact on their well-being.

For the majority of patients at risk for or diagnosed with lymphedema, an exercise regimen typically includes some combination of the following:

- *Flexibility and stretching exercises*: These exercises move the skin, muscle, and other tissues in the affected area, and assist in relieving the feeling of tightness that is often associated with lymphedema. An effective flexibility training program can also improve physical performance and help reduce risk of injury. By improving range of motion, the body requires less energy to make the same movements; it also contributes to more flexible joints and ligaments thus lessening the likelihood of injuries. Deep breathing exercises are beneficial as well (see below). Studies have shown that the venous return and lymphatic drainage in the thoracic lymphatic duct is positively impacted by changes in the intrathoracic pressure caused by deep breathing exercises.[144] The downward and upward movement of the diaphragm in deep abdominal breathing is an essential component for the sufficient return of lymphatic and venous fluid back to the bloodstream. The movement of the diaphragm, combined with the outward and inward movements of the abdomen, ribcage, and lower back, also promotes general well-being, peristalsis, and return of venous blood back to the heart.
- *Strength exercises*: see 4.6.2.
- *Aerobic exercise*: Aerobic conditioning is generally performed in a repetitive fashion using large muscle groups. Some long-term benefits include decrease in resting heart rate, improved muscular strength, weight control, and increased return of venous and lymphatic fluids. Aerobic exercises assist with weight loss and encourage deep breathing, which in turn supports lymphatic and venous return (see also 4.6.3).

Some general rules on exercising with lymphedema:

- *Use common sense:* Lifting heavy weights or running a marathon is not the best way to start a lymphedema exercise regimen. An exercise program should start gradually to avoid sprains and injury to muscles and should be followed by a warm down after active exercises. Studies have shown that a 10- to 15-minute warming down assists the lymphatic system in the removal of excess fluid and metabolites, which have accumulated in the interstitial space.[145,146]
- *Observe:* It is important to monitor the affected extremity during and after exercise activity for any change in comfort level, size, shape, texture, heaviness, or firmness. Any changes could be an indication to adjust a particular activity or to

take a break. If a change persists for more than a few days, the doctor or lymphedema therapist should be consulted.

- *Cooperate with a lymphedema therapist or other health care professional with knowledge in the treatment and management of lymphedema:* In the beginning of an exercise regimen, it is beneficial to work with someone with expertise in lymphedema management who can provide guidance and feedback. In many cases, the exercise program needs to be individualized to take into consideration the stage of lymphedema, possible accompanying medical conditions (heart problems, pulmonary issues, diabetes, etc.), or any medication that has side effects.

Working with instructors and trainers without a medical background and no knowledge of the specific issues regarding lymphedema may have adverse effects, such as increased swelling or injury.

The following exercises serve as guidelines for a decongestive exercise program that incorporate elements of breathing and stretching exercises and can be performed by most patients without difficulties in the self-management phase of therapy. The exercise regimen may be changed to accommodate individual limitations; ideally, the exercises are performed 10 to 15 minutes following the MLD/self-MLD session, and the patient should rest with the extremity elevated for 10 to 15 minutes following the exercise regimen.

Upper Extremity

- Exercises should be performed wearing compression bandages or compression sleeves (except when exercises are performed in the water).
- Tight or restrictive clothing (tight underwear or bra, heavy breast prosthesis) should not be worn while performing the exercises.
- Exercises should be performed twice daily for ~ 10 to 15 minutes. The duration of the program should be increased slowly over a comfortable period of time.
- Movements should be performed in a slow and controlled manner, and the musculature should be relaxed between each individual exercise. The relaxation phase should last at least as long as the time spent during the exercise.

Exercises should be performed sitting on a stool or a chair without leaning back. Many of the exercises, however, may be performed while lying on the floor. Proper breathing techniques should be used throughout the session.

Abdominal breathing (three repetitions):

1. Place both hands on your belly.
2. Inhale deeply through your nose into your belly (feel how you breathe against your hands).
3. Exhale through your mouth.

Perform breathing exercises as often as possible during the day.

Neck exercises (two to three repetitions each):

1. Turn your head slowly and look to the right as far as possible; return to normal position; repeat on the left side.
2. Bend your head to the right and try to touch the shoulder with your ear (do not shrug your shoulder). Return to the starting position and repeat for left side.

Shoulder Exercises

Shoulder rolls (three to five repetitions each):
1. Rotate shoulders alternately on the right and left side.
2. Perform shoulder rolls, forward and backward, using both shoulders.

Shoulder shrug (three to five repetitions each)
1. Shrug both shoulders and inhale. Exhale while relaxing your shoulders.

Arm exercises (three to five repetitions each)

Fingers:

1. Place palms and fingers together.
2. Move little fingers away from each other and back together.
3. Move ring fingers away from each other and back together.

Continue with each finger.

Alternate position:

1. Hold palms out in front of the body with the palms facing up.
2. Move thumb and index finger together, so that the finger pads touch each other; return to open hand.

3. Move thumb and ring finger together, so that the finger pads touch each other; return to open hand.

Continue with each finger.

Hand:

Alternate between hands; the relaxed hand rests on the leg.
1. Make a fist and hold for ~ 3 seconds.
2. Open the fist and relax the hand for ~ 3 seconds.
3. Make a fist and rotate the wrist clockwise and counterclockwise.
4. Make a fist and touch it to the opposite shoulder.

Arm and Hands

Picking Oranges:

1. Stretch out arm and lean forward.
2. Make a fist and return hand to leg.

Climb Up the Ladder

Alternate between arms and continue for ~ 30 to 40 seconds.
1. Hold arms above head.
2. Grasp rungs of imaginary ladder and "climb" as high as possible (remain seated).

Swimming

Use breaststrokes as far as possible to the front, move arms to the side, then to the knees and to the front again.
Hand to Opposite Knee.

Alternate Between Arms

1. Place the palm of one hand on the opposite knee and push down with your hand, then upward with your knee.
2. Hold for 5 seconds.

Exercises with a broomstick (three to five repetitions each)

Climbing up and down the stick:

1. Hold the stick vertically between your knees with your hands.
2. Take the stick at the bottom with one hand and "climb" up and down the stick with alternating hands.

Weight lifting:

1. Hold the stick with both hands horizontally, with the palms up.
2. Lift the stick up and toward your head, then return to the original position.

Wringing the stick:

1. Hold the stick with both hands horizontally, with the palms down and ~ 1 foot apart.
2. Attempt to wring the stick, moving one hand forward and the other back.
3. Hold for ~ 3 to 5 seconds and wring in the other direction.

Canoeing:

1. Hold the stick with both hands horizontally, with the palms down and ~ 1 foot apart.
2. Start to "paddle" to either side with nice, big strokes.

Pendulum:

1. Hold the stick vertically in front of you on one end.
2. Move the stick slowly from one side to the other like a pendulum.
3. Change hands and repeat.

Exercises with a soft ball (three to five repetitions each)

Biceps curl:

1. Hold the ball with one hand, palm up.
2. Curl the ball to your shoulder, then return to the starting position.
3. Alternate hands (the relaxed hand rests on the thigh).

Sponge Squeeze

1. Hold the ball with both hands in your lap and squeeze as hard as you can.
2. Hold the squeeze for ~ 10 seconds.

Roll the Dough

Place the ball on one thigh and roll the ball with your whole hand (fingers and palm) to the knee. Return to the lap, and alternate the hands.

Soft ball circles:

1. Hold the ball in one hand, with the arm extended.

2. Guide the ball with two or three big circles around your body by switching the ball between the hands.
3. Alternate directions.
4. Lift one thigh and guide the ball under the thigh to the other hand; alternate between the hands and legs.

Lower Extremity

- Exercises should be performed while wearing compression bandages or compression garments (except when exercises are performed in the water).
- Tight or restrictive clothing should not be worn while performing the exercises.
- Exercises should be performed twice daily for ~ 10 to 15 minutes. The duration of the program should be increased slowly over a comfortable period of time.
- Movements should be performed in a slow and controlled manner, and the musculature should be relaxed between each individual exercise. The relaxation phase should last at least as long as the time spent during the exercise.

Exercises should be performed while lying supine on the floor, preferably on a cushioned mat or other surface that maintains some firmness. Proper breathing techniques should be used throughout the session. To avoid back strain, a small pillow may be placed under the knees.

Abdominal breathing (three repetitions)

1. Place both hands on your belly.
2. Inhale deeply through your nose into your belly (feel how you breathe against your hands).
3. Exhale through your mouth.

Perform breathing exercises as often as possible during the day.

Foot and leg exercises (three to five repetitions each)

Toe clenches (either alternating or with both feet at the same time):
1. Curl your toes and squeeze for ~ 3 seconds.
2. Relax the toes for ~ 3 seconds.

Spread the toes (either alternating or with both feet at the same time)
1. Spread the toes as far as possible and hold for ~ 3 seconds.

2. Relax the toes for ~ 3 seconds.

Ankle curls (either alternating or with both feet at the same time)

1. Flex the foot as far as possible at the ankle, with the toes pointing away from the body (back of the knee remains on the floor).
2. Hold for ~ 3 seconds.
3. Flex the foot as far as possible at the ankle, with the toes pointing to the shin.
4. Relax for ~ 3 seconds.

Ankle rotation (either alternating or with both feet at the same time)

1. Rotate foot at the ankle, both clockwise and counterclockwise.

Riding the bike (for ~ 1 minute)

While lying on your back, move your legs in the air as if you are riding a bicycle. (If you use a stationary bike, keep it on a low setting to avoid soreness or strain.)

Heel sliding:

1. Move the heel of your foot as close as possible to your buttocks.
2. Return to the starting position, and alternate the legs.

Hand and knee touch:

1. Lift one knee and push the palm of the opposite hand against the knee. Hold for ~ 3 seconds.
2. Relax for ~ 3 seconds, then alternate sides.

Butt lift:

1. Bend the knees and place your feet flat on the floor.
2. Raise your buttocks off the floor and hold for ~ 3 seconds.
3. Bring the buttocks back to the floor and relax for ~ 3 seconds.

Exercises for the lower back (three to four repetitions each)

Knee hugs (keep your head on the floor):

1. Bend one knee and hug the knee with both arms.
2. Bring the knee with your arms as close as possible to your chest.
3. Hold for ~ 3 seconds.
4. Bring the foot back to the floor.
5. Alternate legs.

Back stretch 1 (keep your head and shoulders on the floor and stabilize your body with both palms pressing down on the floor):

1. Bend both knees and move them as close to the chest as possible.
2. Hold for ~ 3 seconds.
3. Bring the feet back to the floor and relax for ~ 3 seconds.

Back stretch 2 (keep your head and shoulders on the floor and stabilize your body with both palms pressing down on the floor):

1. Bend both knees with the foot flat on the floor.
2. Move both knees to the right side as close to the floor as possible, and hold for ~ 3 seconds.
3. Move the knees back to the middle position and relax for ~ 3 seconds.
4. Alternate sides.

Exercises with a soft ball (three to five repetitions each)

Squeeze:

1. Hold the ball between your knees and squeeze together for ~ 3 seconds; relax for ~ 3 seconds.
2. Place the ball under your thigh and squeeze to the floor for ~ 3 seconds; relax for ~ 3 seconds.
3. Alternate legs.

Circles:

1. Bend one knee, and lead the ball behind the thigh and back to the front using both hands.
2. Alternate legs.

Walking:

Walking is a great exercise for lymphedema of the lower extremities. If you use a stair exerciser or treadmill, keep it on a low setting to avoid soreness or strain.

Remember to walk with a normal gait. Do not drag the affected leg, and avoid limping.

5.20.4 Self-MLD

Simple and easy-to-perform MLD techniques are an integral part of the self-management program. In this stage, the patient has completed the intensive phase with the lymphedema therapist and is familiar with the pressures and techniques used in MLD.

Ideally, the self-MLD protocol should be performed at least once a day for ~ 10 to 15 minutes, directly preceding the exercise program, and should be followed by compression therapy.

The following are basic techniques for unilateral upper and lower extremity lymphedema. These techniques may be changed according to specific requirements and physical limitations of the individual patient. It is important that the patient understands the correct pressure to apply with the strokes, and the self-MLD session should not turn into a kneading/massage session.

Upper Extremity

The stationary circles used in this self-treatment are based on the same principles as those performed by the lymphedema therapist. They should be executed using light pressure in the working phase; during the resting phase of the circle, the hand should relax completely. The amount of pressure is sometimes described as the pressure applied while stroking a newborn's head. The circles should be large enough to stretch the skin, but the hand should not slide over the skin. Self-MLD for the arm is performed best in the sitting position. Each stroke should be repeated five to seven times on the same placement, and, if not noted otherwise, the hand of the unaffected side should be used to perform the strokes.

Note: The self-MLD techniques in ▶ Fig. 5.232, ▶ Fig. 5.233, and ▶ Fig. 5.234 depict the sequence used for a lymphedema on the left arm.

Pretreatment

1. Make circles with the fingers lying flat above the collarbone on both sides. The pressure is directed toward the neck. It would be easier for the right hand to manipulate the skin above the left collarbone and vice versa (▶ Fig. 5.232).
2. Make circles in the center of the opposite axilla. Pressure is given with the flat hand of the affected arm and is directed downward (deep) into the axilla (▶ Fig. 5.233).

5

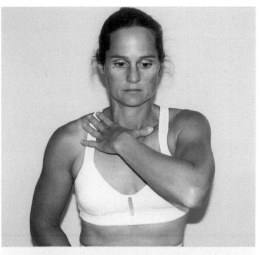

Fig. 5.232 Stationary circles above the collarbone on both sides.

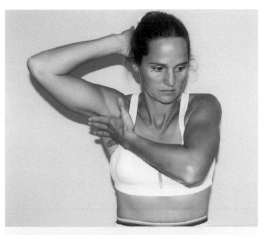

Fig. 5.233 Stationary circles in the axilla on the unaffected side.

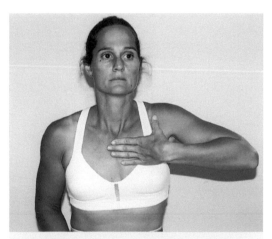

Fig. 5.234 Soft effleurage from the affected axilla to the axilla on the other side.

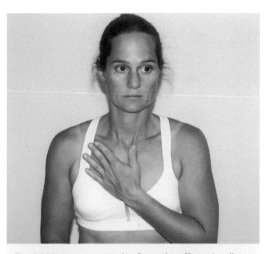

Fig. 5.235 Stationary circles from the affected axilla to the axilla on the other side in several placements.

3. Perform soft effleurage from the affected axilla to the axilla on the other side (▶ Fig. 5.234).
4. Make circles from the affected axilla to the axilla on the other side in several placements. The pressure is directed toward the axilla on the unaffected side (▶ Fig. 5.235).
5. Make circles with the flat hand (use affected arm) in the area of the inguinal lymph nodes on the same side. The hand lies just below the inguinal ligament, and the pressure is directed toward the belly (▶ Fig. 5.236).
6. Make circles with the flat hand from the affected axilla to the inguinal lymph nodes on the same side in several placements. The

pressure is directed toward the inguinal lymph nodes of the same side (▶ Fig. 5.237).

Arm

7. Perform soft effleurage strokes covering the entire arm, beginning on the hand and ending on the top of the shoulder.
8. Make circles covering the deltoid and the shoulder of the affected arm; the pressure is directed toward the neck in several placements (▶ Fig. 5.238; ▶ Fig. 5.239).
9. Make circles with flat fingers from the medial to the lateral upper arm. Work the entire upper arm from the top down to the elbow with this

5

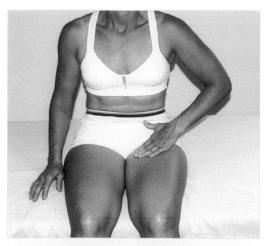

Fig. 5.236 Stationary circles in the area of the inguinal lymph nodes on the same side.

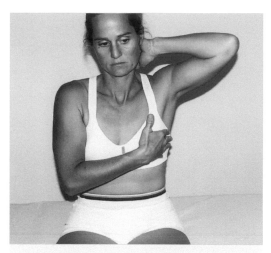

Fig. 5.237 Stationary circles with the flat hand from the affected axilla to the inguinal lymph nodes on the same side in several placements.

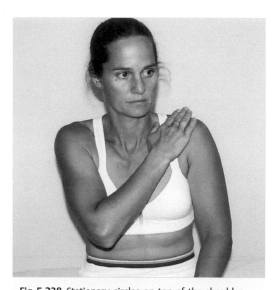

Fig. 5.238 Stationary circles on top of the shoulder.

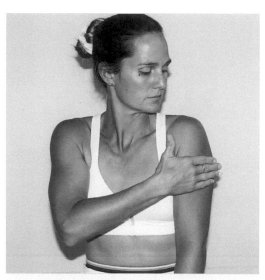

Fig. 5.239 Stationary circles on the lateral upper arm in several placements.

technique. The pressure is directed toward the lateral upper arm (▶ Fig. 5.240).

10.
Rework the lateral upper arm from the elbow to the shoulder with circles. The pressure is directed toward the shoulder.

11.
Make circles in the front of the elbow, the forearm, and the hand. Turn the forearm so that you can reach all aspects of it. The pressure is always

directed to the upper arm (▶ Fig. 5.241;
▶ Fig. 5.242; ▶ Fig. 5.243; ▶ Fig. 5.244).

12.
Rework the upper arm. (You may repeat as many of the hand placements as you wish.)

13.
Repeat steps 1, 2, and 5. (You may repeat as many of the hand placements as you wish.)

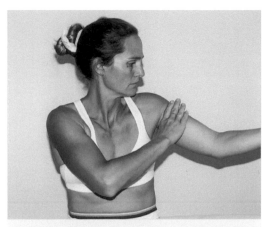

Fig. 5.240 Stationary circles from the medial to the lateral upper arm in several placements.

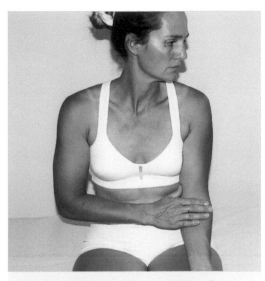

Fig. 5.241 Stationary circles in front of the elbow.

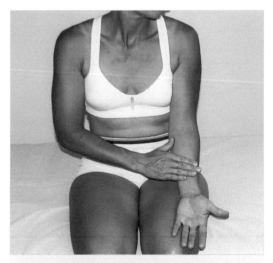

Fig. 5.242 Stationary circles on the anterior forearm.

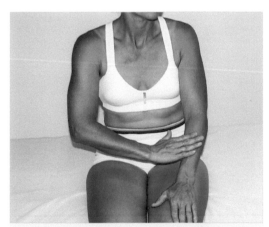

Fig. 5.243 Stationary circles on the posterior forearm.

Lower Extremity

The stationary circles used in this self-treatment are based on the same principles as those performed by the lymphedema therapist. They should be executed using light pressure in the working phase, and the hand should relax completely during the resting phase of the circle. The circles should be large enough to stretch the skin, but the hand should not slide over the skin. Self-MLD for the leg should be performed lying in the supine position. Each stroke should be repeated five to seven times on the same placement.

Note: The self-MLD techniques shown in ▶ Fig. 5.245, ▶ Fig. 5.246, ▶ Fig. 5.247, and ▶ Fig. 5.248 depict the sequence used for a lymphedema on the left leg.

Pretreatment

1. Make circles with the fingers lying flat above the collarbones on each side. Do each side separately, and use the hand of the opposite side. Switch hands to manipulate the other side. The pressure on both sides is directed toward the neck (▶ Fig. 5.245).
2. Make circles in the center of the axilla on the same side. Pressure is given with the flat hand and is directed downward (deep) into the axilla (▶ Fig. 5.246).

5

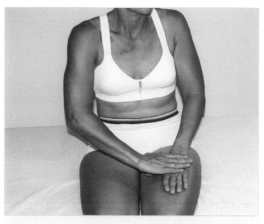

Fig. 5.244 Stationary circles on the back of the hand.

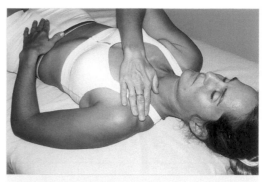

Fig. 5.245 Stationary circles above the collarbones on each side.

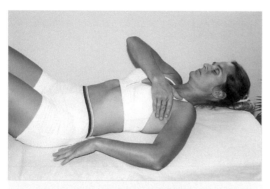

Fig. 5.246 Stationary circles in the axilla on the same side.

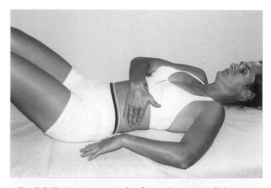

Fig. 5.247 Stationary circles from the waist of the affected side to the axillary lymph nodes on the same side in several placements.

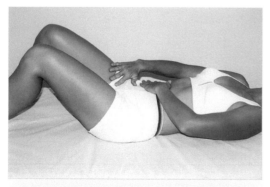

Fig. 5.248 Stationary circles on the inguinal lymph nodes of the unaffected side.

3. Make circles with the flat hand on the side of the trunk, from the waist of the affected side to the axillary lymph nodes on the same side (in several placements). The pressure is directed toward the axillary lymph nodes on the same side (▶ Fig. 5.247).

4. Make circles with the flat hand in the area of the inguinal lymph nodes on the opposite side. The hand lies just below the inguinal ligament, and the pressure is directed toward the belly (▶ Fig. 5.248).

5. Make circles from the inguinal area on the affected side to the inguinal lymph nodes on the other side (in several placements). The pressure is directed to the inguinal lymph nodes on the unaffected side (▶ Fig. 5.249).

6. *Abdominal breathing*: Place both hands flat on your belly and inhale against your hands. The hands follow the belly while you exhale; at the end of the exhalation, both hands press downward and upward (into the thorax). Repeat five times (▶ Fig. 5.250; ▶ Fig. 5.251).

Note: Discuss possible contraindications with your therapist.

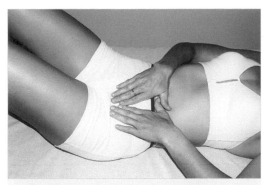

Fig. 5.249 Stationary circles from the inguinal area on the affected side to the inguinal lymph nodes on the other side in several placements.

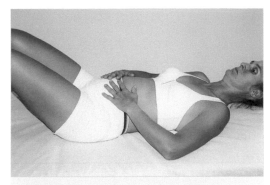

Fig. 5.250 Diaphragmatic breathing: Inhalation.

5

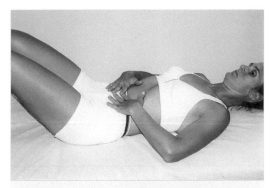

Fig. 5.251 Diaphragmatic breathing: Exhalation.

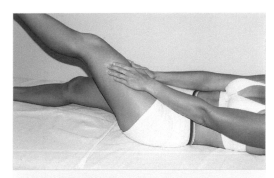

Fig. 5.252 Effleurage on the leg.

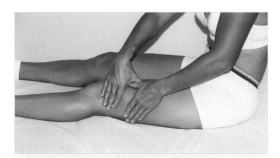

Fig. 5.253 Stationary circles covering the lateral thigh and the hip in several placements.

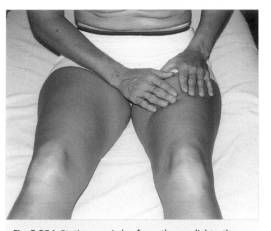

Fig. 5.254 Stationary circles from the medial to the lateral thigh.

Leg

1. Perform soft effleurage strokes covering the entire leg, beginning at the ankles (or the knee) and ending on the lateral waist (▶ Fig. 5.252).
2. Make circles covering the lateral thigh and the hip in several placements. The pressure is directed toward the trunk (▶ Fig. 5.253).
3. Make circles with both flat hands from the medial to the lateral thigh. Work the entire thigh from the top down to the knee with this technique. The pressure is directed toward the lateral thigh (▶ Fig. 5.254).

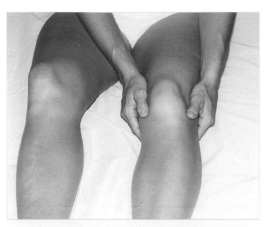

Fig. 5.255 Stationary circles behind the knee.

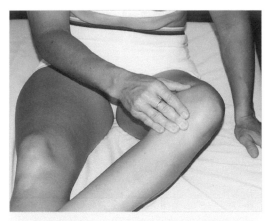

Fig. 5.256 Stationary circles below the medial knee.

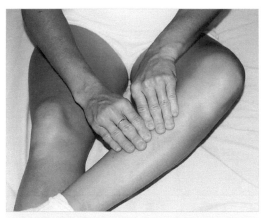

Fig. 5.257 Stationary circles in several placements on the medial lower leg.

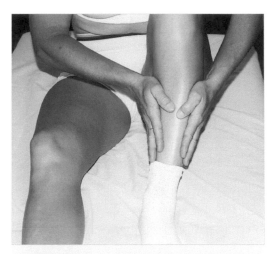

Fig. 5.258 Stationary circles on both sides of the lower leg.

4. Make circles with the flat fingers of both hands behind the knee. The pressure is directed toward the thigh (▶ Fig. 5.255).
5. Make circles with one or both hands in several placements on the medial lower leg, between the knee and the ankle. The pressure is directed toward the thigh (▶ Fig. 5.256; ▶ Fig. 5.257).
6. Make circles with the hands lying flat on both sides of the lower leg. The pressure is directed toward the thigh. Do several placements between the knee and the ankles (▶ Fig. 5.258).
7. Make circles with the fingers of one hand lying flat on the back of the foot. The pressure is directed toward the ankles.
8. Rework the leg. (You may repeat as many of the hand placements as you wish.)
9. Repeat steps 2, 4, and 6. (You may repeat as many of the hand placements as you wish.)

5.20.5 Precautions

Anyone who has undergone lymph node excision and/or radiation therapy is at risk of developing lymphedema. The capacity of the lymphatic system to remove fluid and other substances (lymphatic loads) from the tissues has been reduced by these procedures to a certain degree. Lymphedema may occur directly after the surgery or radiation therapy, may develop months or even years following the procedures, or may never develop.

Certain activities and situations may trigger the onset of lymphedema, or exacerbate the symptoms of existing lymphedema, by further reducing the transport capacity of the lymphatic system or by increasing the amount of lymphatic loads. Individuals who are aware of these risk factors know

5

what can be done to avoid the onset of swelling and infections, which are common in patients suffering from lymphedema as well as those at risk. Knowing the necessary precautions helps prevent aggravation of the symptoms in existing lymphedema.

The following Do's and Don'ts may have a cumulative effect. Whether one or more of these events or situations will be a triggering element depends on other factors, such as overall health (other conditions) and fitness, the extent of the initial procedure (scarring, number of lymph nodes removed), and obesity.

Patients with lymphedema and those at risk of developing it should observe the following precautionary measures. In many cases, modifications to lifestyle are necessary, but a normal activity level should be maintained. In other words, individuals should not refrain from using the affected extremity for fear of developing lymphedema.

There is little evidence-based literature regarding these precautions; most of the following Do's and Don'ts for upper and lower extremity lymphedema are based on knowledge of the pathophysiology of lymphedema and decades of clinical experience among experts in the field of lymphedema management.

Do's and Don'ts for Upper Extremity Lymphedema

- Avoid any injuries to the skin:
  - *Gardening*: Wear gloves.
  - *Pets*: Be careful to avoid scratches when playing with animals; wear gloves.
  - *Mosquito bites*: Use insect repellents, and avoid mosquito-infested areas.
  - *Nail care*: You should keep your fingernails cut short. Do not use scissors to cut your fingernails, and do not cut the cuticles. Do not apply artificial nails.
  - *Shaving*: Use an electric razor to remove hair from the axilla; do not use razor blades
  - *Injections*: Do not allow injections in the swollen or at-risk arm. Instead, take injections in the buttocks, the thigh, or the abdominal area.
  - *Venipunctures*: Do not allow blood to be drawn from the affected (at risk) arm. Have the venipuncture in the other arm, or if both arms are affected, in the lower extremity (certain contraindications may exist). The physician may choose to use vascular access devices (VADs, ports), if appropriate.
  - *Take proper care of minor injuries*: Always carry an alcohol swab, local antibiotic, and a bandage with you.
  - Should you smoke, do not extinguish the cigarette with your affected hand.
  - No piercing or tattoos on the arm or the upper body quadrants.
- Do not have blood pressure readings taken on the affected (at risk) arm:
  - Have the clinician use the other arm; if both arms are affected, an oversize pressure cuff may be used on the thigh or calf (blood pressure taken on the leg may produce a higher reading). If you cannot avoid having the blood pressure taken on the affected arm, make sure that the cuff is inflated only 10 mm Hg above the systolic pressure (this is the point at which the pulse stops) and that only manual equipment is used (automated equipment generally inflates to a very high pressure, which is held for a prolonged period).
- Avoid heat:
  - Avoid hot showers and baths. The arm should not be placed in water temperatures above 102 °F (38.9 °C). Dry thoroughly, but avoid scrubbing or rubbing the skin with a towel.
  - Avoid hot packs and/or ice packs on your arm.
  - Avoid saunas or hot tubs and whirlpools; do not sit too close to a working fireplace.
  - Avoid massage (kneading, stroking, etc.) on the arm and the upper thorax. *Note*: MLD is *not* considered to be a form of massage.
  - Avoid cosmetics that irritate the skin.
  - Avoid getting sunburned. While in the sun, use sunscreen and cover the affected arm with a long-sleeved shirt or a dry towel.
- Clothing/compression sleeve/jewelry:
  - Avoid clothing that is too tight (tight bras, sleeves).
  - You should wear a comfortable bra with wide and padded shoulder straps.
  - Do not wear tight jewelry (rings, bracelets); avoid elastic wristbands.
  - *Prosthesis*: Discuss with your doctor and/or therapist what kind of external breast prosthesis is appropriate in your case (heavier silicone or lighter foam).
  - Wear your compression sleeve all day. See your therapist at least every 6 months to check the condition of the sleeve. Use a rubber glove when applying your compression sleeve. If necessary, apply your bandages at night.
- Exercises:

- ○ Always discuss proper exercises and activities with your therapist.
- ○ Avoid movements that overstrain; should you experience discomfort in the affected arm, reduce the exercise activity and elevate your arm.
- ○ Avoid heavy lifting.
- ○ Gradually increase the intensity and duration of any exercise.
- ○ Monitor the extremity during and after exercise for any changes in size or shape.
- ○ Take frequent rests during exercise to allow your arm to recover.
- Beneficial activities:
  - ○ Swimming, lymphedema exercise program, self-MLD, yoga, water aerobics, walking.
- Medium-risk activities:
  - ○ Jogging/running, biking (use aerobars; minimize gripping), stair exerciser (do not use grips; elevate the arm sometimes), treadmill (use minimal grips), horse riding (hold reins loosely), extreme hiking, mountain climbing.
- High-risk activities:
  - ○ Gardening (wear gloves), tennis/racquet sports, golf, shoveling snow, moving furniture, carrying luggage, carrying heavy grocery bags, scrubbing, weight lifting with the affected arm (not more than 4–6 kg), intense horse riding (gripping reins).

> If you wish to engage in either medium- or high-risk activities, you should discuss additional precautionary measures (extra compression during the activity) with your therapist or doctor.

- Travel:
  - ○ Avoid mosquito-infested regions.
  - ○ Wear an additional bandage or garment on top of your compression sleeve when traveling by car, train, or air (see also Section 5.20.6 later in this chapter). Incorporate frequent stops, or get up from your seat frequently.
- Skin care:
  - ○ Keep your skin meticulously clean.
  - ○ Inspect your skin for any cracks, fungal infections, or rashes.
  - ○ Moisturize your skin daily, especially after taking a shower or bath. Use appropriate ointments or lotions (preferably free of alcohol and fragrance).

- ○ Dry your skin thoroughly after taking a shower or bath (especially in skin creases and web spaces). Use a soft towel, and do not scrub.
- ○ If you undergo radiation therapy, apply the ointments recommended by your physician to any radiation redness on your skin. Avoid chlorinated pools and direct exposure to sunlight.
- Nutrition:
  - ○ Obesity may have a negative effect on swelling; therefore, maintain your ideal body weight.
  - ○ There is no special diet for lymphedema. Keep your diet well balanced. Today most nutritionists recommend a low-salt, low-fat, high-fiber diet.
  - ○ Eating too little protein is not recommended and may cause serious health problems. Reducing protein intake will not reduce the protein component in lymphedema.
- See your doctor if you
  - ○ Have any signs of an infection (fever, chills, red and hot skin).
  - ○ Notice any itching, rash, fungal infections, or any other unusual changes on the skin.
  - ○ Experience an increase in swelling in your fingers, hand, arm, or chest.
  - ○ Experience pain.

Do's and Don'ts for Lower Extremity Lymphedema

- Avoid any injuries to the skin:
  - ○ Do not walk barefoot.
  - ○ *Pets*: Be careful to avoid scratches when playing with animals.
  - ○ *Mosquito bites*: Use insect repellents, and avoid mosquito-infested areas.
  - ○ *Nail care*: You should keep your toenails short, but be careful when cutting your toenails; do not cut the cuticles.
  - ○ *Shaving*: Use an electric razor to remove hair from the leg or lower body quadrant; do not use razor blades.
  - ○ *Injections*: Do not allow injections in the swollen (at risk) leg, in the buttocks on the affected side, or in the abdominal area.
  - ○ *Venipunctures*: Do not allow blood to be drawn from the affected (at risk) leg.
  - ○ *Take care of minor injuries*: Always carry an alcohol swab, local antibiotic, and a bandage with you.
  - ○ Wear solid shoes to avoid ankle injuries.

- No piercing or tattoos on the leg or the lower body quadrants.
- Avoid heat:
  - Avoid hot showers and baths. The leg should not be placed in water temperatures above 102 °F (38.9 °C). Dry thoroughly, but avoid scrubbing or rubbing the skin with a towel.
  - Avoid hot packs and/or ice packs on the affected leg.
  - Avoid saunas or hot tubs and whirlpools. Do not sit too close to a working fireplace.
  - Avoid massage (kneading, stroking, etc.) on the affected leg and the lumbar area. *Note*: MLD is *not* considered to be a form of massage.
  - Avoid cosmetics that irritate the skin.
  - Avoid getting sunburned. While in the sun, use sunscreen, and cover the affected leg with appropriate clothing or a dry towel.
- Clothing/compression stocking/jewelry:
  - Avoid clothing that is too tight (underwear, pants, socks, or stockings that restrict).
  - Do not wear tight jewelry (toe rings); avoid elastic bands around your ankle.
  - Wear your compression stocking/pantyhose all day. Use rubber gloves when applying your compression garment. See your therapist at least every 6 months to check the condition of the garment. If necessary, apply your bandages at night.
- Exercises:
  - Always discuss proper exercises and activities with your therapist.
  - Avoid movements that overstrain. Should you experience discomfort in the affected leg, reduce the exercise activity, and elevate your leg.
  - Elevate your leg as often as possible; avoid prolonged standing, sitting, or crossing legs.
  - Gradually increase the intensity and duration of any exercise.
  - Monitor the extremity during and after exercise for any changes in size or shape.
  - Take frequent rests during exercise to allow your leg to recover.
- Beneficial activities:
  - Swimming, lymphedema exercise program, self-MLD, yoga, water aerobics, walking, treadmill (10–15 minutes, slow walking speed), easy biking (15–20 minutes; use a wide, comfortable saddle), calf pumps, deep breathing exercises.
- Medium-risk activities:
  - Light jogging/running, biking (longer than 30 minutes), stair exerciser (longer than

5 minutes), treadmill (longer than 15 minutes), light horse riding, golfing.
- High-risk activities:
  - Running, tennis/racquet sports, hockey, soccer, wrestling, kickboxing, step aerobics, weight lifting with the affected leg, intense horse riding, sitting or standing over long periods.

If you wish to engage in either medium- or high-risk activities, you should discuss additional precautionary measures (extra compression during the activity) with your therapist or doctor.

- Skin care:
  - Keep your skin meticulously clean (use clean undergarments and socks at all times).
  - Inspect your skin for any cracks, fungal infections, or rashes.
  - Moisturize your skin daily, especially after taking a shower or bath. Use appropriate ointments or lotions (preferably free of alcohol and fragrance).
  - Dry your skin thoroughly after taking a shower or bath (especially in skin creases and web spaces). Use a soft towel, and do not scrub.
  - If you undergo radiation therapy, apply the ointments recommended by your physician to any radiation redness on your skin. Avoid chlorinated pools and direct exposure to sunlight.
- Nutrition:
  - Obesity may have a negative effect on swelling; therefore, maintain your ideal body weight.
  - There is no special diet for lymphedema. Keep your diet well balanced. Today most nutritionists recommend a low-salt, low-fat, high-fiber diet.
  - Eating too little protein is not recommended and may cause serious health problems. Reducing protein intake will not reduce the protein component in lymphedema.
- See your doctor if you
  - Have any signs of an infection (fever, chills, red and hot skin).
  - Notice any itching, rash, fungal infections, or any other unusual changes on the skin.
  - Experience an increase in swelling in your toes, foot, leg, or lower body quadrant.
  - Experience pain.
- Travel:

- Avoid mosquito-infested regions.
- Wear an additional bandage or stocking on top of your compression garment when traveling by car, train, or air (see also 5.20.6 below). Incorporate frequent stops, or get up from your seat frequently; elevate your leg(s) as often as possible.

5.20.6 Traveling with Lymphedema

Air travel may be especially challenging for individuals with lymphedema and those at risk for developing lymphedema. The cabin pressure during flights is lower than the atmospheric pressure on the ground, which causes a change in pressure in the connective tissues. These pressure changes, combined with the pooling of fluid in the tissues, may cause swelling even in normal tissues. It is obvious that these travel-related issues may have even more serious consequences in individuals with a compromised lymphatic system.

To avoid the onset of swelling and to prevent the worsening of preexisting lymphedema, it is recommended that a compression garment be worn during air travel. Compression increases tissue pressure and considerably aids in the prevention of fluid accumulation in the tissues.

While traveling with lymphedema does have some drawbacks and requires more planning, it should not stop those affected by lymphedema from air travel. The following recommendations are intended to help with planning for an enjoyable trip.

5.20.7 Lymphedema and Air Travel

Commercial airline travel is fast, safe, and convenient and in the vast majority of cases without any harmful health effects. However, the aircraft environment and other airline-travel–related factors may cause certain stresses on the patient affected by lymphedema, or the population at risk to develop lymphedema (latent lymphedema). Elements in question include the air pressure (and density), cabin pressure, and the cabin environment (air quality, seating).

Effects of Altitude on Air Pressure

The air's pressure is caused by the weight of the air pressing down on the earth, the body, and the ocean, as well as on the air below. The pressure value depends on the amount of air above the

point where the pressure is measured; if altitude increases, the pressure falls. The exact pressure at a particular altitude depends on weather conditions. To understand the general idea of how pressure decreases with altitude, the following approximation can be used:

As a rule of thumb, the air pressure drops about 1 inch of mercury for each 1,000-foot increase in altitude or about 0.49 pounds per square inch (psi). At sea level, the atmosphere weighs in at about 14.7 psi (101.325 kilopascal or millibar); the pressure of the atmosphere at 8,000 feet is around 10.9 psi (75.156 kilopascal).[147]

Cabin Pressure (Cabin Altitude)

Commercial aircrafts are capable of flying at altitudes that are incompatible with human life and yet the passengers and crew are generally not negatively affected because of the onboard environmental and pressurization systems.[148] Aircraft cabins traveling at high elevations are pressurized and the pressure inside the aircraft has to be kept within the design limits of the fuselage. Although pressurized, the cabin pressure while traveling at altitude is less than that on the ground. The cabin pressure of an aircraft intending to cruise at 40,000 feet is designed to rise gradually from the altitude of the airport of origin to around a maximum of 8,000 ft, and then reduce gently during descent until it matches the air pressure of the destination airport.

Regulations[149] require that commercial aircraft be capable of maintaining a cabin altitude no higher than 8,000 ft at the maximum authorized flight altitude; for most flights, the cabin pressure is maintained at around 7,000 ft when cruising at 40,000 ft. In other words, while flying at that altitude, the atmosphere within the aircraft is like that on a 7,000-ft mountain peak. Referring to the aforementioned information, it is apparent that air pressure (and density) at 7,000 ft are lower than on sea level. Some newer generation airplanes are capable of maintaining a higher cabin pressure.

Effects of Altitude on Air Density

In simple terms, density is the mass of anything divided by the volume it occupies. The density of air is directly proportional to the pressure. With increasing altitude, the pressure decreases, and so does the density of air. Because air is a gas, it can be compressed or expanded. When air is compressed (resulting in increased pressure), a greater amount of air occupies a given volume; thus, the density of air is increased. When pressure is decreased on a given volume of air, the air expands and occupies a greater space; thus, the density of air is decreased. Oxygen accounts for about 21% of the gases in the atmosphere (at sea level as well as at altitude), but because air density decreases with altitude, the amount of oxygen inhaled will decrease with every breath taken. Hence, less oxygen is absorbed into the blood and circulated throughout the body during flight.

Cabin Pressure and the Effects on Lymphedema

Many patients reported that their extremities had started to swell during air travel. In a 1993 study conducted in Australia, 27 of 490 patients reported onset of lymphedema during aircraft flight (15 lower and 12 upper extremities), and worsening of existing lymphedema was reported by 67 patients (44 lower and 23 upper extremities).[150]

The most reasonable explanation for this may be inactivity, especially in lower extremity cases.

Most aircraft are crowded, and passengers are frequently uncomfortable and unable to stretch or easily leave their seats. It is a well-known fact that even people with an intact lymphatic system develop swollen feet and ankles during long flights. Inactivity in combination with a compromised lymphatic drainage can have even more serious consequences.

Inactivity, with the legs in a downward position coupled with the subsequent pooling of venous blood, will lead to an increase in tissue fluid in the lower extremities. This may be enough to trigger the onset of lymphedema in those patients with latent lymphedema, or worsen already existing lymphedema in the legs.

In addition to inactivity, other factors may play a crucial role in those patients traveling with lymphedema.

The decrease in air pressure (the force exerted on the body by the weight of the air) in the cabin, especially in long-haul flights, may trigger the onset of lymphedema, or exacerbate the symptoms of existing lymphedema.

The reduced pressure does have certain effects on those tissues that are or may be affected by lymphedema (suprafascial tissues). Those effects may allow more fluid to be filtered from the blood capillaries into the tissues. Some of this fluid must be removed by the lymphatic system. An increase in the interstitial fluid content as a result of increased filtration may be just enough to trigger the onset of lymphedema in individuals with compromised lymphatic drainage (latency stages) or increase the swelling in individuals affected by upper and/or lower extremity lymphedema. It can also be assumed[150] that the lower pressure in

cabins allows fibrotic capsules in the tissue to become rounded, causing compression and/or distortion of adjacent structures, such as lymphatic collectors and inlet valves of lymph capillaries. This may also result in increased swelling and/or impeded uptake of lymphatic fluid.

In many cases, the elastic fibers in the skin are damaged in lymphedema due to the constant stretch caused by the swelling. This may present an additional factor in the worsening of lymphedema under a low cabin pressure environment.

Air Quality and Humidity in Pressurized Cabins

The environmental system in aircraft provides filtration, controls temperature, and is also responsible for keeping humidity at a reasonable level. In modern aircraft, half of the cabin air consists of fresh air drawn from the engine intakes, and the other half is recirculated and filtered air from the cabin. The filtration systems (some aircrafts are equipped with high efficiency particulate air [HEPA] filters) easily maintain cabin contaminants to low levels. The air is completely exchanged every 2 to 3 minutes, which is far more efficient than environmental systems in a typical home or office building.

Humidity, however, is usually less than 20% in pressurized cabins. This is fairly dry and may cause dehydration, which represents an additional complicating factor in lymphedema. The negative effects of dehydration can be countered by drinking extra water during airplane travel. It must be stressed that alcohol has an additional dehydrating effect and should not be used to replace body fluids.

Ways to Avoid the Onset of Swelling during Flight

Compression therapy seems to be the most effective measure to counter possible negative effects on lymphedema during air travel. Compression therapy (bandages and/or compression garments) increases the tissue pressure. This increase in tissue pressure effectively reduces the accumulation of fluid in the tissues and promotes lymphatic and venous return.

It is highly recommended to perform in-flight exercises. Airlines generally provide a pamphlet or video presentation on in-flight exercises, which are especially beneficial if they are performed while wearing compression bandage or garment.

Following are some recommendations for airline travelers:
- Plan ahead:
  - You should seek the advice of your physician and lymphedema therapist if you have any questions. A note from the physician may help

answer security questions regarding bandages, compression garments, or medication.

- If you are at risk for developing lymphedema, discuss with your physician and/or lymphedema therapist if it may be beneficial to wear a well-fitted compression garment, or short-stretch bandage(s) during the flight.
- You should check the quality of your compression garment. If you have more than one garment, take the extra one with you as a backup. If traveling to high-altitude locations, take the same precautions as for a flight.
- You should ensure that you can manage your own luggage. If traveling with another person or a group, ask someone else to carry the luggage for you. Should you travel on your own, use a suitcase with wheels and do not lift your luggage from the baggage carousel with your swollen arm.
- Carry your prescription medication with you; if necessary, get your prescriptions filled before you leave to make sure they last you through your vacation. If your destination is located in hot or mosquito-infested areas, take precautions (sunscreen, insect repellents, and antibiotics). Should you travel to a tropical country in which filariasis is endemic (especially during the wet season), talk to your doctor about special medication to take with you. Take some antifungal powder with you—the bathrooms and showers in hotel rooms may be a source of infection.
- Carry skin lotion because the air in pressurized cabins is very dry.
- If possible, request an exit seat, which gives you more leg room. Be sure to request an aisle seat so that you can get up periodically without disturbing the person sitting next to you.
- Wear loose, comfortable clothing and comfortable shoes that have been worn previously. If you have lymphedema of the leg, avoid taking off your shoes during the flight.
- Allow ample time to check in and reach your departure gate.
- During the flight:
  - Wear your compression garments. It may also be a good idea to wear an additional short-stretch bandage on top of your garment to counter the effects of low cabin pressure; discuss this with your therapist before you leave.
  - Drink plenty of water or fruit juices and eat lightly—the cabin air is very dry.
  - Ask someone else to place your carry-on luggage in the overhead compartment.

- Stand up and walk around the cabin as often as possible.
- Do not place anything under the seat in front of you, so that you can stretch and exercise your legs.
- Elevate your arms as often as possible if you have lymphedema of the arm and bring a "squeeze" ball for muscle pump exercises.
- If you have an open-toe stocking, it is advisable to apply bandages on your toes and any other part of your foot that may be exposed.
- It may be necessary to wear a glove (or finger/hand bandage) in addition to your arm sleeve. If you have a gauntlet without finger stubs, you may want to bandage your fingers.
- It may also be a good idea to wear an additional short-stretch bandage on top of your garment to counter the effects of low cabin pressure—talk to your therapist.
- Perform some easy-to-remember muscle pump exercises (roll your feet; lift the heels and toes alternating, etc.). Ask your therapist what kind of exercises he or she recommends for during the flight.
- Relax and enjoy your flight.
- Arrival:
  - Do not remove your garment and any additional bandage materials before you reach your final destination.
  - Upon arrival at your destination, a shower and a nap should be your top priority. Make sure you moisturize your skin thoroughly after the shower. A few more exercises with your garments in place would be beneficial.
  - Should you spend a lot of time on the beach, make sure you wear sunscreen and cover your affected limb as often as possible. Wear rubber sandals in the water if you have lymphedema affecting your leg(s).

5.21 Surgical Treatment

5.21.1 Surgical Treatment of Lymphedema

Surgical treatment of lymphedema is currently receiving significant attention in the international lymphedema community. Despite advances in surgical techniques, most clinicians agree that surgery should be reserved primarily for patients in whom more conservative treatment regimens, including CDT, have failed. A recent systematic review of the contemporary medical literature (2004–2011)

Table 5.4 Systematic review findings on surgical treatment of lymphedema

Procedure	Number of studies	Number of patients	Follow-up duration (months)	Volume reduction (%)	Lymphedema assessment	Quality scores, range
Excisional, debulking procedures	6	125	18–72	22[a]	Circumference, infrared Optometric volumetry	2
Liposuction	4	105	6–26	18–118	Water displacement, circumference	6–12
Lymphatic reconstruction	8	2,089	9–87	2–59	Water displacement, circumference	4–8
Tissue transfer	4	61	12–120	+ 13 to 81	Water displacement, circumference	4–11

Source: Adapted from Cormier et al.[151]

[a]Excisional or debulking volume reduction was reported in only one study.

reported on surgical lymphedema treatment and its associated outcomes (▶ Table 5.4).[151]

The first surgical lymphedema treatment was the Charles' procedure, which was described as a limb debulking procedure in 1918. More contemporary adaptations of this procedure have included the preservation of skin bridges and the use of grafted skin to promote improved healing (Sistrunk and Homans-Miller procedures). Serious complications have been associated with these procedures, including bleeding and hematoma, skin necrosis, infection, DVT, pulmonary embolus, poor scar or keloid formation, and posttreatment lymphedema exacerbation or recurrence. In 1935, pedicled flaps were introduced to create connections from anatomic regions with damaged lymphatics to regions with normal lymphatic drainage. The results of these early procedures varied; they were often associated with infections and prolonged hospitalizations. The Thompson procedure was introduced in 1962 to create connections between the dermal and deep lymphatics of the limb by creating a buried dermis flap. However, this procedure was unsuccessful because the skin flap would often not survive and there was no evidence that deep lymphatic connections were created.

Advances in surgical techniques over the past decades have introduced less invasive surgical approaches for lymphedema treatment. These procedures can be categorized as excisional or debulking and include liposuction, lymphatic bypass procedures, and tissue transfer procedures. Excisional procedures involve the radical removal (resection) of skin and soft tissue in the lymphedematous area. The area is then covered by a skin graft for healing. The complications associated with this procedure include bleeding (hematoma), death of grafted skin (necrosis), infection, chronic wounds or delayed healing, blood clots, scarring or poor appearance, destruction of remaining lymphatic vessels, and lymphedema recurrence. In our systematic review, we identified 22 studies of 125 who had undergone excisional procedures (debulking) of the extremities (upper or lower) or genital region (penile or scrotal).[151] The overall volume reduction ranged from 18 to 118%, with a weighted mean reduction of 91%. In a review article on systemic lymphedema treatment, Mehrara et al[152] reported that excisional procedures are typically reserved for patients with lymphostatic elephantiasis.

Liposuction has been introduced as a contemporary technique to remove subcutaneous fat to reduce a limb's overall size. It is considered to result in less morbidity than radical excision; complications include bleeding, infection, skin loss, numbness, and swelling recurrence. From 2004 to 2011, four published studies reviewed 105 patients with liposuction. Although liposuction results in less morbidity than surgical debulking, it does not eliminate the need for compression garments, and lymphedema recurrences have been documented.[151]

Various lymphatic bypass techniques have been proposed for lymphedema treatment, with the goal of creating microscopic connections between lymphatic channels and (most commonly) adjacent veins to "bypass" the lymphatic obstruction. An advantage of microvascular lymphovenous anastomosis procedures is minimal tissue dissection and destruction. However, these procedures are associated with high, early failure rates (e.g., narrowing and scarring of the connections). These procedures should only be performed by highly skilled surgeons who have undergone extensive training in microvascular surgery, which is performed using a microscope.

Tissue transfer procedures include lymph node transplantation and transplanting distant lymph nodes or lymphatic tissue into the area of obstructed lymphatics. Complications associated with tissue transfer procedures include skin flap failure and lymph node or tissue donor site complications. Particularly in lymph node transfer procedures, the remaining lymph nodes at the donor site may be damaged, resulting in lymphedema at the site of lymph node or tissue collection. Four studies that evaluated 61 patients who underwent tissue transfer procedures for upper and lower extremity lymphedema reported a weighted limb volume reduction of 48%, but long-term follow-up data on sustained volume reduction were not reported.[151]

Despite promising reports of significant volume reduction after surgical lymphedema treatment, most studies have found that patients continued to wear compression garments after surgery. Surgical treatment also requires specialty trained physicians, and insurance companies currently consider surgery for lymphedema reduction "investigational." In general, these treatments range in cost from $20,000 to $40,000, not including postsurgical care, continued CDT, garments, and hospitalization. The limited coverage for these procedures often makes surgical treatment an option for only the wealthiest patients.

5.21.2 Lymphedema Surgery as Part of an Integrated Lymphedema Treatment System

Introduction

Nonsurgical management remains the first-line standard of care for lymphedema. Lymphedema surgery, when integrated into a comprehensive lymphedema treatment program for patients, can provide effective and long-term improvements that nonsurgical management alone cannot achieve. Such a treatment program can provide significant improvement for many issues such as recurring cellulitis infections, inability to wear clothing appropriate for the rest of their body size, loss of function of arm or leg, and desire to decrease the amount of lymphedema therapy and compression garment use.

A successful integrated lymphedema treatment program achieves the best results for patients through proper selection of both patient and type of surgery for each patient, lymphedema therapy by an experienced CLT before and after surgery, and a knowledgeable and experienced lymphedema surgeon. Lymphedema surgery is not a "quick fix," and the use of only one type of surgical procedure for all indications or a lack of therapy follow-up produces inconsistent results. Combined or staged lymphedema surgeries also may be used to achieve even better results.

Patient Selection for Lymphedema Surgery

Good candidates for lymphedema surgery are willing to continue with lymphedema therapy before and after any surgical procedure. They appreciate the importance of self-care and continue their compliance with compression as their particular situation requires. These patients are also aware of the importance of replacing their garments as needed in a timely manner. Poor candidates for lymphedema surgery are patients who have never participated in conservative treatment and never worn compression garments. Other unlikely candidates are patients who are unwilling to participate in CDT and are looking for a fast "miracle cure." Additional limiting factors for potential surgical patients are those who smoke and patients who are obese or morbidly obese.

In general, obesity and morbid obesity produces poor surgical outcomes and the same applies with lymphedema surgeries. Meaningful weight loss through a coordinated program that may include behavioral, dietary, and psychosocial counseling and possibly weight reduction surgery should be concluded prior to consideration for lymphedema surgery. The lymphedema in many obese individuals may be permanent even after significant weight loss has taken place.[136,153]

Progression of Lymphedema Swelling Related to Selection of Surgical Procedure

In the earlier stages of the lymphedema disease process, such as stage 0 and stage 1, the swelling of an arm or leg is composed mostly of lymphatic fluid. Here, the swelling is more amenable to conservative treatment with CDT. Patients may also respond well to some types of lymphedema surgery, such as lymphaticovenous anastomosis (LVA) or VLNT, to reverse or greatly decrease the fluid swelling. Over time, the lymphatic channels in the arm or leg break down, sclerose, and lose their ability to effectively clear the excess lymphatic fluid (▶ Fig. 5.259).

The continued accumulation of lymphatic fluid can bring about permanent deposits of solids in the tissues, especially pathologic fat. These solids are permanent, and can easily be visualized with modern, noninvasive methods such as an MRI scan (▶ Fig. 5.260). In such cases, even patients who have CDT administered by an experienced lymphedema therapist still have a remaining measurable volume difference after conservative treatment. This solid-predominant phase corresponds to stage 2 and stage 3 lymphedema swelling.

Lymphedema swelling also greatly increases the risk of dangerous infections, called *cellulitis*, which can be severe in patients with lymphedema. These infections can result in hospitalizations requiring intravenous antibiotics. The arm or leg swelling often causes functional impairments that interfere with work and activities of daily living.

The fluid/solid description of lymphedema swelling is a useful simplification of the overall complex lymphedema disease process. It allows patients and clinicians more easily to communicate the extent of the disease process and better determine which procedures will be most effective for a given patient's presentation. In no way do we intend to use this description to fully or completely describe the lymphedema disease in all of its facets.

The fluid-predominant portion of lymphedema may be treated effectively with physiologic, microvascular surgeries. These include LVAs, VLNT, and lymphaticolymphatic bypass (LB). In LVA surgery, lymphatic channels are directly connected to small veins to bypass a source of obstruction. VLNT surgery involves transplantation of lymphatic tissue from another part of the body to the affected area. LB involves connections directly between the lymphatics and is much less commonly performed. These procedures tend to decrease the amount of therapy and use of garment required, and we have seen even the complete elimination for the need of compression garments in some of our patients.

These procedures tend to have better results when performed when a patient's lymphatic system has less damage. Therefore, the best candidates for LVA or VLNT surgeries are patients with early-stage lymphedema. Less optimal candidates for LVA and VLNT surgeries are patients with more advanced disease with significant amounts of solid present. These are cases in which even the best conservative therapy can no longer decrease the size of the affected arm or leg to match the unaffected side. Such patients are better treated with SAPL to remove this excess solid material first.

It is important to perform physiologic procedures such as VLNT or LVA while the patients are still in the fluid phase of their condition, before the deposition of excess solids occurs. A delay in conservative or surgical lymphedema treatment may allow solids to accumulate and may require patients to undergo SAPL treatment instead. VLNT and LVA may also be used as a second-stage surgery after a SAPL surgery has been performed and

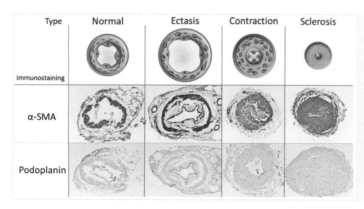

Fig. 5.259 Progression of damage to lymphatic collecting vessels and the corresponding immunostaining findings.[154]

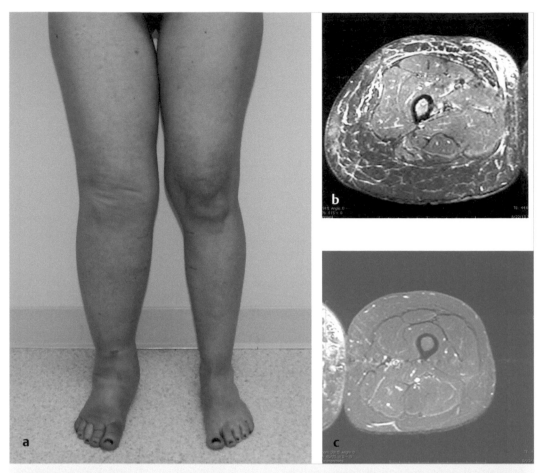

Fig. 5.260 Photos and MRI scans of patient with chronic, solid-predominant, nonpitting edema of right leg. **(a)** Clinical appearance of legs. **(b)** MRI cross-section of right upper leg with lymphedema. Excess lymphedema solids/fat are clearly visualized *(appear as gray)* with lymphedema fluid *(appears as white)* interspersed within and around the solids. **(c)** MRI cross-section of unaffected left upper leg.

healing has occurred. The second-stage VLNT and/or LVA can decrease the amount of compression garment use and therapy required and produce better results than can be achieved with either procedure alone (▶ Fig. 5.261).

Many studies have shown variable results when VLNT or LVA are used to reduce volume.[155,156,157] We find favorable results by using conservative therapy and compression first to reduce the excess fluid volume, and then using VLNT or LVA to reduce the amount of compression and therapy needed to maintain the volume reduction.[158,159]

SAPL best addresses the permanent deposits of solids that are usually found in later, chronic cases. For example, an arm or leg affected by late-stage,

chronic, nonpitting lymphedema which never reduces in size to even close to that of the opposite, unaffected side with a course of lymphedema therapy is very likely to be characterized by solid, rather than fluid swelling. In such a case, application of LVA or VLNT may improve subjective lymphedema symptoms such as fullness or heaviness, but not overall volume.

Significant volume reduction is much less likely with LVA or VLNT, and much more likely with SAPL. For example, in a study by Damstra et al, LVAs performed for patients with solid-predominant lymphedema found little additional improvement in reduction of excess volume[160] (▶ Fig. 5.262).

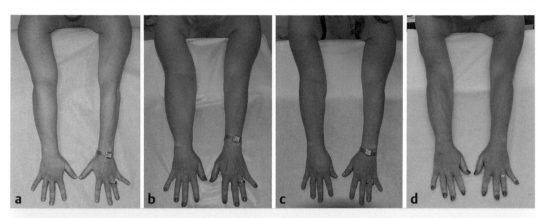

Fig. 5.261 Patient with lymphedema of right arm following right lumpectomy and axillary lymph node dissection and radiation therapy for breast cancer. **(a)** Patient at initial presentation with fluid-predominant, compressible right arm lymphedema. Patient declined surgery at that time. **(b)** Patient 3 years later; lymphedema swelling progressed and volume increased despite conservative therapy to become solid predominant and nonpitting. **(c)** Patient 2 months following suction-assisted protein lipectomy (SAPL). **(d)** Patient 17 months after SAPL and 2 months after staged lymphaticovenous anastomosis and vascularized lymph node transfer surgery. She has a stable excess volume reduction of 98% and wears no compression for an average of 16 hours per day.

5

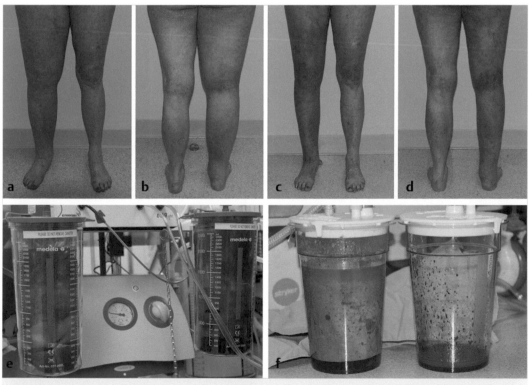

Fig. 5.262 Patient with 4-year history of chronic, noncompressible, nonpitting lymphedema of the right leg following hysterectomy, salpingo-oophorectomy, and lymph node dissection for treatment of ovarian cancer. She was previously treated elsewhere with a vascularized lymph node transfer to the right thigh and lymphaticovenous anastomoses in the right foot and lower leg, which produced mild improvements in symptoms of fullness and heaviness but no reductions in volume excess. **(a,b)** Patient prior to suction-assisted protein lipectomy (SAPL), calculated volume excess 3,554 cm³. **(c,d)** Patient 8 months following SAPL of right leg with stable 82% reduction in volume excess and increased range of motion at knee. **(e,f)** Canisters containing lymphedema solids and fat removed during SAPL.

Treatment

Types of Lymphedema Surgery

Modern lymphedema surgeries such as LVA, VLNT, LB, and SAPL are more precise and less invasive than previous radical attempts at a surgical cure. Previous procedures, such as the Charles' procedure, involved aggressive removal of the skin and deeper tissues down to the level of the muscle fascia, with skin grafts placed over the raw areas. For examples of such procedures, see ▶ Fig. 5.253, ▶ Fig. 5.254, ▶ Fig. 5.255. These invasive procedures are now reserved for a very small number of extreme cases involving thickened, pendulous, and inflamed skin and tissues.[161]

Lymphaticovenous Anastomosis

LVA surgery has been described for many years and involves the direct connection of lymphatic vessels to nearby veins. These connections are usually less than 1 mm in diameter, and require supermicrosurgical expertise. The procedure was first described in 1969 by Yamada and subsequently by O'Brien et al in the 1970s.[162,163] Significant advances in LVA techniques later were described by Koshima et al in Japan and Campisi et al in Italy.[164,165] The connections usually are made into veins with competent valves to allow the one-way movement of excess lymph back into the venous system. In the peripheral parts of the arm or leg, closer to the hands or feet, single or multiple superficial lymphatics are connected to veins. In the proximal areas, closer to the armpit or groin, the lymphatics are larger and fewer, and a smaller number of connections typically are performed (▶ Fig. 5.263, ▶ Fig. 5.264).

Indocyanine green imaging (▶ Fig. 5.265) can help map the lymphatic anatomy and greatly assist the lymphedema surgeon in locating the miniscule lymphatics during surgery. The location and types of connections can vary greatly from patient to patient and are heavily influenced by the patient's anatomy, surgeon's experience, and the progression of the lymphedema disease itself. Because no donor site is required and only a fraction of the lymphatic vessels in the affected arm or leg is connected, LVAs are the least invasive and have the lowest overall surgical risk and recovery among any of the lymphedema surgeries (▶ Fig. 5.266). This also makes LVA ideal for use in the prevention of future lymphedema.[166,167]

Lymphaticolymphatic Bypass

Lymphaticolymphatic bypass was first described in 1986 by Baumeister et al in Germany. The procedure involves the direct connection of lymphatics in the affected arm or leg to lymphatic vessels in a

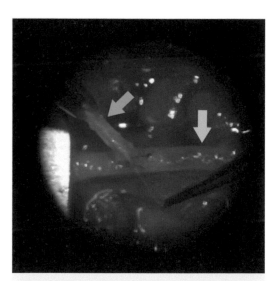

Fig. 5.263 Lymphaticovenous anastomosis (LVA) seen through an operating microscope. The lymphatic vessel (green arrow) has been connected to the side of a small vein (blue arrow). Isosulfan blue dye can be seen draining from the lymphatic vessel to the vein.

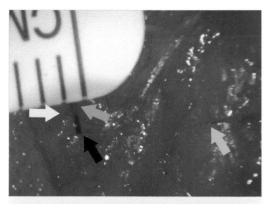

Fig. 5.264 Size of large lymphatic vessel (green arrow, approximately 0.6 mm diameter) as seen through operating microscope during lymphaticovenous anastomosis. Marks on ruler are 1-mm increments. Large black cylinder is 3–0 suture for size reference (black arrow). Two 11–0 sutures used for the lymphatic to vein anastomosis can be seen at left side of lymphatic vessel (yellow arrow). 11–0 needle with suture can also be seen in the surgical field (blue arrow).

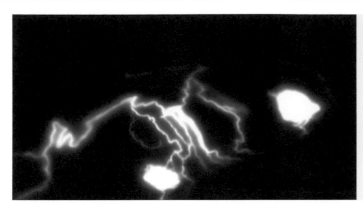

Fig. 5.265 Lymphatic vessels in foot seen with indocyanine green imaging during surgery.

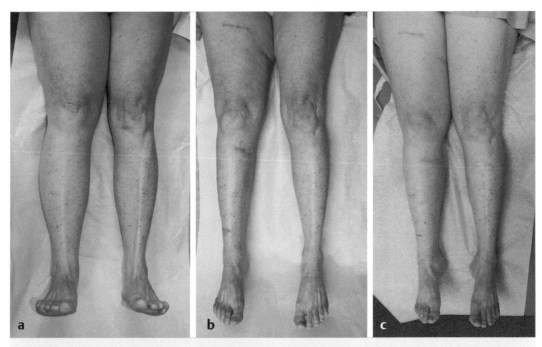

Fig. 5.266 Patient with lymphedema of right leg following hysterectomy, lymph node dissection, and radiation therapy to treat uterine cancer. **(a)** Image before surgery. **(b)** Image 1 week after lymphaticovenous anastomoses of right leg. **(c)** Image of legs 55 months after surgery.

different, healthy portion of the body. Long lymphatic vessels in an unaffected area are mobilized and used as conduits to join the diseased lymphatics with healthy lymphatics past the site of lymphatic obstruction. The authors reported improvements in both limb volumes and the lymphatic transport index. Some reductions in volume were also found with arms decreasing in size more than legs. While the procedure presents a theoretical risk of new lymphedema at the donor harvest site, the risk appears low.[168,169]

Vascularized Lymph Node Transfer

VLNT surgery involves the transfer of a few lymph nodes and surrounding tissue and fat, called *flap*, from an unaffected part of the body, called *donor site*, to the lymphedema-affected area. Many different donor sites have been reported and include the groin, torso, supraclavicular area (near the neck above the collar bone), submental areas (underneath the chin), omentum, and mesentery in the abdomen around the gut. The choice of donor site will be heavily influenced by the

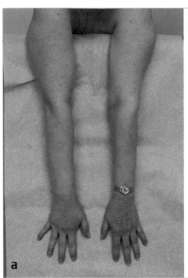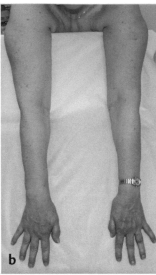

Fig. 5.267 Patient with right arm lymphedema following treatment for breast cancer with bilateral mastectomy, right lymph node dissection, and radiation therapy. (a) Arms prior to surgery. (b) Stable result 4.5 years after vascularized lymph node transfer to right axilla performed together with a deep inferior epigastric perforator flap for breast reconstruction. She requires no daily garment or therapy.

patient's anatomy and the lymphedema surgeon's training and experience. While most surgeons transfer the lymph node flap to the groin or axilla, some prefer to transfer the flap to the wrist or ankle instead.[155,156,170,171,172]

VLNT was first described more than 15 years ago, and many studies have shown VLNT to be effective in improving lymphedema symptoms and swelling. After the LVA or the VLNT procedures, patients typically spend less time in therapy and less time in compression than before surgery. The procedure can greatly decrease and sometimes even eliminate the need for ongoing lymphedema therapy and compression garment use. The incidence of cellulitis and infection in the affected extremity has also been shown to decrease.[158,173] We have found that patients affected by arm lymphedema also can have markedly less hand dorsum swelling following the VLNT procedure to the axilla (▶ Fig. 5.267). As noted previously, patients with less advanced disease tend to have more dramatic improvements with VLNT. Again, patient selection is very important, and VLNT may not be effective in treating the excess solids in chronic lymphedema that are better treated with SAPL (▶ Fig. 5.268).

For patients with lymphedema after breast cancer treatment, a VLNT can be performed at the same time as a breast reconstruction with a deep inferior epigastric perforator (DIEP) flap from the abdomen. The VLNT flap and DIEP flap are harvested together as a single combined flap and transferred together to the chest and axilla as one unit. This achieves both a breast reconstruction

with superior long-term results as well as improvement of the arm and torso lymphedema (▶ Fig. 5.269). The combined procedure is especially effective at treating patients with difficult and complicated presentations, where treatment for cancer has produced extensive scarring and radiation changes in the chest and axillary soft tissues.

VLNT has been shown to improve lymphedema through several different mechanisms. Surgical scar release at the VLNT recipient site, if possible such may be performed in the axilla, can decompress veins and lymphatics constricted by scar. The interposition of the healthy tissue in the VLNT flap prevents the reaccumulation of scar tissue in the area. Spontaneous regrowth of remaining lymphatics in the affected area directly into the transplanted lymphatic tissue has also been shown using different imaging techniques such as lymphoscintigraphy and indocyanine green laser imaging. Also, a direct pumping mechanism that removes lymph fluid buildup has been reported. Additional reductions in tissue fibrosis and increased expression of growth factors such as VEGF-C have also been described.[174,175,176,177] Intraoperative imaging using indocyanine green and/ or Lymphazurin can guide the harvest of lymph nodes in the flap (▶ Fig. 5.270).

Rare cases of lymphedema in the arm or leg after VLNT have been reported in flap donor sites such as the groin, axilla, and supraclavicular (neck) areas.[178,179,180] Minimizing such risks requires an experienced lymphedema surgeon to thoroughly understand the patient's individual lymphatic

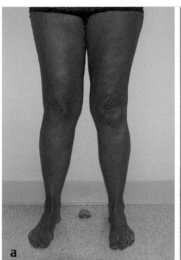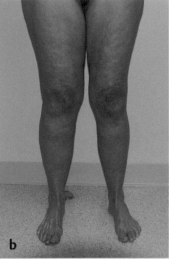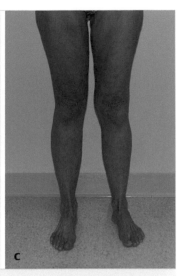

Fig. 5.268 Patient with compressible, fluid-predominant lymphedema of the right leg following hysterectomy and bilateral pelvic lymph node dissection. Treatment recommendation at initial presentation was for continued conservative therapy managed by her home lymphedema therapist including daytime 30- to 40-mm compression garment, nighttime JoViPak, and compression pump use. Symptoms and swelling progressed and patient had vascularized lymph node transfer (VLNT) to the right leg 2.5 years after initial presentation. Following surgery, the symptoms of swelling and fullness have improved significantly and swelling decreases more quickly when it does occur. She no longer requires a nighttime garment or compression pump, and has decreased the frequency of lymphedema therapy. **(a)** Patient at initial presentation. **(b)** Patient 19 months after initial presentation. **(c)** Patient 9 months following VLNT to right leg.

anatomy. While the risk of donor-site lymphedema is present during the surgery and should not be downplayed, there are only isolated cases reported in the medical literature and most lymphedema surgeons believe this risk of new lymphedema to be very low.

The use of reverse lymphatic mapping by the lymphedema surgeon also minimizes donor-site lymphedema risk by mapping the lymph nodes draining the arm or leg closest to the lymph node flap donor site. These imaging techniques include the use of a radioactive tracer similar to that used in lymphoscintigraphy, and/or the use of specialized blue dye such as isosulfan blue (▶ Fig. 5.271) taken up by the peripheral lymphatics.[158,181,182] Reverse mapping uses imaging and lymph node identification techniques similar to those used in standard sentinel lymph node mapping for cancer surgery. This allows the lymphedema surgeon to identify and preserve the lymph nodes that drain the adjacent arm or leg and *avoids* removing or damaging these nodes. We know of no reported cases of lymphedema in a donor limb when reverse lymphatic mapping has been employed.

Suction Assisted Protein Lipectomy

Suction-assisted protein lipectomy (SAPL) surgery permanently removes lymphatic solids and fatty deposits that are typically found later in the disease process and which are otherwise unresponsive to conservative lymphedema therapy, VLNT, or LVA surgeries. The procedure is different from cosmetic liposuction, which is unsuitable to treat lymphedema. SAPL is a derivative of a lymphedema surgery that has been described using various names, including circumferential suction-assisted lipectomy (CSAL), liposuction in lymphedema, and lympho-liposuction.[181,183] First introduced in 1987 by Brorson in Sweden, the original techniques have been refined over the years and have produced significant objective benefit in clinical trials with long-term follow-up.

Medical literature overwhelmingly supports the safety and efficacy of this surgical treatment. These include a 21-year, prospective study of 146 patients with arm involvement treated with SAPL and a 10-year, prospective study of 56 patients with leg involvement treated with SAPL.[184,185] Most significantly, SAPL surgery greatly decreases

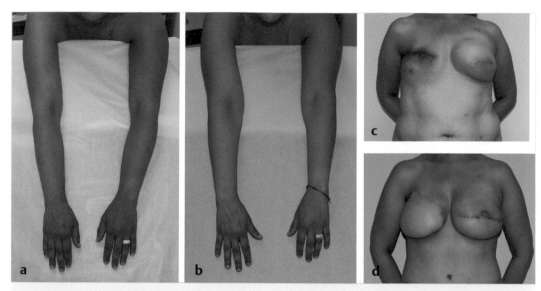

Fig. 5.269 Patient with compressible, right arm lymphedema following bilateral mastectomy, right axillary lymph node dissection, and radiation therapy to the right breast and chest wall to treat right breast cancer. Initial breast reconstruction was with bilateral tissue expanders. The right tissue expander became infected and was removed leaving the right breast irradiated skin densely adherent to the chest wall. The lymphedema was treated with complete decongestive therapy including manual lymph drainage, bandaging, and compression garment placement. She required a 30- to 40-mm compression garment during the day to treat the lymphedema swelling. She was treated with removal of left tissue expander, debridement of right chest wall scar and irradiated skin, and bilateral breast reconstruction with deep inferior epigastric perforator (DIEP) flaps from the abdomen and combined vascularized lymph node transfer to right axilla. Following surgery, symptoms improved significantly and she no longer requires daily compression to treat the lymphedema. **(a)** Arms prior to surgery. **(b)** Arms 20 months following surgery. **(c)** Breasts and chest wall prior to surgery. **(d)** Breasts and chest wall following surgery. Note the left tissue expander was removed at the time of surgery and replaced with a left DIEP flap.

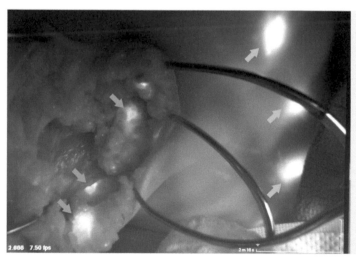

Fig. 5.270 Intraoperative laser imaging of lymph nodes in a vascularized lymph node transfer flap. Indocyanine green dye is injected in the skin *(blue arrows)* and travels with the lymph to be collected in the lymph nodes contained within the fat *(green arrows)*. Together with reverse lymphatic mapping, this imaging is used to design a flap containing lymph nodes that do not drain the adjacent arm or leg.

the incidence of severe extremity cellulitis and hospitalizations requiring intravenous antibiotics to treat such infections. Published studies document a 75% or greater reduction in the incidence of infections and an average 90 to 110% permanent reduction of excess volume. In our own published series, we have reported average infection reductions of about 80% and excess volume reductions of 111% in patients with arms that are affected and 86% in patients who have leg involvement. A

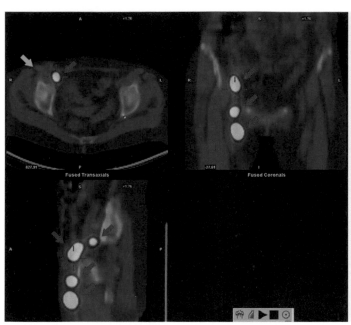

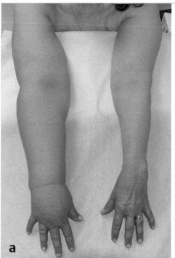

Fig. 5.271 Imaging for planning vascularized lymph node transfer (VLNT) harvest using reverse lymphatic mapping. Images are of Tc-99 tracer mapping overlaid on CT imaging of the same patient. Sentinel lymph nodes (*red arrows*) that take up tracer injected in the leg are clearly visualized and then avoided in the operating room using a standard, handheld Neoprobe. *Green arrow* denotes site of groin VLNT flap harvest away from sentinel nodes.

5

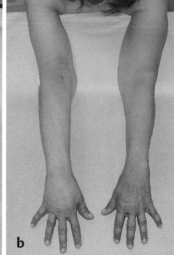

Fig. 5.272 Patient with 12-year history of chronic, solid-predominant lymphedema of the right arm following right mastectomy, axillary dissection, and radiation therapy for breast cancer. (a) Patient prior to suction-assisted protein lipectomy (SAPL). (b) Patient 8 months following SAPL with stable 116% reduction of volume excess (affected right arm smaller than left arm).

reduction in volume excess of greater than 100% indicates that final overall volume of the treated arm or leg is *smaller* than the opposite, unaffected side. A smaller overall treated limb is not uncommon after SAPL, especially in arms (▶ Fig. 5.272). SAPL appears equally effective in treating patient with solid-predominant lymphedema volume excess regardless of the cause of the lymphedema, such as surgery, radiation, trauma, or congenital origin (▶ Fig. 5.273, ▶ Fig. 5.274). Statistically significant reductions in lymphedema, impact on daily activities, the patient's ability to work, improved limb function, reduced lymphedema-

specific emotional distress, and a clear improvement in patient quality of life have also been shown.[158,186,187,188,189]

When performed by an experienced lymphedema surgeon with the support of a CLT, multiple different imaging modalities have shown that SAPL does not further damage lymphatics. Surgery also appears to improve the lymphatic drainage in the arm or leg after healing has occurred. We know of no patients or reports directly or in the medical literature of patients whose lymphedema has become worse after SAPL surgery performed by an experienced lymphedema surgeon.[190,191]

5

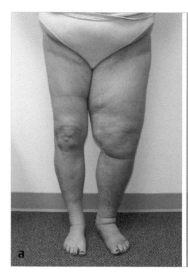
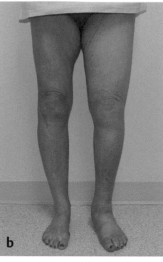

Fig. 5.273 Patient with 46-year history of chronic, congenital, solid-predominant lymphedema of the left leg with prior attempt at direct surgical debulking (Sistrunk procedure) with long residual scar at inner aspect of entire left leg. After suction-assisted protein lipectomy (SAPL), she has a stable 86% reduction in volume excess, improved range of motion, and decreased lymphedema swelling and symptoms. (a) Patient prior to SAPL. (b) Patient 21 months following SAPL.

It must be emphasized that SAPL differs significantly from cosmetic liposuction in many ways, including the procedure technique and instrumentation used, the length and difficulty of the surgery, and solid materials removed. The pathologic lymphedema solids and fat are more firm and difficult to remove than normal fat, and therefore require different surgical instrumentation and technique (▶ Fig. 5.275). Because the lymphatic drainage system of the affected arm or leg previously has been severely damaged by the progression of the lymphedema disease, the ability of an arm or leg affected by lymphedema to clear postoperative swelling and fluid accumulation is greatly impaired. While patients who have had cosmetic liposuction can be adequately treated with the equivalent of class 1 (15–20 mm Hg) compression garments and no lymphedema therapy after surgery, this is not the case after SAPL. In contrast, patients with advanced lymphedema who are treated with SAPL require the use of custom, flat-knit compression garments and MLD performed by an experienced therapist after their surgery.

While SAPL effectively removes excess volume, it does not address the pathophysiology causing the lymphedema swelling and fluid accumulation. Therefore, continuous compression garment use under the care of a CLT following surgery is essential to prevent the redeposition of the pathologic lymphedema solids and fat. As described in the next section, for some patients, requirement for postoperative garment use can be reduced significantly with a VLNT and/or LVA performed at a later time once healing from SAPL is complete.

Lymphedema therapy required before and after the SAPL procedure is intense and cannot be substituted with a simple set of postoperative written instructions to the patient or therapist. Preoperative fitting with custom garments is the first step. The opposite, unaffected arm or leg is used as a general template to order the custom, flat-knit postoperative garments required after surgery. Depending on the patient, compression garments or short-stretch bandages are placed in the operating room at the end of the procedure to minimize postoperative swelling. Additional postoperative therapy and MLD can reduce swelling more rapidly, and new, custom fit flat-knit garments must be remeasured and fit by the lymphedema therapist, as the volume decreases in the months following surgery. Collaboration between the surgical lymphedema therapist and the patient's primary lymphedema therapist is imperative once the patient returns home to continue treatment during their recovery.

The best candidates for SAPL surgery are patients whose lymphedema is chronic, nonpitting, and solid-predominant. These candidates are patients who, after completing a thorough course of CDT, still have a significant volume difference between limbs. While almost all candidates for SAPL already wear compression garments continuously, patients who wish to be considered for SAPL must be willing to continue to wear compression garments after surgery as well. Although the need for lymphedema therapy is greatly reduced after SAPL, patients must be willing to maintain their relationship with their lymphedema therapist. Because of the tremendous and consistent volume

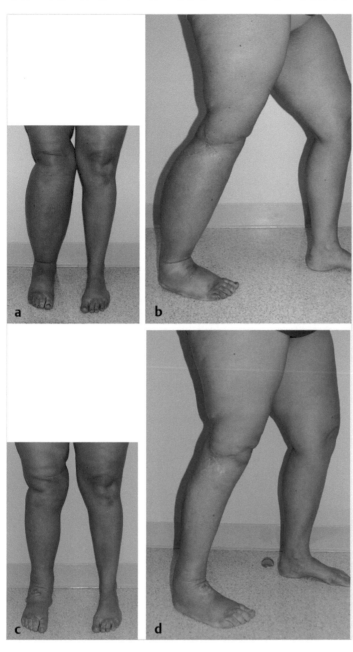

Fig. 5.274 Patient with 30-year history of chronic, solid-predominant lymphedema of the right lower leg following severe trauma requiring multiple surgical reconstructions of bone and soft tissues including multiple skin grafts. **(a,b)** Patient before suction-assisted protein lipectomy (SAPL). **(c,d)** Patient 20 months after SAPL of the right lower leg. She maintains a stable 88% reduction of volume excess in the lower leg following SAPL.

5

reductions and improvements in symptoms and cellulitis attacks, our experience has shown that compression garment use is rarely an issue for patients who have had the surgery. As noted below, VLNT and LVA performed at a later time can reduce this compression requirement.

Poor candidates for SAPL are those who are obese or morbidly obese, unable or unwilling to wear postoperative compression, and unwilling to work with the lymphedema therapist after

surgery. SAPL is not appropriate for patients with fluid-predominant disease including early or mild presentations.

Combined and Staged Lymphedema Surgeries

Lymphedema surgeries may be combined or staged for better patient outcomes. Physiologic procedures such as VLNT and LVA can be combined

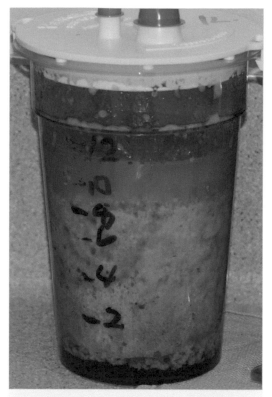

Fig. 5.275 Photo of surgical canister containing the heterogeneous of aspirate of lymphedema solids removed with suction-assisted protein lipectomy.

during the same operation or in sequential operations for increased effectiveness.[181,192]

Staged lymphedema surgeries can also be used to treat both solid and then fluid components of lymphedema separately. For instance, VLNT/LVA can be performed once healing, after the SAPL surgery, is complete to reduce the reaccumulation of lymphatic fluid. Thus, SAPL and VLNT procedures have been combined in a staged approach to manage chronic, solid phase lymphedema. First, SAPL is performed to remove the proteinaceous solids and reduce volume excess. After postoperative swelling stabilizes, VLNT is used to improve lymphatic drainage and address subsequent fluid reaccumulation.

We have documented significant reductions both in excess limb volume and also in the requirement for postoperative garment use in medical literature with the staged SAPL and VLNT combination of procedures (▶ Fig. 5.276). For patients with arm lymphedema, this combined approach has resulted in volume reductions of more than 83% and compression garment use required only in the evenings and at night.[159] Patients with leg lymphedema have similar volume reductions and significant symptomatic improvements as well.

Surgery for Congenital Lymphedema

VLNT and LVA appear to be less effective in patients with congenital, or primary, rather than

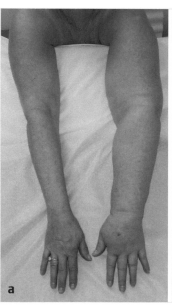
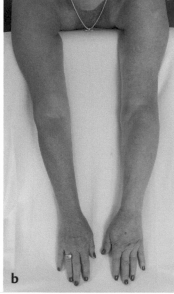

Fig. 5.276 Patient with a 4-year history of lymphedema of the left arm secondary to treatment with left mastectomy, axillary lymph node dissection, and radiation therapy for breast cancer. She was treated with staged suction-assisted protein lipectomy (SAPL) surgery with subsequent deep inferior epigastric perforator (DIEP) flap breast reconstruction and left vascularized lymph node transfer (VLNT). The patient maintains a stable volume reduction of approximately 96% with no compression required for approximately 12 hours per day. (a) Photo of arms after therapy and compression but prior to any surgery. (b) Photo of same patient 59 months after SAPL and 39 months after DIEP and VLNT.

secondary lymphedema. This may be due to the fact that improvements in lymphedema symptoms and swelling achieved by these physiologic procedures appear to relate to the remaining function of the lymphatic system of the affected arm or leg. A lymphatic system in an arm or leg that was normal prior to damage from surgery or radiation therapy may respond better to early intervention with physiologic procedures such as LVA or VLNT compared to a lymphatic system whose function is inherently deficient due to a congenital defect.

In contrast, SAPL is equally effective in treating chronic, solid-predominant lymphedema that results from congenital and as well as secondary lymphedema (▶ Fig. 5.277). In a comparison between congenital and secondary lymphedema patients, there was no statistical difference in the average 12-month improvement in percentage reduction of volume excess between the congenital and secondary groups (95 vs. 83% volume reduction, $p = 0.4$).

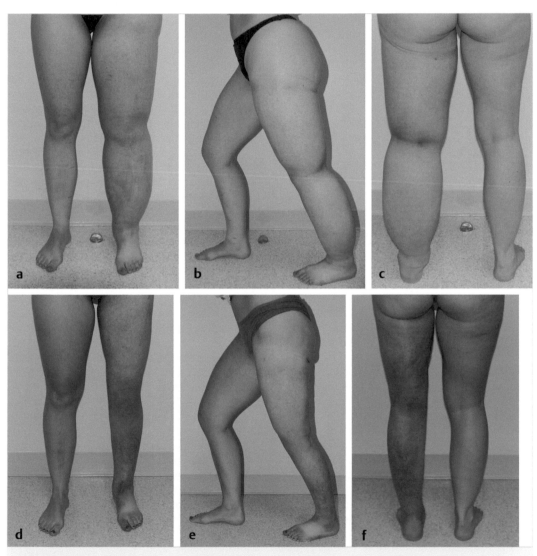

Fig. 5.277 Patient with history of congenital lymphedema of the left leg for 17 years. Patient maintains a stable reduction of excess volume of 123% (affected left leg smaller than right leg) following suction-assisted protein lipectomy (SAPL) surgery. **(a–c)** Patient before SAPL surgery. **(d–f)** Patient 10 months after surgery.

Lymphedema Therapy and Lymphedema Surgery

Lymphedema therapy should be appropriately integrated into any surgical treatment plan as part of an overall lymphedema treatment system. Without lymphedema therapy, most patients treated with lymphedema surgery will not achieve the best result. Postoperative CDT provided by a CLT experienced in caring for lymphedema surgery patients along with self-care performed daily by the patient is important.

The lymphedema surgeon must work closely with a lymphedema therapist to ensure that optimum lymphedema therapy is performed both before and after any lymphedema surgery. This is especially important for SAPL, in which pre- and postoperative planning, measurements, and lymphedema therapy are vital to the success of the surgery. Long-term lymphedema therapy should be administered by the patient's local lymphedema therapist under the direction of the lymphedema surgeon or surgical lymphedema therapist.

Individualized lymphedema therapy integrated into the treatment plan before and after surgery is essential in achieving excellent results. Such therapy includes the foundation of CDT: skin care, MLD, compression bandaging, a home exercise program, and eventually fitting for compression garments. A complete initial evaluation by a CLT is essential. The patient should discuss his or her present garment situation and assess if they are managing their volume effectively and determine if changes need to be made. These changes may require transitioning from a circular knit garment to a flat-knit garment for increased control of the limb volume. After the consultation, it may also be determined that the patient may need to consider increasing the compression class of the garment or possibly require the use of a second garment layer to achieve increased control and stability of their limb volume.

It is also helpful if the CLT is familiar with assessing the patient for any orthopedic needs during postoperative care. This skill set is frequently necessary when a patient has been significantly limited in their range of motion preoperatively due to excess volume from severe lymphedema. Once the volume is reduced, the patient is then able to restore functional joint range of motion as they recover and at times require joint mobilizations to assist with a successful return of mobility. These skills are particularly useful when treating a patient who has had a SAPL surgery for the leg.

Patellar mobilizations as well as addressing the iliotibial band are frequently used to assist the patient with restoring comfortable and functional knee flexion.

The application of lymphedema therapy can vary considerably between lymphedema therapists, and there are different presentations, for example, of what CDT represents in the United States. Even a therapist who has completed instruction from a familiar program may not practice exactly what they have been instructed. In addition, limitations beyond the control of the therapist, such as insurance coverage or clinic regulations, may impose a decreased frequency and intensity with which the therapists are allowed to treat. Prior to surgery, there should be an assessment in terms of the effectiveness of the patient's past and present therapy treatments. Although it is not foolproof, a comprehensive analysis of new patients by both the lymphedema surgeon and therapist allows the gathering of data points of how thorough their care was in the past.

Patients who give CDT a chance and carry it through often still have a remaining measurable volume difference. This volume excess in large part is due to the permanent accumulation of lymphedema solids, especially pathologic fat. Every experienced lymphedema therapist has seen this progression occurring in some patients, especially those who present later in the disease process. Even with the most thorough course of therapy by an experienced lymphedema therapist, CDT cannot change fibrotic tissue into fluid. Unfortunately, there are times when clinicians mistake very concentrated amounts of lymphatic fluid as permanent fibrotic tissue. In these cases, we feel that a mandatory course of CDT is necessary to assess the response of the patient's limb and an attempt to reduce the limb to its fullest.

Some patients no longer respond well to CDT and lymphedema therapy, even if administered by an experienced therapist. Just as a solid sponge can be compressed with well-applied short-stretch bandages only to quickly expand when the bandages are removed, the solid soft tissues rebound after the therapy stops and garments and bandages are temporarily removed. The arm or leg is, indeed, lighter and feels better for a brief time after the treatment because the fluids involved with the spongy solids have been reduced. However, the arm or leg never goes back down to the size of the unaffected side.

Such chronic, solid-predominant cases are effectively treated with SAPL instead.[158] SAPL can remove the permanent solids and achieve results that cannot be achieved with CDT and lymphedema therapy alone, even when the therapy is administered by very experienced lymphedema therapists. The surgical intervention itself reduces the excess solids, rather than the lymphedema therapy, and in such cases the volume reduction achieved with therapy has plateaued prior to the surgery. The lymphedema therapy itself then remains constant both before and after surgery, with the surgery being the only treatment variable.

Summary

Surgery for lymphedema can be very effective when the correctly selected surgery is properly performed in the right patient and lymphedema therapy is involved as an integral component of care. Lymphedema surgery can produce dramatic improvements in symptoms and tremendous reductions in excess volume, even in patients who have found conservative treatments to be ineffective. The aforementioned techniques have been shown to be effective in multiple studies and are no longer considered experimental.

Achieving the best results requires more than just a skilled and experienced lymphedema surgeon, and surgery should be offered as part of a comprehensive treatment system that also includes assessment and treatment by a CLT and appropriate selection of patient and surgical procedure.

Standard lymphedema precautions, such as vigilance with cuts and scratches in the affected arm or leg and bandaging or compression with at-risk activities or flying, should be continued in all lymphedema patients regardless of whether or not they have undergone surgical treatment.

A small but growing number of experienced lymphedema surgeons offer surgical treatment for lymphedema. As is the case with many other disease processes, no overall consensus exists regarding either the exact diagnosis of lymphedema or its surgical management. The training and personal experience of each individual lymphedema surgeon will heavily influence that surgeon's preferred techniques.

Conservative lymphedema therapy should be pursued prior to consideration for surgery and in many cases may be an effective, lower-cost, and noninvasive option for lymphedema management. Surgical treatments are not a "magic bullet." Surgical intervention requires a team effort on the part of the lymphedema surgeon, therapist, and patient. When performed by an experienced lymphedema surgeon as part of an integrated system with expert lymphedema therapy, safe, consistent, and long-term improvements can be achieved.

5.21.3 Breast and Axillary Reconstruction Primer for the Certified Lymphedema Therapist

Introduction

Breast cancer affects nearly 200,000 American women annually.[193] Breast conservation has been accepted as a reasonable treatment option for many early-stage cancers.[194] Novel protocols have incorporated neoadjuvant chemotherapy prior to surgical care as a means to convert previously ineligible candidates.[195] As a result, only 80,000 new breast cancers will be treated with a total mastectomy this year.[193]

Breast reconstruction is a safe and effective means of restoring patients to a sense of "wholeness" after mastectomy.[196] Only 20% of candidates elect to proceed with some form of either immediate (15–20%) or delayed breast reconstruction despite documented high levels of patient satisfaction.[197] The etiology of low rates of breast reconstruction is multifactorial and has been attributed to inadequate patient education, lack of access to care, socioeconomic variables including income and race, physician bias, and health care setting (university vs. private practice). More recently, managed care has influenced this survivorship issue despite federal legislation mandating coverage as defined in the Women's Health Care Act of 1998.[198] Studies by the American Society of Plastic Surgeons suggest that only 30% of American women diagnosed with breast cancer are believed to be appropriately informed of their choices for reconstruction at the time of diagnosis.[199] Data such as these have precipitated newer legislation in New York State, mandating patient education in breast reconstructive options by oncologic surgeons.[134,200]

The majority of breast reconstructions include prosthetic devices at some stage of the reconstructive process, with nearly 60.5% using a permanent saline- or silicone-filled breast implant. Natural breast reconstructions are utilized as a primary reconstruction method in the remaining 39.5%. However, 87.3% of the natural techniques are musculocutaneous reconstructions that sacrifice function compared with the more sophisticated

5

perforator flaps that are composed of only skin and adipose tissue. This is most likely because natural perforator flaps are offered only by reconstructive surgeons with additional microsurgical training and specialization.[201]

Breast Reconstruction Surgical Procedures

Breast reconstruction can be initiated at the time of mastectomy and is referred to as "immediate" breast reconstruction. Reconstructive procedures that occur at any time after the mastectomy healing process is complete are referred to as "delayed" reconstructions. Most methods involve several "stages," where aspects of the reconstruction are addressed in a specific sequence to replace needed skin, mound, nipple, and areolar components.

Breast reconstruction with saline- or silicone-filled implants is the most common method of primary breast reconstruction with rates exceeding 60%.[201] Traditional methods include the placement of an adjustable tissue expander beneath the pectoralis major muscle. Patients undergo "tissue expansion" where saline is injected via a port within the device either weekly or coordinated within a chemotherapy regimen until a desired volume or breast size is achieved. In a staged fashion, the patient returns to the operating room to have the tissue expander removed and replaced with either a saline- or silicone-filled permanent device. Nipple reconstruction is completed several months later, typically with regional tissue flaps requiring only local anesthesia. Areola tattoos complete the process and can be offered as an in-office procedure. "One-step" methods of implant-based breast reconstructions have been popularized given that total skin-sparing mastectomies have been shown to be oncologically sound and acellular dermal matrices have simultaneously been developed to provide support to the inferior pole of the reconstruction site.[202]

Silicone breast implants have been examined closely by the FDA and have been cleared of any association with autoimmune diseases, such as fibromyalgia.[203] Within the context of these clinical investigations, attention has turned to the need for revision surgeries with rates approaching 40% at 10 years in nonirradiated patients and upward of 70% for those with prior regional irradiation.[204] Unplanned reoperations for failed implants in these patients include, but are not limited to, the treatment of capsular contracture, infection, implant exposure, implant deflation/rupture, and pain.[205,206]

Historically, autologous natural breast reconstruction methods have been introduced to address implant reconstruction failures. Latissimus dorsi (LD) myocutaneous rotational flaps were first introduced in the 1970s to add bulk superficially to breast implants to prevent infection or extrusion and as a means to slow capsular contracture.[207] Later in the 1980s, rotational transverse rectus abdominus myocutaneous (TRAM) flaps were popularized in academic centers on the East Coast of the United States as a way to avoid the use of an implanted device during any stage of the reconstructive process.[208,209] TRAM-flap breast reconstruction utilizes excess skin and fat from the lower abdomen to re-create the breast without the need for tissue expansion or a permanent device in appropriately selected patients. TRAM-flap breast reconstruction techniques bear the burden of decreased abdominal strength as the rectus abdominus muscle is sacrificed as a means to provide the vascular pedicle to the reconstruction. With the simultaneous introduction of microsurgery on the West Coast, "free" TRAM-flap breast reconstruction was introduced as a means to preserve muscle strength as only a small portion of the rectus muscle is included in the reconstruction flap region.[210,211] Acceptance of microsurgical free TRAM flap and later the deep inferior epigastric perforator (DIEP) flap[212,213] set the foundation of what we now characterize as the gold standard of muscle-sparing perforator flap breast reconstruction (▶ Table 5.5).[214] Immediate microsurgical natural breast reconstructions with nipple and areolar preservation now define the norm of breast reconstruction with low rates of flap failure reportedly at less than 1% in established centers.[214] Reconstructions such as these provide a superior aesthetic outcome with minimal functional deficits and infrequent unplanned reoperations. Furthermore, they define the reconstruction method of choice for patients treated with regional irradiation.

▶ Fig. 5.278 shows bilateral nipple and areolar sparing prophylactic mastectomies with immediate bilateral DIEP flap natural breast reconstructions. ▶ Fig. 5.278 shows the preoperative appearance of a 64-year-old BRCA-2-positive patient seeking bilateral prophylactic mastectomies and immediate autologous breast reconstructions. Preoperative consultation revealed her desire for a smaller and more youthful appearing reconstruction. Perioperative care included 2 hours of preoperative lymphedema education by a CLT in a hospital setting including bilateral arm measurements and review of risk-reduction practices and daily MLD with continued proactive lymphedema education while hospitalized. The patient was protected intraoperatively with bilateral gray foam-based, short-stretch compression bandaging. The patient was not discharged from hospital until she was proficient in self-bandaging (for air travel). Her reconstruction was completed in two stages and her 6-month postoperative appearance is shown in ▶ Fig. 5.278.

▶ Fig. 5.279 shows *delayed* right breast reconstruction with GAP flap in an irradiated field combined with left *immediate* breast reconstruction with GAP flap. Left panel relates the preoperative appearance of a 42-year-old woman who presents with a past medical history significant for a stage 3 right breast cancer treated with modified radical mastectomy, axillary lymph node resection, adjuvant chemotherapy, and regional irradiation. She elected to proceed with delayed right breast reconstruction with a GAP flap in addition to a prophylactic left mastectomy and immediate GAP flap. Nipple reconstructions were completed with local flaps followed by areolar tattoos. Her postoperative appearance at the time of areolar tattoos is shown in ▶ Fig. 5.279. Note the need for an elliptical skin island on the right to replace skin while the prophylactic mastectomy was completed using a vertical mastopexy design.

Table 5.5 Microsurgical reconstruction flaps and associated donor sites

Muscle-sparing reconstruction flap	Donor site
Deep inferior epigastric perforator (DIEP)	Abdomen
Superficial inferior epigastric artery (SIEA)	Abdomen
Superior gluteal artery perforator (SGAP)	Superior buttock
Inferior gluteal artery perforator (IGAP)	Inferior buttock
Transverse upper gracilis (TUG)	Medial thigh
Anterior lateral thigh (ALT)	Lateral thigh
Profunda artery perforator (PAP)	Posterior thigh
Thoracodorsal artery perforator (TDAP)	Posterior trunk
Intercostal perforator (ICP)	Lateral trunk

Axillary Reconstruction

Sentinel lymph node procedures (SLNP) are now the accepted norm of breast cancer staging.[215] Its acceptance has been fueled by a desire to limit the morbidity of lymphadenectomy. Lymphedema secondary to SLNP occurs at rates of 3 to 8%, whereby full ALND has been associated with a lifetime risk of lymphedema approaching 25%.[103,216,217,218] Regional irradiation added to ALND reportedly has an associated lifetime risk of nearly 50%.[219,220,221] Chronic upper extremity and chest wall pain syndromes have been seen in up to 47% of late stage patients treated with ALND and regional irradiation.[222,223] Commonly, these conditions overlap and many patients confuse pain secondary to radiation-induced brachial plexopathy as a side effect of limb lymphedema.

Recent interest has turned to the surgical treatment of lymphedema and pain syndromes. Built

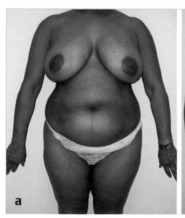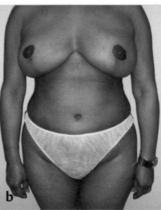

Fig. 5.278 (a,b) Bilateral nipple and areolar sparing prophylactic mastectomies with immediate bilateral deep inferior epigastric perforator flap natural breast reconstructions.

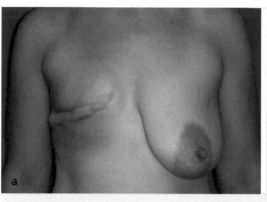 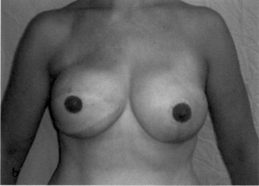

Fig. 5.279 **(a)** *Delayed* right breast reconstruction with gluteal artery perforator (GAP) flap in an irradiated field combined with **(b)** left *immediate* breast reconstruction with GAP flap.

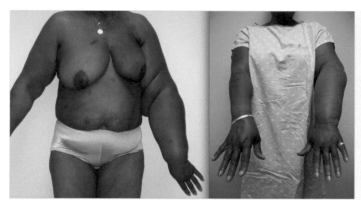

Fig. 5.280 Left axillary reconstruction with vascularized lymph node transfer for secondary lymphedema.

upon an unpopular foundation of debulking and lymphatic bypass procedures, the VLNT has emerged as a possibility for supportive care for individuals who suffer the ill effects of recalcitrant arm lymphedema and pain.[155,170,224,225] VLNT is best understood as a means for axillary reconstruction. Initially, the surgical scar of the axilla is sharply excised re-creating the adenectomy defect. Brachial plexus neuroplasty can be used as an adjunct to this portion of the reconstructive process. An autologous flap containing vascularized lymph nodes and perinodal subcutaneous tissue is then transferred to the axillary reconstruction site, where microsurgical techniques are utilized to reestablish the vascular supply to the transfer. Axillary reconstruction with a VLNT results in improved form of the axilla and lateral chest wall and upper extremity range of motion and function (▶ Fig. 5.280).

▶ Fig. 5.280 shows left axillary reconstruction with VLNT for secondary lymphedema. The left panel shows the preoperative appearance of a 67-year-old woman who presented as a 13-year survivor of a stage 2 left breast cancer treated with breast conservation (lumpectomy, SLNP, ALND, adjuvant chemotherapy, and regional irradiation). She presented with lifestyle-limiting upper extremity lymphedema and osteoradionecrosis of the humeral head in the setting of 15 episodes of cellulitis in the year prior to axillary reconstruction. The patient elected to proceed with a left axillary reconstruction with VLNT (38 g, right groin flap design based on the superficial circumflex artery) without breast reconstruction given her age, comorbidities, and desire for orthopedic reconstructive surgery. Her postoperative appearance at 6 months is shown in the right panel with a 54% reduction in volume of the left arm and improved function. The patient reported only one episode of cellulitis in the first 6 months after reconstruction and was very pleased with her result. She continues with recommended daily MLD, a class II daytime compression garment and nighttime alternative.

Concern from the lymphedema community at large has focused on the possibility of postoperative VLNT donor-site lymphedema. As such, much effort has focused on the refinement of preoperative patient selection criteria, development of intraoperative lymphatic mapping techniques, and defining optimal harvest sites that limit negative long-term consequences in the setting of prospective clinical trials.[226] Initial groin lymph node harvest sites are being replaced with level 5 cervical flaps. Newer flap designs have resulted in lower morbidity with fewer reported cases of donor-site cellulitis, seroma, and cording. Furthermore, focus has been directed toward defining the role of postoperative CDT for this patient population. Given the positive effect of autologous breast reconstruction on arm lymphedema,[110] it will be no surprise that autologous axillary reconstruction may provide some positive effects for these difficult clinical conditions. The larger concern is ensuring that microsurgeons interested in this field of reconstruction gain appropriate training and education from current lymphedema providers, as many fail to seek certification as lymphedema therapists.[227,228,229]

Special Considerations for Lymphedema Patients

1. Proactive Lymphedema Care

Patients having received a diagnosis of breast cancer initially are ill-prepared to assimilate much of the information provided to them regarding the surgical approaches of cancer care, chemotherapy, irradiation therapy, and the associated risk of lymphedema. Many centers have incorporated care extenders, patient educators, and nurse navigators into their care, providing teams to assist in patient education.[230,231] Regrettably, even the most rigorous attempts to address education fall short, as patients internalize a need to move forward with tumor extrication. This commonly results in poorly conceived reconstructive planning and minimal, if any, proactive lymphedema care. Many patients suffering from lymphedema relate that they were never told of the risk of secondary lymphedema due to surgery or irradiation. This may result from information overload and/or selective memory; however, few centers insist on preoperative education by a CLT. Imagine a time when all preoperative patients would receive lymphedema education by a CLT prior to and following all surgical interventions to ensure risk reduction

competence, surveillance, and perioperative compression bandaging.[232] This aspect of lymphedema care is particularly critical for high-risk lymph node–positive patients, as they may undergo sequential surgical procedures many months after diagnosis because chemotherapy and irradiation must be completed prior to completion of the reconstructive process.

2. Implant Failure

Capsular contracture, particularly in an irradiated field, presents as one of the most challenging difficulties a lymphedema therapist may encounter in their clinical practice. Few means of pretreatment or ancillary services promote fluid transport through adherent and immobile irradiated surgical sites. Although a seemingly aggressive approach, severely affected individuals may benefit from removal of their reconstructive breast implants and surgical release of associated adhesions with or without simultaneous autologous reconstruction as a means to support improved lymphatic care.

3. Potential Ill Effect of Latissimus Dorsi Flap Reconstruction

LD flap reconstruction is a common reconstructive choice for patients who have received regional irradiation. Regrettably, plastic surgeons receive no training in the Vodder's method of MLD and fail to appreciate the limitations of anterior mastectomy incisions combined with posterior LD flap donor-site incisions. Given a lifetime risk of lymphedema of 50% for lymph node–positive patients requiring irradiation, LD flaps should be discouraged and most likely replaced with either abdominal or gluteal perforator flaps that preserve superficial and deep lymphatic drainage pathways of the posterior trunk for those patients seeking breast reconstruction.

4. Modified MLD Sequences Incorporating Downstream Breast Reconstruction Sites and Upstream Axillary Lymph Node Transfers

Autologous breast and axillary reconstructions have been shown to support improved lymphatic drainage.[110] Current ongoing investigations suggest that incorporating these regions using the Vodder method MLD may be more useful than rerouting fluid around these regions.[233] Further

5

research must address a means to objectively evaluate the long-term outcome of these novel approaches and to identify the correct sequence of staged breast and axillary reconstruction.

Conclusion

Breast reconstruction has a rich history of surgical procedures, each designed to address the shortcomings of previous methods. Implant-based reconstructions remain popular, given the ease of the surgical procedure for physicians with limited postgraduate training in microsurgical breast reconstruction. Future advances are likely to explore means to improve lymphatic drainage of reconstruction sites that have been injured not only by surgery but also by the additive negative effects of irradiation. The call for excellence in this exciting field will require that surgeons be educated in CDT and participate in ongoing clinical research. Success will depend on open communication between clinicians and lymphedema therapists, all working together to promote better care for these patients.

References

[1] Boris M, Weindorf S, Lasinski BB. The risk of genital edema after external pump compression for lower limb lymphedema. Lymphology. 1998; 31(1):15–20

[2] Feely MA, Olsen KD, Gamble GL, Davis MD, Pittelkow MR. Cutaneous lymphatics and chronic lymphedema of the head and neck. Clin Anat. 2012; 25(1):72–85

[3] Földi E, Földi M. Lymphostatic diseases. In: Földi M, Földi E, Kubik P, et al, eds. Földi's Textbook of Lymphology: For Physicians and Lymphedema Therapists. 2nd ed. Munich, Germany: Urban & Fischer; 2006:224–245

[4] Shenoy RK. Clinical and pathological aspects of filarial lymphedema and its management. Korean J Parasitol. 2008; 46(3):119–125

[5] Mottura AA. Face lift postoperative recovery. Aesthetic Plast Surg. 2002; 26(3):172–180

[6] Kim EY, Eisele DW, Goldberg AN, Maselli J, Kezirian EJ. Neck dissections in the United States from 2000 to 2006: volume, indications, and regionalization. Head Neck. 2011; 33(6):768–773

[7] Ziglinas P, Arnold A, Arnold M, Zbären P. Primary tumors of the submandibular glands: a retrospective study based on 41 cases. Oral Oncol. 2010; 46(4):287–291

[8] Klintworth N, Zenk J, Koch M, Iro H. Postoperative complications after extracapsular dissection of benign parotid lesions with particular reference to facial nerve function. Laryngoscope. 2010; 120(3):484–490

[9] Unlü Y, Becit N, Ceviz M, Koçak H. Management of carotid body tumors and familial paragangliomas: review of 30 years' experience. Ann Vasc Surg. 2009; 23(5):616–620

[10] Kao J, Conzen SD, Jaskowiak NT, et al. Concomitant radiation therapy and paclitaxel for unresectable locally advanced breast cancer: results from two consecutive phase I/II trials. Int J Radiat Oncol Biol Phys. 2005; 61(4):1045–1053

[11] Tribius S, Kronemann S, Kilic Y, et al. Radiochemotherapy including cisplatin alone versus cisplatin + 5-fluorouracil for locally advanced unresectable stage IV squamous cell carcinoma of the head and neck. Strahlenther Onkol. 2009; 185(10):675–681

[12] Guhl G, Diaz-Ley B, Sanchez-Perez J, Jimenez U, Garcia-Diez A. Pemetrexed-induced edema of the eyelid. Lung Cancer. 2010; 69(2):249–250

[13] Deng J, Ridner SH, Dietrich MS, et al. Prevalence of secondary lymphedema in patients with head and neck cancer. J Pain Symptom Manage. 2012; 43(2):244–252

[14] Büntzel J, Glatzel M, Mücke R, Micke O, Bruns F. Influence of amifostine on late radiation-toxicity in head and neck cancer–a follow-up study. Anticancer Res. 2007; 27 4A:1953–1956

[15] Glastonbury CM, Parker EE, Hoang JK. The postradiation neck: evaluating response to treatment and recognizing complications. AJR Am J Roentgenol. 2010; 195(2):W164–71

[16] Baumann DP, Yu P, Hanasono MM, Skoracki RJ. Free flap reconstruction of osteoradionecrosis of the mandible: a 10-year review and defect classification. Head Neck. 2011; 33(6):800–807

[17] Ahlberg A, Nikolaidis P, Engström T, et al. Morbidity of supraomohyoidal and modified radical neck dissection combined with radiotherapy for head and neck cancer: a prospective longitudinal study. Head Neck. 2012; 34(1):66–72

[18] Erdag TK, Guneri EA, Avincsal O, et al. Is elective neck dissection necessary for the surgical management of T2N0 glottic carcinoma? Auris Nasus Larynx. 2013; 40(1):85–88

[19] Klop WM, Veenstra HJ, Vermeeren L, Nieweg OE, Balm AJ, Lohuis PJ. Assessment of lymphatic drainage patterns and implications for the extent of neck dissection in head and neck melanoma patients. J Surg Oncol. 2011; 103(8):756–760

[20] Szolnoky G, Mohos G, Dobozy A, Kemény L. Manual lymph drainage reduces trapdoor effect in subcutaneous island pedicle flaps. Int J Dermatol. 2006; 45(12):1468–1470

[21] Piso DU, Eckardt A, Liebermann A, Gutenbrunner C, Schäfer P, Gehrke A. Early rehabilitation of head-neck edema after curative surgery for orofacial tumors. Am J Phys Med Rehabil. 2001; 80(4):261–269

[22] Piso DU, Eckardt A, Liebermann A, Gehrke A. Reproducibility of sonographic soft-tissue measurement of the head and neck. Am J Phys Med Rehabil. 2002; 81(1):8–12

[23] Katsura K, Hayashi T. Non-neoplastic process after neck dissection demonstrated on enhanced CT in patients with head and neck cancer. Dentomaxillofac Radiol. 2005; 34(5):297–303

[24] Smith BG, Lewin JS. Lymphedema management in head and neck cancer. Curr Opin Otolaryngol Head Neck Surg. 2010; 18(3):153–158

[25] Strossenreuther RHK. Practical instructions for therapists-manual lymph drainage according to Dr. E. Vodder. In: Földi M, Földi E, Kubik P, et al, eds. Földi's Textbook of Lymphology: For Physicians and Lymphedema Therapists. 2nd ed. Munich, Germany: Urban & Fischer; 2006:526–546

[26] Riutta JC, Cheville AL, Trerotola SO. SVC syndrome with a patent SVC: treatment of internal jugular venous occlusion after surgical and radiation therapy of esophageal cancer. J Vasc Interv Radiol. 2005; 16(5):727–731

[27] Lewin JS, Hutcheson KH, Smith BG, Barringer DA, Alvarez CP. Early experience with head and neck lymphedema after treatment for head and neck cancer. Poster presented at: Multidisciplinary Head and Neck Cancer Symposium; February 25–27, 2010; Chandler, AZ

[28] Patterson JM, Hildreth A, Wilson JA. Measuring edema in irradiated head and neck cancer patients. Ann Otol Rhinol Laryngol. 2007; 116(8):559–564

[29] Kubicek GJ, Wang F, Reddy E, Shnayder Y, Cabrera CE, Girod DA. Importance of treatment institution in head and neck cancer radiotherapy. Otolaryngol Head Neck Surg. 2009; 141(2):172–176

[30] Howlader N, Noone AM, Krapcho M, et al. SEER Cancer Statistics Review, 1975–2009 (Vintage 2009 Populations) based on November 2011 SEER data submission, posted to the SEER website. Available at: 2012. http://seer.cancer.gov/csr/1975_2009_pops09/. Accessed April 1, 2012

[31] Strossenreuther RHK, Klose G. Guidelines for the application of MLD/CDT for primary and secondary lymphedema and other selected pathologies. In: Földi M, Földi E, Kubik P, et al, eds. Földi's Textbook of Lymphology: For Physicians and Lymphedema Therapists. 2nd ed. Munich, Germany: Urban & Fischer; 2006:676–683

[32] Smith BG, Hutcheson KA, Little LG, et al. Lymphedema outcomes in patients with head and neck cancer. Otolaryngol Head Neck Surg. 2015; 152(2):284–291

[33] Maus EA, Tan IC, Rasmussen JC, et al. Near-infrared fluorescence imaging of lymphatics in head and neck lymphedema. Head Neck. 2012; 34(3):448–453

[34] Mukherji SK, Armao D, Joshi VM. Cervical nodal metastases in squamous cell carcinoma of the head and neck: what to expect. Head Neck. 2001; 23(11):995–1005

[35] Dietz A, Rudat V, Nollert J, Helbig M, Vanselow B, Weidauer H. Chronic laryngeal edema as a late reaction to radiochemotherapy [in German]. HNO. 1998; 46(8):731–738

[36] Popovtzer A, Cao Y, Feng FY, Eisbruch A. Anatomical changes in the pharyngeal constrictors after chemo-irradiation of head and neck cancer and their dose-effect relationships: MRI-based study. Radiother Oncol. 2009; 93(3):510–515

[37] Lacerda GdeC, Pedrosa RC, Lacerda RC, Santos MC, Brasil AT, Siqueira-Filho AG. Complications related to carotid sinus massage in 502 ambulatory patients. Arq Bras Cardiol. 2009; 92(2):78–87

[38] Rimmer J, Giddings CE, Vaz F, Brooks J, Hopper C. Management of vascular complications of head and neck cancer. J Laryngol Otol. 2012; 126(2):111–115

[39] Strossenreuther R, Asmussen PD. Compression therapy. In: Földi M, Földi E, Strossenreuther RHK, eds. Földi's Textbook of Lymphology: For Physicians and Lymphedema Therapists. 2nd ed. Munich, Germany: Urban & Fischer; 2006:564–627

[40] Ko DS, Lerner R, Klose G, Cosimi AB. Effective treatment of lymphedema of the extremities. Arch Surg. 1998; 133 (4):452–458

[41] Rovig J. The story of JoviPak. Available at: http://www.stepup-speakout.org/ jovi_lymphedema_garments.htm. Accessed March 20, 2012

[42] Shim JY, Lee HR, Lee DC. The use of elastic adhesive tape to promote lymphatic flow in the rabbit hind leg. Yonsei Med J. 2003; 44(6):1045–1052

[43] Rock Tape. Available at: http://www.rocktape.co.uk/downloads/evidenceofefficacy.pdf. Published 2010. Accessed May 24, 2016

[44] Rodrick JR, Poage E, Wanchai A. Management of lymphedema with complementary, alternative, and other non-complete decongestive therapies: a summary of the ALFP. Lymph Link.. 2013; 26(4):S1934–S1482

[45] Malicka I, Rosseger A, Hanuszkiewicz J, Woźniewski M. Kinesiology Taping reduces lymphedema of the upper extremity in women after breast cancer treatment: a pilot study. Przegl Menopauz. 2014; 13(4):221–226

[46] Kase K, Wallis J, Kase T. Clinical Therapeutic Applications of the Kinesio Taping Method. 3rd ed. Kinesio Taping Association; 2013

[47] Parreira PdoC, Costa LdaC, Takahashi R, et al. Kinesio taping to generate skin convolutions is not better than sham taping for people with chronic non-specific low back pain: a randomised trial. J Physiother. 2014; 60(2):90–96

[48] Silva Parreira PdoC, Menezes Costa LdaC, Takahashi R, et al. Do convolutions in Kinesio Taping matter? Comparison of two Kinesio Taping approaches in patients with chronic non-specific low back pain: protocol of a randomised trial. J Physiother. 2013; 59(1):52–, discussion 52

[49] Taradaj J, Halski T, Rosinczuk J, Dymarek R, Laurowski A, Smykla A. The influence of Kinesiology Taping on the volume of lymphoedema and manual dexterity of the upper limb in women after breast cancer treatment. Eur J Cancer Care (Engl). 2016; 25(4):647–660

[50] Pop TB, Karczmarek-Borowska B, Tymczak M, Hałas I, Banaś J. The influence of Kinesiology Taping on the reduction of lymphoedema among women after mastectomy - preliminary study. Contemp Oncol (Pozn). 2014; 18(2):124–129

[51] Smykla A, Walewicz K, Trybulski R, et al. Effect of Kinesiology Taping on breast cancer-related lymphedema: a randomized single-blind controlled pilot study. BioMed Res Int. 2013; 2013:767106

[52] Pekyavaş NÖ, Tunay VB, Akbayrak T, Kaya S, Karataş M. Complex decongestive therapy and taping for patients with postmastectomy lymphedema: a randomized controlled study. Eur J Oncol Nurs. 2014; 18(6):585–590

[53] Gerasimenko MY, Knyazeva TA, Apkhanova TV, Kul'Chitskaya DB. [The application of the method of kinesio-taping technique for the combined non-pharmacological rehabilitation of the patients presenting with lymphedema of the lower extremities]. Vopr Kurortol Fizioter Lech Fiz Kult. 2015; 92(5):22–27

[54] Tsai HJ, Hung HC, Yang JL, Huang CS, Tsauo JY. Could Kinesio tape replace the bandage in decongestive lymphatic therapy for breast-cancer-related lymphedema? A pilot study. Support Care Cancer. 2009; 17(11):1353–1360

[55] Martins JdeC, Aguiar SS, Fabro EA, et al. Safety and tolerability of Kinesio Taping in patients with arm lymphedema: medical device clinical study. Support Care Cancer. 2016; 24 (3):1119–1124

[56] Białoszewski D, Woźniak W, Zarek S. Clinical efficacy of kinesiology taping in reducing edema of the lower limbs in patients treated with the Ilizarov method–preliminary report. Ortop Traumatol Rehabil. 2009; 11(1):46–54

[57] Tozzi U, Santagata M, Sellitto A, Tartaro GP. Influence of Kinesiologic Tape on post-operative swelling After orthognathic Surgery. J Maxillofac Oral Surg. 2016; 15(1):52–58

[58] Bosman J, Piller N. Lymph taping and seroma formation post breast cancer. J Lymphoedema. 2010; 5(2):12–21

[59] Ristow O, Hohlweg-Majert B, Stürzenbaum SR, et al. Therapeutic elastic tape reduces morbidity after wisdom teeth removal-a clinical trial. Clin Oral Investig. 2014; 18 (4):1205–1212

[60] Taradaj J, Halski T, Zduńczyk M, et al. Evaluation of the effectiveness of kinesio taping application in a patient with secondary lymphedema in breast cancer: a case report. Przegl Menopauz. 2014; 13(1):73–77

[61] Lipinska A, Sliwinski Z, Kiebzak W, Senderek T, Kirenko J. The influence of kinesiotaping application on lymphoedema of an upper limb in women after mastectomy. Polish Journal of Physiotherapy. 2007; 7(3):258–269

[62] Kaya S, Akbayrak T, Guney H. Effect of kinesio taping with compression garment on lower extremity volume in

primary lymphedema: a case report. Fizyoterapi Rehabilitasyon. 2008; 19(3):213

[63] Coopee R. Use of "Elastic Taping" in the treatment of head and neck lymphedema. Lymph Link.. 2008; 20(4)

[64] Bosman J. Lymphtaping for lymphoedema: an overview of the treatment and its uses. Br J Community Nurs. 2014; S12 Suppl:S12–, S14, S16–S18

[65] Chou YH, Li SH, Liao SF, Tang HW. Case report: manual lymphatic drainage and kinesio taping in the secondary malignant breast cancer-related lymphedema in an arm with arteriovenous (A-V) fistula for hemodialysis. Am J Hosp Palliat Care. 2013; 30(5):503–506

[66] Sijmonsma, J. Lymph Taping: Theory, Technique, Practice. Tjerk Veen: Fysionair; 2010

[67] Földi M, Földi E, Kubik P. Anatomy of the lymphatic system. In: Földi M, Földi E, Kubik P, et al, eds. Textbook of lymphology: For Physicians and Lymphedema Therapists. Munich, Germany: Urban & Fischer; 2003:20

[68] Földi M, Földi E, Kubik S. Textbook of Lymphology, 3rd ed. Elsevier 2012:323

[69] Browse N, Burnand K, Mortimer P. Principles of surgical treatment. In: Browse N, Burnand K, Mortimer P, eds. Diseases of the Lymphatics. London: Arnold; 2003: Chapter 10

[70] Strossenreuther R. Evaluation. In: Földi M, Földi E, Kubik P, et al, eds. Textbook of Lymphology: For Physicians and Lymphedema Therapists. Munich, Germany: Urban & Fischer; 2003:598

[71] Strossenreuther R. Physiotherapy and other physical therapy techniques. In: Földi M, Földi E, Kubik P, et al, eds. Textbook of Lymphology: For Physicians and Lymphedema Therapists. Munich, Germany: Urban & Fischer; 2003:520–521

[72] Dox I, Melloni J, Eisner G. The Harper Collins Illustrated Medical Dictionary. New York, NY: Harper Collins; 1993

[73] Kaiserling E. Anatomy of the lymphatic system. In: Földi M, Földi E, Kubik P, et al, eds. Földi's Textbook of Lymphology: For Physicians and Lymphedema Therapists. 2nd ed. Munich, Germany: Urban & Fischer; 2006:365

[74] Browse N, Burnand K. Differential diagnosis of chronic swelling. In: Browse N, Burnand K, Mortimer P, eds. Diseases of the Lymphatics. London: Arnold; 2003:163

[75] Weissleder H, Schuchhardt C. Lymphedema in tumor management. In: Weissleder H, Schuchhardt C, eds. Lymphedema Diagnosis and Therapy. 4th ed. Essen, Germany: Viavital Verlag; 2008:217

[76] Földi M, Földi E. Anatomy of the lymphatic system. In: Földi M, Földi E, Kubik P, et al, eds. Földi's Textbook of Lymphology: For Physicians and Lymphedema Therapists. 2nd ed. Munich, Germany: Urban & Fischer; 2006:262

[77] Weissleder H, Schuchhardt C. Lymphedema in tumor management. In: Weissleder H, Schuchhardt C, eds. Lymphedema Diagnosis and Therapy. 4th ed. Essen, Germany: Viavital Verlag; 2008:18

[78] Földi M, Földi E. Anatomy of the lymphatic system. In: Földi M, Földi E, Kubik P, et al, eds. Földi's Textbook of Lymphology: For Physicians and Lymphedema Therapists. 2nd ed. Munich, Germany: Urban & Fischer; 2006:240–242

[79] Cormier JN, Askew RL, Mungovan KS, Xing Y, Ross MI, Armer JM. Lymphedema beyond breast cancer: a systematic review and meta-analysis of cancer-related secondary lymphedema. Cancer. 2010; 116(22):5138–5149

[80] Towers A, Hodgson P, Shay C, Keeley V. Care of the palliative patient with cancer-related lymphedema. Lymphœdema. 2010; 5(1):72–80

[81] McBeth M. Palliative care: providing comfort through lymphedema therapy. Paper presented at the 8th NLN International Conference; September 2008; San Diego, CA

[82] Weissleder H, Schuchhardt C. Lymphedema Diagnosis and Therapy. 3rd ed. Cologne: Viavital Verlag GmbH; 2001:243

[83] Lymphedema Framework. Best Practices for the Management of Lymphoedema: International Consensus Document. London: MEP Ltd; 2006

[84] Weissleder H, Schuchhardt C. Lymphedema Diagnosis and Therapy. 3rd ed. Cologne: Viavital Verlag GmbH; 2001:242

[85] Cheville A. Lymphedema and palliative care. LymphLink. 2002; 14:1–4

[86] Renshaw M. Lymphorrhoea: 'leaky legs' are not just the nurse's problem. Br J Community Nurs. 2007; 12(4):S18–S21

[87] Keeley V. Drugs that may exacerbate and those used to treat lymphedema. Lymphoedema.. 2008; 3(1):57–65

[88] Crooks P, Locke J, Walker J, Keeley V. Palliative bandaging in breast cancer-related arm lymphoedema. J Lymphoedema. 2007; 2(1):50–54

[89] Clein LJ. Edema. In: Al WE, ed. Palliative Medicine. Philadelphia, PA: Saunders Elsevier; 2005: 291–306

[90] Clein LJ, Pugachev E. Reduction of edema of lower extremities by subcutaneous, controlled drainage: eight cases. Am J Hosp Palliat Care. 2004; 21(3):228–232

[91] Stamatakos M, Stefanaki C, Kontzoglou K. Lymphedema and breast cancer: a review of the literature. Breast Cancer. 2011; 18(3):174–180

[92] Kinmonth JB. The Lymphatics. 2nd ed. Baltimore: Arnold; 1982

[93] Browse N, Burnand K, Mortimer P, eds. Diseases of the Lymphatics. London: Arnold; 2003

[94] Zvonik M, Földi E, Felmerer G. The effects of reduction operation with genital lymphedema on the frequency of erysipelas and the quality of life. Lymphology. 2011; 44(3):121–130

[95] Rönkä R, von Smitten K, Tasmuth T, Leidenius M. One-year morbidity after sentinel node biopsy and breast surgery. Breast. 2005; 14(1):28–36

[96] Vitug AF, Newman LA. Complications in breast surgery. Surg Clin North Am. 2007; 87(2):431–451, x

[97] Mayrovitz HN, Brown-Cross D, Mayrovitz BL, Golla AH. Role of truncal clearance as a therapy component. Home Health Care Management Practice OnlineFirst.. 2009; 10 (1177):1–13

[98] Ridner SH, Murphy B, Deng J, et al. A randomized clinical trial comparing advanced pneumatic truncal, chest, and arm treatment to arm treatment only in self-care of arm lymphedema. Breast Cancer Res Treat. 2012; 131(1):147–158

[99] Ridner SH, Murphy B, Deng J, Kidd N, Galford E, Dietrich MS. Advanced pneumatic therapy in self-care of chronic lymphedema of the trunk. Lymphat Res Biol. 2010; 8(4):209–215

[100] Degnim AC, Miller J, Hoskin TL, et al. A prospective study of breast lymphedema: frequency, symptoms, and quality of life. Breast Cancer Res Treat. 2012; 134(3):915–922

[101] Majeski J, Austin RM, Fitzgerald RH. Cutaneous angiosarcoma in an irradiated breast after breast conservation therapy for cancer: association with chronic breast lymphedema. J Surg Oncol. 2000; 74(3):208–212, discussion 212–213

[102] Norman SA, Localio AR, Kallan MJ, et al. Risk factors for lymphedema after breast cancer treatment. Cancer Epidemiol Biomarkers Prev. 2010; 19(11):2734–2746

[103] McLaughlin SA, Wright MJ, Morris KT, et al. Prevalence of lymphedema in women with breast cancer 5 years after sentinel lymph node biopsy or axillary dissection: patient perceptions and precautionary behaviors. J Clin Oncol. 2008; 26(32):5220–5226

5

[104] Clarke D, Martinez A, Cox RS, Goffinet DR. Breast edema following staging axillary node dissection in patients with breast carcinoma treated by radical radiotherapy. Cancer. 1982; 49(11):2295–2299

[105] Boughey JC, Hoskin TL, Cheville AL, et al. Risk factors associated with breast lymphedema. Ann Surg Oncol. 2014; 21 (4):1202–1208

[106] Rönkä RH, Pamilo MS, von Smitten KA, Leidenius MH. Breast lymphedema after breast conserving treatment. Acta Oncol. 2004; 43(6):551–557

[107] Goffman TE, Laronga C, Wilson L, Elkins D. Lymphedema of the arm and breast in irradiated breast cancer patients: risks in an era of dramatically changing axillary surgery. Breast J. 2004; 10(5):405–411

[108] Jones G. The pedicled TRAM flap in breast reconstruction. Clin Plast Surg. 2007; 34(1):83–104, abstract vii

[109] Parrett BM, Sepic J, Pribaz JJ. The contralateral rectus abdominis musculocutaneous flap for treatment of lower extremity lymphedema. Ann Plast Surg. 2009; 62(1):75–79

[110] Chang DW, Kim S. Breast reconstruction and lymphedema. Plast Reconstr Surg. 2010; 125(1):19–23

[111] Perbeck L, Celebioglu F, Svensson L, Danielsson R. Lymph circulation in the breast after radiotherapy and breast conservation. Lymphology. 2006; 39(1):33–40

[112] Brooks C. Radiation therapy: guidelines for physiotherapists. Physiotherapy. 1998; 84:387–395

[113] Fu MR, Guth AA, Cleland CM, et al. The effects of symptomatic seroma on lymphedema symptoms following breast cancer treatment. Lymphology. 2011; 44(3):134–143

[114] O'Toole J, Miller CL, Specht MC, et al. Cording following treatment for breast cancer. Breast Cancer Res Treat. 2013; 140(1):105–111

[115] Torres Lacomba M, Yuste Sánchez MJ, Zapico Goñi A, et al. Effectiveness of early physiotherapy to prevent lymphoedema after surgery for breast cancer: randomised, single blinded, clinical trial. BMJ. 2010; 340:b5396

[116] Kropf N, Macadam SA, McCarthy C, et al. Influence of the recipient vessel on fat necrosis after breast reconstruction with a free transverse rectus abdominis myocutaneous flap. Scand J Plast Reconstr Surg Hand Surg. 2010; 44(2):96–101

[117] Joffe H, Goldhaber S. Review of upper extremity deep venous thrombosis. Am Fam Physician. 2003; 67(6):1345–1346

[118] Finnerty S, Thomason S, Woods M. Audit of the use of kinesiology tape for breast oedema. J Lymphoedema. 2010; 5:38–44

[119] Dirican A, Andacoglu O, Johnson R, McGuire K, Mager L, Soran A. The short-term effects of low-level laser therapy in the management of breast-cancer-related lymphedema. Support Care Cancer. 2011; 19(5):685–690

[120] Ahmed Omar MT, Abd-El-Gayed Ebid A, El Morsy AM. Treatment of post-mastectomy lymphedema with laser therapy: double blind placebo control randomized study. J Surg Res. 2011; 165(1):82–90

[121] Demir T, Kara C, Ozbek E, Kalkan Y. Evaluation of neodymium-doped yttrium aluminium garnet laser, scalpel incision wounds, and low-level laser therapy for wound healing in rabbit oral mucosa: a pilot study. Photomed Laser Surg. 2010; 28(1):31–37

[122] Williams SK, Rabbani F. Complications of lymphadenectomy in urologic surgery. Urol Clin North Am. 2011; 38(4):507–518, vii

[123] Van der Zee AG, Oonk MH, De Hullu JA, et al. Sentinel node dissection is safe in the treatment of early-stage vulvar cancer. J Clin Oncol. 2008; 26(6):884–889

[124] Shon W, Ida CM, Boland-Froemming JM, Rose PS, Folpe A. Cutaneous angiosarcoma arising in massive localized lymphedema of the morbidly obese: a report of five cases and review of the literature. J Cutan Pathol. 2011; 38(7):560–564

[125] Földi M, Földi E, Kubik P, eds. Textbook of Lymphology: For Physicians and Lymphedema Therapists. Munich, Germany: Urban & Fischer; 2003:631

[126] Weissleder H, Schuchhardt C. Lymphedema Diagnosis and Therapy. 3rd ed. Cologne: Viavital Verlag: 2001:277

[127] Partsch H, Flour M, Smith PC, International Compression Club. Indications for compression therapy in venous and lymphatic disease consensus based on experimental data and scientific evidence. Under the auspices of the IUP. Int Angiol. 2008; 27(3):193–219

[128] European Wound Management Association (EWMA). Focus Document: Lymphedema Bandaging in Practice. London: MEP Ltd; 2005

[129] KCI V.A.C. Therapy Clinical Guidelines. A Reference Source for Clinicians. 2014:52

[130] Beidler SK, Douillet CD, Berndt DF, Keagy BA, Rich PB, Marston WA. Inflammatory cytokine levels in chronic venous insufficiency ulcer tissue before and after compression therapy. J Vasc Surg. 2009; 49(4):1013–1020

[131] Kieser DC, Roake JA, Hammond C, Lewis DR. Negative pressure wound therapy as an adjunct to compression for healing chronic venous ulcers. J Wound Care. 2011; 20(1):35–37

[132] Todd M. Managing chronic oedema in the morbidly obese patient. Br J Nurs. 2009; 18(18):1120–1124

[133] Fife CE, Benavides S, Otto G. Morbid Obesity and Lymphedema Management. LymphLink. 2007; 19(3):1–3

[134] Lentol J. Information and access to breast reconstructive surgery law10094-B/S.6993-B; Chapter 354; Health. In: New York State Assembly Committee on Codes: Annual Report 2010. Available at: http://assembly.state.ny.us/comm/Codes/2010Annual/index.pdf. Accessed May 5, 2012

[135] Davies HOB, Popplewell M, Singhal R, Smith N, Bradbury AW. Obesity and lower limb venous disease - the epidemic of phlebesity. Phlebology. 2016; •••:1–7

[136] Greene AK, Grant FD, Slavin SA, Maclellan RA. Obesity-induced lymphedema: clinical and lymphoscintigraphic features. Plast Reconstr Surg. 2015; 135(6):1715–1719

[137] Greene AK, Grant FD, Maclellan RA. Obesity-induced lymphedema non-reversible following massive weight loss. PRS Global Open. Available at: www.PRSGlobalOpen.com p.1–3

[138] Mehrara BJ, Greene AK. Lymphedema and obesity: is there a link? Plast Reconstr Surg. 2014; 134(1):154e–160e

[139] http://www.niddk.nih.gov/health-information/health-topics/weight-control/talking-with-patients-about-weight-loss-tips-for-primary-care/Pages/talking.aspx

[140] Rosenberg AE. Pseudosarcomas of soft tissue. Arch Pathol Lab Med. 2008; 132(4):579–586

[141] Moseley A, Piller N. Exercise for limb lymphedema: evidence that it is beneficial. J Lymphoedema. 2008; 3(1):51–56

[142] Lane K, Jespersen D, McKenzie DC. The effect of a whole body exercise programme and dragon boat training on arm volume and arm circumference in women treated for breast cancer. Eur J Cancer Care (Engl). 2005; 14(4):353–358

[143] Position Statement of the National Lymphedema Network on Exercises. Available at: http://lymphnet.org/pdfDocs/nlnexercise.pdf. Accessed March 4, 2016

[144] Sumner DS. Hemodynamics and pathophysiology of venous disease. In: Rutherford RB, ed. Vascular Surgery. 4th ed. Philadelphia, PA: WB Saunders; 1995;1673–1698

[145] Johannson, et al. Controlled physical training for arm lymphedema patients. Lymphology. 2004; 37 S uppl:37–39

5

[146] Box R, Marnes T, Robertson V, et al. Aquatic Physiotherapy and Breast Cancer Related Lymphoedema. 5th Australasian Lymphology Association Conference Proceedings; 2004:47–9

[147] Pendleton D. Staying alive. AOPA Pilot. 2002; 45(10):121–122

[148] Nagda NL, Koontz MD. Review of studies on flight attendant health and comfort in airliner cabins. Aviat Space Environ Med. 2003; 74:101–109

[149] Electronic Code of Federal Regulations 14 CFR, Chapter 1, Part 25, Section 25–831

[150] Casley-Smith JR, Casley-Smith JR. Lymphedema initiated by aircraft flights. Aviat Space Environ Med. 1996; 67(1):52–56

[151] Cormier JN, Rourke L, Crosby M, Chang D, Armer J. The surgical treatment of lymphedema: a systematic review of the contemporary literature (2004–2010). Ann Surg Oncol. 2012; 19(2):642–651

[152] Mehrara BJ, Zampell JC, Suami H, Chang DW. Surgical management of lymphedema: past, present, and future. Lymphat Res Biol. 2011; 9(3):159–167

[153] Greene AK, Grant FD, Maclellan RA. Obesity-induced lymphedema nonreversible following massive weight loss. Plast Reconstr Surg Glob Open. 2015; 3(6):e426

[154] Mihara M, Hara H, Hayashi Y, et al. Pathological steps of cancer-related lymphedema: histological changes in the collecting lymphatic vessels after lymphadenectomy. PLoS One. 2012; 7(7):e41126

[155] Becker C, Assouad J, Riquet M, Hidden G. Postmastectomy lymphedema: long-term results following microsurgical lymph node transplantation. Ann Surg. 2006; 243(3):313–315

[156] Cheng MH, Chen SC, Henry SL, Tan BK, Lin MC, Huang JJ. Vascularized groin lymph node flap transfer for postmastectomy upper limb lymphedema: flap anatomy, recipient sites, and outcomes. Plast Reconstr Surg. 2013; 131 (6):1286–1298

[157] Gharb BB, Rampazzo A, Spanio di Spilimbergo S, Xu ES, Chung KP, Chen HC. Vascularized lymph node transfer based on the hilar perforators improves the outcome in upper limb lymphedema. Ann Plast Surg. 2011; 67(6):589–593

[158] Granzow JW, Soderberg JM, Kaji AH, Dauphine C. An effective system of surgical treatment of lymphedema. Ann Surg Oncol. 2014; 21(4):1189–1194

[159] Granzow JW, Soderberg JM, Dauphine C. A novel two-stage surgical approach to treat chronic lymphedema. Breast J. 2014; 20(4):420–422

[160] Damstra RJ, Voesten HG, van Schelven WD, van der Lei B. Lymphatic venous anastomosis (LVA) for treatment of secondary arm lymphedema. A prospective study of 11 LVA procedures in 10 patients with breast cancer related lymphedema and a critical review of the literature. Breast Cancer Res Treat. 2009; 113(2):199–206

[161] Granzow JW, Soderberg JM, Kaji AH, Dauphine C. Review of current surgical treatments for lymphedema. Ann Surg Oncol. 2014; 21(4):1195–1201

[162] Yamada Y. The studies on lymphatic venous anastomosis. Nagoya J Med Sci. 1969; 32:1–21

[163] O'Brien BM, Sykes P, Threlfall GN, Browning FS. Microlymphaticovenous anastomoses for obstructive lymphedema. Plast Reconstr Surg. 1977; 60(2):197–211

[164] Campisi C, Eretta C, Pertile D, et al. Microsurgery for treatment of peripheral lymphedema: long-term outcome and future perspectives. Microsurgery. 2007; 27(4):333–338

[165] Koshima I, Inagawa K, Urushibara K, Moriguchi T. Supermicrosurgical lymphaticovenular anastomosis for the treatment

[166] of lymphedema in the upper extremities. J Reconstr Microsurg. 2000; 16(6):437–442

[166] Chang DW. Lymphaticovenular bypass for lymphedema management in breast cancer patients: a prospective study. Plast Reconstr Surg. 2010; 126(3):752–758

[167] Boccardo F, De Cian F, Campisi CC, et al. Surgical prevention and treatment of lymphedema after lymph node dissection in patients with cutaneous melanoma. Lymphology. 2013; 46(1):20–26

[168] Baumeister RG, Siuda S, Bohmert H, Moser E. A microsurgical method for reconstruction of interrupted lymphatic pathways: autologous lymph-vessel transplantation for treatment of lymphedemas. Scand J Plast Reconstr Surg. 1986; 20(1):141–146

[169] Weiss MF, Baumeister RG, Zacherl MJ, Frick A, Bartenstein P, Rominger A. Microsurgical autologous lymph vessel transplantation: does harvesting lymphatic vessel grafts induce lymphatic transport disturbances in the donor limb? [in German]. Handchir Mikrochir Plast Chir. 2015; 47(6):359–364

[170] Lin CH, Ali R, Chen SC, et al. Vascularized groin lymph node transfer using the wrist as a recipient site for management of postmastectomy upper extremity lymphedema. Plast Reconstr Surg. 2009; 123(4):1265–1275

[171] Cheng MH, Huang JJ, Nguyen DH, et al. A novel approach to the treatment of lower extremity lymphedema by transferring a vascularized submental lymph node flap to the ankle. Gynecol Oncol. 2012; 126(1):93–98

[172] Coriddi M, Skoracki R, Eiferman D. Vascularized jejunal mesenteric lymph node transfer for treatment of extremity lymphedema. Microsurgery. 2016

[173] Brorson H, Svensson H. Skin blood flow of the lymphedematous arm before and after liposuction. Lymphology. 1997; 30(4):165–172

[174] Tobbia D, Semple J, Baker A, Dumont D, Johnston M. Experimental assessment of autologous lymph node transplantation as treatment of postsurgical lymphedema. Plast Reconstr Surg. 2009; 124(3):777–786

[175] Cheng MH, Huang JJ, Wu CW, et al. The mechanism of vascularized lymph node transfer for lymphedema: natural lymphaticovenous drainage. Plast Reconstr Surg. 2014; 133 (2):192e–198e

[176] Aschen SZ, Farias-Eisner G, Cuzzone DA, et al. Lymph node transplantation results in spontaneous lymphatic reconnection and restoration of lymphatic flow. Plast Reconstr Surg. 2014; 133(2):301–310

[177] Viitanen TP, Visuri MT, Sulo E, Saarikko AM, Hartiala P. Anti-inflammatory effects of flap and lymph node transfer. J Surg Res. 2015; 199(2):718–725

[178] Vignes S, Blanchard M, Yannoutsos A, Arrault M. Complications of autologous lymph-node transplantation for limb lymphoedema. Eur J Vasc Endovasc Surg. 2013; 45(5):516–520

[179] Pons G, Masia J, Loschi P, Nardulli ML, Duch J. A case of donor-site lymphoedema after lymph node-superficial circumflex iliac artery perforator flap transfer. J Plast Reconstr Aesthet Surg. 2014; 67(1):119–123

[180] Lee M, McClure E, Reinertsen E, Granzow JW. Lymphedema of the upper extremity following supraclavicular lymph node harvest. Plast Reconstr Surg. 2015; 135(6):1079e–1082e

[181] Masia J, Pons G, Nardulli ML. Combined surgical treatment in breast cancer-related lymphedema. J Reconstr Microsurg. 2015

5

[182] Dayan JH, Dayan E, Smith ML. Reverse lymphatic mapping: a new technique for maximizing safety in vascularized lymph node transfer. Plast Reconstr Surg. 2015; 135(1):277–285

[183] Damstra RJ, Voesten HG, Klinkert P, Brorson H. Circumferential suction-assisted lipectomy for lymphoedema after surgery for breast cancer. Br J Surg. 2009; 96(8):859–864

[184] Brorson H. Complete reduction of arm lymphedema following breast cancer - a prospective twenty-one years' study. Plast Reconstr Surg. 2015; 136(4) Suppl:134–135

[185] Brorson H. Liposuction normalizes lymphedema induced adipose tissue hypertrophy in elephantiasis of the leg - a prospective study with a ten-year follow-up. Plast Reconstr Surg. 2015; 136(4) Suppl:133–134

[186] Brorson H, Ohlin K, Olsson G, Karlsson MK. Breast cancer-related chronic arm lymphedema is associated with excess adipose and muscle tissue. Lymphat Res Biol. 2009; 7(1):3–10

[187] Brorson H. From lymph to fat: liposuction as a treatment for complete reduction of lymphedema. Int J Low Extrem Wounds. 2012; 11(1):10–19

[188] Schaverien MV, Munro KJ, Baker PA, Munnoch DA. Liposuction for chronic lymphoedema of the upper limb: 5 years of experience. J Plast Reconstr Aesthet Surg. 2012; 65(7):935–942

[189] Boyages J, Kastanias K, Koelmeyer LA, et al. Liposuction for advanced lymphedema: a multidisciplinary approach for complete reduction of arm and leg swelling. Ann Surg Oncol. 2015; 22 Suppl 3:S1263–S1270

[190] Brorson H, Svensson H, Norrgren K, Thorsson O. Liposuction reduces arm lymphedema without significantly altering the already impaired lymph transport. Lymphology. 1998; 31 (4):156–172

[191] Granzow J, Andersen G, Soderberg J. Lymphatic anatomy is not damaged by suction assisted protein lipectomy (SAPL) Surgery. Submitted, NLN Conference

[192] Qiu SS, Chen HY, Cheng MH. Vascularized lymph node flap transfer and lymphovenous anastomosis for Klippel-Trenaunay syndrome with congenital lymphedema. Plast Reconstr Surg Glob Open. 2014; 2(6):e167

[193] Jemal A, Siegel R, Xu J, Ward E. Cancer statistics, 2010. CA Cancer J Clin. 2010; 60(5):277–300

[194] Jacobson JA, Danforth DN, Cowan KH, et al. Ten-year results of a comparison of conservation with mastectomy in the treatment of stage I and II breast cancer. N Engl J Med. 1995; 332(14):907–911

[195] Lee MC, Rogers K, Griffith K, et al. Determinants of breast conservation rates: reasons for mastectomy at a comprehensive cancer center. Breast J. 2009; 15(1):34–40

[196] Bezuhly M, Temple C, Sigurdson LJ, Davis RB, Flowerdew G, Cook EF, Jr. Immediate postmastectomy reconstruction is associated with improved breast cancer-specific survival: evidence and new challenges from the Surveillance, Epidemiology, and End Results database. Cancer. 2009; 115 (20):4648–4654

[197] Yueh JH, Slavin SA, Adesiyun T, et al. Patient satisfaction in postmastectomy breast reconstruction: a comparative evaluation of DIEP, TRAM, latissimus flap, and implant techniques. Plast Reconstr Surg. 2010; 125(6):1585–1595

[198] Reuben BC, Manwaring J, Neumayer LA. Recent trends and predictors in immediate breast reconstruction after mastectomy in the United States. Am J Surg. 2009; 198(2):237–243

[199] American Society of Plastic Surgeons. Are breast cancer patients being kept in the dark? Available at: http://www. plasticsurgery.org/ News-and-Resources/Press-Release-Archives/2009-Press-Release-Archives/Are-Breast-Cancer-Patients-Being-Kept-In-The-Dark.html. Accessed May 5, 2012

[200] Hartocollis A. Before breast is removed, a discussion on options. The New York Times, 2010:A23. Available at: http:// www.nytimes. com/2010/08/19/nyregion/10surgery.html. Accessed May 5, 2012

[201] Albornoz CR, Bach PB, Pusic AL, et al. The influence of sociodemographic factors and hospital characteristics on the method of breast reconstruction, including microsurgery: a U.S. population-based study. Plast Reconstr Surg. 2012; 129 (5):1071–1079

[202] Niemeyer M, Paepke S, Schmid R, Plattner B, Müller D, Kiechle M. Extended indications for nipple-sparing mastectomy. Breast J. 2011; 17(3):296–299

[203] US Department of Health & Human Services. Silicone gel-filled breast implants. Available at: http://www.fda.gov/ MedicalDevices/ProductsandMedicalProcedures/Implantsand Prosthetics/Breast-Implants/ucm063871.htm. Accessed May 5, 2012

[204] US Department of Health & Human Services. Update on the safety of silicone gel-filled breast implants (2011) - Executive Summary. Available at: http://www.fda.gov/MedicalDevices/Productsand-MedicalProcedures/ImplantsandProsthetics/BreastImplants/ucm259866.htm. Accessed May 5, 2012

[205] US Department of Health & Human services. Breast implant complications booklet. Available at: http://www.fda.gov/ MedicalDevices/ProductsandMedicalProcedures/Implantsand Prosthetics/BreastImplants/ucm259296.htm. Accessed May 5, 2012

[206] US Department of Health & Human Services. Risks of breast implants. Available at: http://www.fda.gov/MedicalDevices/ Productsand-MedicalProcedures/ImplantsandProsthetics/ BreastImplants/ucm064106.htm. Accessed May 5, 2012

[207] Schneider WJ, Hill HL, Jr, Brown RG. Latissimus dorsi myocutaneous flap for breast reconstruction. Br J Plast Surg. 1977; 30(4):277–281

[208] Dinner MI, Hartrampf CR, Jr. Re: Drever: lower abdominal transverse rectus abdominis myocutaneous flap for breast reconstruction. Ann Plast Surg. 1983; 11(5):453–454

[209] Bunkis J, Walton RL, Mathes SJ, Krizek TJ, Vasconez LO. Experience with the transverse lower rectus abdominis operation for breast reconstruction. Plast Reconstr Surg. 1983; 72 (6):819–829

[210] Schusterman MA, Kroll SS, Weldon ME. Immediate breast reconstruction: why the free TRAM over the conventional TRAM flap? Plast Reconstr Surg. 1992; 90(2):255–261, discussion 262

[211] Alpert BS, Buncke HJ, Jr, Mathes SJ. Surgical treatment of the totally avulsed scalp. Clin Plast Surg. 1982; 9(2):145–159

[212] Allen RJ, Treece P. Deep inferior epigastric perforator flap for breast reconstruction. Ann Plast Surg. 1994; 32(1):32–38

[213] Blondeel PN, Boeckx WD. Refinements in free flap breast reconstruction: the free bilateral deep inferior epigastric perforator flap anastomosed to the internal mammary artery. Br J Plast Surg. 1994; 47(7):495–501

[214] Massey MF, Spiegel AJ, Levine JL, et al. Group for the Advancement of Breast Reconstruction. Perforator flaps: recent experience, current trends, and future directions based on 3974 microsurgical breast reconstructions. Plast Reconstr Surg. 2009; 124(3):737–751

[215] D'Angelo-Donovan DD, Dickson-Witmer D, Petrelli NJ. Sentinel lymph node biopsy in breast cancer: a history and current clinical recommendations. Surg Oncol. 2012; 21 (3):196–200

5

[216] Golshan M, Martin WJ, Dowlatshahi K. Sentinel lymph node biopsy lowers the rate of lymphedema when compared with standard axillary lymph node dissection. Am Surg. 2003; 69 (3):209–211, discussion 212

[217] Boneti C, Korourian S, Bland K, et al. Axillary reverse mapping: mapping and preserving arm lymphatics may be important in preventing lymphedema during sentinel lymph node biopsy. J Am Coll Surg. 2008; 206(5):1038–1042, discussion 1042–1044

[218] Goldberg JI, Riedel ER, Morrow M, Van Zee KJ. Morbidity of sentinel node biopsy: relationship between number of excised lymph nodes and patient perceptions of lymphedema. Ann Surg Oncol. 2011; 18(10):2866–2872

[219] Deo SV, Ray S, Rath GK, et al. Prevalence and risk factors for development of lymphedema following breast cancer treatment. Indian J Cancer. 2004; 41(1):8–12

[220] Shah C, Vicini FA. Breast cancer-related arm lymphedema: incidence rates, diagnostic techniques, optimal management and risk reduction strategies. Int J Radiat Oncol Biol Phys. 2011; 81(4):907–914

[221] Tsai RJ, Dennis LK, Lynch CF, Snetselaar LG, Zamba GK, Scott-Conner C. The risk of developing arm lymphedema among breast cancer survivors: a meta-analysis of treatment factors. Ann Surg Oncol. 2009; 16(7):1959–1972

[222] Andersen KG, Kehlet H. Persistent pain after breast cancer treatment: a critical review of risk factors and strategies for prevention. J Pain. 2011; 12(7):725–746

[223] Gärtner R, Jensen MB, Nielsen J, Ewertz M, Kroman N, Kehlet H. Prevalence of and factors associated with persistent pain following breast cancer surgery. JAMA. 2009; 302 (18):1985–1992

[224] Becker C, Pham DN, Assouad J, Badia A, Foucault C, Riquet M. Postmastectomy neuropathic pain: results of microsurgical lymph nodes transplantation. Breast. 2008; 17(5):472–476

[225] Saaristo AM, Niemi TS, Viitanen TP, Tervala TV, Hartiala P, Suominen EA. Microvascular breast reconstruction and lymph node transfer for postmastectomy lymphedema patients. Ann Surg. 2012; 255(3):468–473

[226] National Institute of Lymphology. Ongoing clinical research at our centers of excellence in the care of lymphedema: ICG lymph node mapping in the setting of VLNTx. Available at: http://www.nilymph.com/ongoing-clinical-research-our-centers-excellence-care-lymphedema. Accessed May 5, 2012

[227] Kasseroller RG. The Vodder school: the Vodder method. Cancer. 1998; 83(12) Suppl American:2840–2842

[228] Cheville AL, McGarvey CL, Petrek JA, Russo SA, Taylor ME, Thiadens SR. Lymphedema management. Semin Radiat Oncol. 2003; 13(3):290–301

[229] Cohen SR, Payne DK, Tunkel RS. Lymphedema: strategies for management. Cancer. 2001; 92(4) Suppl:980–987

[230] Thiadens SR. Current status of education and treatment resources for lymphedema. Cancer. 1998; 83(12) Suppl American:2864–2868

[231] Alderman AK, Hawley ST, Waljee J, Mujahid M, Morrow M, Katz SJ. Understanding the impact of breast reconstruction on the surgical decision-making process for breast cancer. Cancer. 2008; 112(3):489–494

[232] National Institute of Lymphology. Proactive "protect the limb" protocol. Available at: http://www.nilymph.com/proactive. Accessed May 6, 2012

[233] US National Institutes of Health. Outcomes after perforator flap reconstruction for breast reconstruction and/or lymphedema treatment. Clinical Trials.gov website. Available at: http://clinicaltrials.gov/ ct2/show/NCT01273909. Accessed June 28, 2012

Recommended Reading

Białoszewski D, Woźniak W, Zarek S. Clinical efficacy of kinesiology taping in reducing edema of the lower limbs in patients treated with the Ilizarov method–preliminary report. Ortop Traumatol Rehabil. 2009; 11(1):46–54

Bringezu G, Schreiner O. Die Therapieform manuelle Lymphdrainage: ein aktuelles Lehrbuch einer erfolgreichen Behandlungsmethode. Lübeck, Germany: Haase; 1987

Brown JC, Schmitz KH. Weight lifting and physical function among survivors of breast cancer: a post hoc analysis of a randomized controlled trial. J Clin Oncol. 2015; 33(19):2184–2189

Browse N, Burnand K, Mortimer P. Diseases of the Lymphatics. London: Arnold; 2003:175–207

Brorson H, Ohlin K, Olsson G, Långström G, Wiklund I, Svensson H. Quality of life following liposuction and conservative treatment of arm lymphedema. Lymphology. 2006; 39(1):8–25

Cherry KJ, Gloviczki P, Stanson AW. Persistent sciatic vein: diagnosis and treatment of a rare condition. J Vasc Surg. 1996; 23(3):490–497

Cohen MM, Jr. Klippel-Trenaunay syndrome. Am J Med Genet. 2000; 93(3):171–175

Coopee R. Use of "Elastic Taping" in the treatment of head and neck lymphedema. Lymph Link.. 2008; 20(4)

Damstra RJ, Voesten HG, Klinkert P, Brorson H. Circumferential suction-assisted lipectomy for lymphoedema after surgery for breast cancer. Br J Surg. 2009; 96(8):859–864

Driscoll D, Gloviczki P, Hussmann D, et al. Paper presented at: K-T Support Group Meeting; July 18–19, 2008; Rochester, MN

Földi M. Treatment of lymphedema. [editorial]. Lymphology. 1994; 27(1):1–5

Foeldi M, Foeldi E. Foeldi's Textbook of Lymphology for Physicians and Lymphedema Therapists. 3rd ed. Munich: Elsevier; 2012

Funayama E, Sasaki S, Oyama A, Furukawa H, Hayashi T, Yamamoto Y. How do the type and location of a vascular malformation influence growth in Klippel-Trénaunay syndrome? Plast Reconstr Surg. 2011; 127(1):340–346

Getz DH. The primary, secondary, and tertiary nursing interventions of lymphedema. Cancer Nurs. 1985; 8(3):177–184

Gleim IN, Gleim GW. Pilot Handbook: A Comprehensive Text/Reference for All Pilots. 8th ed. Gainesville, FL: Gleim; 2008

Gloviczki P, Driscoll DJ. Klippel-Trenaunay syndrome: current management. Phlebology. 2007; 22(6):291–298

Grotting JC, Urist MM, Maddox WA, Vasconez LO. Conventional TRAM flap versus free microsurgical TRAM flap for immediate breast reconstruction. Plast Reconstr Surg. 1989; 83(5):828–841, discussion 842–844

Hocutt JE, Jr. Cryotherapy. Am Fam Physician. 1981; 23(3):141–144

Hutzschenreuter P, Ehlers R. Effect of manual lymph drainage on the autonomic nervous system [in German]. Z Lymphol. 1986; 10 (2):58–60

Jacob AG, Driscoll DJ, Shaughnessy WJ, Stanson AW, Clay RP, Gloviczki P. Klippel-Trénaunay syndrome: spectrum and management. Mayo Clin Proc. 1998; 73(1):28–36

Janniger CK. Klippel-Trénaunay-Weber syndrome. 2012. Available at: http://emedicine.medscape.com/article/1084257-overview. Accessed June 28, 2012

Kaya S, Akbayrak T, Guney H. Effect of kinesio taping with compression garment on lower extremity volume in primary lymphedema: a case report. [in Turkish]. Fizyoterapi Rehabilitasyon. 2008; 19(3):213

Kinmonth J. The Lymphatics; Diseases, Lymphography and Surgery. London: Arnold; 1972

Klippel-Trénaunay Support Group. Description of Klippel-Trénaunay syndrome. Available at: http://www.k-t.org/ description.html. Accessed August 9, 2008

Lawrance P. Innovations in the management of chronic oedema. Br J Community Nurs. 2009 S uppl:S14–S21

Lee A, Driscoll D, Gloviczki P, Clay R, Shaughnessy W, Stans A. Evaluation and management of pain in patients with Klippel-Trenaunay syndrome: a review. Pediatrics. 2005; 115(3):744–749

Lipinska A, Sliwinski Z, Kiebzak W, Senderek T, Kirenko J. The influence of kinesio taping application on lymphoedema of an upper limb in women after mastectomy [in Polish]. Fizjoterapia Polska. 2007; 7(3):258–269

Liu NF, Lu Q, Yan ZX. Lymphatic malformation is a common component of Klippel-Trenaunay syndrome. J Vasc Surg. 2010; 52 (6):1557–1563

Liu Q, Zhou X, Wei Q. Treatment of upper limb lymphedema after radical mastectomy with liposuction technique and pressure therapy [in Chinese]. Zhongguo Xiu Fu Chong Jian Wai Ke Za Zhi. 2005; 19(5):344–345

Lymphology Association of North America (LANA). Certified lymphedema therapist candidate information brochure. Available at: http://www.clt-lana.org. Accessed June 28, 2012

Mattassi R, Vaghi M. Management of the marginal vein: current issues. Phlebology. 2007; 22(6):283–286

Moodie D, Driscoll D, Salvatore D. Peripheral vascular disease in children—Klippel-Trénaunay syndrome. In: Young JR, Olin JW, Bartholomew JR. eds. Peripheral Vascular Diseases. 2nd ed. St. Louis, MO: Mosby; 1996:541–552

Mulliken JB, Young AE. Vascular Birthmarks: Hemangiomas and Malformations. Philadelphia, PA: Saunders; 1988

Muscari-Lin E. Truncal lymphedema. LymphLink 2004;16(1):1–2, 21

Nagda NL, Koontz MD. Review of studies on flight attendant health and comfort in airliner cabins. Aviat Space Environ Med. 2003; 74 (2):101–109

National Cancer Institute (US), Office of Cancer Communications. The breast cancer digest: a guide to medical care, emotional support, educational programs, and resources. 2nd ed. Bethesda, MD: US Dept. of Health, Education, and Welfare, Public Health Service, National Institute of Health, National Cancer Institute; 1984:78

NLN. 2010 Position Statement of the National Lymphedema Network. Training of Lymphedema Therapists. Available at: http://wwwlymphnet.org/pdfDocs/nlntraining.pdf. Accessed June 28, 2012

North American Lymphedema Education Association. Available at: http://lymphedemaeducationassociation.org/about.html. Accessed June 28, 2012

Oduber CE, Khemlani K, Sillevis Smitt JH, Hennekam RC, van der Horst CM. Baseline Quality of Life in patients with Klippel-Trenaunay syndrome. J Plast Reconstr Aesthet Surg. 2010; 63(4):603–609

Olszewski W. Lymph Stasis: Pathophysiology, Diagnosis and Treatment. Florida: CRC Press; 1991:387–388

Pendleton L. Staying alive. Available at: http://www.qopa.org/careerpilot/tastaying_alive.html. Accessed September 5, 2012

Qi F, Gu J, Shi Y, Yang Y. Treatment of upper limb lymphedema with combination of liposuction, myocutaneous flap transfer, and lymph-fascia grafting: a preliminary study. Microsurgery. 2009; 29 (1):29–34

Rayman RB. Cabin air quality: an overview. Aviat Space Environ Med. 2002; 73(3):211–215

Rönkä RH, Pamilo MS, von Smitten KA, Leidenius MH. Breast lymphedema after breast conserving treatment. Acta Oncol. 2004; 43 (6):551–557

Rosenfeld RG, Tesch LG, Rodriguez-Rigau LJ, et al. Recommendations for diagnosis, treatment and management of individuals with Turner syndrome. Endocrinologist. 1994; 4(5):351–358

Ruggiero FP, Mitzner R, Samant S, et al. Neck dissection classification. Emedicine. Available at: http://emedicine.medscape.com/article/849834-overview. Accessed June 28, 2012

Schook CC, Mulliken JB, Fishman SJ, Alomari AI, Grant FD, Greene AK. Differential diagnosis of lower extremity enlargement in pediatric patients referred with a diagnosis of lymphedema. Plast Reconstr Surg. 2011; 127(4):1571–1581

Senderek T, Breitenbach S, Halas I. Kinesio taping: new opportunities in physiotherapeutic treatment of pregnant women [in Polish]. Fizjoterapia Polska. 2005; 5(2):266–271

Servelle M. Klippel and Trénaunay's syndrome. 768 operated cases. Ann Surg. 1985; 201(3):365–373

Silverstein MD, Heit JA, Mohr DN, Petterson TM, O'Fallon WM, Melton LJ, III. Trends in the incidence of deep vein thrombosis and pulmonary embolism: a 25-year population-based study. Arch Intern Med. 1998; 158(6):585–593

Tsai HJ, Hung HC, Yang JL, Huang CS, Tsauo JY. Could Kinesio tape replace the bandage in decongestive lymphatic therapy for breast-cancer-related lymphedema? A pilot study. Support Care Cancer. 2009; 17(11):1353–1360

US Department of Transportation, Federal Aviation Administration. Pilot's handbook of aeronautical knowledge. FAA-H-8083–25A. Oklahoma City, OK: United States Department of Transportation, Federal Aviation Administration, Airman Testing Standards Branch; 2008. Available at: http://www.faa.gov. Accessed June 28, 2012

Williams A. Breast and trunk oedema after treatment for breast cancer. Lymphoedema. 2006; 1(1):32–39

Weissleder H, Schuchhardt C. Lymphedema Diagnosis and Therapy.4th ed. Essen: Viavital Verlag; 2008

5

Chapter 6

Administration

6 Administration

6.1 Introduction

Health care professionals working in the field of lymphedema management see patients who may suffer from primary or secondary lymphedema, venous insufficiencies, or other conditions that may benefit from complete decongestive therapy (CDT). Cases may be relatively simple, or they may involve complicating factors, such as skin alterations, genital involvement, or additional pathologies exacerbating already existing symptoms. Some patients suffer from lymphedema for decades prior to seeing a certified lymphedema therapist, and in many cases the involved extremity has reached proportions so enormous that it is difficult to comprehend how it was possible for the swelling to get so out of control. However simple or complicated the case may be, the best results in lymphedema management are achieved if the patient is seen on a daily basis and treatments are given until the limb is decongested. Treatments given two or three times per week may cause more problems than benefit. Compression bandages slide if they are not renewed daily, causing tourniquet effects, or the patient may remove the bandages, leading to re-accumulation of lymph fluid in the extremity. The therapist is then forced to spend part of the treatment session removing this fluid for a second time, which seriously hampers treatment progress.

Reducing the size of a lymphedematous extremity back to a normal or near normal volume is rewarding for both the patient and the therapist. This rewarding and clinically challenging experience is payback for the hardship the patient has had to endure and any obstacles a health care professional may have had to overcome prior to establishing a lymphedema clinic.

This chapter focuses on some key points in the establishment of a lymphedema clinic, whether it is a freestanding treatment center or part of an existing clinic or department.

6.2 Setting Up a Lymphedema Clinic

Among the factors influencing the establishment of a well-run lymphedema clinic are the selection of personnel, the determination of required space and equipment, and marketing issues in promoting the clinic.

6.2.1 Personnel

A high level of competency and skill is needed to master all components of CDT and to provide patients with the proper degree of intervention. The quality of training will have a great impact on the level of care the patients receive.

To provide a high standard of care, it is necessary that the therapists are specifically educated and trained in lymphedema management. It is highly recommended that therapists complete a training program in CDT, consisting of 135 classroom hours attained from one training program. The training should consist of one-third theoretical instruction and two-thirds practical hands-on work.

Successful lymphedema management requires daily treatments in the intensive phase; it is therefore desirable to employ two lymphedema therapists to cover for absence and for professional exchange and support. In a freestanding treatment center, it is also necessary to have at least one more person covering the phone and reception area, as well as dealing with insurance and billing issues.

6.2.2 Required Space

Regulations concerning minimum space and design requirements for health care facilities (health centers, suites, or clinics) may vary from state to state. Regulations can be obtained from professional associations.

It is desirable to have two treatment rooms per therapist, two bathrooms, a shower, an exercise room, a reception area (to include a waiting room), and a storage room.

Treatment Room

Treatment room should be approximately 80 to 100 ft^2 (~ 7–9 m^2) per room with the following equipment: treatment table (adjustable in height and able to support patients' weight), chair, clothes hanger, rolling stool, shelf with bandaging and padding materials, and patient education materials.

The best patient scheduling is achieved by having two therapy rooms per therapist. If you allow ample time between patients, you may be able to function well with one room per therapist.

Bathroom/Shower

A bathroom/shower should be approximately 50 ft^2 (~ 5 m^2), and wheelchair should be accessible. For appropriate patient hygiene, a shower within the treatment center is desirable. Patients have to wear the compression bandages between the daily treatment sessions and often remove the bandages at home before taking a shower. It is imperative for treatment success that the bandages are not removed at the patient's home (except if they cause pain or numbness in the extremity). Patients taking a shower at their home should protect the bandaged extremity with either a cast shield or a large trash bag. If a shower is not available in the treatment facility, patients should shower at home with the covered bandages in place, remove the bandages in the clinic, and wash the extremity with a washcloth at the clinic's sink.

Exercise Room

An exercise room should be approximately 300 to 500 ft^2 (~ 28–46 m^2) to accommodate exercise mats. For group exercises or support group meetings, a room size of approximately 1,000 ft^2 (~ 305 m^2) is appropriate.

Reception Area

Reception area should be approximately 400 ft^2 (~ 37 m^2) to accommodate patient waiting room, record storage, documentation space, and other materials

If the treatment facility provides twice-a-day treatment, a patient lounge area of approximately 400 ft^2 (~ 37 m^2) in addition to the reception area, containing a refrigerator, microwave, coffee/tea maker, audiovisual equipment, and comfortable rest area, is desirable.

Storage Room

Storage room should be approximately 50 ft^2 (~ 5 m^2) to accommodate bandaging materials and other items.

6.2.3 Equipment

The basic equipment needed for a well-run lymphedema clinic includes the following:
- Furniture for the reception area and treatment rooms.
- Adjustable treatment tables.
- Compression materials (see Section 6.3).
- Audiovisual equipment and other materials for patient education.
- Computer(s) and software (limb measurement program).
- Digital camera(s).
- Measuring tape(s) and documentation forms.
- Manual sphygmomanometer(s).
- Exercise equipment (soft balls, sticks, therabands, etc.).
- Basic office supplies.

6.2.4 Marketing Issues

Whether the lymphedema treatment center is freestanding or part of an existing clinic or department, referral sources must be developed to ensure success. The following suggestions should be considered to make the clinic's presence known to the lymphedema community and to physicians.

Direct Mailings or Visits to Physicians in the Community

The information source should contain a brochure outlining the clinic's services. When designing the brochure, it should be kept in mind that physicians are busy and prefer information that is precise, short, and to the point. A photo depicting a lymphedema patient before and after treatment with manual lymph drainage and CDT on the cover page of the brochure is always helpful to bring the point across.

Certified Therapist Listing on Websites

Training centers for CDT generally offer a listing of their graduates on their websites, which can be accessed by patients seeking certified therapists. Several organizations established "therapist locators" on their websites. These provide assistance in locating a qualified therapist, who meets recommended training standards. The National Lymphedema Networks resource can be located on their website (www.lymphnet.org, accessed March 4, 2016). The Lymphology Association of North America provides a link at their website as well (www.clt-lana.org, accessed March 4, 2016). The American Lymphedema Framework Project (ALFP) developed a mobile web application software labeled Look4LE, which provides a common directory of trained lymphedema specialists with an

6

online registration and validation system. Patients are able to install this free web application to search for certified lymphedema specialists worldwide

Certified Therapist Listings in Publications Relevant to Lymphedema

The National Lymphedema Network distributes a quarterly publication. This publication contains valuable information for lymphedema patients and therapists. For a fee, therapists and clinics may be listed in the resource guide of this publication.

Brochures

Brochures outlining the services provided should be distributed at health fairs and breast cancer–related/lymphedema-related events and at the offices of oncologists and vascular and plastic surgeons.

In-Service Presentations

Presentations can be given at local clinics and health care facilities. It is helpful to bring educational materials (posters, slides) to support each presentation.

Advertisements

Local newspapers and other media are appropriate vehicles for advertising services.

Insurance Companies

The provider relations department of insurance companies offering coverage in the service area should be contacted and be made aware of the services the facility offers.

6.3 Suggested Materials to Start Up a Lymphedema Program

An adequate inventory of supplies should be on hand before the lymphedema program opens. The treatment center should keep a sufficient quantity of compression materials in stock, or the patients themselves should be told to order the materials needed directly from a distributor before the initial treatment. The approximate quantity of compression materials needed for each individual patient during the decongestive phase is determined during the evaluation.

A detailed description of the materials used in lymphedema management and a listing of recommended materials used for upper and lower extremity lymphedema bandaging are given in Chapter 5, Required Materials.

The initial expense to keep a sufficient amount of lymphedema bandaging supply in stock is approximately $2,500 to $3,000 (this should cover ~ 10–15 patients).

- Short-stretch bandages:
  - Ten rolls of 4 cm.
  - Twenty rolls of 6 cm.
  - Twenty rolls of 8 cm.
  - Forty rolls of 10 cm.
  - Five rolls of 10 cm × 10 m (double length).
  - Forty rolls of 12 cm.
  - Five rolls of 12 cm × 10 m (double length).
- Wide-width short-stretch bandages (white bandages):
  - Five rolls of 15 cm.
  - Five rolls of 20 cm.
- Padding bandages:
  - Thirty rolls of 10 cm.
  - Forty rolls of 15 cm.
- Soft foam:
  - (Best is 0.25-in [6-mm] and 0.5-in [12-mm] thickness with a recommended density of approximately 1.6 lb [725 g]/ft^3, one sheet each).
- High-density foam:
  - Ten pieces small Komprex kidney (size 0).
  - Two pad rolls (8 cm × 2 m × 1 cm).
  - Four sheets (100 cm × 50 cm × 1 cm).
- *Foam padding rolls* (Rosidal soft) can be used instead of gray foam:
  - Thirty rolls of 10 cm.
  - Fifteen rolls of 15 cm.
- *Gauze bandages* (finger and toe bandages):
  - *Mollelast*: 10 boxes (200 rolls) of 4 cm × 4 m, or 8 bags of Elastomull 1 in × 4.1 yd (2.5 cm × 3.7 m).
  - Ten boxes (200 rolls) of 6 cm × 4 m, or 17 bags of Elastomull 2 in × 4.1 yd (5 cm × 3.7 m).
  - Translast (skin colored): 10 boxes (200 rolls) of 6 cm × 4 m.
- *Stockinettes* (tubular gauze):
  - Two boxes for small arms or children's legs (Lohmann size 5 or Tricofix D5).
  - Two boxes for "normal" arms and lower legs (Lohmann size 6 or Tricofix E6).
  - Four boxes for big arms and "normal" legs (Lohmann size 7 or Tricofix E6).

- Five boxes for very big arms and bigger legs (Lohmann size 9 or Tricofix F7/G9).
- Two boxes for very big legs, small trunk (Lohmann size K1).
- Two boxes for extremely large legs and trunk (Lohmann size K2).
- Lotion:
  - Bottles of 10 to 15 × 8 ounce (236 mL), or 5 × 32 ounce (946 ml) bottles (Lymphoderm, Eucerin, etc.).
- Other:
  - Five bandage winders.
  - Educational materials (posters, etc.).

Some distributors offer prepacked bandage kits for lymphedema management. These kits are available for either upper or lower extremity lymphedema bandaging and typically contain two complete sets of short-stretch bandages, stockinettes, padding, and gauze bandages. Foam generally is not included and must be ordered separately. Ordering kits instead of separate items may simplify the ordering process, but distributors typically charge an additional amount for the packaging process.

6.4 Reimbursements and Billing

If providers work on a private pay basis, a reasonable charge will have to be established, covering all expenses (including bandages, padding materials, etc.), plus profit. A price list detailing all parts of the treatment should be posted in the treatment center.

Health care reimbursement is an ever-changing and very complex issue. Lymphedema management services are provided by physical therapists, physical therapist assistants, occupational therapists, occupational therapist assistants, massage therapists, and nurses. Insurance reimbursement may vary depending on providers and practice settings. Providers should confer with insurance companies to inquire about reimbursement policies for their individual professional group. It is also advisable to consult respective professional associations for the most current updates and regulations.

During the past few years, the Women's Health and Cancer Rights Act (WHCRA) of 1998 has had a positive impact on reimbursement for lymphedema management. This federal law, which became effective on October 21, 1998, requires group health plans (as well as payers providing individual coverage) that provide coverage for mastectomies to also cover reconstructive surgery and prostheses following mastectomies. The treatment and management of physical complications resulting from mastectomies, such as lymphedema, are also covered under this act.

Not included in the statutes of this act is the type of treatment that must be provided. This decision is left to the individual insurance provider to determine.

Patients who had problems getting insurance coverage before the WHCRA became effective should contact their insurance company and ask the following questions:
- Does the WHCRA of 1998 affect my coverage for lymphedema treatment?
- Does my insurance policy cover manual lymph drainage and CDT (Current Procedural Terminology [CPT] code 97140) for the treatment of my lymphedema?
- Is it necessary that a physical therapist perform the manual lymph drainage/CDT to be reimbursed, or can an occupational therapist, registered nurse, or massage therapist administer the therapy?

Patients should also contact their state's insurance department to find out whether the WHCRA will apply to the coverage if they are part of an insured group plan or individual health insurance.

Payers generally do not cover compression bandages and compression garments. Recent improvement has been seen in the coverage for gradient compression garments. Effective as of October 1, 2003, the Centers for Medicare and Medicaid Services (CMS) approved coverage for compression garments in the treatment of venous stasis ulcerations. Coverage may be provided for garments delivering compression between 30 and 50 mmHg and if the patient has an open venous stasis ulcer that has been treated by a physician or another health care professional.

The CMS article states in part that compression garments that serve a therapeutic or protective function may be covered if certain requirements are met. Because successful long-term lymphedema management depends on gradient compression garments as well, the lymphedema community should advocate for extended coverage to include lymphedema care.

Lymphedema clinics obtain their compression materials from vendors specialized in the distribution of lymphedema management materials. Depending on the individual practice setting, patients may reimburse the providers for materials used or order the necessary supplies directly from vendors.

6

6.4.1 Current Procedural Terminology Codes

Correct coding is one of the most important, and often one of the most frustrating, aspects of successfully operating a practice for lymphedema management. Correct coding is something of a science, made even more complex by frequent changes in the definitions of the codes and the approved methods of combining them.

The five-digit codes apply to medical services or procedures performed by health care providers. The CPT codes are established by the CPT editorial panel of the American Medical Association and have become the industry's coding standard for reporting.

The following CPT codes are commonly used in billing for lymphedema management; health care providers should be aware that the interpretation of these codes by various payers might vary.

- Timed codes:
  - When billing Medicare for any of the timed codes, the providers must follow appropriate CMS guidelines regarding unit of service requirements.
    - Evaluation codes.
    - 97001: physical therapy evaluation.
    - 97003: occupational therapy evaluation.
- Therapy codes:
  - 97140: manual therapy techniques (e.g., mobilization/manipulation, manual lymphatic drainage [MLD], manual traction), one or more regions. Charge is based on 15-minute increments.
  - Depending on the condition, the MLD portion of the treatment may last between 30 minutes and 1 hour.
  - 97530: therapeutic activities, direct (one-on-one) patient contact by the provider (use of dynamic activities to improve functional performance). Based on 15-minute increments.
  - Can be used with or without bandages on the affected extremity.
  - 97110: therapeutic procedure, one or more areas. Based on 15-minute increments. Therapeutic exercises to develop strength and endurance, range of motion, and flexibility.
  - Can be used with or without bandages on the affected extremity (theraband, ball, etc.).
  - 97535: self-care/home management training. Self-care management, patient education in self-MLD for home program, self-bandaging, Dos and Don'ts, and appropriate activity

guidelines. Charge is based on 15-minute increments.
  - 97750: physical performance test, measurements. Circumferential and/or volumetric measurements, with written report (measurement forms, volume programs). Charge is based on 15-minute increments.
  - 97504: orthotics fitting and training. Pressure garment measurements for upper or lower extremity and trunk.
  - 97039: unlisted therapeutic procedure. Skin care, breathing exercises, deep abdominal techniques, and therapist's application of low-pH skin lotion, antibiotic ointment, or other skin treatments on the affected limb prior to bandaging.

6.4.2 ICD-10 Codes

The Health Insurance Portability and Accountability Act (HIPAA) mandates that health care providers use a standard code set to specify diagnoses and procedures for reimbursement of services by health plans. ICD stands for international classification of diseases; the codes within this system are used to translate medical diagnoses or terms into a coding system. This coding system is currently used within the medical community and updated every October. ICD-10 is the 10th revision of the international classification of diseases and related health problems (ICD), a medical classification list developed by the World Health Organization (WHO). It contains codes for diseases, signs and symptoms, abnormal findings, complaints, social circumstances, and external causes of injury or diseases. It is a system of coding that distinguishes each diagnosis by an alphanumerical classification. The new ICD-10 contains over 69,000 different codes that state diagnosis or condition. More than 100 countries use the ICD system to report and monitor death and disease rates worldwide. The United States developed a clinical modification (ICD-10-CM) for medical diagnoses based on WHO's ICD-10. The formerly used ICD-9-CM coding system, in use since 1979, was outdated and not descriptive enough and was replaced on October 1, 2015, by the new and restructured ICD-10-CM code set. This updated set of codes provides a marked improvement in the specificity and clinical information of the reporting, thus allowing more information to be conveyed in one code (▸ Table 6.1).

6

Table 6.1 ICD-10-CM codes relevant for lymphedema.

I89.0	Lymphedema, not elsewhere classified
I89.1	Lymphangitis
I89.8	Other specified noninfective disorders of lymphatic vessels and lymph nodes (chylous disorders)
I97.2	Postmastectomy lymphedema syndrome
Q82.0	Hereditary lymphedema (lower extremities)
M79.89	Other specified soft tissue disorders (swelling of limb)
N90.89	Other specified noninflammatory disorders of vulva and perineum (vulvar edema)
R60.0	Localized edema
R60.1	Generalized edema
R60.9	Edema, unspecified
I87.019	Postthrombotic syndrome with ulcer of unspecified lower extremity
I87.029	Postthrombotic syndrome with inflammation of unspecified lower extremity
I87.039	Postthrombotic syndrome with ulcer and inflammation of unspecified lower extremity

6.5 Sample Forms and Templates

▶ Fig. 6.1, ▶ Fig. 6.2, ▶ Fig. 6.3, ▶ Fig. 6.4, ▶ Fig. 6.5, ▶ Fig. 6.6, ▶ Fig. 6.7, ▶ Fig. 6.8, ▶ Fig. 6.9, ▶ Fig. 6.10, ▶ Fig. 6.11 are a compilation of sample forms that may be helpful in the process of establishing a lymphedema clinic.

6

Patient Information

Date: _____

Patient's Name: _____

Address: _____

City: _____ State: _____ Zip Code: _____

Date of Birth: _____

Phone: (___) _____ (Res.)

(___) _____ ext. _____ (Business)

Marital Status: (M)   (S)   (O)ther

Social Security No.: _____

Patient's Employer: _____

Address: _____

City: _____ State: _____ Zip Code: _____

Phone: (___) _____

Name of Spouse/Parent/Significant Other: _____

Address (if different than patient): _____

City: _____ State: _____ Zip Code: _____ Phone: _____

PLEASE HAVE INSURANCE CARD(S) AVAILABLE TO BE COPIED

Insurance Company: _____

Policy Holder's Name: _____ Policy Holder's Date of Birth: _____

Primary Care Physician: _____

Physician's Address: _____

Phone: (___) _____ UPIN#: _____

How did you hear about our facility?: _____

Did you receive our brochure by mail? _____ YES _____ NO

I HAVE RECEIVED A COPY OF THE NOTICE OF PRIVACY PRACTICES _____ Yes _____ No

Fig. 6.1 Patient information form.

Lymphedema Evaluation

Name: _____ Date: _____

1. For how long have you had lymphedema? _____

2. Have you ever had any lymphedema infections? _____

3. Do you ever leak fluid? _____

4. Do you take prophylactic antibiotics? _____

5. Do you take diuretics for lymphedema? _____

6. Do you take benzopyrones for lymphedema? _____

7. Do you take any other drugs for lymphedema? _____

8. Does anyone in your family have lymphedema? _____

9. Which extremity has lymphedema?
   (check all that apply)   Left Arm _____ Right Arm _____
                             Left Leg _____ Right Leg _____

10. Have you had prior treatment for lymphedema?
   (check all that apply)   Surgery _____ Compression Garment _____
                             Antibiotics _____ Pneumatic Pump _____
                             Manual Lymph Drainage _____

11. Do you have bronchial asthma? _____

12. Do you have hypertension? _____

13. Do you have diabetes? _____

14. Do you have allergies? _____

15. Do you have any cardiac problems? _____

16. Do you have any kidney problems? _____

17. Do you have any circulatory problems? _____

18. What medication(s) are you currently taking? _____

19. Have you ever had radiation therapy? _____

20. Have you ever received chemotherapy? _____

21. What operation(s) have you had? _____

(over)

Fig. 6.2 Lymphedema evaluation. *(continued)*

Lymphedema Evaluation
(continued)

22. Which physician referred you to our facility? _____

    Name: _____

    Address: _____

    Phone: (   ) _____

23. Can we write to or discuss your lymphedema problem with this physician?
    YES _____ NO _____

24. If you are treated at this office, you will then be asked to follow a maintenance program at home.
    This consists of:
    a) Elastic sleeve or stocking worn during the day.
    b) Bandaging of limb overnight.
    c) Meticulous skin care to avoid infections.
    d) Remedial exercises to accelerate lymph flow.

    Are you prepared to follow such a program? _____

Fig. 6.2 *(cont.)* Lymphedema evaluation.

Physical Examination

Patient's name: _____ Date: _____

Date of birth: _____

General appearance: _____   Genitalia: _____

_____   _____

_____   _____

_____   _____

_____   Musculo/skeletal: _____

Skin: _____   _____

_____   _____

_____   _____

HEENT: Head _____

       Ears _____   Neurological: _____

       Eyes _____   _____

       Nose _____   _____

       Throat _____

Neck: _____   Other: _____

_____   _____

_____   _____

Chest/lungs: _____

_____

_____

Cardiac: _____

_____

_____

Abdomen/back: _____

_____

_____

_____

_____

Right   Left   Left   Right

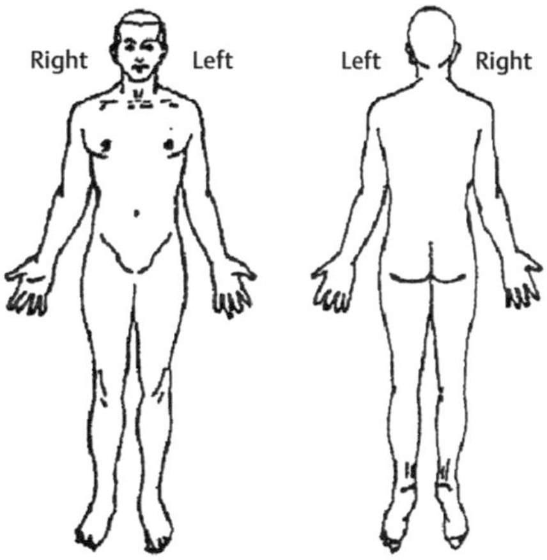

Fig. 6.3 Physical evaluation form.

6

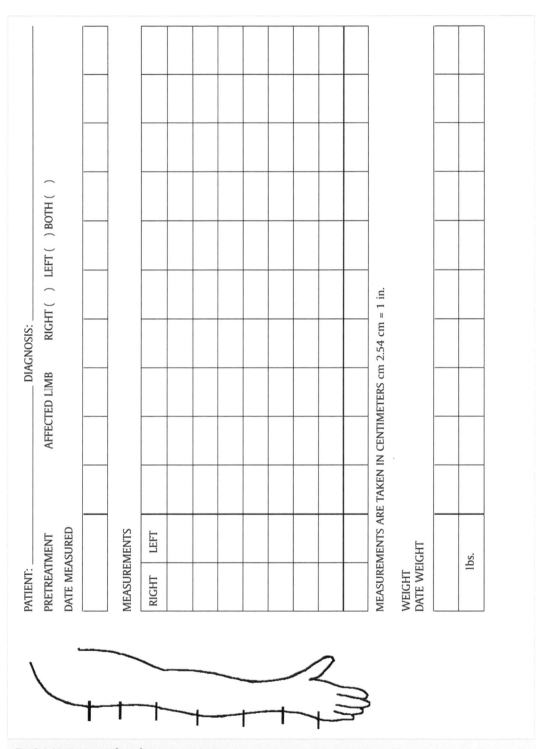

PATIENT: _____ DIAGNOSIS: _____

PRETREATMENT   AFFECTED LIMB   RIGHT ( )   LEFT ( )   BOTH ( )

DATE MEASURED

MEASUREMENTS

RIGHT	LEFT									

MEASUREMENTS ARE TAKEN IN CENTIMETERS cm 2.54 cm = 1 in.

WEIGHT

DATE WEIGHT

lbs.

Fig. 6.4 Measurement form for upper extremity.

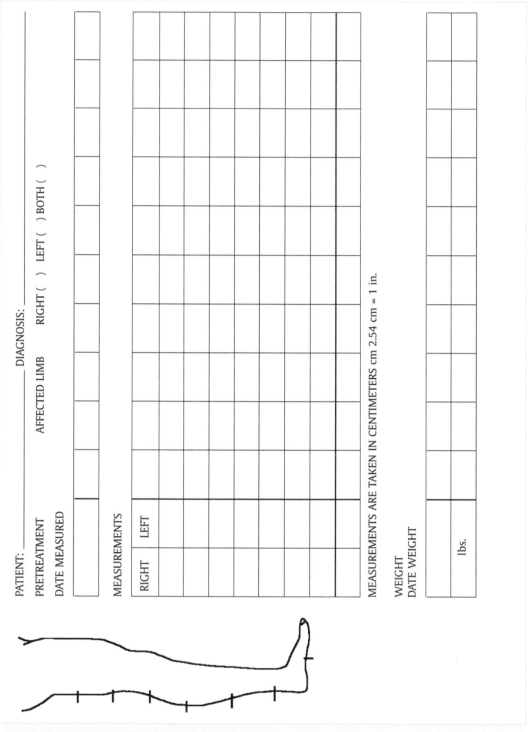

Fig. 6.5 Measurement form for lower extremity.

Progress Notes

PATIENT: _____

Date of birth: _____

Date	

6

Fig. 6.6 Progress notes form.

Photography Release Form

I _____ hereby give the
Facility's Name and Address the absolute and irrevocable right to take and permission to use photographs of me, or in which I may be included with others.

a) To copyright the same in said organization's own name or any name that they choose, and/or

b) To use, re-use, publish and republish the same in whole or in parts, individually or in conjunction with other photographs, in any medium and for the purpose of medical information of the public, medical staff of clinic employees, including (but not by the way of limitation) illustration, promotion, and advertising and trade, and/or

c) To use my name in connection therewith if they so choose Yes _____ No _____

d) Restrictions: _____ No facial photographs _____ Other _____

_____

I hereby release and discharge the   from any and all claims and demands arising out of or in conjunction with the use of photographs, including but not limited to any and all claims of libel, invasion of privacy, etc.

This authorization and release shall also ensure to the benefit of the legal representatives, licensees and assigns of the

I am over the age of eighteen, have read the foregoing, and fully understand the contents thereof.

ADULT RELEASE   MINOR RELEASE

_____   _____
(Participant's Name)   (Minor's Name)

_____   _____
(Signature)   (Signature – Parent, Guardian)

                                            _____
                                            (Relationship to Participant)

_____   _____
(Witness)   (Date)

Fig. 6.7 Photography release form.

Notice of Privacy Practices
Patient Consent Form

Name of Practice: _____

The Department of Health and Human Services has established a "Privacy Rule" to help ensure that personal health care information is protected for privacy. The Privacy Rule was also created in order to provide a standard for certain health care providers to obtain their patients' consent for uses and disclosures of health information about the patient to carry out treatment, payment or health care operations. As our patient, we want you to know that we respect the privacy of your personal medical records and that we will do all we can to secure and protect that privacy. We strive to always take reasonable precautions to protect your privacy. When it is appropriate and necessary, we provide the minimum necessary information to only those we feel are in need of your health care information and information about treatment, payment or health care operations, in order to provide health care that is in your best interest.

We also want you to know that we support your full access to your personal medical records. We may have indirect treatment relationships with you (such as laboratories that only interact with physicians and not patients), and may have to disclose personal health information for purposes of treatment, payment or health care operations. These entities are most often not required to obtain patient consent.

You may refuse to consent to the use or disclosure of your personal health information, but this must be in writing.

Receipt of Notice of Privacy Practices
Written Acknowledgment Form

I, (Patient's Name) _____, have received and

reviewed a copy of (Name of Practice) _____ 's Notice of Privacy Practices.

Signature of the patient or the patient's guardian: _____

Date: _____

Fig. 6.8 Privacy rules consent form.

Patient Authorization for Use and Disclosures of Protected Health Information to Third Parties

Name of Practice: _____

Section A: Must be completed for all authorizations

I hereby authorize the use of disclosure of my individually identifiable health information as described below. I understand that this authorization is voluntary. I understand that if the organization authorized to receive the information is not a health plan or health care provider, the released information may no longer be protected by federal privacy regulations.

Patient's Name: _____ ID Number: _____

Persons/organizations providing information:

_____

Persons/organizations receiving the information:

_____

Specific description of information (including date(s)):

_____

_____

Section B: Must be completed only if a health plan or health care provider has requested the authorization

1. The provider must complete the following statement:
   will the health care provider requesting the authorization receive financial or in-kind compensation in exchange for using or disclosing the health information described above? Yes _____ No _____

2. The patient must read and initial the following statement:
   I understand that I will receive a copy of this form once I have signed it. Patient's initials: _____

Section C: Must be completed for all authorizations

The patient or the patient's representative must read and initial the following statements:
1. I understand that this authorization will expire on _____/_____/_____ (DD/MM/YYYY) Initials: _____

2. I understand that I may revoke this authorization at any time by notifying the practice in writing. I understand that this revocation will not have any effect on any actions they took before they received the revocation. Initials: _____

Signature of the patient or the patient's representative: _____

Printed name of the patient or the patient's representative: _____

Relationship to the patient: _____

Fig. 6.9 Health information consent form.

Letter of Medical Necessity

Date:

RE:

To Whom It May Concern:

I had the pleasure of seeing Mr./Mrs. _____ on _____

He/she was found to have Primary/Secondary Lymphedema of the _____ following

_____

I believe he/she will benefit from _____ treatments of Complete Decongestive Therapy, given daily for a total of _____ weeks.

Complete Decongestive Therapy:

Each CDT treatment consists of four steps:

1. Meticulous skin and nail care, including the eradication of any infection

2. Manual Lymph Drainage, a manual treatment technique that stimulates lymph vessels to contract more frequently and that channels lymph and edema fluid toward adjacent, functioning lymph systems. Manual Lymph Drainage begins with stimulation of the lymph vessels and nodes in adjacent basins (neck, contralateral/ipsilateral axilla and/or groin), which is followed by manual decongestion, in segmental order, of the involved trunk, upper part, lower part of the extremity, wrist (ankle),and hand (foot). Edema fluid and obstructed lymphatics are made to drain toward the venous angle, toward functioning lymph basins across the midline of the body, down toward the groin, over the top of the shoulder, around the back,and so forth.

3. Compression Bandaging is done immediately after Manual Lymph Drainage. Bandages are applied from the distal to the proximal aspect of the extremity with maximal pressure distally and minimal pressure proximally. This is done by using several layers of cotton bandages or foam materials to ensure uniform pressure distribution or to increase pressure in areas that are particularly fibrotic. The bandages do not constrict blood flow but increase diminished skin and interstitial pressures. This prevents any reaccumulation of excavated edema fluid and also prevents the ultrafiltration of additional fluid into the interstitial space.

4. The bandaged patient is next guided through a series of decongestive exercises with the muscles and joints functioning within closed space. The exercises increase lymph flow in all available lymph channels and in collateral pathways that are used to make the passage to the venous angle.

This should reduce his/her swelling and stabilize his/her condition. Without this therapy, his/her swelling can be expected to progress and lead to complications.

The patient will also be instructed in a home maintenance program so that he/she can continue treatment on his/her own at home.

Sincerely,

Fig. 6.10 Example of letter of medical necessity.

6

Information on Lymphedema

Fig. 6.11 Information on lymphedema for patients. *(continued)*

What Is Lymphedema?

Lymphedema is a swelling of a body part, most often the extremities. It may also occur in the face, the trunk, the abdomen or the genital area. Lymphedema is the result of an accumulation of protein-rich fluid in the superficial tissues, which can have significant pathological and clinical consequences for the patient if left untreated. Once present, this chronic and progressive condition will not disappear again.

Causes of Lymphedema

Lymphedema is classified as either primary or secondary. Primary lymphedema is caused by congenital malformations of the lymphatic system and may be present at birth or develop later in life, often in puberty or during pregnancy. Primary forms usually affect the lower extremities but may also be present in upper extremities.

Secondary lymphedema is more common and often the result of surgery or radiation therapy for cancer. Surgical procedures in combination with the removal of lymph nodes, such as mastectomies or lumpectomies with the removal and/or irradiation of axillary lymph nodes, are a very common reason for the onset of secondary lymphedema in the United States. Other causes include trauma or infection of the lymphatic system. Severe venous insufficiencies may also contribute to the onset of lymphedema (phlebolymphostatic edema).

Primary and secondary lymphedema may affect the upper or lower extremity. In general it can be said that the legs are more often involved in primary lymphedema whereas secondary forms are more commonly found in the upper extremities.

Symptoms of Lymphedema

Early stages of lymphedema (stage I) may be temporarily reduced by simple elevation of the limb. Without proper treatment, however, the protein-rich swelling causes a progressive hardening, of the affected tissues; this condition is known as lymphostatic fibrosis and is present in stage II lymphedema. Other complications such as fungal infections, additional hardening, and very often an extreme increase in volume of the swollen extremity are typical for stage III lymphedema.

Primary and secondary lymphedema usually affect one extremity only; if both extremities, for example, both legs, are involved, the swelling appears asymmetrically.

Treatment Methods

Medication: Diuretics are often prescribed in order to control lymphedema but are proven to have very poor long-term results in the treatment of this condition. Diuretics decrease the water content of the swelling while the protein molecules remain in the tissues. As soon as the diuretic loses its effectiveness, these proteins continue to draw water to the edematous area.

Surgery: Several surgical procedures for lymphedema are described. It is safe to say that not a single one of these surgeries performed during the past century showed consistent results.

Pneumatic Compression Pumps: This mechanical device works with sleeves containing compressed air, which are applied to the patient's swollen extremity. Inappropriate use of these devices can cause serious complications in lymphedema patients. In some cases pumps may be applied under the supervision of specially trained therapists and in combination with other treatment modalities (see below).

Complete Decongestive Therapy (CDT): Since there is no cure for lymphedema, the goal of the therapy is to reduce the swelling and to maintain the reduction. For the majority of the patients this can be achieved by the skillful application of this therapy, which is safe, reliable, and noninvasive. CDT shows good long-term results in both primary and secondary lymphedema; it consists of two phases and the following combined modalities:

Manual Lymph Drainage (MLD): this gentle manual treatment technique increases the activity of certain lymph vessels and manually moves interstitial fluid. Applied correctly, a series of MLD treatments decreases the volume of the affected extremity to a normal or near normal size and is applied daily in the first phase of the therapy.

Compression Therapy: the elastic fibers in the skin are damaged in lymphedema. In order to prevent reaccumulation of fluid it is necessary to apply sufficient compression to the affected extremity.

Compression therapy also improves the function of the muscle pumps, helps to reduce fibrotic tissue, and promotes venous and lymphatic return.

In the first phase of CDT, compression therapy is achieved with the application of special short-stretch bandages. These bandage materials are used between MLD treatments and prevent the reaccumulation of lymph fluid, which has been moved out of the extremity during the MLD session. Once the extremity is decongested, the patient wears compression garments during the day. In some cases it may be necessary for the patient to additionally wear bandages at night. In order to achieve best results, specially trained personnel should take measurements for these elastic support garments; incorrectly fitted sleeves or stockings will have negative effects. The type of garments (round or flat-knit style) and the compression class depend on many factors such as the patient's age and the severity of the swelling. For upper extremity lymphedema, compression classes I (20–30 mmHg) or II (30–40 mmHg); for lymphedema of the lower extremities, compression classes II, III (40–50 mmHg) or IV (> 50 mmHg) are suitable. In some cases it may be necessary to apply compression class III to an upper extremity or an even greater compression than class IV to a lower extremity lymphedema. This can be achieved by wearing two stockings on top of each other, or by the application of bandages on top of a stocking.

To have the maximum effect, garments must be worn every day and replaced after 6 months.

Exercises: a customized exercise program is designed by the therapist for each patient. These decongestive exercises aid the effects of the joint and muscle pumps and should be performed by the patient wearing the compression bandage or garment. Vigorous movements or exercises causing pain must be avoided. Exercises should be performed slowly and with both the affected and nonaffected extremity.

Skin care: the skin in lymphedema is very susceptible to infections and usually dry. A low-pH lotion, free of alcohol and fragrances, should be used to maintain the moisture of the skin and to avoid infections. You should consult your physician if there are any fungal infections present in your affected extremity.

Do's and Don'ts

Your lymphedema therapist will explain to you in detail how to avoid infections and other conditions, which could lead to a worsening of your lymphedema. Listed below are just a few general guidelines:

Avoid any injuries to the skin – be careful working in the garden, playing with your pets or doing housework. Avoid the use of scissors to cut your nails and don't cut your cuticles. Injuries, even small ones, may cause infections.

Avoid mosquito bites – wear insect repellents when outdoors. A single mosquito bite can cause an infection.

Use caution when exercising – avoid movements that overstrain; discuss proper exercises and activities with your therapist.

Avoid heat – very hot showers, hot packs on your extremity, sunbathing, and the use of saunas could have a negative effect on your lymphedema. Avoid extreme changes in temperature (hot/cold), massages ("Swedish") on your affected extremity or any cosmetics that irritate the skin.

Inform all health care personnel that you have lymphedema – injections or acupuncture in your affected extremity should be avoided. Blood pressure should be taken on the extremity free of lymphedema.

Nutrition is important – there is no special diet for lymphedema. Today most nutritionists recommend a low-salt, low-fat diet. Obesity may have a negative effect on your swelling.

Travel – avoid mosquito-infested areas; when traveling by airplane apply an additional bandage on top of your garment.

Clothing – clothing that is too tight may restrict the proper flow of lymph. Avoid tight bras, panties or socks and make sure your jewelry fits loosely.

See your doctor – if you have any signs of an infection (fever, chills, red and hot skin), fungal infections or if you notice any other unusual changes that may be related to your lymphedema.

General tips – always wear your compression garments during the day and if necessary your bandages at night; elevate your extremity as often as possible during the daytime; perform your exercises daily and always consult your doctor or therapist should you have any questions about your lymphedema.

Fig. 6.11 *(cont.)* Information on lymphedema for patients.

6

Recommended Reading

American Medical Association. CPT Look Up Page. Accessed September 5, 2012. https://ocm. ama-assn.org/OCM/CPTRelativeValue-Search.do? submit button = accept

Centers for Medicare and Medicaid Services. Accessed September 5, 2012. http://www.cms.gov

Centers for Medicare and Medicaid Services. The Women's Health and Cancer Rights Act.. Accessed September 5, 2012. https://www.cms.gov/Regulations-and-Guidance/Health-Insurance-Reform/ HealthInsReformforConsume/downloads/WHCRA-Helpful_-Tips_2010_06_14.pdf

Electronic Code of Federal Regulations 14 CFR, Chapter 1, part 25, section 25–831. http://ecfr.gpoaccess.gov/cgi/t/text/ text-idx? c=ecfr&tpl=/ecfrbrowse/Title14/14tab_02

Electronic Code of Federal Regulations 14 CFR, Chapter 1, part 25, section 25–841. http://ecfr.gpoaccess.gov/cgi/t/text/ text-idx? c=ecfr&tpl=/ecfrbrowse/Title14/14tab_02

Lymphology Association of North America Certified Lymphedema Therapist Candidate information brochure. Accessed June 29, 2012. http:// www.clt-lana.org

6

Index

6

6

6